diFIORE'S ATLAS OF HISTOLOGY WITH FUNCTIONAL CORRELATIONS

ELEVENTH EDITION

W9-AYB-204

diFIORE'S ATLAS OF HISTOLOGY WITH FUNCTIONAL CORRELATIONS

ELEVENTH EDITION

Victor P. Eroschenko, PhD

Professor of Anatomy
WWAMI Medical Program
University of Idaho
Moscow, Idaho

Wolters Kluwer | Lippincott Williams & Wilkins
Health

Philadelphia · Baltimore · New York · London
Buenos Aires · Hong Kong · Sydney · Tokyo

Acquisitions Editor: Crystal Taylor
Managing Editor: Kelly Horvath
Marketing Manager: V. Sanders
Production Editor: Gina Aiello
Designer: Steve Druding
Compositor: Aptara, Inc.

Copyright © 2008 Lippincott Williams & Wilkins

351 West Camden Street
Baltimore, MD 21201

530 Walnut Street
Philadelphia, PA 19106

All rights reserved. This book is protected by copyright. No part of this book may be reproduced in any form or by any means, including photocopying, or utilized by any information storage and retrieval system without written permission from the copyright owner.

The publisher is not responsible (as a matter of product liability, negligence, or otherwise) for any injury resulting from any material contained herein. This publication contains information relating to general principles of medical care that should not be construed as specific instructions for individual patients. Manufacturers' product information and package inserts should be reviewed for current information, including contraindications, dosages, and precautions.

Printed in the United States of America

Tenth Edition, 2005

Library of Congress Cataloging-in-Publication Data

Eroschenko, Victor P.
  Di Fiore's atlas of histology with functional correlations. — 11th ed. /
Victor P. Eroschenko.
     p. ; cm.
  Includes index.
  ISBN-13: 978-0-7817-7057-6
  ISBN-10: 0-7817-7057-2
  1. Histology—Atlases. I. Fiore, Mariano S. H. di. Atlas de histlogía
normal. English. II. Title. III. Title: Atlas of histology with functional
correlations.
  [DNLM: 1. Histology—Atlases. QS 517 E71d 2008]
  QM557.F5513 2008
  611'.018—dc22

                              2007040302

The publishers have made every effort to trace the copyright holders for borrowed material. If they have inadvertently overlooked any, they will be pleased to make the necessary arrangements at the first opportunity.

To purchase additional copies of this book, call our customer service department at (800) 638-3030 or fax orders to (301) 223-2320. International customers should call (301) 223-2300.

Visit Lippincott Williams & Wilkins on the Internet: http://www.LWW.com. Lippincott Williams & Wilkins customer service representatives are available from 8:30 am to 6:00 pm, EST.

                                      07 08 09 10
                              1 2 3 4 5 6 7 8 9 10

Dedicated

To those who matter so much

Ian
McKenzie
Sarah
Shannon

      and
      Diane
      Kathryn
      Tatiana
      Sharon

            and
            Todd
            Shaun

            and most especially and always
            Elke

The publication of the 11th edition of *Atlas of Histology* comes after a thorough and critical review by numerous external reviewers. The author carefully evaluated all of the reviewers' comments and suggestions. Many of the valuable suggestions that fit the design and purpose of the atlas were implemented in preparing the new edition.

Basic Approach

Although the research in numerous and different areas of science continues to produce valuable new results, histology remains one of the fundamental sciences that is essential in understanding and interpreting this new knowledge. In preparing the 11th edition of the atlas, the author maintained its unique and traditional approach, namely, providing the student with realistic, full-color composite and idealized illustrations of histologic structures. Added to the illustrations are actual photomicrographs of similar structures. This unique approach has become a popular trademark of the atlas. In addition, all structures have been directly correlated with the most important and essential functional correlations. This approach allows the student to learn histologic structure and their major functions at the same time, without spending additional time on reference books. The images and information presented in this format in the atlas have served the needs of undergraduate, graduate, medical, veterinary, and biologic science students in numerous previous editions. The present edition continues to address the needs of present or future students of histology.

Changes in the 11th Edition

Several significant changes that have been incorporated into this atlas are presented in detail below.

- All introductory chapters and all sections with functional correlations have been updated and expanded to reflect the new scientific information and interpretations.
- Each chapter is followed by a comprehensive summary in the form of an easy-to-follow outline.
- All remaining old illustrations from previous editions have been replaced with new, original, and digitized color illustrations. All other illustrations that were not originally digitized have been recolorized to improve their appearance.
- Transmission electron micrographs of skeletal muscle have been added to the muscle chapter to illustrate the details of individual muscle fibers and their sarcomeres.
- Scanning and transmission electron micrographs of the podocytes and their unique associations with the capillaries in the renal corpuscles have been added to the chapter on the kidney.

Electronic Atlas

Currently, there is an increased use of various computer-based technologies in histology instruction. As a result, the 11th edition of the atlas allows the student access via an electronic code to an interactive electronic atlas and a histology image library with each copy of the book. The interactive atlas is specifically designed to allow the students to further test their knowledge of histologic illustrations and photomicrographs that are found in the atlas. Specific features of the electronic atlas include a labels on/labels off feature, rollover "hot spots," and rollover labels. In addition, a self-testing feature allows the students to practice identifying the features on the images. In addition to the interactive atlas, the students will have access to a histology library that contains more than 475 digitized histology photomicrographs. All histology images have been separated into chapters that match those in the atlas, with each chapter containing an average of 20 images. The library images are specifically designed for use by the students to reinforce the material that was previously learned in laboratory or lecture. Consequently, these images do not have any labels and are identified only by a figure number for each chapter.

For the instructors, a separate histology image library has been prepared, with more than 950 improved and digitized photomicrograph images. These images have also been separated into corresponding chapters, with each image identified with abbreviations only. There are no labels on the images and each image can be imported into Microsoft PowerPoint and labeled by the instructors to provide necessary information during lectures or laboratory exercises. Because there are multiple images of the similar structures, instructors can use different images for lectures or laboratories of the same structures without repetition.

Thus, the current edition of the atlas should serve as a valuable supplement in histology laboratories where traditional histology is taught with microscopes and glass slides, or where computer-based images are used as a substitute for microscopes, or in which a combination of both technologies are used simultaneously.

ACKNOWLEDGMENTS

As in previous editions of this atlas, I have been very fortunate to be associated with numerous professional individuals, who were very instrumental in assisting me in preparing and improving this edition of the atlas.

Dr. E. Roland Brown (tueztuez@yahoo.com), freelance artist, prepared all of the new histology illustrations and recolorized the remaining images that were not computer-generated.

Sonja L. Gerard of Oei Graphics, Bellevue, Washington, corrected or improved the lead-in art for each chapter of the atlas.

Dr. Mark DeSantis, a long-time colleague and Professor Emeritus of the WWAMI Medical Education Program and Department of Biology, University of Idaho, Moscow, Idaho, provided constructive suggestions and corrections for improving the chapters on the nervous system.

Mr. Carter Rowley, Fort Collins, Colorado, a friend and a colleague of many years, graciously provided the transmission electron micrographs of the skeletal muscles from his own personal collection.

Assistant Professor Christine Davitt, School of Biological Sciences, Washington State University, Pullman, Washington, assisted me in scanning the negative images of the kidney corpuscles and their contents.

As a special acknowledgment, I want to express my sincere appreciation to Dr. Sergei Yakovlevich Amstislavsky, Novosibirsk State University, Institute of Cytology and Genetics, Russian Academy of Sciences, Siberian Division, Novosibirsk, Russia. As a dear friend and a highly valuable research partner, Sergei Yakovlevich graciously provided me with images from the ovaries of the European mink.

I also acknowledge the able assistance of Crystal Taylor and Kelly Horvath of Lippincott Williams & Wilkins. Their major efforts in initiating and continuing the process for preparing the new edition of the atlas are greatly appreciated.

Finally, to all who assisted me in this endeavor in the past, I express my sincere appreciation.

Victor P. Eroschenko, Ph.D.
Moscow, Idaho
June 2007

CONTENTS

PART II ◼ ORGANS 169

Introduction

Interpretation of Histologic Sections

Histologic sections are thin, flat slices of fixed and stained tissues or organs mounted on glass slides. Such sections are normally composed of cellular, fibrous, and tubular structures. Their cells exhibit a variety of shapes, sizes, and layers. Fibrous structures are solid and found in connective, nervous, and muscle tissues. Tubular structures are hollow and represent various types of blood vessels, ducts, and glands of the body.

In tissues and organs the cells, fibers, and tubes have a random orientation in space and are a part of a three-dimensional structure. During the preparation of histology slides, the thin sections do not have depth. In addition, the plane of section does not always cut these structures in exact transverse or cross section. This produces a variation in the appearance of the cells, fibers, and tubes, depending on the angle of the plane of section. As a result of these factors, it is difficult to correctly perceive the three-dimensional structure from which the sections were prepared on a flat slide. Therefore, correct visualization and interpretation of these sections in their proper three-dimensional perspective on the slide becomes an important criterion for mastering histology. Figures I.1 and I.2 illustrate how the appearance of cells and tubes changes with the plane of section.

FIGURE I.1 ■ Planes of Section of a Round Object

To illustrate how the shape of a three-dimensional cell can be altered in a histologic section, a hard-boiled egg has been sectioned in longitudinal and transverse (cross) planes. The composition of a hard-boiled egg serves as a good example of a cell, with the yellow yolk representing the nucleus and the surrounding egg white (pale blue) representing the cytoplasm. Enclosing these structures are the soft eggshell membrane and a hard eggshell (red). At the rounded end of the egg is the air space (blue).

The **midline** sections of the egg in the **longitudinal (a)** and **transverse planes (d)** disclose its correct shape and size, as they appear in these planes of section. In addition, these two planes of section reveal the correct appearance, size, and distribution of the internal contents within the egg.

Similar but more **peripheral** sections of the egg in the **longitudinal (b)** and **transverse planes (e)** still show the external shape of the egg. However, because the sections were cut peripheral to the midline, the internal contents of the egg are not seen in their correct size or distribution within the egg white. In addition, the size of the egg appears smaller.

The **tangential planes (c and f)** of section graze or only pass through the outermost periphery of the egg. These sections reveal that the egg is oval (c) or a small round (f) object. The egg yolk is not seen in either section because it was not located in the plane of section. As a result, such tangential sections do not reveal sufficient detail for correct interpretation of the egg size or of its contents or their distribution within the internal membrane.

Thus, in a histologic section, individual structure shape and size may vary depending on the plane of section. Some cells may exhibit full cross sections of their nuclei, and they appear prominent in the cells. Other cells may exhibit only a fraction of the nucleus, and the cytoplasm appears large. Still other cells may appear only as clear cytoplasm, without any nuclei. All these variations are attributable to different planes of section through the nuclei. Understanding these variations in cell and tube morphology will result in a better interpretation of the histologic sections.

FIGURE I.2 ■ Planes of Section of a Tube

Tubular structures are often seen in histologic sections. Tubes are most easily recognized when they are cut in transverse (cross) sections. However, if the tubes are sectioned in other planes, they must first be visualized as three-dimensional structures to be recognized as tubes. To illustrate how a blood vessel, duct, or glandular structure may appear in a histologic section, a curved tube with a simple (single) epithelial cell layer is sectioned in longitudinal, transverse, and oblique planes.

A **longitudinal (a)** plane of section that cuts the tube in the midline produces a U-shaped structure. The sides of the tube are lined by a single row of cuboidal (round) cells around an empty lumen except at the bottom, where the tube begins to curve; in this region the cells appear multilayered.

Transverse (d and e) planes of section of the same tube produce round structures lined by a single layer of cells. The variations that are seen in the cytoplasm of different cells are related to the planes of section through the individual cells, as explained above. A transverse section of a straight tube can produce a single image (e). The double image (d) of the same structure can represent either two tubes running parallel to each other or a single tube that has curved in the space of the tissue or organ that is sectioned.

A **tangential (b)** plane of section through the tube produces a solid, multicellular, oval structure that does not resemble a tube. The reason for this is that the plane of section has grazed the outermost periphery of tube as it made a turn in space; the lumen was not present in the plane of section. An **oblique (c)** plane of section through the tube and its cells produces an oval structure that includes an oval lumen in the center and multiple cell layers at the periphery.

A **transverse (f)** section in the region of a sharp curve in the tube grazes the innermost cell layer and produces two round structures connected by a multiple, solid layer of cells. These sections of the tube also contain round lumen, indicating that the plane of section passed perpendicular to the structure.

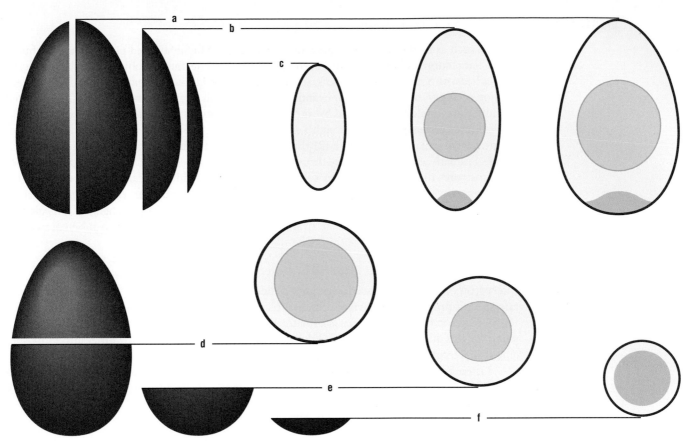

FIGURE I.1 ■ Planes of section of a round object.

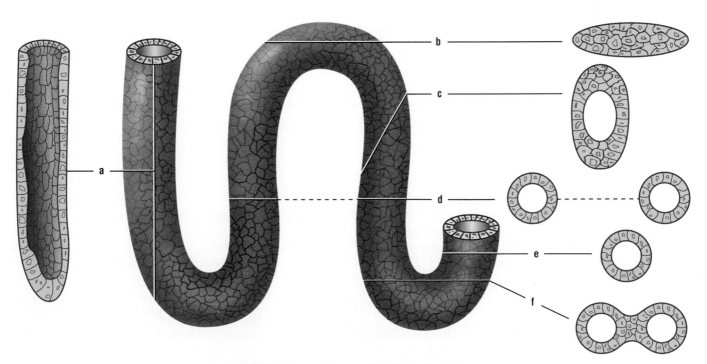

FIGURE I.2 ■ Planes of section of a tube.

FIGURE I.3 ■ Tubules of the Testis in Different Planes of Section

Organs such as the testes and kidneys consist primarily of highly twisted or convoluted tubules. When flat sections of such organs are seen on a histology slide, the cut tubules exhibit a variety of shapes because of the plane of section. To show how twisted tubules appear in a histologic slide, a portion of a testis was prepared for examination. Each testis consists of numerous, highly twisted seminiferous tubules that are lined by multilayered or stratified germinal epithelium.

A **longitudinal plane** (1) through a seminiferous tubule produces an elongated tubule with a long lumen. A **transverse plane** (2) through a single seminiferous tubule produces a round tubule. Similarly, a **transverse plane through a curve** (3, 5) of a seminiferous tubule produces two oval structures that are connected by solid layers of cells. An **oblique plane** (4) through a tubule produces an oval structure with an oval lumen in the center and multiple cell layers at the periphery. A **tangential plane** (6) of a seminiferous tubule passes through its periphery. As a result, this plane produces a solid, multicellular, oval structure that does not resemble a tube because the lumen is not seen.

Interpretation of Structures Prepared by Different Types of Stains

Interpretation of histologic sections is greatly aided by the use of different stains, which stain certain specific properties in different cells, tissues, and organs. The most prevalent stain that is used for preparation of histology slides is hematoxylin and eosin (H&E) stain. Most of the images prepared for this atlas were taken from slides stained with H&E stain. To show other and more specific characteristic features of different cells, tissues, and organs, other stains are used.

Listed below are the stains that were used to prepare the slides and their specific staining characteristics.

Hematoxylin and Eosin Stain
- Nuclei stain blue
- Cytoplasm stains pink or red
- Collagen fibers stain pink
- Muscles stain pink

Masson's Trichrome Stain
- Nuclei stain black or blue black
- Muscles stain red
- Collagen and mucus stain green or blue
- Cytoplasm of most cells stains pink

Periodic Acid-Schiff Reaction (PAS)
- Glycogen stains deep red or magenta
- Contents of goblet cells in digestive organs and respiratory epithelia stain magenta red
- Basement membranes and brush borders in kidney tubules stain positive, or pink

Verhoeff's Stain for Elastic Tissue
- Elastic fibers stain jet black
- Nuclei stain gray
- Remaining structures stain pink

Mallory-Azan Stain
- Fibrous connective tissue, mucus, and hyaline cartilage stain deep blue
- Erythrocytes stain red-orange
- Cytoplasm of liver and kidney stains pink
- Nuclei stain red

Wright's or Giemsa's Stain
- Erythrocyte cytoplasm stains pink
- Lymphocyte nuclei stain dark purple-blue with pale blue cytoplasm
- Monocyte cytoplasm stains pale blue and nucleus stains medium blue
- Neutrophil nuclei stain dark blue
- Eosinophil nuclei stain dark blue and the granules stain bright pink

- Basophil nuclei stain dark blue or purple, cytoplasm stains pale blue, and granules stain deep purple
- Platelets stain light blue

Cajal's and Del Rio Hortega's Methods (Silver and Gold Methods)
- Myelinated and unmyelinated fibers and neurofibrils stain blue-black
- General background is nearly colorless
- Astrocytes stain black
- Depending on the methods used, the end product can stain black, brown, or gold

Osmic Acid (Osmium Tetroxide) Stain
- Lipids in general stain black
- Lipids in myelin sheath of nerves stain black

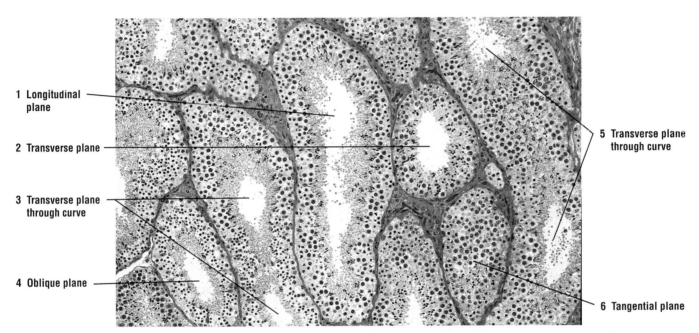

1 Longitudinal plane

2 Transverse plane

3 Transverse plane through curve

4 Oblique plane

5 Transverse plane through curve

6 Tangential plane

FIGURE 1.3 ■ Tubules of the testis in different planes of section. Stain: hematoxylin and eosin (plastic section). × 30.

PART I

TISSUES

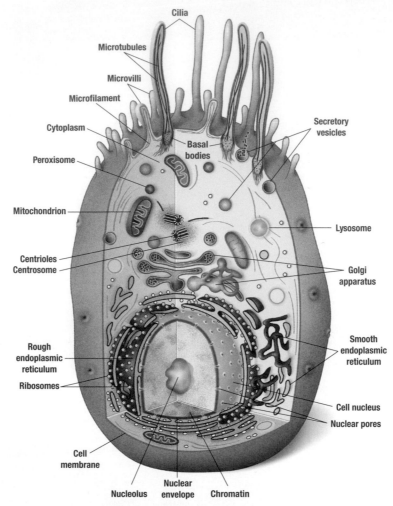

Cilia

Microtubules

Microvilli

Microfilament

Cytoplasm

Peroxisome

Basal
bodies

Secretory
vesicles

Mitochondrion

Lysosome

Centrioles
Centrosome

Golgi
apparatus

Rough
endoplasmic
reticulum

Smooth
endoplasmic
reticulum

Ribosomes

Cell nucleus

Nuclear pores

Cell
membrane

Nucleolus

Nuclear
envelope

Chromatin

OVERVIEW FIGURE 1.1 ■ Composite illustration of a cell, its cytoplasm, and its organelles.

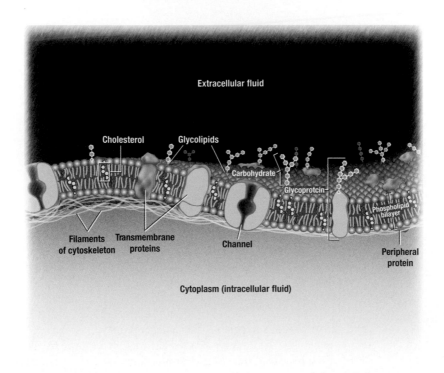

Extracellular fluid

Cholesterol

Glycolipids

Carbohydrate

Glycoprotein

Phospholipid
bilayer

Filaments
of cytoskeleton

Transmembrane
proteins

Channel

Peripheral
protein

Cytoplasm (intracellular fluid)

OVERVIEW FIGURE 1.2 ■ Composition of cell membrane.

The Cell and the Cytoplasm

Introduction—Light and Electron Microscopy

Histology, or microscopic anatomy, is a visual, colorful science. The light source for the early microscopes was sunlight. In modern microscopes, an electric light bulb with tungsten filaments serves as the main light source.

With the simplest light microscopes, examination of mammalian cells showed a nucleus and a cytoplasm, surrounded by some sort of a border or cell membrane. As microscopic techniques evolved, the use of various histochemical, immunocytochemical, and staining techniques revealed that the cytoplasm of different cells contained numerous subcellular elements called **organelles.** Although much initial information in histology was gained by examining tissue slides with a light microscope, its resolving power was too limited. To gain additional information called for increased resolution.

With the advent of transmission electron microscopy, superior resolution, and higher magnification of cells, examination of the contents of the cytoplasm became possible. Histologists are now able to describe the ultrastructure of the cell, its membrane, and the numerous organelles that are present in the cytoplasm of different cells.

The Cell

All living organisms contain a multitude of cell types, whose main functions are to maintain a proper **homeostasis** in the body, which is maintaining the internal environment of the body in a relatively constant state. To perform this task, the cells possess certain structural features in their cytoplasm that are common to all. As a result, it is possible to illustrate a cell in a more generalized, composite form with various cytoplasmic organelles. It is essential to remember, however, that the quantity, appearance, and distribution of the cytoplasmic organelles within a given cell depend on the cell type and its function.

The Cell Membrane

Except for the mature red blood cells, all mammalian cells contain a **cytoplasm** and a **nucleus.** In addition, all cells are surrounded by a **cell** or a **plasma membrane,** which forms an important barrier or boundary between the internal and the external environments. Internal to the cell membrane is the **cytoplasm,** a dense, fluidlike medium that contains numerous **organelles,** microtubules, microfilaments, and membrane-bound secretory granules or ingested material. In most cells, the nucleus is also located within the cytoplasm.

The membrane that surrounds the cell consists of a **phospholipid bilayer,** a double layer of **phospholipid molecules.** Interspersed within and embedded in the phospholipid bilayer of the cell membrane are the **integral membrane proteins** and **peripheral membrane proteins,** which make up almost half of the total mass of the membrane. The integral proteins are incorporated within the lipid bilayer of the cell membrane. Some of the integral proteins span the entire thickness of the cell membrane. These are the **transmembrane proteins** and they are exposed on the outer and the inner surface of the cell membrane. The peripheral proteins do not protrude into the phospholipid bilayer and are not embedded within the cell membrane. Instead, they are associated with the cell membrane on both its extracellular (outer) and intracellular (inner) surfaces. Some of the peripheral proteins are anchored to the network of tiny **microfilaments** of the cytoskeleton of the cell and are held firmly in place. Also present within the plasma membrane is the lipid molecule **cholesterol.** Cholesterol stabilizes the cell membrane, makes it more rigid, and regulates the fluidity of the phospholipid bilayer.

Located on the external surface of the cell membrane is a delicate, fuzzy cell coat called the **glycocalyx,** composed of carbohydrate molecules that are attached to the integral proteins of the cell membrane and that project from the external cell surface. The glycocalyx is seen primarily with electron microscopic images of the cells. The glycocalyx has an important role in cell recognition, cell-to-cell attachments or adhesions, and as receptor or binding sites for different blood-borne hormones.

Molecular Organization of the Cell Membrane

The lipid bilayer of the cell membrane has a fluid consistency, and, as a result, the compositional structure of the cell membrane is characterized as a **fluid mosaic model.** The phospholipid molecules of the cell membrane are distributed as two layers. Their **polar heads** are arranged on both the inner and outer surfaces of the cell membrane. The **nonpolar tails** of the lipid layers face each other in the center of the membrane. In electron micrographs, however, the cell membrane appears as three layers, consisting of outer and inner electron-dense layers, and a less dense or lighter middle layer. This discrepancy is owing to the osmic acid (osmium tetroxide) that is used to fix and stain tissues for electron microscopy. Osmic acid binds to the polar heads of the lipid molecules in the cell membrane and stains them very densely. The nonpolar tails in the middle of the cell membrane remain light and unstained.

Cell Membrane Permeability and Membrane Transport

The phospholipid bilayer of the cell membrane is permeable to certain substances and impermeable to others. This property of the cell membrane is called **selective permeability.** Selective permeability forms an important barrier between the internal and external environments of the cell, which then maintains a constant intracellular environment.

The phospholipid bilayer is permeable to such molecules as oxygen, carbon dioxide, water, steroids, and other lipid-soluble chemicals. Other substances, such as glucose, ions, or proteins, cannot pass through the cell membrane and cross it only by specific **transport mechanisms.** Some of these substances are transported through the integral membrane proteins using pump molecules or through protein channels that allow the passage of specific molecules. A process called **endocytosis** performs the uptake and transfer of molecules and solids across the cell membrane into the cell interior. In contrast, the release of material from the cell cytoplasm across the cell membrane is called **exocytosis.**

Pinocytosis is the process by which cells ingest small molecules of extracellular fluids or liquids. **Phagocytosis** refers to the ingestion or intake of large particles by the cells, such as bacteria, worn out cells, or cellular debris. **Receptor-mediated endocytosis** is the more selective form of pinocytosis or phagocytosis. In this process, specific molecules in the extracellular fluid bind to receptors on the cell membrane and are then taken into the cell cytoplasm. The receptors cluster on the membrane, and the membrane indents at this point to form a pit that is coated with peripheral membrane proteins called **clathrin.** The pit pinches off and forms a clathrin-coated vesicle that enters the cytoplasm. Examples of receptor-mediated endocytosis include uptake of low-density lipoproteins and insulin from the blood.

Cellular Organelles

Each cell cytoplasm contains numerous organelles, each of which performs a specialized metabolic function that is essential for maintaining cellular homeostasis and cell life. A membrane similar to the cell membrane surrounds such important cytoplasmic organelles as nucleus, mitochondria, endoplasmic reticulum, Golgi complex, lysosomes, and peroxisomes. Organelles that are not surrounded by membranes include ribosomes, basal bodies, centrioles, and centrosomes.

Mitochondria

Mitochondria are round, oval, or elongated structures whose variability and number depend on cell function. Each mitochondrion (singular) consists of an outer and inner membrane. The inner membrane exhibits numerous folds called **cristae.** In protein-secreting cells, these cristae project into the interior of the organelle like shelves. In steroid-secreting cells, such as the adrenal cortex or interstitial cells in the testes, the mitochondria cristae are tubular.

Endoplasmic Reticulum

The **endoplasmic reticulum** in the cytoplasm is an extensive network of sacs, vesicles, and interconnected flat tubules called **cisternae.** Endoplasmic reticulum may be rough or smooth. Their predominance and distribution in a given cell depends on cell function.

Rough endoplasmic reticulum is characterized by numerous flattened, interconnected cisternae, whose cytoplasmic surfaces are covered or studded with dark-staining granules called **ribosomes.** The presence of ribosomes distinguishes the rough endoplasmic reticulum, which extends from the nuclear envelope around the nucleus to sites throughout the cytoplasm. In contrast, **smooth endoplasmic reticulum** is devoid of ribosomes, and it consists primarily of anastomosing or connecting tubules. In most cells, smooth endoplasmic reticulum is continuous with rough endoplasmic reticulum.

Golgi Apparatus

The **Golgi apparatus** is also composed of a system of membrane-bound, smooth, flattened, stacked, and slightly curved **cisternae.** These cisternae, however, are separate from those of endoplasmic reticulum. In most cells, there is a polarity in the Golgi apparatus. Near the Golgi apparatus, numerous small vesicles with newly synthesized proteins bud off from the rough endoplasmic reticulum and move to the Golgi apparatus for further processing. The Golgi cisternae nearest the budding vesicles are the forming, convex, or the *cis* **face** of the Golgi apparatus. The opposite side of the Golgi apparatus is the maturing inner concave side or the *trans* face. Vesicles from the endoplasmic reticulum move through the cytoplasm to the *cis* side of the Golgi apparatus and bud off from the *trans* side to transport proteins to different sites in the cell cytoplasm.

Ribosomes

The **ribosomes** are small, electron-dense granules found in the cytoplasm of the cell; a membrane does not surround ribosomes. In a given cell, there are both **free ribosomes** and **attached ribosomes,** as seen on the endoplasmic reticulum cisternae. Ribosomes have an important role in **protein synthesis** and are most abundant in the cytoplasm of protein-secreting cells. Ribosomes perform an essential role in decoding or translating the **coded genetic messages** from the nucleus for amino acid sequence of proteins that are then synthesized by the cell. The unattached or free ribosomes synthesize proteins for use within the cell cytoplasm. In contrast, ribosomes that are attached to the membranes of the endoplasmic reticulum synthesize proteins that are packaged and stored in the cell as lysosomes, or are released from the cell as secretory products.

Lysosomes

Lysosomes are organelles produced by the Golgi apparatus that are highly variable in appearance and size. They contain a variety of hydrolyzing or digestive enzymes called **acid hydrolases.** To prevent the lysosomes from digesting the cytoplasm and cell contents, a membrane separates the lytic enzymes in the lysosomes from the cytoplasm. The main function of lysosomes is the **intracellular digestion** or **phagocytosis** of substances taken into the cells. Lysosomes digest phagocytosed microorganisms, cell debris, cells, and damaged, worn-out, or excessive cell organelles, such as rough endoplasmic reticulum or mitochondria. During intracellular digestion, a membrane surrounds the material to be digested. The membrane of the lysosome then fuses with the ingested material, and their hydrolytic enzymes are emptied into the formed vacuole. After digestion of the lysosomal contents, the indigestible debris in the cytoplasm is retained in large membrane-bound vesicles called **residual bodies.** Lysosomes are very abundant in such phagocytic cells as tissue macrophages and specific white blood cells (leukocytes).

Peroxisomes

Peroxisomes are cell organelles that appear similar to lysosomes, but are smaller. They are found in nearly all cell types. Peroxisomes contain several types of **oxidases,** which are enzymes that oxidize various organic substances to form hydrogen peroxide, a highly cytotoxic product. Peroxisomes also contain the enzyme **catalase,** which eliminates excess hydrogen peroxide by breaking it down into water and oxygen molecules. Because the degradation of hydrogen peroxide takes place within the same organelle, peroxisomes protect other parts of the cells from this cytotoxic product. Peroxisomes are abundant in the cells of the liver and kidney, where much of the toxic substances are removed from the body.

The Cytoskeleton of the Cell

The **cytoskeleton** of a cell consists of a network of tiny protein filaments and tubules that extend throughout the cytoplasm. It serves the cell's structural framework. Three types of filamentous proteins, microfilaments, intermediate filaments, and microtubules, form the cytoskeleton of a cell.

Microfilaments, Intermediate Filaments, and Microtubules

Microfilaments are the thinnest structures of the cytoskeleton. They are composed of the protein **actin** and are most prevalent on the peripheral regions of the cell membrane. These structural proteins shape the cells, and are involved in cell movement and movement of the cytoplasmic organelles. The microfilaments are distributed throughout the cells and are used as anchors at cell junctions. The actin microfilaments also form the structural **core** of microvilli and the **terminal web** just inferior to the plasma membrane. In muscle tissues, the actin filaments fill the cells and are associated with myosin proteins to induce muscle contractions.

Intermediate filaments are thicker than microfilaments, as their name implies. Several cytoskeletal proteins that form the intermediate filaments have been identified and localized. The intermediate filaments vary among cell types and have specific distribution in different cell types. Epithelial cells contain the intermediate filaments **keratin.** In skin cells, these filaments terminate at cell junctions, where they stabilize the shape of the cell and their attachments to adjacent cells. **Vimentin** filaments are found in many mesenchymal cells. **Desmin** filaments are found in both smooth and striated muscles. **Neurofilament** proteins are found in the nerve cells and their processes. **Glial filaments** are found in astrocytic glial cells of the nervous system. **Lamin** intermediate filaments are found on the inner layer of the nuclear membrane.

Microtubules are found in almost all cell types except red blood cells. They are the largest elements of the cytoskeleton. Microtubules are hollow, unbranched structures composed of the two-protein subunit, α and β **tubulin.** All microtubules originate from the microtubule-organizing center, the **centrosome** in the cytoplasm, which contains a pair of **centrioles.** In the centrosome, the tubulin subunits polymerize and radiate from the centrioles in a starlike pattern from the center. Microtubules determine cell shape and function in intracellular movement of organelles and secretory granules and form spindles that guide the movement of chromosomes during cell division or mitosis. These tubules are most visible and are predominant in **cilia** and **flagella,** where they are responsible for the beating movements.

Centrosome and Centrioles

The **centrosome** is an area of the cytoplasm located near the nucleus. Within the centrosome are two small cylindrical structures called **centrioles** and the surrounding matrix; the centrioles are perpendicular to each other. Each centriole consists of nine evenly spaced clusters of three microtubules arranged in a circle. The microtubules have longitudinal orientation and are parallel to each other.

Before mitosis, the centrioles in the centrosome replicate and form two pairs. During mitosis, each pair moves to the opposite poles of the cell, where they become microtubule-organizing centers for **mitotic spindles** that control the distribution of chromosomes to the daughter cells.

Cytoplasmic Inclusions

The **cytoplasmic inclusions** are temporary structures that accumulate in the cytoplasm of certain cells. **Lipids**, **glycogen**, **crystals**, **pigment**, or byproducts of metabolism are inclusions and represent the nonliving parts of the cell.

The Nucleus and the Nuclear Envelope

The **nucleus** is the largest organelle of a cell. Most cells have a single nucleus, but other cells may exhibit multiple nuclei. Skeletal muscle cells have multiple nuclei, whereas mature red blood cells of mammals do not have a nucleus, or are nonnucleated.

The nucleus consists of **chromatin,** one or more **nucleoli** (singular, nucleolus), and **nuclear matrix.** The nucleus contains the cellular genetic material **deoxyribonucleic acid** (DNA), which encodes all cell structures and functions. A double membrane called the **nuclear envelope** surrounds the nucleus. Both the inner and outer layers of the nuclear envelope have a structure similar to the lipid bilayer of the cell membrane. The outer nuclear membrane is studded with ribosomes and is continuous with the rough endoplasmic reticulum. At intervals around the periphery of the nucleus, the outer and inner membranes of the nuclear envelope fuse to form numerous **nuclear pores.** These pores function in controlling the movement of metabolites, macromolecules, and ribosomal subunits between the nucleus and cytoplasm.

FIGURE 1.1 ■ Apical Surfaces of Ciliated and Nonciliated Epithelium

A low-magnification electron micrograph shows alternating ciliated and nonciliated cells in the epithelium of the efferent ductules of the testis. The **cilia (1)** in the ciliated cells are attached to the dense **basal bodies (2)** at the cell apices, from which they extend into the **lumen (7)** of the duct. In contrast to cilia, the **microvilli (8)** in the nonciliated cells are much shorter.

Note also the dense structures in the apices between the adjacent epithelial cells. These are the **junctional complexes (3)** that hold the cells together. Distinct **cell membranes (10)** separate the individual cells. Located in the cytoplasm of these cells are numerous, elongated or rod-shaped **mitochondria (5),** a few stacked **cisternae** of the **rough endoplasmic reticulum (11),** numerous light-staining **vesicles (4),** and some secretory products in the form of **dense bodies (6).** Each cell also contains various-shaped **nuclei (12)** with dispersed, dense-staining nuclear **chromatin (13)** arranged around the nuclear periphery.

FIGURE 1.2 ■ Junctional Complex Between Epithelial Cells

A high-magnification electron micrograph illustrates a junctional complex between two adjacent epithelial cells. In the upper or apical region of the cells, the opposing cell membranes fuse to form a **tight junction** or **zonula occludens (2a),** which extends around the cell peripheries like a belt. Inferior to the zonula occludens (2a) is another junction called the **zonula adherens (2b).** It is characterized by a dense layer of proteins on the inside of the plasma membranes of both cells, which attach to the cytoskeleton filaments of each cell. A small intercellular space with transmembrane adhesion proteins separates the two membranes. This type of junction also extends around the cells like a belt. Below the zonula adherens is a **desmosome (2c).** Desmosomes (2c) do not encircle the cells, but are spotlike structures that have random distribution in the cells. The cytoplasmic side of each desmosome exhibits dense areas composed of attachment proteins. Transmembrane glycoproteins extend into the intercellular space between opposing cells membranes of the desmosome and attach the cells to each other.

Note also in the micrograph the distinct **cell membranes (3)** of each cell, the numerous **mitochondria (1)** in cross section, and a variety of **vesicular structures (6)** in their cytoplasm. Visible on the cell apices are sections of **cilia (5)** with a core of **microtubules** and a few **microvilli (4).**

FUNCTIONAL CORRELATIONS: Junctional Complex

Junctional complexes have a variety of functions, depending on their morphology or shape. In the epithelium that lines the stomach, intestines, and urinary bladder, the **zonulae occludentes** or tight junctions prevent the passage of corrosive chemicals or waste products between cells and into the bloodstream. In this manner, the cells form an epithelial barrier. The tight junctions consist of **transmembrane proteins** that fuse the outer membranes of adjacent cells. Similarly, the **zonula adherens** assists these cells in resisting separation, such that the transmembrane proteins attach to the cytoskeleton proteins and bind adjacent cells. **Desmosomes** are spotlike structures that are most commonly seen in the epithelium of the skin and in cardiac muscle fibers. Here, the cells are subjected to great mechanical stresses. In these organs, desmosomes prevent skin cells from separating and cardiac muscle cells from pulling apart during heart contractions. The desmosomes have transmembrane proteins that extend into the intercellular space between adjacent cell membranes to anchor the cells together.

Other junctional complexes are **hemidesmosomes** and **gap junctions.** Hemidesmosomes are one half of the desmosome and are present at the base of epithelial cells. Here, hemidesmosomes anchor the epithelial cells to basement membrane and the adjacent connective tissue. Basement membrane consists of a basal lamina and reticular fibers of the connective tissue (see Figure 1.3).

Gap junctions are also spotlike in structure. The plasma membranes at gap junctions are closely apposed, and tiny fluid channels called **connexons** connect the adjacent cells. Ions and small molecules can easily diffuse through these connexons from one cell to another. These fluid channels are vital for very rapid communication between cells, especially in cardiac muscle cells and nerve cells, where fast impulse transmission through the cells or axons is essential for synchronization of normal functions.

1 Cilia

2 Basal bodies

3 Junctional complexes

4 Vesicles

5 Mitochondria

6 Dense bodies

7 Lumen

8 Microvilli

9 Basal bodies

10 Cell membranes

11 Rough endoplasmic reticulum

12 Nuclei

13 Chromatin

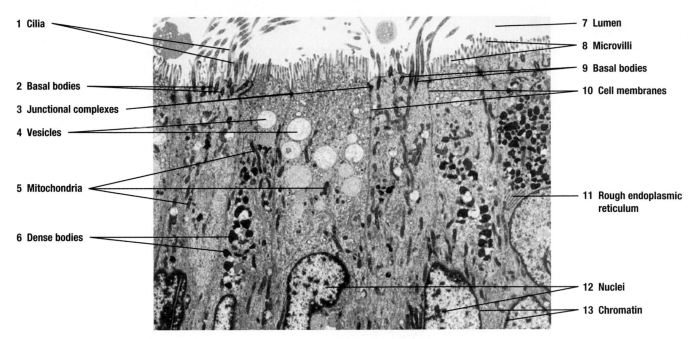

FIGURE 1.1 ■ Apical surfaces of ciliated and nonciliated epithelium. ×10,600.

1 Mitochondria

2 Junctinal complex
   a. Tight junction
   b. Zonula adherens
   c. Desmosome

3 Cell membranes

4 Microvilli

5 Cilia with microtubules

6 Vesicles

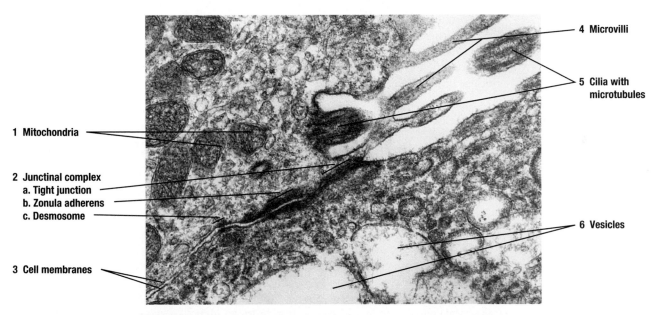

FIGURE 1.2 ■ Junctional complex between epithelial cells. ×31,200.

FIGURE 1.3 ■ Basal Regions of Epithelial Cells

A medium-magnification electron micrograph illustrates the appearance of the basal region or the base of epithelial cells. Note that the basal regions of the cells are attached to a thin, moderately electron-dense layer called the **basal lamina (3)**. Deep to the basal lamina (3) is a **connective tissue (2)** layer of fine reticular fibers. The basal lamina (3) is seen only with the electron microscope. Basal lamina (3) and the reticular fibers of connective tissue (2) are seen under the light microscope as a basement membrane.

Inferior to the epithelial cells is an elongated, spindle-shaped **fibroblast (4)** with its **nucleus (4)** and dispersed **chromatin (5)**, surrounded by numerous connective tissue fibers (2) produced by the fibroblasts. In the cytoplasm of one of the epithelial cells is also seen a **nucleus (8)**, dispersed **chromatin (9)**, and a dense, round **nucleolus (7)**. **Cisternae** of **rough endoplasmic reticulum (11)**, elongated **mitochondria (14)**, and various types of **dense bodies (6)** are visible in different cells. Between the individual epithelial cells is a distinct **cell membrane (1, 10)**. Hemidesmosomes are not illustrated (see Figure 1.4), but attach the basal membrane of the cells to the basal lamina (3).

FIGURE 1.4 ■ Basal Region of an Ion-Transporting Cell

A medium-magnification electron micrograph illustrates the basal region of a cell from the distal convoluted tubule of the kidney. In contrast to the basal regions of epithelial cells, the basal regions of cells in convoluted kidney tubules are characterized by numerous and complex **infoldings** of the **basal cell membrane (5)**. These infoldings then form numerous **basal membrane interdigitations (11)** with the similar infoldings of the neighboring cell. Numerous and long **mitochondria (4, 10)** with vertical or apical-basal orientations are located between the cell membrane infoldings. Also, numerous, dark-staining spotlike **hemidesmosomes (6, 12)** attach the highly infolded basal cell membrane to the electron-dense **basal lamina (7, 13)**.

A portion of a large **nucleus (1)** is visible with its dispersed **chromatin (9)**. Surrounding the nucleus is a distinct **nuclear envelope (2)**, which consists of a double membrane. Both the outer and inner membranes of the nuclear envelope (2) fuse at intervals around the periphery of the nucleus to form numerous **nuclear pores (3)**.

FUNCTIONAL CORRELATIONS: Infolded Basal Regions of the Cell

The deep **infoldings** of the basal and lateral cell membranes are seen only with electron microscopy. These infoldings are found in certain cells of the body, whose main function is to transport **ions** across the cell membrane. The cells in the tubular portions of the kidney (proximal convoluted tubules and distal convoluted tubules) selectively absorb useful or nutritious components from the glomerular filtrate and retain them in the body. At the same time, these cells eliminate toxic or nonuseful metabolic waste products such as urea and drug metabolites.

Because these cells transport numerous ions across their membranes, increased amounts of energy are needed, which is generated by **Na$^+$/K$^+$ ATPase pumps** embedded in the infolded basal and lateral cell membranes. To perform these vital functions, considerable amount of chemical energy is needed. The numerous **mitochondria** located in these basal infoldings continually supply the cells with the energy source (ATP) that operates these pumps for membrane transport. Similar basal cell membrane infoldings are seen in the striated ducts of the salivary glands. These glands produce saliva, which is then modified by selective transport of various ions across the cell membrane as it moves through these ducts to the larger excretory ducts.

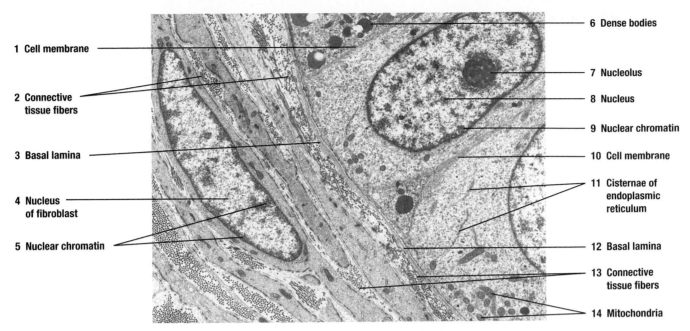

1 Cell membrane

2 Connective
 tissue fibers

3 Basal lamina

4 Nucleus
 of fibroblast

5 Nuclear chromatin

6 Dense bodies

7 Nucleolus

8 Nucleus

9 Nuclear chromatin

10 Cell membrane

11 Cisternae of
 endoplasmic
 reticulum

12 Basal lamina

13 Connective
 tissue fibers

14 Mitochondria

FIGURE 1.3 ■ Basal regions of epithelial cells. ×9,500.

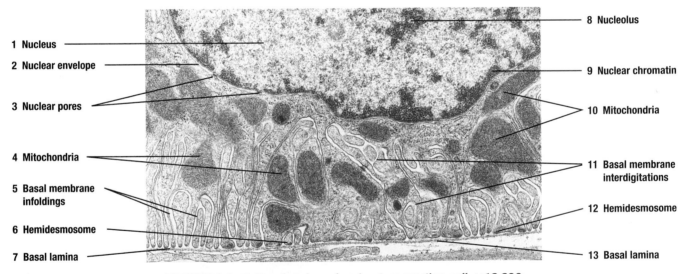

1 Nucleus

2 Nuclear envelope

3 Nuclear pores

4 Mitochondria

5 Basal membrane
 infoldings

6 Hemidesmosome

7 Basal lamina

8 Nucleolus

9 Nuclear chromatin

10 Mitochondria

11 Basal membrane
 interdigitations

12 Hemidesmosome

13 Basal lamina

FIGURE 1.4 ■ Basal region of an ion-transporting cell. ×16,600.

FIGURE 1.5 ■ Cilia and Microvilli

This high-magnification electron micrograph illustrates the ultrastructural differences between cilia (singular, cilium) and microvilli (singular, microvillus). Both **cilia (1)** and **microvilli (2)** project from the apical surfaces of certain cells in the body. The cilia (1) are long, motile structures, with a core of uniformly arranged **microtubules (3)** in longitudinal orientation. The core of each cilium contains a constant number of nine microtubule doublets located peripherally and two single microtubules in the center. Each cilium is attached to and extends from the **basal body (4)** in the apical region of the cell. Instead of nine microtubule doublets, the basal bodies exhibit nine microtubule triplets and no central microtubules.

In contrast to cilia, microvilli (2) are smaller, shorter, closely packed fingerlike extensions that greatly increase the surface area of certain cells. Microvilli (2) are nonmotile and exhibit a core of thin microfilaments called actin. The actin filaments extend from the microvilli (2) into the apical cytoplasm of the cell to form a terminal web, a complex network of actin filaments.

FIGURE 1.6 ■ Nuclear Envelope and Nuclear Pores

A high-magnification electron micrograph illustrates in detail part of a **nucleus (8)** and the surrounding membrane, the **nuclear envelope (3),** which consists of an **outer nuclear membrane (3a)** and an **inner nuclear membrane (3b).** Between the two nuclear membranes (3a, 3b) is a space. The outer nuclear membrane (3a) is in contact with the **cell cytoplasm (4),** whereas the inner nuclear membrane (3b) is associated with the **nuclear chromatin (7).** The nuclear envelope is continuous with the **rough endoplasmic reticulum (1),** and the outer nuclear membrane (3a) usually contains ribosomes. At certain intervals around the nucleus, the two membranes of the nuclear envelope (3) fuse and form numerous **nuclear pores (2, 6).**

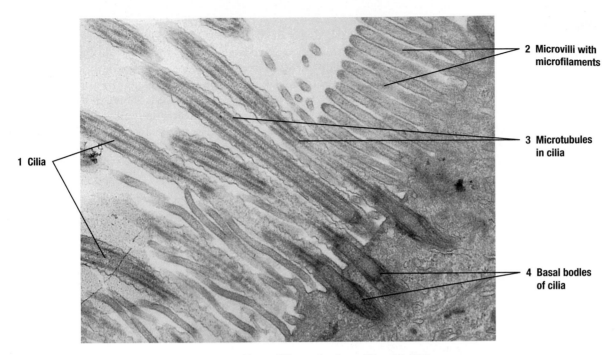

2 **Microvilli with microfilaments**

3 **Microtubules in cilia**

1 **Cilia**

4 **Basal bodles of cilia**

FIGURE 1.5 ■ Cilia and microvilli. ×20,000.

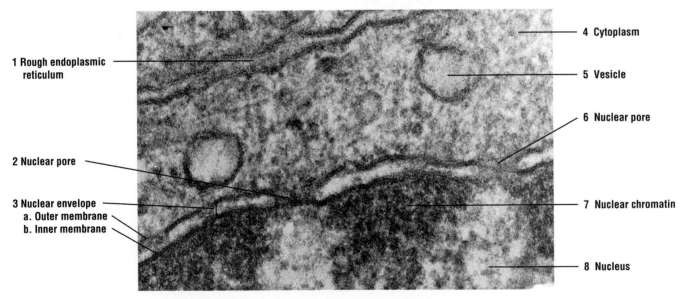

4 **Cytoplasm**

1 **Rough endoplasmic reticulum**

5 **Vesicle**

6 **Nuclear pore**

2 **Nuclear pore**

3 **Nuclear envelope**
   a. **Outer membrane**
   b. **Inner membrane**

7 **Nuclear chromatin**

8 **Nucleus**

FIGURE 1.6 ■ Nuclear envelope and nuclear pores. ×110,000.

FIGURE 1.7 ■ Mitochondria

A high-magnification electron micrograph illustrates the ultrastructure of **mitochondria (1, 4)** in a **longitudinal section (1)** and in **cross section (4).** Note that the mitochondria (1, 4) also exhibit two membranes. The **outer mitochondrial membrane (5, 9)** is smooth and surrounds the entire organelle. The inner mitochondrial membrane is highly folded, surrounds the matrix of the mitochondria, and projects inward into the organelle to form the numerous, shelflike **cristae (6).** Some mitochondrial matrix may contain dense-staining granules. Also visible in the **cytoplasm (8)** of the cell are variously sized, light-staining **vacuoles (7),** a section of **rough endoplasmic reticulum (2),** and free **ribosomes (3).** This type of mitochondria with shelflike cristae (6) is normally found in protein-secreting cells and muscle cells.

FUNCTIONAL CORRELATIONS

Cilia

Cilia are highly motile surface modifications in cells that line the respiratory organs, oviducts or uterine tubes, and efferent ducts in the testes. Cilia are inserted into the **basal bodies.** The main function of cilia is to sweep or move fluids, cells, or particulate matter across cell surfaces. In the lungs, the cilia rid the air passages of particulate matter or mucus. In the oviduct, cilia move eggs and sperm along the passageway, and in the testes, cilia move mature sperm into the epididymis.

The motility exhibited by cilia is caused by the sliding of adjacent microtubule doublets in the core of the cilia. Each of the nine doublets in the cilia consists of two subfibers called A and B. Extending from the A subfiber are two armlike filaments containing the **motor protein dynein,** which exhibits ATPase activity. This protein uses the energy of ATP hydrolysis to move cilia. Dynein extensions from one doublet bind to subfiber B of the adjacent doublet, producing a sliding force between the doublets and causing cilia motility.

Microvilli

In contrast to cilia, **microvilli** are nonmotile. Microvilli are highly developed on the apical surfaces of epithelial cells of small intestine and kidney. Here, the main functions of the microvilli are to absorb nutrients from the digestive tract of the small intestine or the glomerular filtrate in the kidney.

Nucleus, Nucleolus, and Nuclear Pores

The **nucleus** is the control center of the cell; it stores and processes most of the cell's genetic information. The nucleus directs all of the activities of the cell through the process of protein synthesis and ultimately controls the structural and functional characteristics of each cell. The cell's genetic material, **deoxyribonucleic acid (DNA),** is visible in the cell in the form of **chromatin.** When the cells are not actively producing protein, the DNA is not condensed and does not stain.

The **nucleolus** is a dense-staining, nonmembrane-bound structure within the nucleus. One or more nucleoli may be visible in a given cell. The nucleolus functions in synthesis, processing, and assembly of **ribosomes.** In nucleoli, the ribosomal **ribonucleic acid (RNA)** is produced and combined with proteins to form ribosomal subunits. These ribosomal subunits are then transported to the cell cytoplasm through the nuclear pores to form complete ribosomes. Consequently, nucleoli are prominent in cells that synthesize large amounts of proteins.

Nuclear pores control the transport of macromolecules into and out of the nucleus. The nuclear pore membrane, like other cell membranes, shows selective permeability. As a result, some of the larger molecules travel through the pores via an active transport mechanism.

Mitochondria

These organelles produce most of the high-energy molecule **adenosine triphosphate (ATP)** present in cells and are, therefore, considered the powerhouses of the cells. The numerous cristae in the mitochondria increase the surface area of the inner membrane. The cristae contain most of the respiratory chain enzymes as well as ATP synthetase, which is responsible for cell respiration (oxidative phosphorylation) and production of cell ATP. Surrounding the cristae is an amorphous **mitochondrial matrix.** It contains enzymes, ribosomes, and a small, circular DNA molecule called **mitochondrial DNA.**

Cells that are highly active metabolically, such as those in the skeletal and cardiac muscles, contain increased number of mitochondria. These cells need and use ATP at a very high rate. Also, in these high-energy cells, the mitochondria exhibit large numbers of closely packed cristae, whereas in cells with low-energy metabolism, there are fewer mitochondria with less extensively developed cristae.

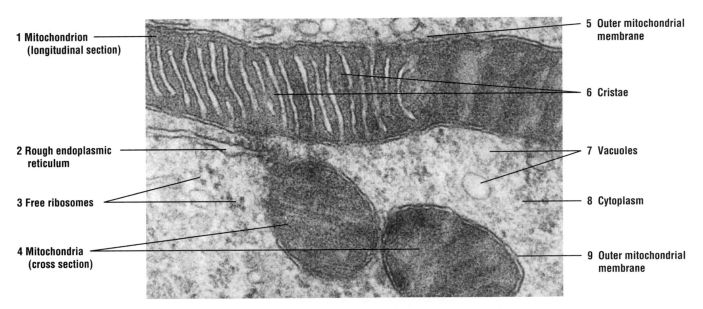

1 Mitochondrion (longitudinal section)
2 Rough endoplasmic reticulum
3 Free ribosomes
4 Mitochondria (cross section)
5 Outer mitochondrial membrane
6 Cristae
7 Vacuoles
8 Cytoplasm
9 Outer mitochondrial membrane

FIGURE 1.7 ■ Mitochondria (longitudinal and cross section). ×49,500.

FIGURE 1.8 ■ Rough Endoplasmic Reticulum

A high-magnification electron micrograph illustrates the components of the **rough endoplasmic reticulum (3)** in the cytoplasm of a cell. It consists of stacked layers of membranous cavities called **cisternae (3)**. In the rough endoplasmic reticulum, ribosomes are attached to the outer surface of the membranes. Also present in the cytoplasm are **free ribosomes (4, 13)**, some of which attach to other ribosome and form ribosome groups called **polyribosomes (4, 13)**. Visible in the cytoplasm are also numerous **mitochondria (2, 10)**, in both **longitudinal (10)** and **cross section (2)**, **dense secretory granules (8)**, and very thin strands of **microfilaments (5, 11)**. In the lower right corner of the micrograph the smooth cisternae and associated vesicles of the **Golgi apparatus (14)** are visible. Note the **cell membranes (1, 9)** of adjacent cells, **nuclear envelope (6)**, and portions of the **nucleus (7)** and nuclear **chromatin (12)**.

FIGURE 1.9 ■ Smooth Endoplasmic Reticulum

This high magnification electron micrograph illustrates the structure of the **smooth endoplasmic reticulum (2)** in two adjacent cells. Smooth endoplasmic reticulum (2) is devoid of ribosomes and consists primarily of smooth, anastomosing tubules. In this micrograph, the tubules of the smooth endoplasmic reticulum (2) are primarily seen in cross section. In other sections, the smooth endoplasmic reticulum (2) can be seen as flattened vesicles. In some cells, smooth endoplasmic reticulum is continuous with **cisternae** of the **rough endoplasmic reticulum (7)**, as seen in this micrograph.

Also seen in the micrograph are the **cell membranes (6, 11)** of the two cells, the **cell membrane interdigitations (10)**, and the **extracellular matrix (9)** between the two cell membranes. A section of the **nucleus (4, 5)**, **nuclear envelope (8)**, **nuclear chromatin (3)**, and **mitochondrion (1)** in cross section are also visible in the two cells. The mitochondria (1) in these cells contain tubular cristae, indicating that the cells synthesize products other than proteins.

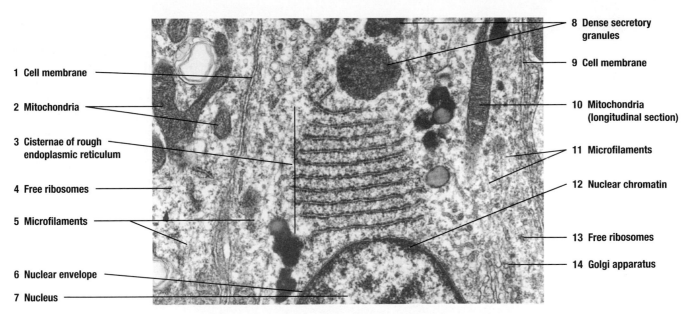

1 Cell membrane

2 Mitochondria

3 Cisternae of rough
   endoplasmic reticulum

4 Free ribosomes

5 Microfilaments

6 Nuclear envelope

7 Nucleus

8 Dense secretory
   granules

9 Cell membrane

10 Mitochondria
    (longitudinal section)

11 Microfilaments

12 Nuclear chromatin

13 Free ribosomes

14 Golgi apparatus

FIGURE 1.8 ■ Rough endoplasmic reticulum. ×32,000.

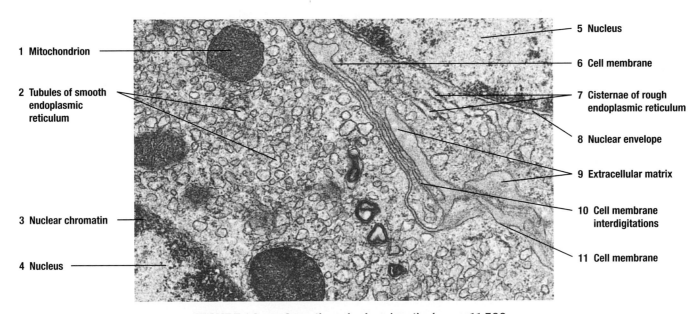

1 Mitochondrion

2 Tubules of smooth
   endoplasmic
   reticulum

3 Nuclear chromatin

4 Nucleus

5 Nucleus

6 Cell membrane

7 Cisternae of rough
   endoplasmic reticulum

8 Nuclear envelope

9 Extracellular matrix

10 Cell membrane
    interdigitations

11 Cell membrane

FIGURE 1.9 ■ Smooth endoplasmic reticulum. ×11,500.

FIGURE 1.10 ▪ Golgi Apparatus

A high-magnification electron micrograph illustrates the components of the **Golgi apparatus (2).** This apparatus consists of membrane-bound **Golgi cisternae (2)** with numerous membranous **Golgi vesicles (1)** located near the end of the cisternae. The Golgi apparatus (2) usually exhibits a crescent shape. Its convex side is called the *cis* **face (3),** and the opposite, concave side is the *trans* face (9) of the Golgi apparatus (2). This micrograph illustrates the Golgi apparatus (2) in the seminiferous tubule of the testis, where a spermatid is undergoing transformation into a sperm. At this stage of the transformation, the Golgi apparatus (2) is packaging and condensing the secretory product into an electron-dense **acrosome granule (7).** The acrosome granule (7) is located in the **acrosomal vesicle (8)** that adheres to the **nuclear envelope (6)** at the anterior pole of the spermatid. In the left corner of the micrograph, note a short cisterna of the **granular (rough) endoplasmic reticulum (4)** and some **free ribosomes (5)** in the **cytoplasm (11)** of the spermatid. A **cell membrane (10)** surrounds the cell.

FUNCTIONAL CORRELATIONS

Rough Endoplasmic Reticulum

Cells that synthesize large amounts of protein for export, such as pancreatic acinar cells or salivary gland cells, exhibit a highly developed and extensive **rough endoplasmic reticulum** with numerous stacks of flattened cisternae. Thus, the main function of rough endoplasmic reticulum is **protein synthesis.** Proteins that will be transported or exported either to the outside of the cell or packaged in organelles such as lysosomes are synthesized by the ribosomes attached to the surface of the rough endoplasmic reticulum. In addition, **integral membrane proteins** and **phospholipid molecules** are synthesized by the rough endoplasmic reticulum and inserted into the cell membrane. In contrast, proteins for the cytoplasm, nucleus, and mitochondria are synthesized by the **free ribosomes** located within the cell cytoplasm.

Smooth Endoplasmic Reticulum

Although the **smooth endoplasmic reticulum** is continuous with the rough endoplasmic reticulum, its membranes lack ribosomes, and, therefore, its functions are completely different and unrelated to protein synthesis. Smooth endoplasmic reticulum is found in abundance in cells that synthesize **phospholipids, cholesterol,** and **steroid hormones,** such as estrogens, testosterone, and corticosteroids. When liver cells are exposed to potentially harmful drugs and chemicals, smooth endoplasmic reticulum proliferates and inactivates or **detoxifies** the chemicals. Skeletal and cardiac muscle fibers also exhibit an extensive network of smooth endoplasmic reticulum for **calcium storage** between contractions and from which calcium is released to initiate muscular contractions.

Golgi Apparatus

The **Golgi apparatus** is present in almost all cells. Its size and development varies, depending on the cell function; however, it is most highly developed in **secretory cells.** Most of the proteins synthesized by the cisternae of the rough endoplasmic reticulum are transported in the cell cytoplasm to the *cis* face of the Golgi apparatus, which faces the rough endoplasmic reticulum. Within the Golgi cisternae are different types of enzymes that modify, sort, and package proteins for different destinations in the cell. As the protein molecules move through the different Golgi cisternae, sugars are added to the proteins and lipids to form **glycoproteins** and **glycolipids.** Also, proteins are added to lipids to form **lipoproteins.** As the secretory molecules near the exit or *trans* face of the Golgi cisternae, they are further modified, sorted, and packaged as membrane-bound vesicles, which then separate from the Golgi cisternae. Some secretory vesicles become lysosomes. Others migrate to the cell membrane and are incorporated into the cell membrane itself, thus contributing proteins and phospholipids to the membrane. Still other secretory granules become vesicles filled with a secretory product destined for export to the outside of the cell.

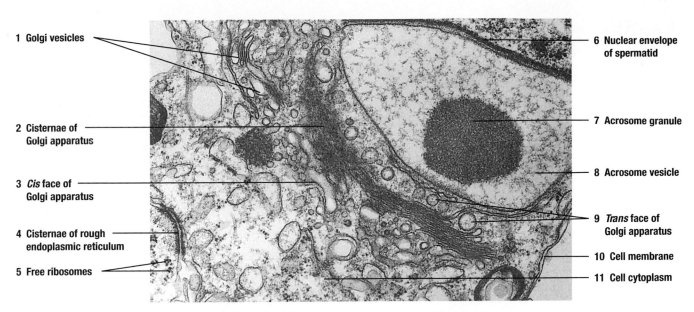

1 Golgi vesicles

2 Cisternae of
   Golgi apparatus

3 *Cis* face of
   Golgi apparatus

4 Cisternae of rough
   endoplasmic reticulum

5 Free ribosomes

6 Nuclear envelope
   of spermatid

7 Acrosome granule

8 Acrosome vesicle

9 *Trans* face of
   Golgi apparatus

10 Cell membrane

11 Cell cytoplasm

FIGURE 1.10 ■ Golgi apparatus. ×23,000.

CHAPTER 1 ■ Summary

Cell and Cytoplasm

- Cells maintain proper homeostasis of the body
- Certain structural features common to all cells

The Cell Membrane

- Consists of phospholipid bilayer and integral (transmembrane) membrane proteins
- Peripheral membrane proteins located on external and internal cell surfaces
- Peripheral proteins anchored to microfilaments of cytoskeleton
- Cholesterol molecules within the cell membrane stabilize the cell membrane
- Carbohydrate glycocalyx covers cell surfaces
- Glycocalyx important for cell recognition, cell adhesion, and receptor binding sites

Molecular Organization of Cell Membrane

- Lipid bilayer in fluid state, hence the fluid mosaic model
- Phospholipids distributed in two layers with polar heads on inner and outer surfaces
- Nonpolar tails in center of membrane

Cell Membrane Permeability and Transport

- Cell membrane shows selective permeability and forms a barrier between internal and external cell environments
- Permeable to oxygen, carbon dioxide, water, steroids, and lipid-soluble chemicals
- Larger molecules enter cell by specialized transport mechanisms
- Endocytosis is ingestion of extracellular material into the cell
- Exocytosis is release of material from the cell
- Pinocytosis is ingestion of extracellular fluid
- Phagocytosis is uptake of large, solid particles
- Receptor-mediated endocytosis involves pinocytosis or phagocytosis via receptors on cell membrane and formation of clathrin-coated pits
- Uptake of low-density lipoproteins and insulin as example of receptor-mediated endocytosis

Cellular Organelles

Mitochondria

- Surrounded by cell membrane
- Shelflike cristae in protein-secreting cells and tubular cristae in steroid-secreting cells
- Present in all cells, especially numerous in highly metabolic cells
- Produce high-energy ATP molecules
- Cristae contain respiratory chain enzymes for ATP production
- Matrix contains enzymes, ribosomes, and circular mitochondrial DNA

Rough Endoplasmic Reticulum

- Exhibits interconnected cisternae with ribosomes
- Highly developed in protein-synthesizing cells
- Synthesizes proteins for export or lysosomes
- Synthesizes integral membrane proteins and phospholipids

Smooth Endoplasmic Reticulum

- Devoid of ribosomes and consists of anastomosing tubules
- Found in cells that synthesize phospholipids, cholesterol, and steroid hormones
- In liver cells, proliferates to deactivate or detoxify harmful chemicals
- In skeletal and cardiac muscle fibers, stores calcium between contractions

Golgi Apparatus

- Present in all cells, highly developed in secretory cells
- Consists of stacked, curved cisternae with convex side as the *cis* face
- Mature concave side is the *trans* face
- Cisternae enzymes modify, sort, and package proteins
- Adds sugars to proteins and lipids to form glycoproteins, glycolipids, and lipoproteins
- Secretory granules are modified, sorted, and packaged in membranes for export outside of cell or for lysosomes

Ribosomes

- Appear as free and attached (as to endoplasmic reticulum)
- Most abundant in protein-synthesizing cells
- Decode genetic messages from nucleus for amino acid sequence of protein synthesis
- Free ribosomes synthesize proteins for cell use
- Attached ribosomes synthesize proteins that are packaged for export or lysosomes use

Lysosomes

- Filled with hydrolyzing or digesting enzymes
- Separated from cytoplasm by membrane
- Functions in intracellular digestion or phagocytosis
- Digest microorganisms, cellular debris, worn-out cells, or cell organelles
- Residual bodies seen after phagocytosis
- Very abundant in phagocytic and certain white blood cells

Peroxisomes

- Contain oxidases that form cytotoxic hydrogen peroxide
- Contain enzyme catalase to eliminate excess hydrogen peroxide
- Abundant in liver and kidney cells, which remove much of the toxic material

The Cytoskeleton of the Cell

Microfilaments

- Thinnest microfilaments in the cytoskeleton
- Composed of protein actin
- Distributed throughout cell and used as anchors at cell junctions
- Form core of microvilli and terminal web at cell apices

Intermediate Filaments

- Thicker than microfilaments
- Epithelial cells contain keratin filaments
- Vimentin filaments found in mesenchymal cells
- Desmin filaments found in smooth and skeletal muscles
- Glial filaments found in astrocytic cells of the nervous system
- Lamin filaments found in nuclear membrane

Microtubules

- Largest filaments in cytoskeleton
- Composed of α and β tubulin
- Originate from centrosome
- Most visible in cilia and flagella

Centrosome and Centrioles

- Centrosome located near nucleus; contains two centrioles
- Centrioles perpendicular to one another; contain nine clusters of three microtubules each
- Before mitosis, centrioles replicate
- During mitosis, centrioles form mitotic spindles

Cytoplasmic Inclusions

- Temporary structures such as lipids, glycogen, crystals, and pigment

Nucleus and Nuclear Envelope

- Nucleus contains chromatin, nucleoli, nuclear matrix, and cellular DNA
- Double membrane called the nuclear envelope surrounds the nucleus
- Outer membrane of nuclear envelope contains ribosomes
- Nuclear pores at intervals in the nuclear envelope
- Nuclear pores control movements of material between nucleus and cytoplasm

Surfaces of Cells

Junctional Complex

- Tight junctions form an effective epithelial barrier
- Transmembrane proteins fuse the outer membranes of adjacent cells to form tight junctions
- In zonula adherens, transmembrane proteins attach to cytoskeleton and bind adjacent cells
- Desmosomes are spotlike structures, very prominent in skin and cardiac cells
- Desmosomes anchor cells through extension of transmembrane proteins into intercellular space between adjacent cells
- Gap junctions are spotlike structures with fluid channels called connexons
- Ions and chemicals diffuse through connexons from cell to cell
- Gap junctions allow rapid communications between cells for synchronized action

Basal Regions of Cells

Infolded Basal Regions of the Cell

- Infolded basal and lateral cell membranes function in ionic transport
- Found in kidney and salivary gland cells
- Na^+/K^+ ATPase pumps embedded in infolded membranes
- Numerous mitochondria in infoldings supply ATP for ion transport

Cilia

- Motile apical surface modifications
- Line cells in the respiratory organs, uterine tubes, and efferent ducts in testes
- Motility caused by sliding microtubule doublets
- Motor protein dynein uses ATP to move cilia

Microvilli

- Nonmotile apical surface modifications
- Well developed in small intestines and kidney
- Main function is absorption

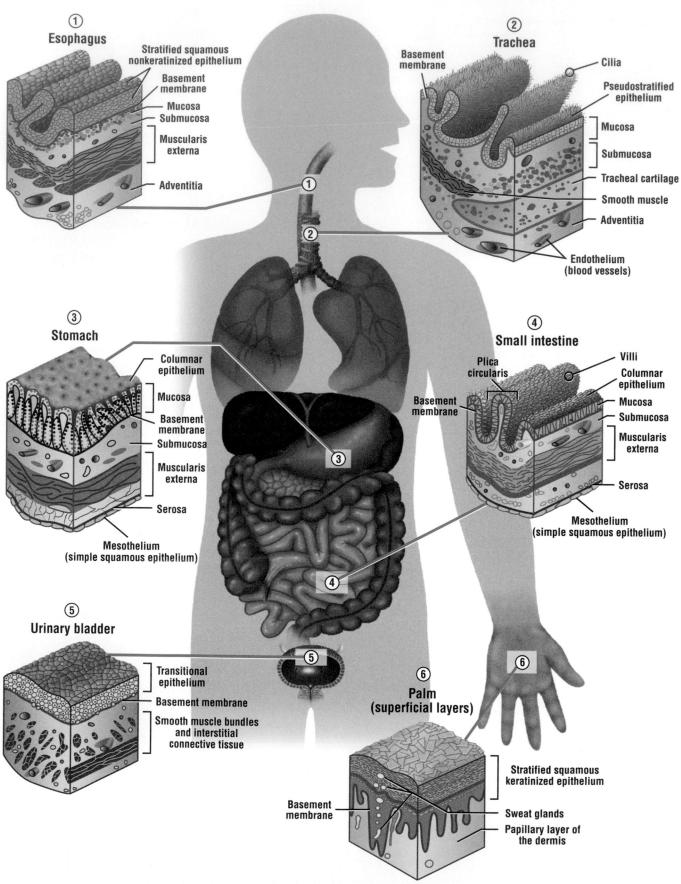

① Esophagus

Stratified squamous nonkeratinized epithelium
Basement membrane
Mucosa
Submucosa
Muscularis externa
Adventitia

② Trachea

Basement membrane
Cilia
Pseudostratified epithelium
Mucosa
Submucosa
Tracheal cartilage
Smooth muscle
Adventitia
Endothelium (blood vessels)

③ Stomach

Columnar epithelium
Mucosa
Basement membrane
Submucosa
Muscularis externa
Serosa
Mesothelium (simple squamous epithelium)

④ Small intestine

Plica circularis
Villi
Columnar epithelium
Basement membrane
Mucosa
Submucosa
Muscularis externa
Serosa
Mesothelium (simple squamous epithelium)

⑤ Urinary bladder

Transitional epithelium
Basement membrane
Smooth muscle bundles and interstitial connective tissue

⑥ Palm (superficial layers)

Stratified squamous keratinized epithelium
Sweat glands
Basement membrane
Papillary layer of the dermis

OVERVIEW FIGURE 2 ■ Different types of epithelia in selected organs.

Epithelial Tissue

SECTION 1 ■ Classification of Epithelial Tissue

Location of Epithelium

The four basic tissue types in the body are the epithelial, connective, muscular, and nervous tissue. These tissues exist and function in close association with one another.

The **epithelial tissue,** or **epithelium,** consists of sheets of cells that cover the **external surfaces** of the body, line the **internal cavities,** form various **organs** and **glands,** and line their **ducts.** Epithelial cells are in contact with each other, either in a single layer or multiple layers. The structure of lining epithelium, however, differs from organ to organ, depending on its location and function. For example, epithelium that covers the outer surfaces of the body and serves as a protective layer differs from the epithelium that lines the internal organs.

The overview illustration shows different types of epithelia in selected organs.

Classification of Epithelium

Epithelium is classified according to the number of **cell layers** and the **morphology** or structure of the **surface cells.** A **basement membrane** is a thin, noncellular region that separates the epithelium from the underlying **connective tissue.** This membrane is easily seen with a light microscope. An epithelium with a single layer of cells is **simple,** and that with numerous cell layers is **stratified.** A **pseudostratified** epithelium consists of a single layer of cells that attach to a **basement membrane,** but not all cells reach the surface. An epithelium with flat surface cells is called **squamous.** When the surface cells are round, or as tall as they are wide, the epithelium is **cuboidal.** When the cells are taller than they are wide, the epithelium is called **columnar.** Epithelium is **nonvascular,** that is, it does not have blood vessels. Oxygen, nutrients, and metabolites **diffuse** from the blood vessels located in the underlying connective tissue to the epithelium.

Special Surface Modifications on Epithelial Cells

Epithelial cells in different organs exhibit special cell membrane modifications on their **apical** or upper **surfaces.** These modifications are cilia, stereocilia, or microvilli. **Cilia** are motile structures found on certain cells in the **uterine tubes, uterus,** and conducting tubes of the **respiratory system. Microvilli** are small, nonmotile projections that cover all absorptive cells in the small intestine and proximal convoluted tubules in the kidney. **Stereocilia** are long, nonmotile, branched microvilli that cover the cells in the **epididymis** and **vas deferens.** The function of microvilli and stereocilia is absorption.

Types of Epithelia

Simple Epithelium

Simple squamous epithelium that covers the external surfaces of the digestive organs, lungs, and heart is called **mesothelium.** Simple squamous epithelium that covers the lumina of the heart chambers, blood vessels, and lymphatic vessels is called **endothelium.**

Simple cuboidal epithelium lines small excretory ducts in different organs. In the proximal convoluted tubules of the kidney, the apical surfaces of the simple cuboidal epithelium are lined with a **brush border** consisting of **microvilli.**

Simple columnar epithelium covers the **digestive organs** (stomach, small and large intestines, and gallbladder). In the small intestine, simple columnar absorptive cells that cover the **villi** also exhibit **microvilli.** Villi are fingerlike structures that project into the lumen of the small intestine. In the female reproductive tract, the simple columnar epithelium is lined with motile cilia.

Pseudostratified Columnar Epithelium

Pseudostratified columnar epithelium lines the **respiratory passages** and lumina of the **epididymis** and **vas deferens.** In trachea, bronchi, and larger brochioles, the surface cells exhibit motile **cilia;** in the epididymis and vas deferens, the surface cells exhibit nonmotile **stereocilia,** which are branched or modified microvilli.

Stratified Epithelium

Stratified squamous epithelium contains multiple cell layers. The basal cells are cuboidal to columnar; these cells give rise to cells that migrate toward the surface and become squamous. There are two types of stratified squamous epithelia: nonkeratinized and keratinized.

Nonkeratinized epithelium exhibits live surface cells and covers moist cavities such as the mouth, pharynx, esophagus, vagina, and anal canal. **Keratinized epithelium** lines the external surfaces of the body. The surface layers contain nonliving, keratinized cells that are filled with the protein **keratin.** The exposed epithelium that covers the palms and soles exhibits especially thick layers of keratinized cells.

Stratified cuboidal epithelium and **stratified columnar epithelium** have a limited distribution in the body. Both types of epithelia line the larger **excretory ducts** of the pancreas, salivary glands, and sweat glands. In these ducts, the epithelium exhibits two or more layers of cells.

Transitional epithelium lines the minor and major calyxes, pelvis, ureter, and bladder of the **urinary system.** This type of epithelium changes shape and can resemble either stratified squamous or stratified cuboidal epithelia, depending on whether it is stretched or contracted. When transitional epithelium is **contracted,** the surface cells appear **dome-shaped;** when **stretched,** the epithelium appears **squamous.**

FIGURE 2.1 ■ Simple Squamous Epithelium: Surface View of Peritoneal Mesothelium

To visualize the surface of the simple squamous epithelium, a small piece of mesentery was fixed and treated with silver nitrate and then counterstained with hematoxylin. The cells of the simple squamous epithelium (**mesothelium**) appear flat, adhere tightly to each other, and form a sheet with the thickness of a single cell layer. The irregular **cell boundaries (1)** of the epithelium stain dark and are highly visible owing to silver deposition between the cell boundaries, and they form a characteristic mosaic pattern. The blue-gray **cell nuclei (2)** are centrally located in the yellow- to brown-stained **cytoplasm (3).**

Simple squamous epithelium is common in the body. It covers the surfaces that allow passive transport of gases or fluids, and lines the pleural (thoracic), pericardial (heart), and peritoneal (abdominal) cavities.

FIGURE 2.2 ■ Simple Squamous Epithelium: Peritoneal Mesothelium Surrounding Small Intestine (Transverse Section)

The simple squamous epithelium that lines different organs in pleural and peritoneal cavities is called mesothelium. A transverse section of a wall of the small intestine illustrates **mesothelium (1),** a thin layer of spindle-shaped cells with prominent and oval nuclei. A thin **basement membrane (2)** is located directly under the mesothelium (1). In a surface view, the dispositon of these cells would appear similar to those shown in Figure 2.1.

Mesothelium (1) and the underlying irregular **connective tissue (5)** form the serosa of the peritoneal cavity. Serosa is attached to a layer of **smooth muscle fibers (6)** called the muscularis externa **serosa** (overview illustration, parts 3 and 4). In this illustration, the bundles of smooth muscle fibers (6) are cut in the transverse plane. Also present in the connective tissue are small **blood vessels (4),** lined also by a simple squamous epithelium called the **endothelium (4),** and numerous **fat (adipose) cells (3).**

FUNCTIONAL CORRELATIONS: Simple Squamous Epithelium

In the peritoneal cavity, simple squamous epithelium **reduces friction** between visceral organs by producing lubricating fluids and **transports fluid.** In the cadiovascular system, this epithelium or endothelium allows for passive **transport** of fluids, nutrients, and metabolites across the thin capillary walls. In the lungs, the simple squamous epithelium provides for an efficient means of **gas exchange** or **transport** across the thin-walled capillaries and alveoli.

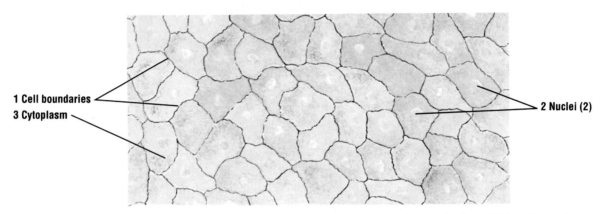

1 Cell boundaries

3 Cytoplasm

2 Nuclei (2)

FIGURE 2.1 ■ Simple squamous epithelium: surface view of peritoneal mesothelium. Stain: silver nitrate with hematoxylin. High magnification.

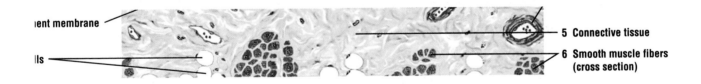

ient membrane

lls

5 Connective tissue

6 Smooth muscle fibers (cross section)

FIGURE 2.2 ■ Simple squamous epithelium: peritoneal mesothelium surrounding small intestine (transverse section). Stain: hematoxylin and eosin. High magnification.

FIGURE 2.3 ■ Different Epithelial Types in the Kidney Cortex

This high-power photomicrograph of the kidney illustrates the different types of epithelia that are present in the kidney cortex (peripheral region). **Simple squamous epithelium (1)** lines the outer portion of the double-layered epithelial capsule called **Bowman's capsule (5).** The inner layer of the capsule surrounds the **capillaries (3)** of the **glomerulus (2).** The glomerulus (2) is a tuft of capillaries (3) where blood filtration takes place. Simple squamous epithelium called **endothelium (4, 9)** also lines the capillaries (3) and all **blood vessels (8). Simple cuboidal epithelium (6)** lines the lumina of the surrounding **convoluted tubules (7).** The blue-staining fibers surrounding Bowman's capsule (5), convoluted tubules (7), and blood vessels (8) in the kidney cortex are the collagen fibers of the **connective tissue (10).**

FIGURE 2.4 ■ Simple Columnar Epithelium: Stomach Surface

The surface of the stomach is covered by a tall **simple columnar epithelium (1).** The illustration shows the light-staining **apical cytoplasm (1a)** and the dark-staining **basal nuclei (1b)** of the simple columnar epithelium (1). The epithelial cells are in close contact with each other and are arranged in a single row. A thin, connective tissue **basement membrane (2, 9)** separates the surface epithelium (1) from the underlying collagen fibers and cells of the **connective tissue (3, 10),** called the **lamina propria.** Small **blood vessels (5),** lined with endothelium, are present in the connective tissue (3, 10).

In some areas the surface epithelium has been sectioned in transverse or oblique plane. When a plane of section passes close to the free surface of the epithelium, the sectioned **apices (6)** of the epithelium resemble a layer of stratified enucleated polygonal cells. When a plane of section passes through **bases (7)** of the epithelial cells, the nuclei resemble a stratified epithelium.

The surface cells of the stomach secrete a protective coat of mucus. The pale appearance of cytoplasm is caused by the routine histologic preparation of the tissues. The mucigen droplets that filled the apical cytoplasm (1a) were lost during section preparation. The more granular cytoplasm is located basally (1b) and stains more acidophilic.

In an empty stomach, the stomach wall exhibits numerous **temporary folds (8)** that disappear when the stomach is filled with solid or fluid material. Also, the surface epithelium extends downward to form numerous indentations or pits in the surface of the stomach called **gastric pits (11),** seen in both logitudinal and transverse section.

FUNCTIONAL CORRELATIONS: Simple Cuboidal Epithelium and Simple Columnar Epithelium

Simple cuboidal epithelium lines various ducts of glands and organs, where it covers the surface for sturdiness and protection. In kidneys, this epithelium functions in transport and absorption of filtered substances. Simple columnar epithelium covers the surface of the stomach. These cells are **secretory** and produce **mucus.** The mucus covers the stomach surface and **protects** its surface lining from the corrosive gastric secretions normally found in the stomach during food processing and digestion.

1 Simple squamous
  epithelium

2 Glomerulus

3 Capillaries

4 Endothelium

5 Bowman's
  capsule

6 Simple cuboidal
  epithelium

7 Convoluted
  tubules

8 Blood vessels

9 Endothelium

10 Connective
   tissue

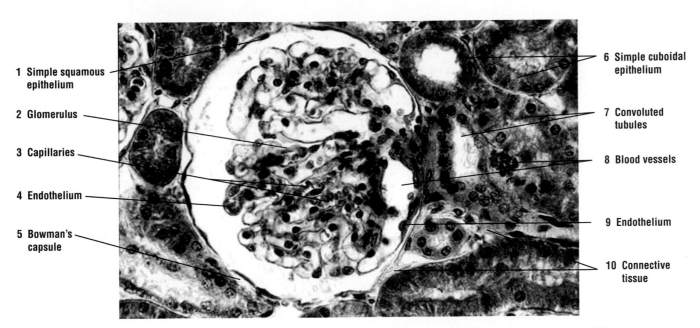

FIGURE 2.3 ■ Different epithelial types in the kidney cortex. Stain: Masson's trichrome. ×120.

1 Simple columnar
  surface epithelium
  a. Apical cytoplasm
  b. Basal nuclei

2 Basement membrane

3 Connective tissue
  (lamina propria)

4 Connective tissue cells

5 Blood vessel

6 Apices of epithelium
  (cytoplasm, oblique
  section)

7 Bases of epithelium
  (nuclei, oblique
  section)

8 Temporary folds

9 Basement membrane

10 Connective tissue
   (lamina propria)

11 Gastric pits
   (longitudinal and
   transverse sections)

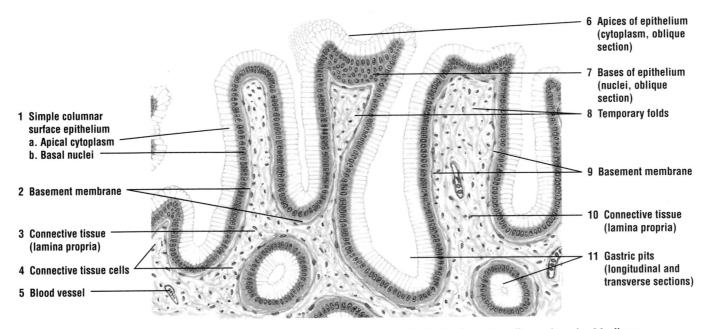

FIGURE 2.4 ■ Simple columnar epithelium: surface of stomach. Stain: hematoxylin and eosin. Medium magnification.

The intestinal **villi** (1), illustrated in transverse section and longitudinal section, are covered by simple columnar epithelium. In the small intestine, the epithelium consists of two cell types: columnar cells with **striated borders** (5, 7) and oval-shaped **goblet cells** (6, 13). The striated border (5, 7) is seen as a reddish outer cell layer with faint vertical striations; these striations represent microvilli on the apices of columnar cells.

Pale-staining goblet cells (6, 13) are interspersed among the columnar cells. During routine histologic preparation, the mucus is lost; hence, the goblet cell cytoplasm appears clear or only lightly stained (6, 13). Normally, the mucigen droplets occupy **cell apices** (4) and the nucleus cell **bases** (4).

When the epithelium at the tip of a villus is sectioned in an oblique plane, the cell apices (4) of the columnar cells appear as a mosaic of enucleated cells, while the cell bases (4) appear as stratified epithelium.

A thin connective tissue **basement membrane** (8) is visible directly under the epithelium. The connective tissue **lamina propria** (12) contains an empty lymphatic vessel with a very thin endothelium called the **central lacteal** (2, 9). Also present in the lamina propria (12) are numerous **blood vessels** (10) and a **capillary** (14) lined with endothelium. **Smooth muscle fibers** (3, 11) extend into the villi. In this illustration, smooth muscle fibers (3, 11) are cut in transverse section (3) and longitudinal section (11).

The lamina propria also contains numerous other connective tissue cells, such as plasma cells, lymphocytes, macrophages, and fibroblasts. These cells are normally seen with higher magnification.

FUNCTIONAL CORRELATIONS: Epithelium With Striated Borders (Small Intestine) and Brush Borders (Kidney)

The main function of the epithelium in the small intestine is **absorption.** This function is enhanced by the presence of fingerlike **villi,** which increase the absorptive surface area and which are covered by simple columnar epithelium with **striated borders** or **microvilli.** These microvilli absorb nutrients and fluids from the intestinal contents. The intestinal epithelium also contains numerous **goblet cells.** These cells secrete **mucus,** which **protects** the surface lining from corrosive secretions that enter the small intestine from the stomach during digestion.

Production of urine by the kidney involves filtration, absorption, and excretion. The apical surfaces of the simple cuboidal epithelium in the proximal convoluted tubules of the kidney are also covered with **brush borders** or **microvilli.** The main function of these microvilli is to **absorb** the nutrient material and fluid from the filtrate that passes through the tubules.

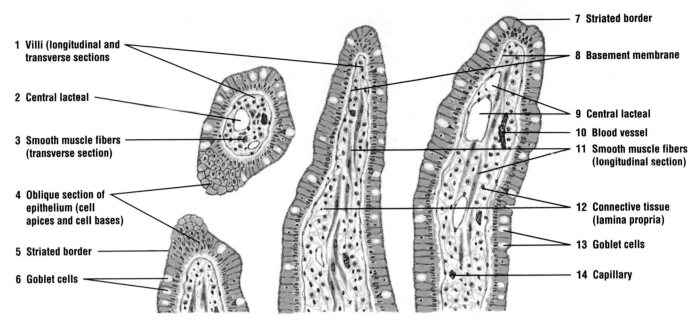

1 **Villi (longitudinal and transverse sections**

2 **Central lacteal**

3 **Smooth muscle fibers (transverse section)**

4 **Oblique section of epithelium (cell apices and cell bases)**

5 **Striated border**

6 **Goblet cells**

7 **Striated border**

8 **Basement membrane**

9 **Central lacteal**

10 **Blood vessel**

11 **Smooth muscle fibers (longitudinal section)**

12 **Connective tissue (lamina propria)**

13 **Goblet cells**

14 **Capillary**

FIGURE 2.5 ■ Simple columnar epithelium on villi in small intestine: cells with striated borders (microvilli) and goblet cells. Stain: hematoxylin and eosin. Medium magnification.

FIGURE 2.6 ■ Pseudostratified Columnar Ciliated Epithelium: Respiratory Passages—Trachea

Pseudostratified columnar ciliated epithelium lines the upper respiratory passages, such as the trachea and bronchi. In this type of epithelium, the cells appear to form several layers. Serial sections show that all cells reach the **basement membrane (4, 13)**; however, because the epithelial cells are of different shapes and heights, not all reach the surface. For this reason, this type of epithelium is called pseudostratified rather than stratified.

Numerous motile and closely spaced **cilia (1, 8)** (cilium, singular) cover all cell apices of the ciliated cells, except those of the light-staining, oval **goblet cells (3, 11)** that are interspersed among the ciliated cells. Each cilium arises from a **basal body (9),** whose internal morphology is identical to the centriole. The basal bodies (9) are located directly beneath the apical cell membrane and are adjacent to each other; they often give the appearance of a continuous dark, apical membrane (9).

In pseudostratified epithelium, the deeper nuclei belong to the intermediate and short **basal cells (12).** The more superficial, oval nuclei belong to the columnar ciliated cells (1, 8). The small, round, heavily stained nuclei, without any visible surrounding cytoplasm, are those of **lymphocytes (2, 10).** These cells migrate from the underlying **connective tissue (5)** through the epithelium.

A clearly visible basement membrane (4, 13) separates the pseudostratified epithelium from the underlying connective tissue (5). Visible in the connective tissue (5) are **fibrocytes (5a),** dense **collagen fibers (5b),** scattered lymphocytes, and small **blood vessels (14).** Deeper in the connective tissue are glands with **mucous acini (6)** and **serous acini (7, 15).** These provide secretions that moisten the respiratory passages.

FUNCTIONAL CORRELATIONS: Epithelium With Cilia or Stereocilia

In most **respiratory passages** (trachea and bronchi), **psedostratified epithelium** contains both **goblet cells** and **ciliated cells.** Ciliated cells cleanse the inspired air and transport **mucus** and **particulate material** across the cell surfaces to the oral cavity for expulsion.

Simple columnar ciliated cells in the **uterine tubes** facilitate the conduction of oocyte and sperm across their surfaces. In the **efferent ductules** of the **testes,** ciliated cells assist in **transporting** sperm out of the testis and into ducts of the epididymis.

The **epididymis** and **vas deferens** are lined by pseudostratified epithelium with **stereocilia.** The major function of stereocilia in these organs is to absorb fluid produced by cells in the testes.

FIGURE 2.7 ■ Transitional Epithelium: Bladder (Unstretched or Relaxed)

Transitional epithelium (1) is found exclusively in the excretory passages of the urinary system. It covers the lumina of renal calyces, pelvis, ureters, and bladder. This stratified epithelium is composed of several layers of similar cells. The epithelium changes its shape in response to either stretching, as a result of fluid accumulation, or contraction during voiding of urine.

In a relaxed, unstretched condition, the **surface cells (7)** are usually cuboidal and bulge out. Frequently, **binucleate (two nuclei) cells (6)** are visible in the superficial layers or surface cells (7) of the bladder.

Transitional epithelium (1) rests on a **connective tissue (3, 8)** layer, composed primarily of **fibroblasts (8a)** and **collagen fibers (8b).** Between the connective tissue (3, 8) and the transitional epithelium (1) is a thin **basement membrane (2).** The base of the epithelium is not indented by connective tissue papillae, and it exhibits an even contour.

Small **blood vessels, venules (4, 11),** and **arterioles (9)** of various sizes are present in the connective tissue (3, 8). Deeper in the connective tissue are strands of **smooth muscle fibers (5, 10),** sectioned in both cross (5) and longitudinal (10) planes. The muscle layers in the bladder are located deep to the connective tissue (3, 8).

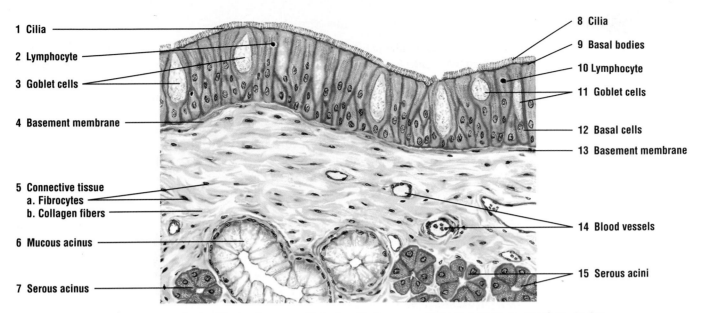

1 Cilia
2 Lymphocyte
3 Goblet cells
4 Basement membrane
5 Connective tissue
   a. Fibrocytes
   b. Collagen fibers
6 Mucous acinus
7 Serous acinus

8 Cilia
9 Basal bodies
10 Lymphocyte
11 Goblet cells
12 Basal cells
13 Basement membrane
14 Blood vessels
15 Serous acini

FIGURE 2.6 ■ Pseudostratified columnar ciliated epithelium: respiratory passages—trachea. Stain: hematoxylin and eosin. High magnification.

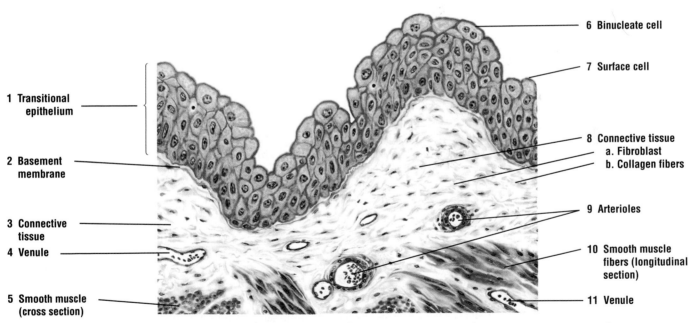

1 Transitional
  epithelium
2 Basement
  membrane
3 Connective
  tissue
4 Venule
5 Smooth muscle
  (cross section)

6 Binucleate cell
7 Surface cell
8 Connective tissue
   a. Fibroblast
   b. Collagen fibers
9 Arterioles
10 Smooth muscle
   fibers (longitudinal
   section)
11 Venule

FIGURE 2.7 ■ Transitional epithelium: bladder (unstretched or relaxed). Stain: hematoxylin and eosin. High magnification.

FIGURE 2.8 ■ Transitional Epithelium: Bladder (Stretched)

When fluid begins to fill the bladder, the **transitional epithelium** (1) changes its shape. Increased volume in the bladder appears to reduce the number of cell layers. This is because the **surface cells** (5) flatten to accommodate increasing surface area. In the stretched condition, the transitional epithelium (1) may resemble stratified squamous epithelium found in other regions of the body. Note also that the folds in the bladder wall dissapear, and the **basement membrane** (2) is smoother. As in the empty bladder (Figure 2.7), the underlying **connective tissue** (6) contains **venules** (3) and **arterioles** (7). Below the connective tissue (6) are **smooth muscle fibers** (4, 8), sectioned in cross (4) and longitudinal (8) planes. (Compare transitional epithelium with stratified squamous epithelium of the esophagus, Figure 2.9.)

FUNCTIONAL CORRELATIONS: Transitional Epithelium

Transitional epithelium allows **distension** of the urinary organs (calyces, pelvis, ureters, bladder) during urine accumulation and **contraction** of these organs during the emptying process without breaking the cell contacts in the epithelium. This change in cell shape is owing to the unique feature of the cell membrane in the transitional epithelium. Here are found specialized regions called **plaques.** When the bladder is empty, the plaques are folded into irregular contours. During bladder filling and stretching of the epithelium the plaques disappear. In addition, because plaques appear impermeable to fluids and salts, transitional epithelium forms a **protective osmotic barrier** between urine in the bladder and the underlying connective tissue.

FIGURE 2.9 ■ Stratified Squamous Nonkeratinized Epithelium: Esophagus

Stratified squamous epithelium is characterized by numerous cell layers, with the outermost layer consisting of flat or squamous cells, which contain nuclei and are alive. The thickness of the epithelium varies among different regions of the body, and, as a result, the composition of the epithelium also varies. Illustrated in this figure is an example of a moist, **nonkeratinized stratified squamous epithelium** (1) that lines the oral cavity, esophagus, vagina, and anal canal.

Cuboidal or low columnar **basal cells** (5) are located at the base of the stratified epithelium. The cytoplasm is finely granular, and the oval, chromatin-rich nucleus occupies most of the cell. Cells in the intermediate layers of the epithelium are **polyhedral** (4) with round or oval nuclei, and more visible cell cytoplasm and membranes. **Mitoses** (6) are frequently observed in the deeper cell layers and in the basal cells (5). Cells and their nuclei become progressively flatter as the cells migrate toward the free surface of the epithelium. Above the polyhedral cells (4) are several rows of flattened or **squamous cells** (3).

A fine **basement membrane** (7) separates the epithelium (1) from the underlying **connective tissue,** the **lamina propria** (2). **Papillae** (10) or extensions of connective tissue indent the lower surface of the epithelium (1), giving it a characteristic wavy appearance. The connective tissue (2) contains **collagen fibers** (11), **fibrocytes** (9), **capillaries** (12), and **arterioles** (8).

In areas where stratified squamous epithelium is exposed to increased wear and tear, the outermost layer, called the stratum corneum, becomes thick and keratinized, as illustrated in the epidermis of the palm in Figure 2.10.

An example of thin, stratified squamous epithelium without connective tissue papillae indentation is found in the cornea of the eye; the surface underlying the epithelium is smooth. This type of epithelium is only a few cell layers thick, but it has the characteristic arrangement of basal columnar, polyhedral, and superficial squamous cells.

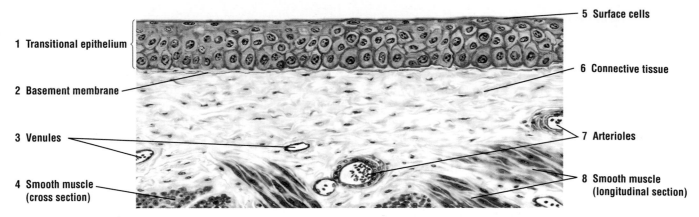

1 Transitional epithelium
5 Surface cells
2 Basement membrane
6 Connective tissue
3 Venules
7 Arterioles
4 Smooth muscle (cross section)
8 Smooth muscle (longitudinal section)

FIGURE 2.8 ■ Transitional epithelium: bladder (stretched). Stain: hematoxylin and eosin. High magnification.

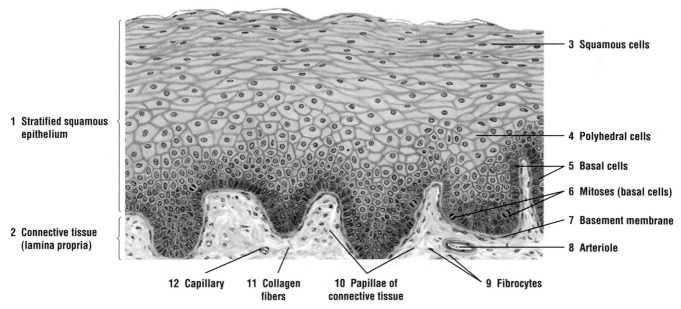

1 Stratified squamous epithelium
2 Connective tissue (lamina propria)
3 Squamous cells
4 Polyhedral cells
5 Basal cells
6 Mitoses (basal cells)
7 Basement membrane
8 Arteriole
12 Capillary
11 Collagen fibers
10 Papillae of connective tissue
9 Fibrocytes

FIGURE 2.9 ■ Stratified squamous nonkeratinized epithelium: esophagus. Stain: hematoxylin and eosin. Medium magnification.

FIGURE 2.10 ■ Stratified Squamous Keratinized Epithelium: Palm of the Hand

The skin is covered with **stratified squamous keratinized epithelium (1)**. The outermost layer of the skin contains dead cells and is called the **stratum corneum (5)**. In the palms and soles, the stratum corneum (5) is thick, whereas in the rest of the body, it is thinner. Inferior to the stratum corneum (5) are the different cell layers that give rise to the stratum corneum (5).

This medium-power photomicrograph illustrates the stratified squamous keratinized epithelium (1) of the palm and the cell layers **stratum granulosum (6), stratum spinosum (7)**, and the basal cell layer, **stratum basale (8)**. The epithelium is attached to the underlying **connective tissue (3)** layer composed of dense collagen fibers and fibroblasts. The underlying surface of the epithelium (1) is indented by connective tissue (3) extensions called **papillae (2)** that form the characteristic wavy boundary between the epithelium (1) and the connective tissue (3). Passing through the connective tissue (3) and the epithelium (1) are **excretory ducts of the sweat glands (4)** that are located deep to the epithelium.

FIGURE 2.11 ■ Stratified Cuboidal Epithelium: Excretory Duct in Salivary Gland

The stratified cuboidal epithelium has a limited distribution and is seen in only a few organs. The larger excretory ducts in the salivary glands and in the pancreas are lined with stratified cuboidal epithelium. This figure illustrates a high-power photomicrograph of a large excretory duct of a salivary gland. The luminal lining consists of two layers of cuboidal cells, forming the **stratified cuboidal epithelium (1)**. Surrounding the excretory duct are collagen fibers of the **connective tissue (2, 7)** and **blood vessels (3, 5)** that are lined by simple squamous epithelium called **endothelium (4, 6)**.

FUNCTIONAL CORRELATIONS: Stratified Epithelium

Stratified squamous epithelium is well suited to withstand increased wear and tear in the moist cavities of the esophagus, vagina, and oral cavity. Its multilayered cellular composition protects the surfaces of these organs. In the larger excretory ducts of kidney, salivary glands, and pancreas, another cell layer is added to form either stratified cuboidal or stratified columnar epithelium for even more protection (see Figure 2.11).

Formation of dead **keratin layers** or keratinization on the skin surface provides additional protection from abrasion, desiccation, and bacterial invasion.

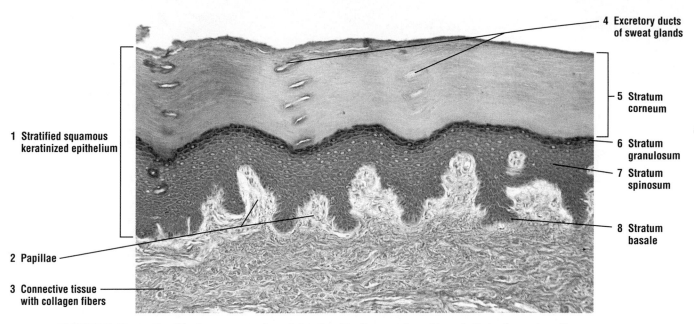

1 Stratified squamous keratinized epithelium

2 Papillae

3 Connective tissue with collagen fibers

4 Excretory ducts of sweat glands

5 Stratum corneum

6 Stratum granulosum

7 Stratum spinosum

8 Stratum basale

FIGURE 2.10 ■ Stratified squamous keratizined epithelium: palm of hand. Stain: hematoxylin and eosin. ×40.

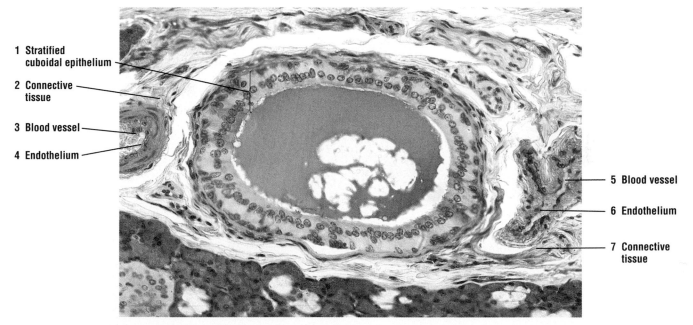

1 Stratified cuboidal epithelium

2 Connective tissue

3 Blood vessel

4 Endothelium

5 Blood vessel

6 Endothelium

7 Connective tissue

FIGURE 2.11 ■ Stratified cuboidal epithelium: excretory duct in salivary gland. Stain: hematoxylin and eosin. ×100.

SECTION 1 ■ Classification of Epithelial Tissue

Epithelial Tissue

Major Features

- Classification based on number of cell layers and cell morphology
- Basement membrane separates epithelium from connective tissue
- All epithelia are nonvascular; delivery of nutrients to cells and removal of metabolic waste occurs via diffusion
- Surface modifications include motile cilia, microvillli, and stereocilia

Types of Epithelia

Simple Squamous Epithelium

- Single layer of flat or squamous cells, includes mesothelium and endothelium
- Mesothelium lines external surfaces of digestive organs, lung, and heart
- Endothelium lines inside of heart chambers, blood vessels, and lymphatic vessels
- Functions in filtration, diffusion, transport, secretion, and reduction of friction

Simple Cuboidal Epithelium

- Single layer of round cells
- Lines small ducts and kidney tubules
- Protects ducts; transports and absorbs filtered material in kidney tubules

Simple Columnar Epithelium

- All cells are tall, some lined by microvilli
- Lines the lumina of digestive organs
- Secretes protective mucus for stomach lining
- Absorption of nutrients in small intestine

Pseudostratified Columnar Epithelium, Epithelium with Cilia or Stereocilia

- All cells reach basement membrane, but not all reach the surface
- Ciliated cells interspersed among mucus-secreting goblet cells
- In respiratory passages, ciliated cells clean inspired air and transport particulate matter across cell surfaces
- In female reproductive tract and efferent ducts of testes, ciliated cells transport oocytes and sperm across cell surfaces
- In epididymis and vas deferens, the lining stereocilia absorb testicular fluid

Stratified Epithelium

- Formed by multiple layers of cells, the superficial cell layer determining epithelial type
- Nonkeratinized squamous epithelium contains live superficial cell layer
- Nonkeratinized squamous forms moist and protective layer in esophagus, vagina, and oral cavity
- Keratinized epithelium contains dead superficial cell layer
- Keratinized epithelium provides protection against abrasion, bacterial invasion, and desiccation
- Cuboidal epithelium lines large excretory ducts in different organs
- Cuboidal epithelium provides protection for the ducts

Transitional Epithelium

- Found exclusively in renal calyces, renal pelvis, ureters, and bladder
- Changes shape in response to stretching caused by fluid accumulation
- During extension or contraction, cell contact unbroken
- Forms protective barrier between urine and underlying tissue

SECTION 2 ■ Glandular Tissue

The body contains a variety of glands. They are classified as either **exocrine glands** or **endocrine glands.** The cells or parenchyma of these glands develop from epithelial tissue. Exocrine glands secrete their products into **ducts,** whereas endocrine glands deliver their secretory products into the **circulatory system.**

Exocrine Glands

Exocrine glands are either **unicellular** or **multicellular.** Unicellular glands consist of single cells. The mucus-secreting **goblet cells** found in the epithelia of the small and large intestines and in the respiratory passages are the best examples of unicellular glands.

Multicellular glands are characterized by a **secretory portion,** an end piece where the epithelial cells secrete a product, and an epithelium-lined **ductal portion,** through which the secretion from the secretory regions is delivered to the exterior of the gland. Larger ducts are usually lined by stratified epithelium.

Simple and Compound Exocrine Glands

Multicellular exocrine glands are divided into two major categories depending on the structure of their ductal portion. A **simple exocrine gland** exhibits an unbranched duct, which may be straight or coiled. Also, if the terminal secretory portion of the gland is shaped in the form of a tube, the gland is called a **tubular gland.**

An exocrine gland that shows a repeated branching pattern of the ducts that drain the secretory portions is called a **compound exocrine gland.** Furthermore, if the secretory portions of the gland are shaped like a flask or a tube, the glands are called **acinar (alveolar) glands** or **tubular glands,** respectively. Certain exocrine glands exhibit a mixture of both tubular and acinar secretory portions. Such glands are called **tubuloacinar glands.**

Exocrine glands may also be classified on the basis of the secretory products of their cells. Glands that contain cells that produce a viscous secretion that lubricates or protects the inner lining of the organs are **mucous glands.** Glands with cells that produce watery secretions often rich in enzymes are **serous glands.** Certain glands in the body contain a mixture of both mucous and serous secretory cells; these are **mixed glands.**

Merocrine and Holocrine Glands

Exocrine glands may also be classified according to the method by which their secretory product is discharged. **Merocrine glands,** such as pancreas, release their secretion by exocytosis without any loss of cellular components. Most exocrine glands in the body secrete their product in this manner. In **holocrine glands,** such as the sebaceous glands of the skin, the cells themselves become the secretory product. Gland cells accumulate lipids, die, and degenerate to become **sebum,** the secretory product. Another type of gland, called apocrine glands (mammary glands), discharge part of the secretory cell as the secretory product. However, almost all glands once classified as apocrine are now regarded as merocrine glands.

Endocrine Glands

Endocrine glands differ from exocrine glands in that they do not have ducts for their secretory products. Instead, endocrine glands are highly vascularized, and their secretory cells are surrounded by rich **capillary networks.** The close proximity of the secretory cells to the capillaries allows for efficient release of the secretory products into the **bloodstream** and their distribution to different organs via the systemic circulation.

The endocrine glands can be either **individual cells** (unicellular glands) as seen in the digestive organs as enteroendocrine cells, **endocrine tissue** in mixed glands (both endocrine and exocrine) as seen in pancreas and male and female reproductive organs, or as separate **endocrine organs** as the pituitary gland, thyroid glands, parathyroid glands, and adrenal glands. Individual

43

endocrine cells, called enteroendocrine cells, are found in the digestive organs. Endocrine tissues are seen in such mixed glands as the pancreas and the reproductive organs of both sexes.

FIGURE 2.12 ■ Unbranched Simple Tubular Exocrine Glands: Intestinal Glands

Unbranched simple tubular glands without excretory ducts are best represented by the **intestinal glands** (crypts of Lieberkühn) in the **large intestine** (A and B) and **rectum.** The **surface epithelium** and the **secretory cells** of the glands in the intestines are lined with numerous goblet cells; these are unicellular exocrine glands. Similar but shorter intestinal glands with goblet cells are also found in the small intestine.

FIGURE 2.13 ■ Simple Branched Tubular Exocrine Glands: Gastric Glands

Simple or slightly branched tubular glands without excretory ducts are found in the stomach. These are the **gastric glands** (A and B). In the fundus and body of the stomach, they are lined with modified columnar cells that are highly specialized for secreting hydrochloric acid and the precursor for the proteolytic enzyme pepsin.

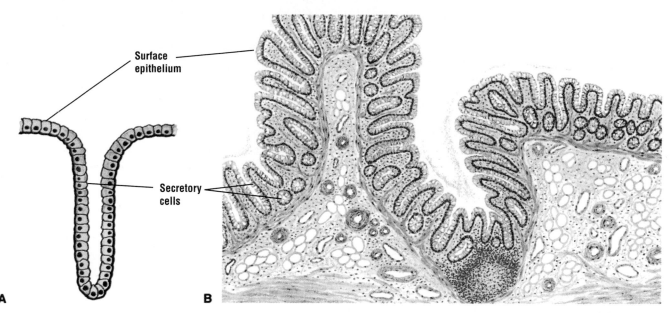

FIGURE 2.12 ■ Unbranched simple tubular exocrine glands: intestinal glands. (A) Diagram of gland. (B) Transverse section of large intestine. Stain: hematoxylin and eosin. Medium magnification.

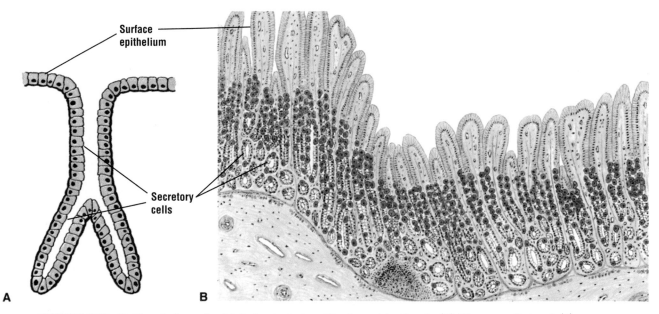

FIGURE 2.13 ■ Simple branched tubular exocrine gland: gastric glands. (A) Diagram of gland. (B) Transverse section of stomach. Stain: hematoxylin and eosin. Low magnification.

FIGURE 2.14 ■ Coiled Tubular Exocrine Glands: Sweat Glands

Sebaceous glands in the skin are coiled tubular glands with long, unbranched ducts (A and B). Note the **secretory cells** of the gland and the **excretory duct,** lined by stratified cuboidal epithelium, which delivers the secretory product to the surface.

FIGURE 2.15 ■ Compound Acinar (Exocrine) Gland: Mammary Glands

The mammary gland is an example of a **compound acinar (alveolar) gland** (A and B). The lactating mammary gland contains enlarged **secretory acini (alveoli)** with large lumina that are filled with milk. Draining these acini (alveoli) are **excretory ducts,** some of which contain secretory material and are lined by stratified epithelium.

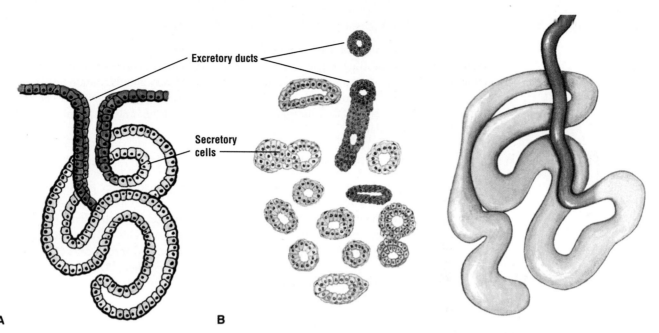

Excretory ducts

Secretory cells

A   B

FIGURE 2.14 ■ Coiled tubular exocrine glands: sweat glands. (A) Diagram of gland. (B) Transverse and three-dimensional view of coiled sweat gland. Stain: hematoxylin and eosin. Medium magnification.

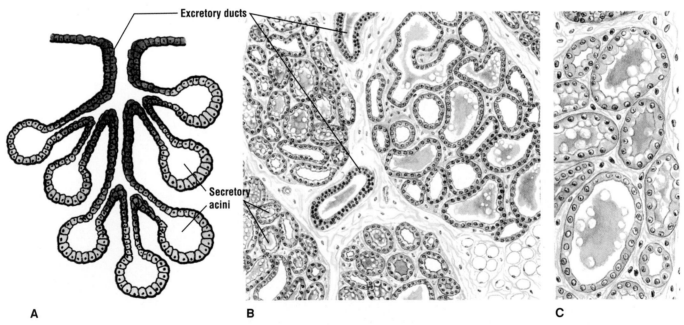

Excretory ducts

Secretory acini

A   B   C

FIGURE 2.15 ■ Compound acinar exocrine gland: mammary gland. (A) Diagram of gland. (B and C) Mammary gland during lactation. Stain: hematoxylin and eosin. (B) Low magnification. (C) Medium magnification.

FIGURE 2.16 ■ Compound Tubuloacinar (Exocrine) Gland: Salivary Glands

The salivary glands (parotid, submandibular, and sublingual) best illustrate **compound tubuloacinar glands** (A and B). The glands contain **secretory acinar elements** and **secretory tubular elements.** In addition, the submandibular and sublingual salivary glands contain both serous and mucous acini. Details and comparisons of these acini are described in Chapter 11. The **excretory ducts** are lined with cuboidal, columnar, or stratified epithelium, and are named according to their location in the gland.

FIGURE 2.17 ■ Compound Tubuloacinar (Exocrine) Gland: Submaxillary Salivary Gland

A photomicrograph of a submaxillary salivary gland shows the secretory units of a compound tubuloacinar gland. The grapelike **secretory acinar elements** (1) are circular in transverse section and are distinguished from the longer **secretory tubular elements** (7) of the gland. Empty lumina can be seen in some sections of both types of secretory elements. This salivary gland is a mixed gland and contains both the **mucous cells (4),** which stain light, and **serous cells (5),** which stain dark. Draining the secretory elements of the gland are **excretory ducts (3, 6, 8).** The small excretory ducts are lined by simple cuboidal epithelium and surrounded by **connective tissue (2),** which also surrounds all of the secretory elements.

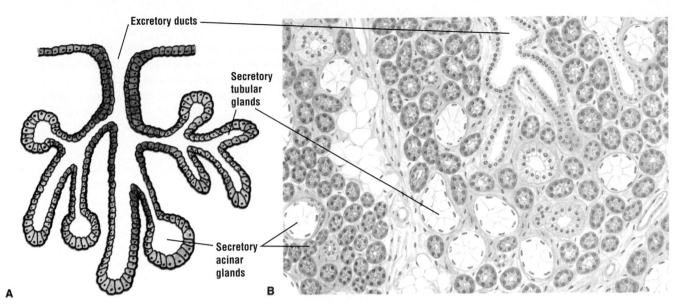

FIGURE 2.16 ■ Compound tubuloacinar (exocrine) gland: salivary gland. (A) Diagram of gland. (B) Submandibular salivary gland. Stain: hematoxylin and eosin. Low magnification.

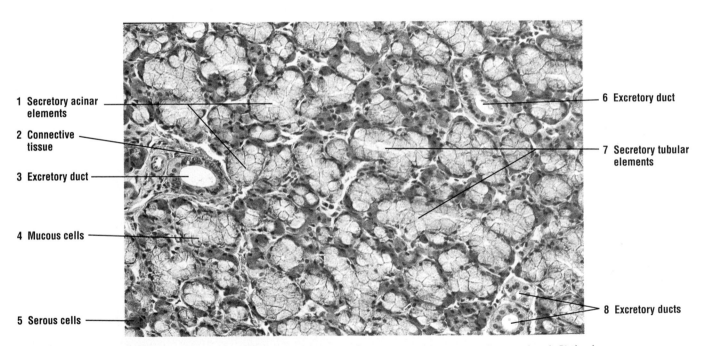

1 Secretory acinar elements

2 Connective tissue

3 Excretory duct

4 Mucous cells

5 Serous cells

6 Excretory duct

7 Secretory tubular elements

8 Excretory ducts

FIGURE 2.17 ■ Compound tubuloacinar (exocrine) gland: submaxillary salivary gland. Stain: hematoxylin and eosin. ×64.

FIGURE 2.18 ■ Endocrine Gland: Pancreatic Islet

An example of an endocrine gland is illustrated as a pancreatic islet from the pancreas. The pancreas is a mixed gland, containing both an **exocrine portion** and **endocrine portion.** In the pancreas, the exocrine acini surround the endocrine pancreatic islets (A and B).

The structure and function of other endocrine organs (glands) are presented in greater detail in Chapter 18.

FIGURE 2.19 ■ Endocrine and Exocrine Pancreas

A photomicrograph of pancreas shows a mixed gland with both endocrine and exocrine portions. The **exocrine pancreas (3)** consists of numerous secretory acini that deliver their secretory material into the **excretory duct (1),** which is lined by simple cuboidal epithelim and surrounded by a layer of connective tissue. The **endocrine pancreas (5)** is called the pancreatic islet (5) because it is separated from the cells of the exocrine pancreas (3) by a thin **connective tissue capsule (4).** The endocrine pancreatic islet (5) does not contain excretory ducts. Instead, it is highly vascularized, and all of the secretory products leave the pancreatic islet via numerous **blood vessels (capillaries) (2).**

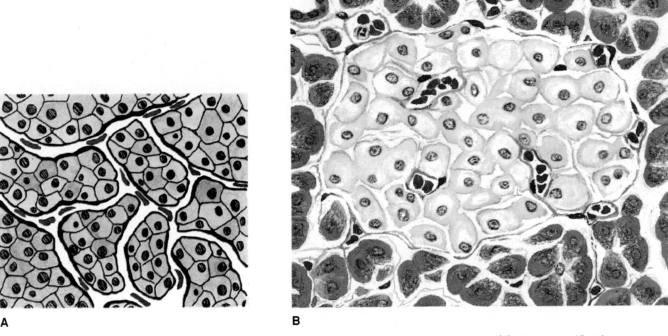

A   B

FIGURE 2.18 ■ Endocrine gland: plancreatic islet. (A) Diagram of pancreatic islet. (B) High magnification of endocrine and exocrine pancreas. Stain: hematoxylin and eosin. High magnification.

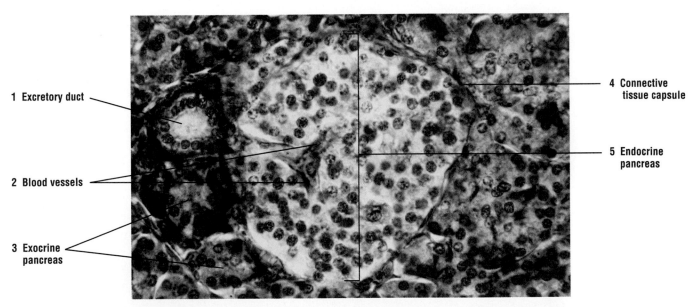

1 Excretory duct

2 Blood vessels

3 Exocrine pancreas

4 Connective tissue capsule

5 Endocrine pancreas

FIGURE 2.19 ■ Endocrine and exocrine pancreas. Stain: Mallory-Azan. ×100.

CHAPTER 2 ■ Summary

Glandular Tissue

Exocrine Glands

- Can be unicellular or multicellular
- Multicellular glands contain secretory portion and ductal portion
- Secretions enter the ductal system
- Simple tubular glands exhibit unbranched duct; found in intestinal glands
- Coiled tubular glands seen in sweat glands
- Compound glands exhibit repeated ductal branching with either acinar (alveolar) or tubular secretory portions
- Compound acinar glands seen in mammary glands
- Compound tubuloacinar glands seen in salivary glands
- Mucous glands lubricate and protect inner linings of organs
- Serous glands produce watery secretions that contain enzymes

- Mixed glands contain both serous and mucous cells
- Merocrine glands, like pancreas, release secretion without cell loss
- Holocrine glands, like sebaceous skin glands, release secretion with cell components

Endocrine Glands

- Are individual cells as enteroendocrine cells in digestive organs
- Are endocrine portions in organs such as pancreatic islets in pancreas
- Are endocrine glands such as pituitary, thyroid, or adrenal glands
- Do not have ducts
- Are highly vascularized
- Secretory products enter bloodstream (capillaries) for systemic distribution

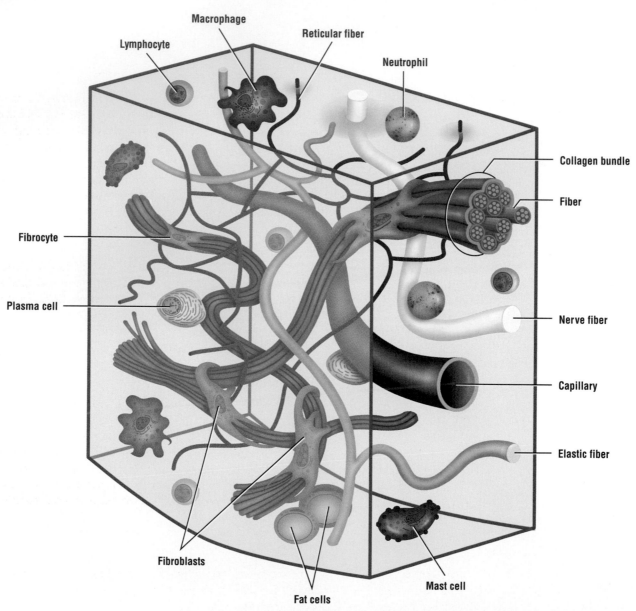

Lymphocyte

Macrophage

Reticular fiber

Neutrophil

Collagen bundle

Fiber

Fibrocyte

Nerve fiber

Plasma cell

Capillary

Elastic fiber

Fibroblasts

Mast cell

Fat cells

OVERVIEW FIGURE 3 ■ Composite illustration of loose connective tissue with its predominant cells and fibers.

CHAPTER 3

Connective Tissue

Classification of Connective Tissue

Connective tissue develops from mesenchyme, an embryonic type of tissue. Embryonic connective tissue is present in the umbilical cord and in the pulp of the developing teeth. With the exceptions of blood and lymph, **connective tissue** consists of **cells** and **extracellular material** called **matrix.** The extracelluar matrix consists of connective **tissue fluid, ground substance** within which are embedded the different protein **fibers** (collagen, reticular, and elastic). The connective tissue binds, anchors, and supports various cells, tissues, and organs of the body. The connective tissue is classified as either loose connective tissue or dense connective tissue, depending on the amount, type, arrangement, and abundance of cells, fibers, and ground substance.

Loose Connective Tissue

Loose connective tissue is more prevalent in the body than dense connective tissue. It is characterized by a loose, irregular arrangement of connective tissue fibers and abundant ground substance. Numerous connective tissue cells and fibers are found in the matrix. **Collagen fibers, fibroblasts, adipose cells, mast cells,** and **macrophages** predominate in loose connective tissue, with fibroblasts being the most common cell types. The overview figure shows the various types of cells and fibers that are present in the loose connective tissue.

Dense Connective Tissue

In contrast, **dense connective tissue** contains thicker and more densely packed collagen fibers, with fewer cell types and less ground substance. The collagen fibers in **dense irregular connective tissue** exhibit a random and irregular orientation. Dense connective tissue is present in the dermis of skin, in capsules of different organs, and in areas that need strong support. In contrast, **dense regular connective tissue** contains densely packed collagen fibers that exhibit a regular and parallel arrangement. This type of tissue is found in the **tendons** and **ligaments.** In both connective tissue types, **fibroblasts** are the most abundant cells, which are located between the dense collagen bundles.

Cells of the Connective Tissue

The two most common cell types in the connective tissue are the active **fibroblasts** and the inactive or resting fibroblasts, the **fibrocytes.** Fusiform-shaped fibroblasts synthesize all of the connective tissue fibers and the extracellular ground substance.

Adipose (fat) cells, which may occur singly or in groups, are seen frequently in the connective tissue; these cells store fat. When adipose cells predominate, the connective tissue is called an **adipose tissue.**

Macrophages or **histiocytes** are phagocytic cells and are most numerous in loose connective tissue. They are difficult to distinguish from fibroblasts, unless they are performing phagocytic activity and contain ingested material in their cytoplasm.

Mast cells, usually closely associated with blood vessels, are widely distributed in the connective tissue of the skin and in the digestive and respiratory organs. Mast cells are spherical cells filled with fine, regular dark-staining and basophilic granules.

Plasma cells arise from the lymphocytes that migrate into the connective tissue. These cells are found in great abundance in loose connective tissue and lymphatic tissue of the respiratory and digestive tracts.

Leukocytes, or white blood cells, neutrophils, and eosinophils, migrate into the connective tissue from the blood vessels. Their main function is to defend the organism against bacterial invasion or foreign matter.

Fibroblasts and adipose cells are permanent or resident connective tissue cells. Neutrophils, eosinophils, plasma cells, mast cells, and macrophages migrate from the blood vessels and take residence in the connective tissue of different regions of the body.

Fibers of the Connective Tissue

There are three types of connective tissue fibers: **collagen, elastic,** and **reticular.** The amount and arrangement of these fibers depend on the function of the tissues or organs in which they are found. Fibroblasts synthesize all of the collagen, elastic, and reticular fibers.

Type of Collagen Fibers

Collagen fibers are tough, thick, fibrous proteins that do not branch. They are the most abundant fibers and are found in almost all connective tissue of all organs. The most frequently recognized fibers in histologic slides are the following:

- **Type I** collagen fibers. These are found in the dermis of skin, tendons, ligaments, and bone. They are very strong and offer great resistance to tensil stresses.
- **Type II** collagen fibers. These are present in hyaline cartilage and elastic cartilage. The fibers provide resistance to pressure.
- **Type III** collagen fibers. These are the thin, branching reticular fibers that form the delicate supporting meshwork in such organs as the lymph nodes, spleen, and bone marrow.
- **Type IV** collagen fibers. These are present in the basal lamina of the basement membrane, to which the basal regions of the cells attach.

Reticular Fibers

Reticular fibers, consist maily of type III collagen, are thin and form a delicate netlike framework in the liver, lymph nodes, spleen, hemopoietic organs, and other locations where blood and lymph are filtered. Reticular fibers also support capillaries, nerves, and muscle cells. These fibers become visible only when the tissue or organ is stained with silver stain.

Elastic Fibers

Elastic fibers are thin, small, branching fibers that allow stretch. They have less tensile strength than collagen fibers, and are composed of microfibrils and the protein **elastin.** When stretched, elastic fibers return to their original size (recoil) without deformation. Elastic fibers are found in abundance in the lungs, bladder, and skin. In the walls of the aorta and pulmonary trunk, the presence of elastic fibers allows for stretching and recoiling of these vessels during powerful blood ejections from the heart ventricles. In the walls of the large vessels, the smooth muscle cells synthesize the elastic fibers.

FIGURE 3.1 ■ Loose Connective Tissue (Spread)

The plate illustrates a composite image of a mesentery that was stained to show different fibers and cells. Mesentery is a thin sheet composed of loose connective tissue.

The pink **collagen fibers (3)** are the thickest, largest, and most numerous fibers. In this connective tissue preparation, the collagen fibers (3) course in all directions.

The **elastic fibers (5, 10)** are thin, fine, single fibers that are usually straight; however, after tissue preparation, the fibers may become wavy as a result of the release of tension. Elastic fibers (5, 10) form branching and anastomosing networks. Fine reticular fibers are also present in loose connective tissue, but these are not included in this illustration.

The fixed permanent cells of connective tissues are the **fibroblasts (2).** The fibroblasts (2) are flattened cells with an oval nucleus, sparse chromatin, and one or two nucleoli. Fixed **macrophages,** or **histiocytes (12),** are always present in the connective tissue. When inactive, they appear similar to fibroblasts, although their processes may be more irregular and their nuclei smaller. Phagocytic inclusions, however, alter the cytoplasm of the macrophages. In this illustration, the cytoplasm of different macrophages (12) is filled with dense-staining particles that were ingested by these cells.

Mast cells (1, 9) are also present in loose connective tissue and are seen as single or grouped cells along small blood vessels (**capillary, 7**). The mast cells (1, 9) are usually ovoid, with a small, centrally placed nucleus and cytoplasm filled with fine, closely packed granules that stain dense or deep red with neutral red stain.

Numerous different blood cells are also seen in the loose connective tissue. **Small lymphocytes (6)** exhibit a dense-staining nucleus that occupies most of the cell cytoplasm. **Large lymphocytes (8)** also exhibit a dense nucleus with more cytoplasm. Loose connective tissue also contains blood cells such as eosinophils and neutrophils, and adipose cells. These are illustrated in greater detail below in Figure 3.2, and in loose connective tissue in Figure 3.4 and mesentery of an intestine in Figure 3.11, respectively.

The faint background around the fibers and cells is the ground substance.

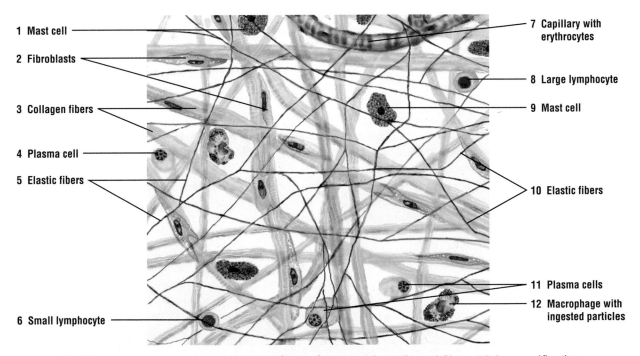

1 Mast cell
2 Fibroblasts
3 Collagen fibers
4 Plasma cell
5 Elastic fibers
6 Small lymphocyte
7 Capillary with erythrocytes
8 Large lymphocyte
9 Mast cell
10 Elastic fibers
11 Plasma cells
12 Macrophage with ingested particles

FIGURE 3.1 ■ Loose connective tissue (spread). Stained for cells and fibers. High magnification.

FIGURE 3.2 ■ Individual Cells of Connective Tissue

The main cells of connective tissue are the fibroblasts and fibrocytes. The **fibroblast (1)** is an elongated cell with cytoplasmic projections, an ovoid nucleus with sparse chromatin, and one or two nucleoli. The **fibrocyte (6)** is a more mature, smaller spindle-shaped cell without cytoplasmic projections; the nucleus is similar but smaller than that in the fibroblast.

The **plasma cell (2)** exhibits a smaller, eccentrically placed nucleus with condensed, coarse chromatin clumps distributed peripherally in a characteristic radial (cartwheel) pattern and one central mass. A prominent, clear area in the cytoplasm is adjacent to the nucleus.

The large **adipose cell (3)** exhibits a narrow rim of cytoplasm and a flattened, eccentric nucleus. In histologic sections, the large fat globules of adipose cells have been dissolved by different chemicals, leaving a large, highly characteristic empty space.

The **large lymphocyte (4)** and **small lymphocyte (10)** are spherical cells that differ primarily in the greater amount of cytoplasm that is present in the large lymphocyte (4). The dense-staining nuclei of all lymphocytes have condensed chromatin but no nucleoli.

The free **macrophage (5)** usually appears round with irregular cell outlines, but exhibits a variable appearance. In the illustration, the macrophage exhibits a small nucleus rich in chromatin and cytoplasm filled with dense, ingested particles.

Eosinophil (7) is a large blood cell with a bilobed nucleus and large, eosinophilic cytoplasmic granules that fill the cytoplasm.

Neutrophil (8) is also a large blood cell, characterized by a multilobed nucleus and a lack of stained granules in the cytoplasm.

Cells with **pigment granules (9)** may be seen in the connective tissue. Also, the basal epithelial cells of the skin contain brown-staining pigment or melanin granules.

Mast cell (11) is usually ovoid, with a small, centrally placed nucleus. The cytoplasm is normally filled with fine, closely packed, and dense-staining granules.

FUNCTIONAL CORRELATIONS: Individual Cells in Connective Tissue

Fibroblasts are the dominant cells in the connective tissue. These highly active cells, with irregularly branched cytoplasm, synthesize **collagen, reticular**, and **elastic fibers**, as well as carbohydrates such as glycosaminoglycans, proteoglycans, and glycoproteins of the **extracellular matrix.** The spindle-shaped *fibrocytes* are smaller than the fibroblasts and are mature and less active cells of the fibroblast line.

Macrophages or histiocytes are **phagocytes** that ingest bacteria, dead cells, cell debris, and other foreign matter in the connective tissue. These cells also enhance immunologic activities of the lymphocytes. Macrophages are **antigen-presenting cells** to lymphocytes and perform an important function in the immune response. These cells are derived from circulating blood monocytes that take up residence in the connective tissue. Macrophages have specific names in different organs. In liver, the macrophages are called **Kupfer cells,** in bone, **osteoclasts,** and in the central nervous system, **microglia.**

Lymphocytes are the most numerous cells in the loose connective tissue of the respiratory and gastrointestinal tracts. They mediate immune responses to antigens that enter these organs by producing antibodies and kill virus-infected cells by inducing cell death or apoptosis.

Plasma cells are derived from lymphocytes that have been exposed to antigens. They synthesize and secrete **antibodies** that destroy specific antigens and defend the body against infections.

Adipose cells **store fat** (lipid) and provide protective packing material in and around numerous organs.

Neutrophils are active and powerful phagocytes; they engulf and destroy bacteria at sites of infections.

Eosinophils become active and increase in number after parasitic infections or allergic reactions. They phagocytize antigen-antibody complexes formed during allergic reactions.

Mast cells synthesize and release **histamine** and **heparin.** Exposure of mast cells to allergens causes rapid release of histamine and other vasoactive chemicals. Histamine is a potent mediator of inflammation. It dilates blood vessels, increases their permeability to fluid thereby causing edema, and induces signs and symptoms of immediate hypersensitive (allergic) reactions. In contrast, heparin is a weak anticoagulant.

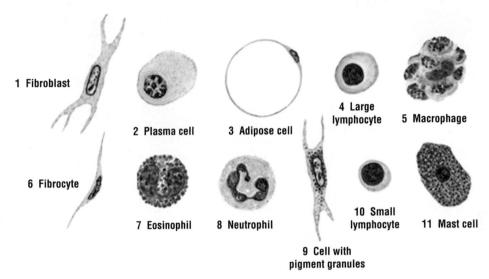

FIGURE 3.2 ■ Cells of the connective tissue. Stain: hematoxylin and eosin. High magnification or oil immersion.

FIGURE 3.3 ■ Embryonic Connective Tissue

The embryonic connective tissue resembles the mesenchyme or mucous connective tissue; this is loose and irregular connective tissue. The difference in ground substance (semifluid versus jelly-like) is not apparent in these sections.

The **fibroblasts (4)** are numerous, and fine **collagen fibers (1)** are found between them, some coming in close contact with fibroblasts. Embryonic connective tissue is vascular. **Capillaries (3)** lined with endothelium and filled with **red blood cells (2)** are visible in the ground substance.

At higher magnification, primitive **fibroblasts (5)** are seen as large, branching cells with cytoplasm, prominent cytoplasmic processes, an ovoid nucleus with fine chromatin, and one or more nucleoli. The widely separated **collagen fibers (6)** are more apparent at this magnification.

FIGURE 3.4 ■ Loose Connective Tissue

Collagen fibers (9) predominate in loose connective tissue, course in different directions, and form a loose fiber meshwork. In the illustration, collagen fibers (9) are sectioned in various planes, and transverse ends may be seen. The fibers are acidophilic and stain pink with eosin. Thin elastic fibers are also present in loose connective tissue, but are difficult to distinguish with this stain and at this magnification.

The **fibroblasts (2)** are the most numerous cells in the loose connective tissue and may be sectioned in various planes, so that only parts of the cells may be seen. Also, during section preparation, the cytoplasm of these cells may shrink. A typical fibroblast (2) shows an oval nucleus with sparse chromatin and lightly acidophilic cytoplasm, with few short processes.

Also present in loose connective tissue are various blood cells such as the **neutrophils (6)** with lobulated nuclei, **eosinophils (3)** with red-staining granules, and small **lymphocytes (7)**, with dense-staining nuclei and sparse cytoplasm. The **fat** or **adipose cells (5)** appear characteristically empty with a thin rim of cytoplasm and peripherally displaced flat **nuclei (4)**.

The connective tissue is highly vascular; **capillaries (8)** sectioned in different planes (t.s., transverse section; l.s., longitudinal section) are visible. Larger blood vessels, such as an **arteriole (1)** with blood cells, are also seen in the loose connective tissue.

FIGURE 3.5 ■ Dense Irregular and Loose Irregular Connective Tissue (Elastin Stain)

This figure illustrates a section of connective tissue that shows a transition zone between loose irregular connective tissue in the upper region and a more dense irregular connective tissue in the lower region of the illustration. In addition, the tissue section has been specially prepared to show the presence and destribution of elastic fibers in the connective tissue.

The **elastic fibers (1, 7)** have been selectively stained a deep blue using Verhoeff's method. Using Van Gieson's as a counterstain, acid fuchsin stains **collagen fibers** red **(2, 6)**. Cellular details of fibroblasts are not obvious, but the **fibroblast nuclei (3, 5)** stain deep blue. **Blood vessels (4)** are also present.

The characteristic features of dense irregular and loose connective tissues become apparent with this staining technique. In dense irregular connective tissue the collagen fibers (6) are larger, more numerous, and more concentrated. Elastic fibers are also larger and more numerous (7). In contrast, in the loose connective tissue, both fiber types are smaller (1, 2) and more loosely arranged. Fine elastic networks are seen in both types of connective tissue.

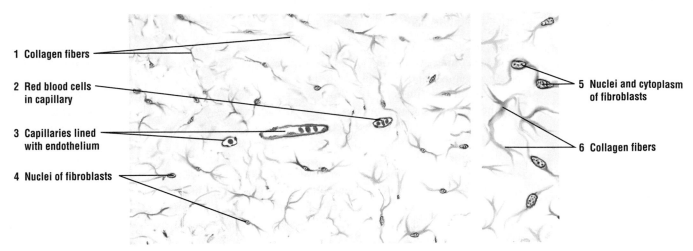

1 Collagen fibers

2 Red blood cells in capillary

3 Capillaries lined with endothelium

4 Nuclei of fibroblasts

5 Nuclei and cytoplasm of fibroblasts

6 Collagen fibers

FIGURE 3.3 ■ Embryonic connective tissue. Stain: hematoxylin and eosin. Left, low magnification; right, high magnification.

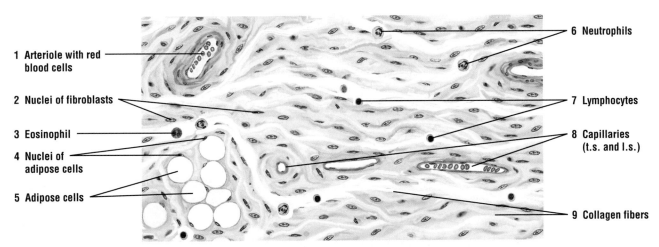

1 Arteriole with red blood cells

2 Nuclei of fibroblasts

3 Eosinophil

4 Nuclei of adipose cells

5 Adipose cells

6 Neutrophils

7 Lymphocytes

8 Capillaries (t.s. and l.s.)

9 Collagen fibers

FIGURE 3.4 ■ Loose connective tissue with blood vessels and adipose cells. Stain: hematoxylin and eosin. High magnification.

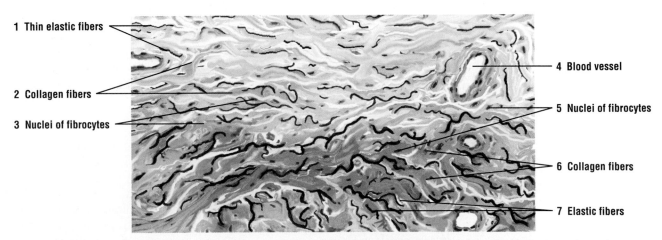

1 Thin elastic fibers

2 Collagen fibers

3 Nuclei of fibrocytes

4 Blood vessel

5 Nuclei of fibrocytes

6 Collagen fibers

7 Elastic fibers

FIGURE 3.5 ■ Dense irregular and loose irregular connective tissue. Stain: Verhoeff's elastin stain and Van Gieson's. Medium magnification.

FIGURE 3.6 ■ Loose Irregular and Dense Irregular Connective Tissue

This figure illustrates a gradual transition from **loose irregular connective tissue (5)** to **dense irregular connective tissue (1).** Where firmer support and more strength are required, dense irregular connective tissue replaces the loose type.

The **collagen fibers (2, 9)** in both types of tissue are large, typically found in bundles, and sectioned in several planes because they course in various directions. Also present here are thin, wavy elastic fibers that form fine networks. However, these fibers are not obvious in routine histologic preparations.

In the dense connective tissue (1), the **fibroblasts (3)** are often found compressed among the collagen fibers (2). In the loose connective tissue (5), the collagen fibers (9) are less compressed, and the fibroblasts **(10)** are more visible. Also illustrated in the connective tissue are **capillaries (4),** a small **venule (11),** an **eosinophil (6)** with lobulated nucleus, **lymphocytes (7)** with large round nuclei without visible cytoplasm, a **plasma cell (8),** and numerous **adipose cells (12).**

FIGURE 3.7 ■ Dense Irregular Connective Tissue and Adipose Tissue

Illustrated in this photomicrograph is a deep section of the skin called the dermis. This region contains **dense irregular connective tissue (1)** and the collagen-producing **fibroblasts (3).** In this type of connective tissue, the **collagen fibers (2)** show a very random and irregular orientation. Adjacent to the dense irregular connective tissue (1) is a region of **adipose tissue (4)** with its numerous **adipose cells (5).** Because of the tissue preparation with different chemicals, the individual adipose cells appear empty, and only their flattened, dense-staining nuclei are visible. Deep in the skin are also found numerous sweat glands. The light-staining regions are the **secretory cells of the sweat gland (7).** The dark staining cells form a **stratified cuboidal epithelium** of the **excretory duct of the sweat gland (6, 8).** The excretory duct **(6, 8)** continues through the connective tissue and the stratified squamous epithelium of the skin, and exits on the surface of the skin (see Figure 3.9).

FUNCTIONAL CORRELATIONS: Ground Substance and Connective Tissue

The **ground substance** in connective tissue consists primarily of amorphous, transparent, and colorless **extracellular matrix,** which has the properties of a semifluid gel and a high water content. The matrix supports, surrounds, and binds all of the connective tissue cells and fibers. The ground substance contains different types of mixed, unbranched polysaccharide chains of **glycosaminoglycans, proteoglycans,** and **adhesive glycoproteins. Hyaluronic acid** constitutes the principal glycosaminoglycan of connective tissue. Except for hyaluronic acid, the various glycosaminoglycans are bound to a core protein to form much larger molecules called **proteoglycan aggregates.** These proteoglycans attract large amounts of water, which forms the hydrated gel of the ground substance.

The semifluid consistency of the ground substance in the connective tissue facilitates **diffusion** of oxygen, electrolytes, nutrients, fluids, metabolites, and other water-soluble molecules between the cells and the blood vessels. Similarly, waste products from the cells diffuse through the ground substance back into the blood vessels. Also, because of its viscosity, the ground substance serves as an efficient **barrier.** It prevents movement of large molecules and the spread of pathogens from the connective tissue into the bloodstream. However, certain bacteria can produce hyaluronidase, an enzyme that hydrolyzes hyaluronic acid and reduces the viscosity of the gellike ground substance, allowing pathogens to invade the surrounding tissues.

The density of ground substance depends on the amount of extracellular tissue fluid or water that it contains. Mineralization of ground substance, as a result of increased calcium deposition, changes its density, rigidity, and permeability to diffusion, as seen in normal developing cartilage models and bones.

In addition to proteoglycans, connective tissue also contains several cell **adhesive glyco-proteins,** which bind cells to the fibers. One glycoprotein, **fibronectin,** is the adhesion protein. It binds connective tissue cells, collagen fibers, and proteoglycans, thereby interconnecting all three components of the connective tissue. Integral proteins of the plasma membrane, called **integrins,** bind to extracellular collagen fibers and to actin filaments in the cytoskeleton, thus establishing a structural continuity between the cytoskeleton and the extracellular matrix. **Laminin** is a large glycoprotein and a major component of the cell basement membrane. This protein binds epithelial cells to the basal lamina.

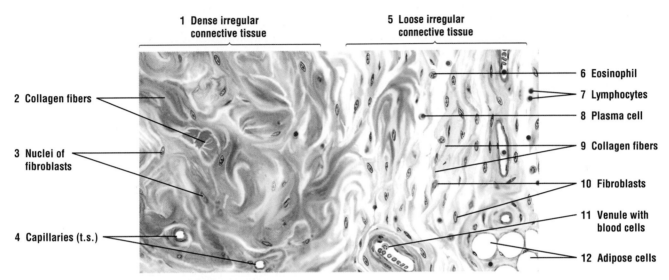

FIGURE 3.6 ■ Dense irregular and loose irregular connective tissue. Stain: hematoxylin and eosin. High magnification.

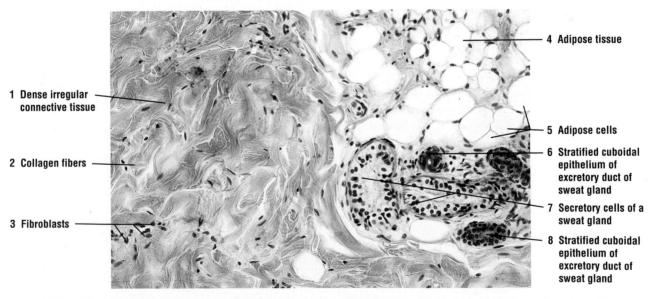

FIGURE 3.7 ■ Dense irregular connective tissue and adipose tissue. Stain: hematoxylin and eosin. ×64.

FIGURE 3.8 ■ Dense Regular Connective Tissue: Tendon (Longitudinal Section)

Dense regular connective tissue is present in ligaments and tendons. A section of a tendon in longitudinal plane is illustrated in which some of the collagen fibers are stretched and some are relaxed.

The **collagen fibers (2, 5, 8)** are arranged in compact, parallel bundles. Between collagen bundles (2, 5, 8) are thin partitions of looser connective tissue that contain parallel rows of **fibroblasts (1, 3)**. The fibroblasts (1, 3) have short processes (not visible here) and nuclei that appear ovoid when seen in **surface view (3)** or flat and rodlike in **lateral view (1)**. When the tendon is stretched, the bundles of collagen fibers (2) are straight. When the tendon is relaxed, the bundles of collagen fibers (8) become wavy.

Dense irregular connective tissue with less regular fiber arrangement than in the tendon also surrounds and partitions the collagen bundles as the **interfascicular connective tissue (4)**. Here are also found **fibroblasts (6)** and numerous blood vessels, such as this **arteriole (7)**, that supply the connective tissue cells.

FIGURE 3.9 ■ Dense Regular Connective Tissue: Tendon (Longitudinal Section)

A photomicrgraph of dense regular connective tissue of a tendon shows that it has a compact, regular, and parallel arrangement of **collagen fibers (1)**. Between the densely packed collagen fibers are seen flattened nuclei of the **fibroblasts (2)**. A small **blood vessel (3)** with blood cells courses between the dense bundles of collagen fibers to supply the connective tissue cells of the tendon.

FUNCTIONAL CORRELATIONS: Dense Irregular Connective Tissue

Dense irregular connective tissue consists primarily of **collagen fibers** with minimal amounts of surrounding ground substance. Except for the **fibroblasts**, cells in this type of connective tissue are sparse. Collagen fibers exhibit great **tensile strength**, and their main function is **support**. Collagen fibers also exhibit **random orientation** and are most highly concentrated in those areas of the body where strong support is needed to resist pulling forces from different directions.

FUNCTIONAL CORRELATIONS: Dense Regular Connective Tissue

Dense regular connective tissue is present where **great tensile strength** is required, such as in **ligaments** and **tendons**. The parallel and dense arrangements of collagen fibers offer strong resistance to forces pulling along a **single axis or direction.**

Tendons and ligaments are attached to bones and are constantly subjected to strong pulling forces. Because of the dense arrangement of collagen fibers, little ground substance is present, and the predominant cell types are the **fibroblasts**, which are located between rows of collagen fibers.

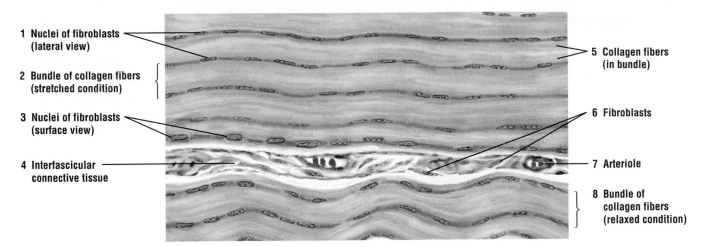

1 **Nuclei of fibroblasts (lateral view)**

2 **Bundle of collagen fibers (stretched condition)**

3 **Nuclei of fibroblasts (surface view)**

4 **Interfascicular connective tissue**

5 **Collagen fibers (in bundle)**

6 **Fibroblasts**

7 **Arteriole**

8 **Bundle of collagen fibers (relaxed condition)**

FIGURE 3.8 ■ Dense regular connective tissue: tendon (longitudinal section). Stain: hematoxylin and eosin. Medium magnification.

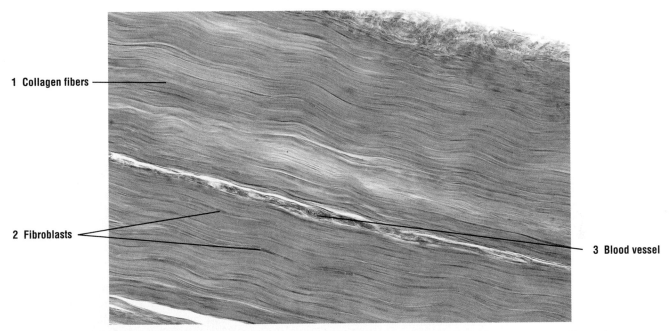

1 **Collagen fibers**

2 **Fibroblasts**

3 **Blood vessel**

FIGURE 3.9 ■ Dense regular connective tissue: tendon (longitudinal section). Stain: hematoxylin and eosin. ×64.

FIGURE 3.10 ■ Dense Regular Connective Tissue: Tendon (Transverse Section)

A transverse section of a tendon is illustrated at a lower magnification (left side) and a higher magnification (right side). Within each large bundle of **collagen fibers (3, 7)** are **fibroblasts (nuclei) (1, 8)** sectioned transversely. The fibroblasts are located between the bundles of collagen fibers (3, 7). These fibroblasts (8) are better distinguished at the higher magnification on the right side, which shows bundles of collagen fibers (7) and the branched shape of fibroblasts (8) in transverse section.

Between the large collagen bundles are the interfascicular **connective tissue (2)** partitions. These partitions contain blood vessels, **arteriole** and **venules (6)**, nerves, and, occasionally, the sensitive pressure receptors **Pacinian corpuscles (9)**.

Also illustrated in the left side of the figure is a transverse section of several **skeletal muscle fibers (4)**. These are adjacent to the tendon, but are separated from it by connective tissue partition. Note that the **nuclei (5)** of skeletal muscles fibers (4) are located on the periphery of the fibers, whereas the fibroblasts (1, 8) are located between bundles of collagen fibers (3, 7).

FIGURE 3.11 ■ Adipose Tissue: Intestine

A small section of a mesentery of the intestine is illustrated, in which large accumulations of **adipose (fat) cells (4, 8)** are organized into an adipose tissue. The **connective tissue (9)** that surrounds the adipose tissue is covered by a simple squamous epithelium called **mesothelium (10)**.

Adipose cells (4, 8) are closely packed and separated by thin strips of **connective tissue septa (3)**, in which are found compressed **fibroblasts (7)**, **arterioles (1)**, **venules (2, 6)**, nerves, and **capillaries (5)**.

Individual adipose cells appear as empty cells (4) because the fat was dissolved by chemicals used during routine histologic preparation of the tissue. The **adipose cell nuclei (8)** are compressed to the peripheral rim of the cytoplasm, and in certain sections, it is difficult to distinguish between fibroblast nuclei (7) and adipose cell nuclei (8).

FUNCTIONAL CORRELATIONS: Adipose Tissue

The two distinct types of adipose tissues in the body are **white adipose tissue** and **brown adipose tissue.** These adipose tissues represent the main sites of **lipid storage** and **metabolism** in the body.

Cells of the white adipose tissue are large and store lipids as a single large droplet. The lipids stored in adipose cells are primarily triglycerides. White adipose tissue exhibits a wider distribution than brown adipose tissue. White adipose tissue is distributed throughout the body, with the distribution pattern showing variations that are dependent on the sex and age of the individual. In addition to serving as an energy source, white adipose tissue provides **insulation** under the skin and forms cushioning **fat pads** around organs. Adipose tissue is also highly vascularized as a result of its high metabolic activity. The adipose cells also have receptors for insulin, glucocorticoids, growth hormone, and other factors that influence adipose tissue to accumulate and release lipids. Furthermore, white adipose tissue also secretes a hormone called **leptin,** which increases carbohydrate and lipid metabolism in cells while inhibiting or suppressing appetite and food intake.

The cells of brown adipose tissue are smaller than white adipose tissue and store lipids as multiple small droplets. Brown adipose tissue is found in all mammals, but is best developed in animals that **hibernate.** The main function of brown adipose tissue is to supply the body with **heat.** In newborn humans exposed to cold or in fur-bearing animals emerging from hibernation, the brown adipose tissue is especially used to generate and increase body heat during these critical periods. The production of heat by the brown adipose tissue is regulated by the sympathetic nervous system, which releases norepinephrine to promote hydrolysis of lipids. The amount of brown adipose tissue gradually decreases in older individuals, and is mainly found around the adrenal glands, great vessels, and in the neck region.

1 Fibroblasts

2 Interfascicular
connective tissue

3 Bundles of
collagen fibers

4 Skeletal muscle fibers

5 Nuclei of skeletal
muscles

6 Arteriole and venules

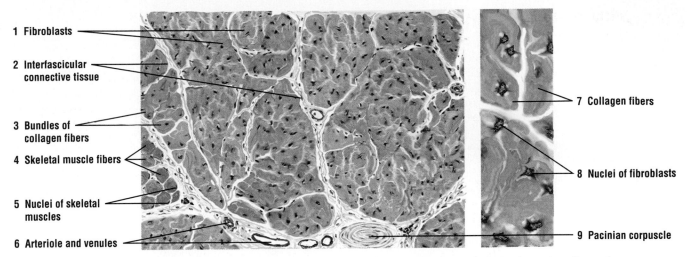

7 Collagen fibers

8 Nuclei of fibroblasts

9 Pacinian corpuscle

FIGURE 3.10 ■ Dense regular connective tissue: tendon (transverse section). Stain: hematoxylin and eosin. Left, low magnification; right: high magnification.

1 Arteriole

2 Venule

3 Connective
tissue septa

4 Adipose cells

5 Capillary

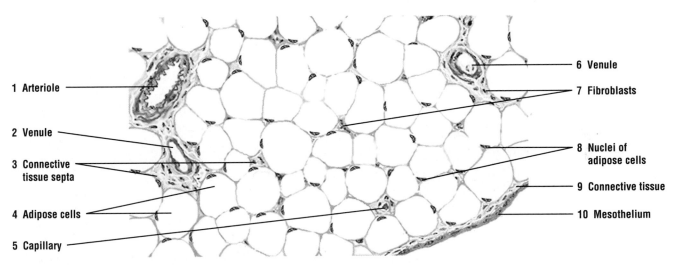

6 Venule

7 Fibroblasts

8 Nuclei of
adipose cells

9 Connective tissue

10 Mesothelium

FIGURE 3.11 ■ Adipose tissue in the intestine. Stain: hematoxylin and eosin. Medium magnification.

Connective Tissue

Classification

- Develops from mesenchyme and consists of cells and ground substance
- Embryonic connective tissue is present in umbilical cord and developing teeth
- Classified as loose or dense connective tissue

Loose Connective Tissue

- More prevalent in body and exhibits loose, irregular arrangement of cells and fibers
- Abundant ground substance
- Collagen fibers, fibroblasts, adipose cells, mast cells, and macrophages predominate

Dense Irregular Connective Tissue

- Consists primarily of fibroblasts, and thick and densely packed collagen fibers
- Fewer other cell types and minimal ground substance
- Collagen fibers exhibit random orientation and provide strong tissue support
- Concentrated in areas where resistance to forces from differernt directions is needed

Dense Regular Connective Tissue

- Fibers densely packed with regular, parallel orientation
- Present in tendons and ligaments that are attached to bones
- Great resistance to forces pulling along single axis or direction
- Minimal ground substance; predominant cell is fibroblast

Cells of Connective Tissue

Fibroblasts

- Are active permanent cells that synthesize all collagen, reticular, and elastic connective tissue fibers
- Synthesize glycosaminoglycans, proteoglycans, and glycoproteins of ground substance

Fibrocytes

- Smaller than fibroblasts
- Inactive or resting connective tissue cells

White Adipose (Fat) Cells

- Occur singly or in groups
- When adipose cells predominate, the connective tissue is adipose tissue
- Store fat (lipid) as single large droplet primarily as tryglycerides

- Appear as empty cells because lipid is dissolved during tissue preparation
- Distributed throughout body, serves as insulation, and forms fat pads for organ protection
- Highly vascularized owing to high metabolic activity
- Exhibit numerous receptors for different hormones that influence accumulation and release of lipid
- Secrete hormone leptin to increase lipid metabolism and to inhibit appetite

Brown Adipose Cells

- Cells smaller than white adipose cells; store lipid as multiple droplets
- Best developed in hibernating animals
- In newborns or animals emerging from hibernation, generates body heat
- Norepinephrine from sympathetic nervous system promotes hydrolysis of lipids

Macrophages

- Most numerous in loose connective tissue
- Ingest bacteria, dead cells, cell debris, and foreign matter
- Are antigen-presenting cells to lymphocytes for immunologic response
- Derived from circulating blood monocytes
- Called Kupfer cells in liver, osteoclasts in bone, and microglia in central nervous system

Lymphocytes

- Most numerous in loose connective tissue of respiratory and gastrointestinal tracts
- Produce antibodies and kill virus-infected cells

Plasma Cells

- Characterized by chromatin distributed in radial pattern
- Derived from lymphocytes exposed to antigens
- Produce antibodies to destroy specific antigens

Mast Cells

- Closely associated with blood vessel
- Found in skin, respiratory, and digestive system connective tissue
- Spherical cells with fine, regular basophilic granules
- Release histamine when exposed to allergens, causing allergic reactions

Neutrophils

- Active phagocytes; engulf and destroy bacteria

Eosinophils

- Increase after parasitic infestation
- Phagocytize antigen–antibody complexes during allergic reactions

Collagen Fibers

- Type I found in skin, tendons, ligaments, and bone
- Type II found in hyaline and elastic cartilage
- Type III forms meshwork in liver, lymph node, spleen, and hemopoietic organs
- Type IV found in basal lamina of basement membrane

Ground Substance

- Consists of extracellular matrix, a semifluid gel with high water content
- Contains polysaccharide chains of glycosaminoglycans, proteoglycans, and adhesive glycoproteins
- Hyaluronic acid is main glycosaminoglycan
- Other glycosaminoglycans form proteoglycan aggregates, which attract water
- Facilitates diffusion between cells and blood vessels
- Barrier to spread of pathogens
- Bacteria can hydrolyze hyaluronic acid and reduce barrier viscocity
- Contains several adhesive glycoproteins, such as fibronectin, that bind cells to fibers

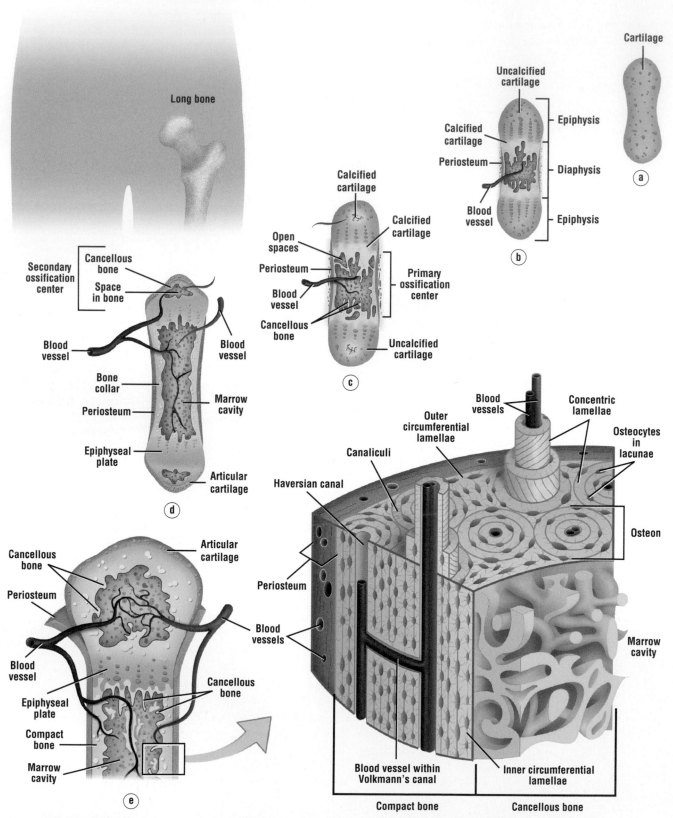

OVERVIEW FIGURE 4 ■ Endochondral ossification illustrating the progressive stages of bone formation, from a cartilage model to bone, including the histology of a section of formed compact bone.

Cartilage and Bone

SECTION 1 ■ Cartilage

Characteristics of Cartilage

Cartilage is a special form of connective tissue that also develops from the **mesenchyme.** Similar to the connective tissue, cartilage consists of cells and **extracellular matrix** composed of connective tissue fibers and ground substance. In contrast to connective tissue, cartilage is **nonvascular** (avascular) and receives its nutrition via diffusion through the extracellular matrix.

Cartilage exhibits tensile strength, provides firm structural support for soft tissues, allows flexibility without distortion, and is resilient to compression. Cartilage consists mainly of cells called **chondrocytes** and **chondroblasts** that synthesize the extensive extracellular matrix. There are three main types of cartilage in the body: hyaline, elastic, and fibrocartilage. Their classification is based on the amount and types of connective tissue fibers that are present in the extracellular matrix.

Cartilage Types

Hyaline Cartilage

Hyaline cartilage is the most common type. In embryos, hyaline cartilage serves as a skeletal model for most bones. As the individual grows, the cartilage bone model is gradually replaced with bone by a process called **endochondral ossification.** In adults, most of the hyaline cartilage model has been replaced with bone, except on the articular surfaces of bones, ends of ribs (costal cartilage), nose, larynx, trachea, and in bronchi. Here, the hyaline cartilage persists throughout life and does not calcify.

Elastic Cartilage

Elastic cartilage is similar in appearance to hyaline cartilage, except for the presence of numerous branching elastic fibers within its matrix. Elastic cartilage is highly flexible and occurs in the external ear, walls of the auditory tube, epiglottis, and larynx.

Fibrocartilage

Fibrocartilage is characterized by large amounts of irregular and dense bundles of coarse collagen fibers in its matrix. In contrast to hyaline and elastic cartilage, fibrocartilage consists of alternating layers of cartilage matrix and thick dense layers of **type I collagen** fibers. The collagen fibers normally orient themselves into the direction of functional stress. Fibrocartilage has a limited distribution in the body and is found in the intervertebral disks, symphysis pubis, and certain joints.

Perichondrium

Most of the hyaline and elastic cartilage is surrounded by a peripheral layer of vascularized, dense, irregular connective tissue called the **perichondrium.** Its outer fibrous layer contains type I collagen fibers and fibroblasts. The inner layer of perichondrium is cellular and **chondrogenic.** Chondrogenic cells form the chondroblasts that secrete the cartilage matrix. Hyaline cartilage on the articulating surfaces of bones is not lined by perichondrium. Similarly, because fibrocartilage is always associated with dense connective tissue fibers, it does not exhibit an identifiable perichondrium.

Cartilage Matrix

Cartilage matrix is produced and maintained by chondrocytes and chondroblasts. The collagen or elastic fibers give cartilage matrix its firmness and resilience. Similar to loose connective tissue, the extracellular **ground substance** of cartilage contains sulfated glycosaminoglycans and hyaluronic acid that are closely associated with the elastic and collagen fibers within the ground substance. Also, cartilage matrix is highly hydrated because of its high water content, which allows for diffusion of molecules to and from the chondrocytes. Cartilage is a semirigid tissue and can act as a shock absorber. Embedded within its matrix are varying proportions of collagen and elastic fibers. The presence of these fibers characterizes cartilage as hyaline cartilage, elastic cartilage, or fibrocartilage.

Hyaline cartilage matrix consists of the fine **type II collagen fibrils** embedded in a firm amorphous hydrated matrix rich in proteoglycans and structural glycoproteins. Most of the proteoglycans in cartilage matrix exist as large **proteoglycan aggregates,** which contain sulfated glycosaminoglycans linked to core proteins and molecules of nonsulfated glycosaminoglycan hyaluronic acid. The proteoglycan aggregates bind to the thin fibrils of the collagen matrix.

In addition to type II collagen fibrils and proteoglycans, cartilage matrix also contains an adhesive glycoprotein called **chondronectin.** These macromolecules bind to glycosaminoglycans and collagen fibers, providing adherence of chondroblasts and chondrocytes to collagen fibers of surrounding matrix.

FIGURE 4.1 ■ Fetal Hyaline Cartilage

This figure illustrates hyaline cartilage in an early stage of development. Superficial **mesenchyme (1)** with **blood vessels (5)** surrounds the nonvascular fetal cartilage. At this stage, lacunae around the **fetal chondroblasts (4, 7)** are not visible, and the chondroblasts (4, 7) resemble superficial mesenchymal cells (1). Fetal chondroblasts (4, 7) are randomly distributed without forming isogenous groups and secrete the **intercellular cartilage matrix (8).**

During development, mesenchyme cells (1) concentrate on the periphery of the cartilage and their nuclei become elongated. This region develops into **perichondrium (2, 6),** a sheath of dense irregular connective tissue with fibroblasts (2, 6) that surrounds hyaline and elastic cartilage. The inner layer of the perichondrium (2, 6) becomes the **chondrogenic layer (3)** that gives rise to chondroblasts (4, 7).

FIGURE 4.2 ■ Hyaline Cartilage and Surrounding Structures: Trachea

This illustration depicts a section of a hyaline cartilage plate from the trachea. **Perichondrium (5)** with **fibroblasts (7)** surround the cartilage. The inner **chondrogenic layer (4)** produces **chondroblasts (8)** that differentiate into chondrocytes. **Chondrocytes** in lacunae appear either singly or in **isogenous groups (3).** Lacunae and chondrocytes (3) in the middle of the cartilage plate are large and spherical, but become progressively flatter toward the periphery, where these cells are differentiating chondroblasts (8). The **interterritorial** (intercellular) **matrix (1)** stains lighter, whereas the **territorial matrix (2)** around the lacunae stains darker.

Vascular (9) connective tissue (10) and tracheal glands with grapelike secretory units called acini are visible near the cartilage. **Serous acini (11)** produce watery secretions, whereas **mucous acini (12)** secrete a lubricating mucus. An **excretory duct (6)** delivers these secretions into the tracheal lumen.

FUNCTIONAL CORRELATIONS: Cartilage Cells

Cartilage develops from primitive **mesenchyme cells** that differentiate into **chondroblasts.** These cells divide mitotically and synthesize the cartilage **matrix** and **extracellular material.** As the cartilage model grows, the individual chondroblasts are surrounded by extracellular matrix and become trapped in compartments called **lacunae** (singular, *lacuna*). In the lacunae are mature cartilage cells called **chondrocytes.** The main function of chondrocytes is to maintain the cartilage matrix. Some lacunae may contain more than one chondrocyte; these groups of chondrocytes are called **isogenous groups.**

Mesenchyme cells can also differentiate into fibroblasts that form the **perichondrium,** a dense, irregular connective tissue layer that invests the cartilage. The inner cellular layer of perichondrium contains chondrogenic cells, which can differentiate into chondroblasts, secrete cartilage matrix, and become trapped in lacunae as chondrocytes.

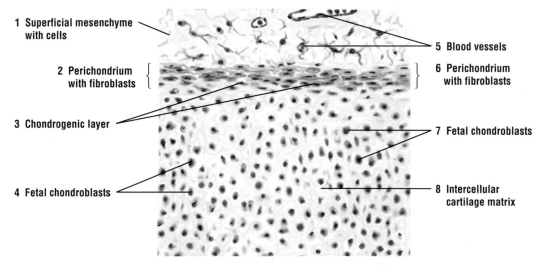

1 Superficial mesenchyme with cells
2 Perichondrium with fibroblasts
3 Chondrogenic layer
4 Fetal chondroblasts
5 Blood vessels
6 Perichondrium with fibroblasts
7 Fetal chondroblasts
8 Intercellular cartilage matrix

FIGURE 4.1 ■ Developing fetal hyaline cartilage. Stain: hematoxylin and eosin. Medium magnification.

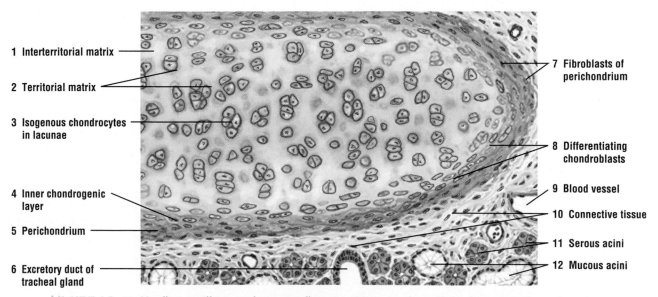

1 Interterritorial matrix
2 Territorial matrix
3 Isogenous chondrocytes in lacunae
4 Inner chondrogenic layer
5 Perichondrium
6 Excretory duct of tracheal gland
7 Fibroblasts of perichondrium
8 Differentiating chondroblasts
9 Blood vessel
10 Connective tissue
11 Serous acini
12 Mucous acini

FIGURE 4.2 ■ Hyaline cartilage and surrounding structures: trachea. Stain: hematoxylin and eosin. Medium magnification.

FIGURE 4.3 ◼ Cells and Matrix of Mature Hyaline Cartilage

Higher magnification illustrates an interior or central region of mature hyaline cartilage. Distributed throughout the homogeneous ground substance, the **matrix (4, 5)**, are ovoid spaces called **lacunae (3)** containing mature cartilage cells, the **chondrocytes (1, 2)**. In intact cartilage, chondrocytes fill the lacunae. Each chondrocyte has a granular cytoplasm and a **nucleus (1)**. During histologic preparations, chondrocytes (1, 2) shrink, and the lacunae (3) appear as clear spaces. Cartilage cells in the matrix are seen either singly or in isogenous groups.

Hyaline cartilage matrix (4, 5) appears homogeneous and usually basophilic. The lighter-staining matrix between chondrocytes (2) is called **interterritorial matrix (5)**. The more basophilic or darker matrix adjacent to the chondrocytes is the **territorial matrix (4)**.

FIGURE 4.4 ◼ Hyaline Cartilage: Developing Bone

A photomicrograph of a section through a developing bone shows a portion of the hyaline cartilage and its characteristic homogenous **matrix (1)**. Located within the matrix (1) are the mature hyaline cartilage cells **chondrocytes (3)** in their **lacunae (2)**. Surrounding the hyaline cartilage is the dense, irregular connective tissue **perichondrium (5)**. On the inner surface of the perichondrium (5) is the **chondrogenic layer (4)**.

FUNCTIONAL CORRELATIONS: Cartilage (Hyaline, Elastic, and Fibrocartilage)

Cartilage is nonvascular, but it is surrounded by the vascular connective tissue **perichondrium.** Because of the high water content in the cartilage, all nutrients enter and metabolites leave the cartilage by diffusing through the matrix. Also, cartilage matrix is soft and pliable and not as hard as bone. As a result, cartilage can simultaneously grow by two different processes: interstitial and appositional.

Interstitial growth of cartilage involves mitosis of chondrocytes within the matrix and deposition of new matrix between and around the cells. This growth process increases cartilage size from within. **Appositional growth** occurs on the periphery of the cartilage. Here, chondroblasts differentiate from the inner cellular layer of the perichondrium and deposit a layer of cartilage matrix that is apposed to the existing cartilage layer. This growth process increases cartilage width.

Hyaline cartilage provides a firm structural and flexible support. Elastic cartilage, owing to the numerous branching elastic fibers in its matrix, confers structural support as well as increased flexibility. In contrast to hyaline cartilage, which can calcify with aging, the matrix of elastic cartilage does not calcify. The main function of fibrocartilage is to provide tensile strength, bear weight, and resist stretch or compression.

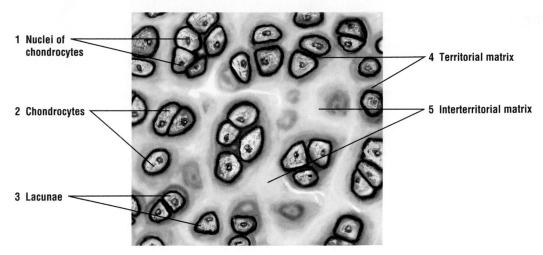

1 Nuclei of chondrocytes

2 Chondrocytes

3 Lacunae

4 Territorial matrix

5 Interterritorial matrix

FIGURE 4.3 ■ Cells and matrix of mature hyaline cartilage. Stain: hematoxylin and eosin. High magnification.

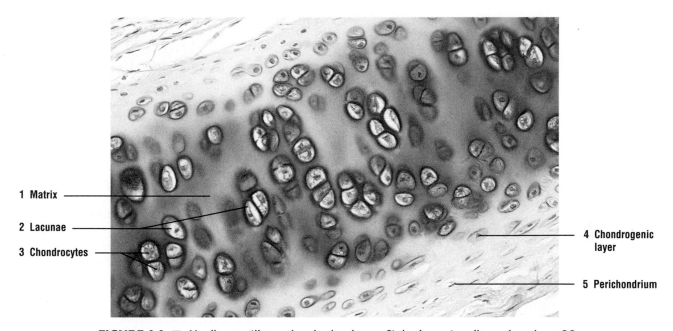

1 Matrix

2 Lacunae

3 Chondrocytes

4 Chondrogenic layer

5 Perichondrium

FIGURE 4.4 ■ Hyaline cartilage: developing bone. Stain: hematoxylin and eosin. ×80.

FIGURE 4.5 ■ Elastic Cartilage: Epiglottis

Elastic cartilage differs from hyaline cartilage principally by the presence of numerous **elastic fibers (4)** in its **matrix (7).** Staining the cartilage of the epiglottis with silver reveals the thin elastic fibers **(4).** Elastic fibers **(4, 7)** enter the cartilage matrix from the surrounding connective tissue **perichondrium (1)** and become distributed as branching and anastomosing fibers of various sizes. The density of the fibers varies among elastic cartilages as well as among different areas of the same cartilage.

As in hyaline cartilage, larger **chondrocytes** in **lacunae (3, 8)** are more prevalent in the interior of the plate. The smaller and flatter chondrocytes are located peripherally in the inner **chondrogenic layer** of **perichondrium (2),** from which chondroblasts develop to synthesize the cartilage matrix. Also visible in the perichondrium **(1)** are the connective tissue **fibrocytes (5)** and a **venule (6).**

FIGURE 4.6 ■ Elastic Cartilage: Epiglottis

A photomicrograph of a section of an epiglottis shows that this type of structure is characterized by the presence of a cartilage with fine, branching **elastic fibers (2)** in its **matrix (5),** in addition to distinct **chondrocytes (3)** and **lacunae (4).** The presence of elastic fibers **(2)** gives this cartilage flexibility, in addition to support. Surrounding the elastic cartilage is a layer of dense, irregular connective tissue **perichondrium (1).**

FIGURE 4.7 ■ Fibrous Cartilage: Intervertebral Disk

In fibrous cartilage, the **matrix (5)** is filled with dense **collagen fibers (2, 6),** which frequently exhibit parallel arrangement, as seen in tendons. Small **chondrocytes (1, 4)** in **lacunae (3)** are usually distributed in **rows (4)** within the fibrous cartilage matrix **(5),** rather than at random or in isogenous groups, as is seen in hyaline or elastic cartilage. All chondrocytes and lacunae (1, 3, 4) are of similar size; there is no gradation from larger central chondrocytes to smaller and flatter peripheral cells.

A perichondrium, normally present around hyaline cartilage and elastic cartilage, is absent because fibrous cartilage usually forms a transitional area between hyaline cartilage and tendon or ligament.

The proportion of collagen fibers (2, 6) to cartilage matrix (5), the number of chondrocytes, and their arrangement in the matrix (5) may vary. Collagen fibers (2, 6) may be so dense that the matrix (5) is invisible. In such case, chondrocytes and lacunae will appear flattened. Collagen fibers within a bundle are normally parallel but collagen bundles may course in different directions.

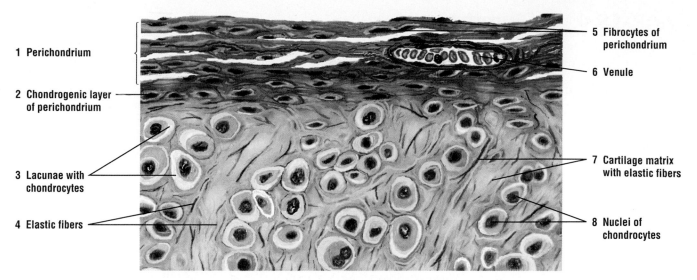

1 Perichondrium

2 Chondrogenic layer
   of perichondrium

3 Lacunae with
   chondrocytes

4 Elastic fibers

5 Fibrocytes of
   perichondrium

6 Venule

7 Cartilage matrix
   with elastic fibers

8 Nuclei of
   chondrocytes

FIGURE 4.5 ■ Elastic cartilage: epiglottis. Stain: silver. High magnification.

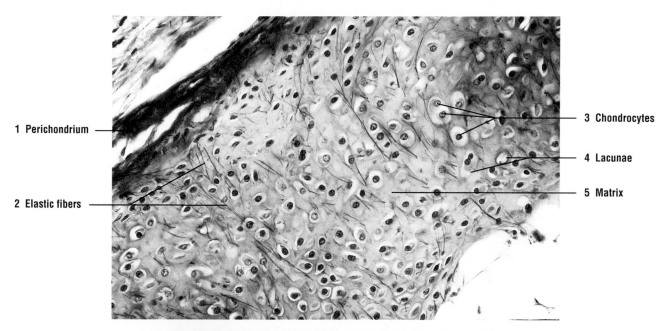

1 Perichondrium

2 Elastic fibers

3 Chondrocytes

4 Lacunae

5 Matrix

FIGURE 4.6 ■ Elastic cartilage: epiglottis. Stain: silver. ×80.

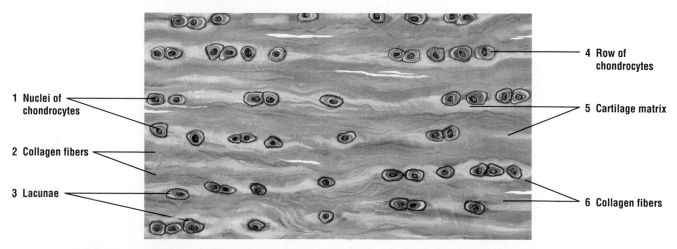

1 Nuclei of
   chondrocytes

2 Collagen fibers

3 Lacunae

4 Row of
   chondrocytes

5 Cartilage matrix

6 Collagen fibers

FIGURE 4.7 ■ Fibrous cartilage: intervertebral disk. Stain: hematoxylin and eosin. High magnification.

CHAPTER 4 ■ **Summary**

SECTION 1 ■ Cartilage

Characteristics of Cartilage

- Develops from mesenchyme and consists of cells, connective tissue fibers, and ground substance
- Nonvascular, gets nutrients via diffusion through ground substance
- Performs numerous supportive functions
- Cells include chondrocytes and chondroblasts
- Three types of cartilage are the hyaline, elastic, and fibrocartilage

Hyaline Cartilage

- Most common in the body and serves as a skeletal model for most bones
- Replaced by bone during endochondral ossification
- Contains type II collagen fibrils
- In adults, present on articular surfaces of bones, ends of ribs, nose, larynx, trachea, and bronchi

Elastic Cartilage

- Contains branching elastic fibers in matrix and is highly flexible
- Found in external ear, auditory tube, epiglottis, and larynx

Fibrocartilage

- Filled with dense bundles of type I collagen fibers that alternate with cartilage matrix
- Provides tensile strength, bears weight, and resists compression
- Found in intervertebral disks, symphysis pubis, and certain joints

Perichondrium

- Found on peripheries of hyaline and elastic cartilage
- Peripheral layer is dense vascular connective tissue with type I collagen
- Inner layer is chondrogenic and gives rise to chondroblasts that secrete cartilage matrix
- Articular hyaline cartilage of bones and fibrocartilage not lined by perichondrium

Cartilage Matrix

- Produced and maintained by chondrocytes and chondroblasts
- Contains large proteoglycan aggregates and is highly hydrated
- Allows diffusion and is semirigid shock absorber
- Adhesive glycoprotein chondronectin binds cells and fibrils to surrounding matrix
- Elastic cartilage provides structural support and increased flexibility

Cartilage Cells

- Primitive mesenchyme cells differentiate into chondroblasts that synthesize the matrix
- Mature cartilage cells, chondrocytes, become enclosed in lacunae
- Inner layer of surrounding connective tissue perichondrium is chondrogenic
- Chondroblasts enlarge the cartilage by both interstitial and appositional growth

SECTION 2 ■ Bone

Characteristics of Bone

Similar to cartilage, **bone** is also a special form of connective tissue and consists of **cells, fibers, and extracellular matrix.** Because of mineral deposition in the matrix, bones become calcified. As a result, bones become hard and can bear more weight than cartilage, serve as a rigid skeleton for the body, and provide attachment sites for muscles and organs.

Bone also protects the brain in the skull, heart and lungs in the thorax, and urinary and reproductive organs between the pelvic bones. In addition, bones function in **hemopoiesis** (blood cell formation), and serve as crucial **reservoirs** for calcium, phosphate, and other minerals. Almost all (99%) of the calcium in the body is stored in bones, from which the body receives its daily calcium supply.

The Process of Bone Formation (Ossification)

Bone development begins in the embryo by two distinct processes: endochondral ossification and intramembranous ossification. Although the bones are produced by two different methods, they exhibit the same histologic structures (Overview Figure 4).

Endochondral Ossification

Most bones in the body develop by the process of **endochondral ossification,** in which a temporary hyaline cartilage model precedes bone formation. This cartilage model continues to grow by both interstitial and appositional means, and primarily is used to form the short and long bones. As development progresses, the chondrocytes divide, hypertrophy (enlarge), and mature, and the hyaline cartilage model begins to calcify. As calcification of the cartilage model continues, diffusion of nutrients and gases through the calcified matrix decreases. Consequently, chondrocytes die, and the fragmented calcified matrix serves as a structural framework for the deposition of bony material.

As soon as a layer of bony material is deposited around the calcifying cartilage, the inner perichondrial cells exhibit their osteogenic potential, and a thin periosteal collar of bone forms around the midpoint of the shaft of the bone. This external surrounding connective tissue is now called the **periosteum.** Mesenchyme cells differentiate into **osteoprogenitor cells** from the inner layer of periosteum, and blood vessels from the periosteum invade the calcified and degenerating cartilage model. Osteoprogenitor cells proliferate and differentiate into **osteoblasts** that secrete the osteoid matrix, a soft initially collagenous tissue that lacks minerals but is quickly mineralized into the bone. The osteoblasts are then surrounded by bone in the cavelike **lacunae** and are now called **osteocytes;** there is one osteocyte per lacuna. Osteocytes establish a complex cell-to-cell connection through tiny canals in the bone called **canaliculi;** these eventually open into channels that house the blood vessels. Osteoprogenitor cells also arise from the inner surface of bone called **endosteum.** Endosteum lines all internal cavities in the bone and consists of a single layer of osteoprogenitor cells.

Mesenchyme tissue, osteoblasts, and blood vessels form a **primary ossification center** in the developing bone that first appears in the **diaphysis** or the shaft of the long bone, followed by a **secondary ossification center** in the **epiphysis** or the articular surface of the expanded end. In all developing long bones, cartilage in the diaphysis and epiphysis is replaced by bone, except in the **epiphyseal plate** region, which is located between the diaphysis and epiphysis. Growth in this region continues and is responsible for lengthening the bone until bone growth stops. Expansion of the two ossification centers eventually replaces all cartilage with bone, including the epiphyseal plate. The only exceptions are the free or articulating ends of long bones. Here, a layer of permanent hyaline cartilage covers the bone and is called the **articular cartilage.**

Intramembranous Ossification

In **intramembranous ossification,** bone development is not preceded by a cartilage model. Instead, bone develops from the connective tissue **mesenchyme.** Some mesenchyme cells differentiate directly into osteoblasts that produce the surrounding **osteoid matrix,** which quickly calcifies. Numerous ossification centers are formed, anastomose, and produce a network of **spongy bone** that consists of thin rods, plates, and spines called **trabeculae.** The osteoblasts then become surrounded by bone in the cavelike **lacunae** and become **osteocytes.** As in endochondral ossification, once osteocytes are in the lacunae, they establish a complex cell-to-cell connection through the **canaliculi.**

The **mandible, maxilla, clavicles,** and most of the **flat bones of the skull** are formed by the intramembranous method. In the developing skull, the centers of bone development grow radially, replace the connective tissue, and then fuse. In newborns, the **fontanelles** in the skull represent the soft membranous regions where intramembranous ossification of skull bones is in the process of ossification.

Bone Types

Examination of bone in cross section shows two types, **compact bone** and **cancellous (spongy) bone** (see Overview Figure 4). In long bones, the outer cylindrical part is the dense compact bone. The inner surface of compact bone adjacent to the marrow cavity is the cancellous (spongy) bone. Cancellous bone contains numerous interconnecting areas and is not dense; however, both types of bone have the same microscopic appearance. In newborns, the marrow cavities of long bones are red and produce blood cells. In adults, the marrow cavities of long bones normally are yellow and filled with adipose (fat) cells.

In compact bone, the collagen fibers are arranged in thin layers of bone called **lamellae** that are parallel to each other in the periphery of the bone, or concentrically arranged around a blood vessel. In a long bone, the **outer circumferential lamellae** are deep to the periosteum. **Inner circumferential lamellae** surround the bone marrow cavity. **Concentric lamellae** surround the canals with blood vessels, nerves, and loose connective tissue called the **osteons (Haversian systems).** The space in the osteon that contains blood vessels and nerves is the **central (Haversian) canal.** Most of the compact bone consists of **osteons.** Lacunae with osteocytes and connected via canaliculi are found between the lamellae in each osteon (see Overview Figure 4).

Bone Matrix

The bone matrix consists of living cells and extracellular material. Because the bone matrix is calcified or mineralized, it is harder than cartilage. Diffusion is not possible through the calcified matrix; therefore, bone matrix is highly vascularized. Bone matrix contains both organic and inorganic components. The organic components enable bones to resist tension, while the mineral components resist compression.

The major organic components of bone matrix are the coarse **type I collagen fibers,** which are the predominant proteins. The other organic components are sulfated glycosaminoglycans and hyaluronic acid that form larger proteoglycan aggregates. Glycoproteins osteocalcin and osteopontin bind tightly to calcium crystals during mineralization of bone. Another matrix protein, sialoprotein, binds osteoblasts to the extracellular matrix through the integrins of the plasma membrane proteins.

The inorganic component of bone matrix consists of the minerals calcium and phosphate in the form of hydroxyapatite crystals. The association of coarse collagen fibers with hydroxyapatite crystals provides the bone with its hardness, durability, and strength. In addition, as the need arises, hormones such as parathyroid hormone from the parathyroid gland and **calcitonin** from the thyroid gland maintain a proper mineral content in the blood.

FIGURE 4.8 ■ Endochondral Ossification: Development of a Long Bone (Panoramic View, Longitudinal Section)

During endochondral ossification, the bone is first formed as a model of embryonic hyaline cartilage. As bone development progresses, the cartilage model is replaced by bone. The process of endochondral ossification can be followed by examining the upper part of the illustration and proceeding downward.

In the upper part, the hyaline cartilage is surrounded by connective tissue **perichondrium (13).** The **zone** of **reserve cartilage (1)** shows chondrocytes in their lacunae distributed singly or in small groups. Below this region is the **zone** of **proliferating chondrocytes (2)** where the chondrocytes divide and become arranged in vertical columns. **Chondrocytes** in **lacunae (14)** increase in size in the **zone** of **chondrocyte hypertrophy (3)** as a result of swelling of the nucleus and cytoplasm. The hypertrophied chondrocytes degenerate, forming thin **plates** of **calcified cartilage** matrix (15). Below this region is the **zone of ossification** (4), where a bony material is deposited on the plates of calcified cartilage matrix (15).

Blood sinusoids (20) or capillaries invade the calcifying cartilage. Lacunar walls and the calcified cartilage (15) are eroded, and the **red bone marrow cavity (16)** is formed. The connective tissue around the newly formed bone is called **periosteum (5, 6, 17)**, and this region is now the **zone of ossification (4)**. In this illustration, bone is stained dark red. Osteoprogenitor cells from the **inner periosteum (6)** continue to differentiate into osteoblasts, deposit **osteoid** and **bone (8)** around the remaining plates of calcified cartilage (15), and form the **periosteal bone collar (7)**.

Formation of new periosteal bone (7) keeps pace with the formation of new endochondral bone. The bone collar (7) increases in thickness and compactness as development of bone proceeds. The thickest portion of the bone collar (7) is seen in the central part of the developing bone called the diaphysis. The primary center of ossification is located in the diaphysis, where the initial periosteal bone collar (7) is formed.

Red bone marrow (16) fills the cavity of newly formed bone with hemopoietic (blood forming) cells. Fine reticular connective tissue fibers in the bone marrow (16) are obscured by masses of developing erythrocytes, granulocytes, **megakaryocytes (12)**, **bony spicules (11, 22)**, numerous blood sinusoids (20), capillaries, and blood vessels.

Surrounding the shaft of the developing bone are the soft tissues. The **epidermis (18)** of skin is lined by stratified squamous epithelium. Below the epidermis (18) is the subcutaneous **connective tissue** of the **dermis (19)**, in which are seen **hair follicles (9)**, **blood vessels (10)**, **adipose cells (21)**, and **sweat glands (23)**.

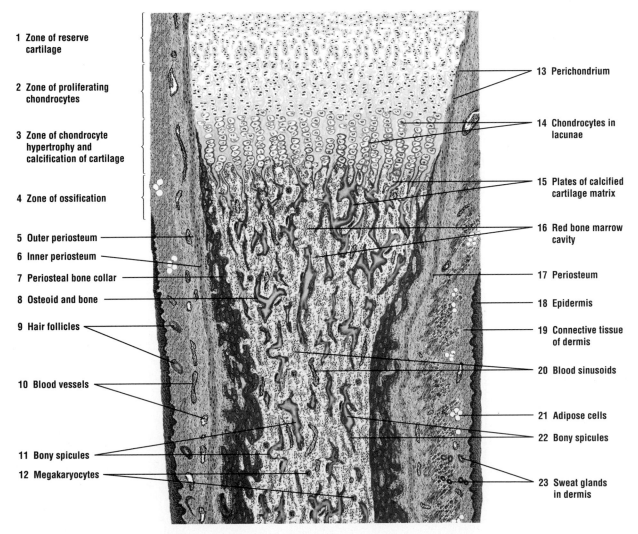

1 Zone of reserve cartilage

2 Zone of proliferating chondrocytes

3 Zone of chondrocyte hypertrophy and calcification of cartilage

4 Zone of ossification

5 Outer periosteum

6 Inner periosteum

7 Periosteal bone collar

8 Osteoid and bone

9 Hair follicles

10 Blood vessels

11 Bony spicules

12 Megakaryocytes

13 Perichondrium

14 Chondrocytes in lacunae

15 Plates of calcified cartilage matrix

16 Red bone marrow cavity

17 Periosteum

18 Epidermis

19 Connective tissue of dermis

20 Blood sinusoids

21 Adipose cells

22 Bony spicules

23 Sweat glands in dermis

FIGURE 4.8 ■ Endochondral ossification: development of a long bone (panoramic view, longitudinal section). Stain: hematoxylin and eosin. Low magnification.

FIGURE 4.9 ■ Endochondral Ossification: Zone of Ossification

This figure shows endochondral ossification at higher magnification and in greater detail and corresponds to the upper region of Figure 4.8.

Proliferating **chondrocytes (1, 14)** are arranged in distinct vertical columns. Below is the zone of **hypertrophied chondrocytes (2, 15).** Chondrocytes and lacunae undergo hypertrophy as a result of increased glycogen and lipid accumulations in their cytoplasm and nuclear swelling. The cytoplasm of hypertrophied chondrocytes **(2, 15)** becomes **vacuolized (16),** the nuclei become pyknotic, and the thin cartilage plates become surrounded by **calcified matrix (5, 17).**

Osteoblasts (6, 20) line up along remaining plates of calcified cartilage **(5, 17)** and lay down a layer of **osteoid (19)** and bone. Osteoblasts trapped in the osteoid or bone become **osteocytes (9, 21). Capillaries (8, 18)** from the **marrow cavity (10)** invade the newly ossified area.

The developing marrow cavity **(10)** contains numerous **megakaryocytes (13, 24)** and pluripotential stem cells that give rise to erythrocytic and granulocytic **blood cells (23).** Multinucleated **osteoclasts (11, 22)** lie in shallow depressions called **Howship's lacunae (11, 22)** and are adjacent to bone that is being resorbed.

The left side of the illustration shows an area of **periosteal bone (7)** with osteocytes **(9)** in their lacunae. The new bone is added peripherally by osteoblasts **(6),** which develop from osteoprogenitor cells of the **inner periosteum (12).** The outer layer of periosteum continues as the connective tissue **perichondrium (3).**

FIGURE 4.10 ■ Endochondral Ossification: Zone of Ossification

This photomicrograph illustrates the transformation of hyaline cartilage into bone through the process of endochondral ossification. The **hyaline cartilage matrix (6)** contains **proliferating chondrocytes (7)** and **hypertrophied chondrocytes (1)** with **vacuolated cytoplasm (2).** Below these cells are plates or **spicules** of **calcified cartilage (3)** surrounded by **osteoblasts (4).** As the cartilage calcifies, a **marrow cavity (5)** is formed with blood vessels, **hemopoietic tissue (10),** osteoprogenitor cells, and osteoblasts **(4).** The hyaline cartilage is surrounded by the connective tissue **perichondrium (8).** The marrow cavity in the new bone is surrounded by the connective tissue **periosteum (9).**

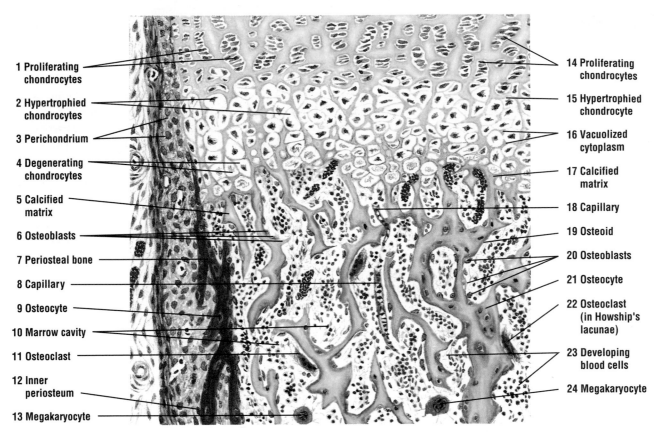

1 Proliferating chondrocytes

2 Hypertrophied chondrocytes

3 Perichondrium

4 Degenerating chondrocytes

5 Calcified matrix

6 Osteoblasts

7 Periosteal bone

8 Capillary

9 Osteocyte

10 Marrow cavity

11 Osteoclast

12 Inner periosteum

13 Megakaryocyte

14 Proliferating chondrocytes

15 Hypertrophied chondrocyte

16 Vacuolized cytoplasm

17 Calcified matrix

18 Capillary

19 Osteoid

20 Osteoblasts

21 Osteocyte

22 Osteoclast (in Howship's lacunae)

23 Developing blood cells

24 Megakaryocyte

FIGURE 4.9 ■ Endochondral ossification: zone of ossification. Stain: hematoxylin and eosin. Medium magnification.

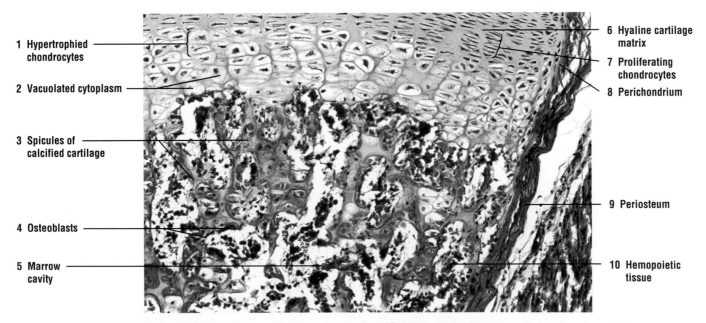

1 Hypertrophied chondrocytes

2 Vacuolated cytoplasm

3 Spicules of calcified cartilage

4 Osteoblasts

5 Marrow cavity

6 Hyaline cartilage matrix

7 Proliferating chondrocytes

8 Perichondrium

9 Periosteum

10 Hemopoietic tissue

FIGURE 4.10 ■ Endochondral ossification: zone of ossification. Stain: hematoxylin and eosin. ×50.

FIGURE 4.11 ■ Endochondral Ossification: Formation of Secondary (Epiphyseal) Centers of Ossification and Epiphyseal Plate in Long Bones (Longitudinal Section, Decalcified Bone)

The hyaline cartilage in epiphyseal ends of two developing bones is illustrated. Both bones exhibit **secondary centers of ossification (5, 11).** Although cartilage is nonvascular, numerous **blood vessels (1, 6),** sectioned in a different plane, pass through the cartilage matrix to supply the osteoblasts and osteocytes in the secondary centers of ossification (5, 11). **Articular cartilage (4, 12)** covers both articulating ends of the future bone. A **synovial** or **joint cavity (3)** separates the two cartilage models. The inner synovial membrane of squamous cells lines the synovial cavity (3), except over the articular cartilages (4, 12). A synovial membrane, together with the connective tissue, may extend into the joint cavity as **synovial folds (2, 13).** The synovial cavity (3) is covered by a connective tissue capsule.

In the lower bone, an active **epiphyseal plate (16)** is seen between the secondary ossification center (5) and the developing shaft of the bone. A **zone** of **proliferating chondrocytes (7)** and a **zone of chondrocyte hypertrophy** and **calcification** of **cartilage (8)** are clearly visible in the epiphyseal plate (16). Small **spicules** of **calcified cartilage (9, 15)** surrounded by red-stained bony material and **primitive bone marrow cavities** with **hemopoiesis (14, 17)** are seen in the shaft of the bone and secondary center of ossification (5). A **megakaryocyte (18)** is also visible in the lower bone marrow cavity (17). A connective tissue **periosteum (19)** surrounds the compact **bone (10).**

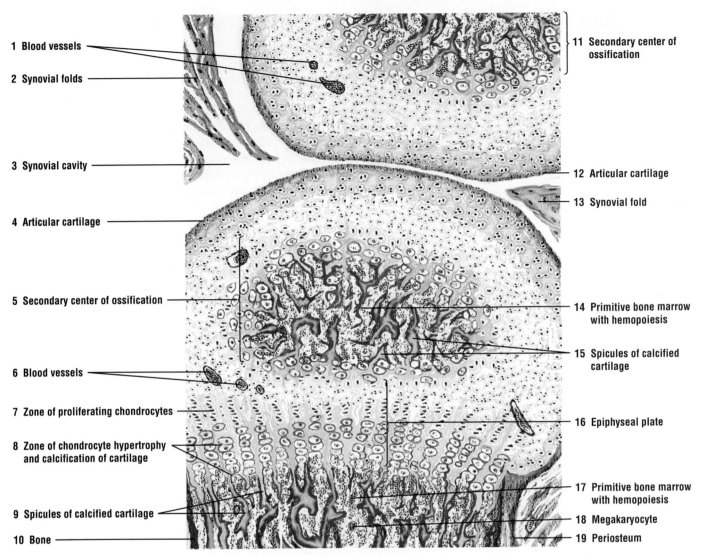

1 Blood vessels

2 Synovial folds

3 Synovial cavity

4 Articular cartilage

5 Secondary center of ossification

6 Blood vessels

7 Zone of proliferating chondrocytes

8 Zone of chondrocyte hypertrophy and calcification of cartilage

9 Spicules of calcified cartilage

10 Bone

11 Secondary center of ossification

12 Articular cartilage

13 Synovial fold

14 Primitive bone marrow with hemopoiesis

15 Spicules of calcified cartilage

16 Epiphyseal plate

17 Primitive bone marrow with hemopoiesis

18 Megakaryocyte

19 Periosteum

FIGURE 4.11 ■ Endochondral ossification: formation of secondary (epiphyseal) centers of ossification and epiphyseal plate in long bone (decalcified bone, longitudinal section). Stain: hematoxylin and eosin. Low magnification.

FIGURE 4.12 ■ Bone Formation: Development of Osteons (Haversian Systems; Transverse Section, Decalcified)

This illustration shows the **primitive bone marrow (15)** and developing osteons in a compact bone. Vascular tufts of connective tissue from the periosteum or endosteum invade and erode the bone and form primitive osteons. Bone reconstruction or remodeling will continue as the initial osteons, and then later ones, are broken down or eroded, followed by the formation of new osteons.

The new **bone matrix (11)** and **bone spicule (12)** of an immature compact bone are stained deep red with eosin owing to the presence of collagen fibers in the matrix. Numerous primitive osteons are visible in transverse section, with large **central (Haversian) canals (2, 9)** surrounded by a few concentric **lamellae (9)** of bone and **osteocytes** in **lacunae (10).** The central (Haversian) canals (2, 9) contain **primitive osteogenic connective tissue (13)** and **blood vessels (2).** Bone deposition is continuing in some of the primitive osteons (2, 9), as indicated by the presence of **osteoblasts (1, 14)** around the central (Haversian) canals (2, 9) and the margin of the innermost bone lamella. In some osteons, the multinucleated **osteoclasts (6)** have formed and eroded shallow depressions called **Howship's lacunae (5)** in the bone. Osteoclasts (6) continue to resorb and remodel the bone as it forms.

Primitive osteogenic connective tissue (13) passes through the bone, from which arise tufts of vascular connective tissue that give rise to new central (Haversian) canals (2, 9). Osteoblasts (1, 14) are located along the periphery of the developing central canals.

In the lower left corner of the figure is the primitive bone marrow (15), in which hemopoiesis (blood cell formation) is in progress; this is the red marrow. Also present in the bone marrow cavity (15) are developing erythrocytes and granulocytes, **megakaryocytes (4, 8), blood sinusoids (vessels) (3, 7),** and osteoclasts (6) in the eroded Howship's lacunae (5). Some megakaryocytes (4, 8) are adjacent to the blood sinusoids. Their cytoplasmic processes protrude into these blood sinusoids, where they eventually fragment and enter the blood stream as platelets.

FUNCTIONAL CORRELATIONS: Bone Cells

Developing and adult bones contain four different cell types: osteoprogenitor cells, osteoblasts, osteocytes, and osteoclasts.

Osteoprogenitor cells are undifferentiated, pluripotential stem cells derived from the connective tissue **mesenchyme.** These cells are located on the inner layer of connective tissue periosteum and in the single layer of internal endosteum that lines the marrow cavities, osteons (Haversian system), and perforating canals in the bone (see Overview Figure 4). The main functions of periosteum and endosteum are nutrition of bone and to provide continuous supply of new osteoblasts for growth, remodeling, and bone repair. During bone development, osteoprogenitor cells proliferate by mitosis and differentiate into osteoblasts, which then secrete collagen fibers and the bony matrix.

Osteoblasts are present on the surfaces of bone. They synthesize, secrete, and deposit osteoid, the organic components of new bone matrix. Osteoid is uncalcified and does not contain any minerals; however, shortly after its deposition, it is rapidly mineralized and becomes bone.

Osteocytes are the mature form of osteoblasts and are the principal cells of the bone; they are also smaller then osteoblasts. Like the chondrocytes in cartilage, osteocytes are trapped by the surrounding bone matrix that was produced by osteoblasts. Osteocytes lie in the cavelike lacunae and are very close to a blood vessel. In contrast to cartilage, only one osteocyte is found in each lacuna. Also, because mineralized bone matrix is much harder than cartilage, nutrients and metabolites cannot freely diffuse through it to the osteocytes. Consequently, bone is very vascular and possesses a unique system of channels or tiny canals called canaliculi, which open into the osteons.

Osteocytes are branched cells. Their cytoplasmic extensions enter the canaliculi, radiate in all directions from each lacuna, and make contact with neighboring cells through gap junctions. These connections allow passage of ions and small molecules from cell to cell. The canaliculi contain extracellular fluid, and the gap junctions in the cytoplasmic extensions allow individual osteocytes to communicate with adjacent osteocytes and with materials in the nearby blood vessels. In this manner, the canaliculi form complex connections around the blood vessels in the osteons and constitute an efficient exchange mechanism: nutrients are brought to the osteocytes, gaseous exchange takes place between the blood and cells, and metabolic wastes are removed from the osteocytes. The canaliculi keep the osteocytes alive, and the osteocytes, in turn, maintain the homeostasis of the surrounding bone matrix and blood concentrations of calcium and phosphates. When an osteocyte dies, the surrounding bone matrix is reabsorbed by osteoclasts.

Osteoclasts are large, multinucleated cells found along bone surfaces where resorption (removal of bone), remodeling, and repair of bone take place. They do not belong to the osteoprogenitor cell line. Instead, the osteoclasts originate from the fusion of blood or hemopoietic progenitor cells that belong to the mononuclear macrophage-monocyte cell line of the bone marrow. The main function of osteoclasts is bone resorption during remodeling (renewal or restructuring). Osteoclasts are often located on the resorbed surfaces or in shallow depressions in the bone matrix called Howship's lacunae. Lysosomal enzymes released by osteoclasts erode these depressions.

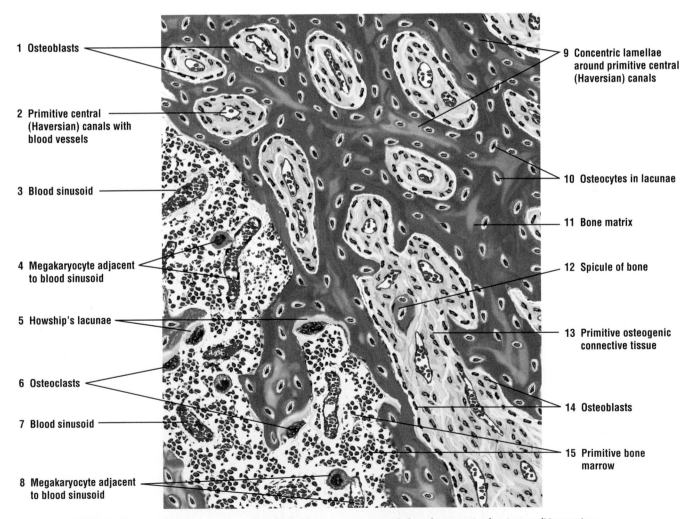

1 Osteoblasts

2 Primitive central (Haversian) canals with blood vessels

3 Blood sinusoid

4 Megakaryocyte adjacent to blood sinusoid

5 Howship's lacunae

6 Osteoclasts

7 Blood sinusoid

8 Megakaryocyte adjacent to blood sinusoid

9 Concentric lamellae around primitive central (Haversian) canals

10 Osteocytes in lacunae

11 Bone matrix

12 Spicule of bone

13 Primitive osteogenic connective tissue

14 Osteoblasts

15 Primitive bone marrow

FIGURE 4.12 ■ Bone formation: primitive bone marrow and development of osteons (Haversian systems; decalcified bone, transverse section). Stain: hematoxylin and eosin. Medium magnification.

FIGURE 4.13 ■ Intramembranous Ossification: Developing Mandible (Decalcified Bone, Transverse Section)

This illustration depicts a section of mandible in the process of intramembranous ossification. External to the developing bone is the stratified squamous keratinized epithelium of the **skin (1)**. Inferior to the skin (1), the embryonic mesenchyme has differentiated into the highly vascular primitive **connective tissue (2)** with **nerves** and **blood vessels (9),** and a denser connective tissue **periosteum (3, 10).**

Below the periosteum (3, 10) is the developing bone. The cells in the periosteum (3, 10) have differentiated into **osteoblasts (6, 10)** and formed numerous anastomosing **trabeculae** of **bone (7, 11)** that surround the primitive **marrow cavities (8, 15).** In the marrow cavities (8, 15) are embryonic connective tissue cells and fibers, **blood vessels (4), arterioles (12),** and nerves. Peripherally, collagen fibers of the periosteum (3, 10) are in continuity with the fibers of the embryonic connective tissue of adjacent marrow cavities (3) and with collagen fibers within the trabeculae of bone (7, 11).

Osteoblasts (6, 10) actively deposit the bony matrix and are seen in linear arrangement along the developing trabeculae of bone (7, 11). **Osteoid (14),** the newly synthesized bony matrix, is seen on the margins of certain bone trabeculae. The **osteocytes (5)** are located in lacunae of the trabeculae (7, 11). **Osteoclasts (13)** are multinucleated large cells that associated with bone resorption and remodeling during bone formation.

Although collagen fibers embedded in the bony matrix are obscured, the continuity with embryonic connective tissue fibers in the marrow cavities may be seen at the margins of numerous trabeculae (3).

Formation of new bone is not a continuous process. Inactive areas appear where ossification has temporarily ceased. Osteoid and osteoblasts are not present in these areas. In some primitive marrow cavities, fibroblasts differentiate into osteoblasts (3, 10).

FIGURE 4.14 ■ Intramembranous Ossification: Developing Skull Bone

A higher-power photomicrograph illustrates the development of skull bone by the process of intramembranous ossification. The connective tissue **periosteum (5)** surrounds the developing bone and gives rise to the **osteoblasts (1, 6)** that form the **bone (7).** Osteoblasts (1, 6) are located along the developing **bony trabeculae (3).** Trapped within the formed bone (7) and the bony trabeculae (3) are the **osteocytes (2)** in their lacunae. Also associated with the bony trabeculae (3) are the multinuclear **osteoclasts (8)** that remodel the developing bone. A primitive **marrow cavity (4)** with **blood vessels (9), blood cells (9),** and hemopoietic tissue is located between the formed bony trabeculae (3).

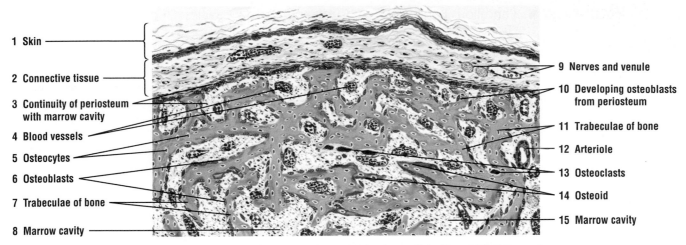

1 Skin

2 Connective tissue

3 Continuity of periosteum with marrow cavity

4 Blood vessels

5 Osteocytes

6 Osteoblasts

7 Trabeculae of bone

8 Marrow cavity

9 Nerves and venule

10 Developing osteoblasts from periosteum

11 Trabeculae of bone

12 Arteriole

13 Osteoclasts

14 Osteoid

15 Marrow cavity

FIGURE 4.13 ■ Intramembranous ossification: developing mandible (decalcified bone, transverse section). Stain: Mallory-Azan. Low magnification.

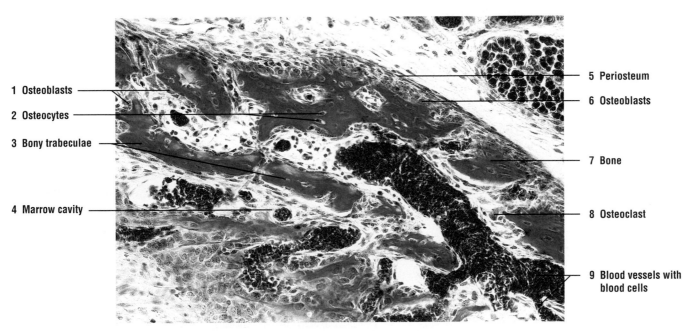

1 Osteoblasts

2 Osteocytes

3 Bony trabeculae

4 Marrow cavity

5 Periosteum

6 Osteoblasts

7 Bone

8 Osteoclast

9 Blood vessels with blood cells

FIGURE 4.14 ■ Intramembranous ossification: developing skull bone. Stain: Mallory-azan. ×64.

FIGURE 4.15 ■ Cancellous Bone With Trabeculae and Marrow Cavities: Sternum (Transverse Section, Decalcified)

Cancellous bone consists primarily of slender bone **trabeculae (5)** that ramify, anastomose, and enclose irregular **marrow cavities** with **blood vessels (4)**. The **periosteum (2, 7)** that surrounds the trabeculae (5) of cancellous bone merges with adjacent dense irregular **connective tissue** with **blood vessels (1)**. Inferior to the periosteum (2, 7), the bone trabeculae (5) merge with a thin layer of **compact bone (9)** that contains a forming or **primitive osteon (6)** and a mature **osteon (Haversian system) (8)** with concentric lamellae.

Except for concentric lamellae in the primitive osteon (6) and mature osteon (8), the bone inferior to periosteum (2, 7) and the bone trabeculae (5) exhibit parallel lamellae. **Osteocytes (3)** in lacunae are visible in trabeculae (5) and compact bone (9).

Between bone trabeculae (5) are the marrow cavities with blood vessels (4) and **hemopoeitic tissue (11)** that gives rise to new blood cells. Because of the low magnification, individual red and white blood cells are not recognizable. Lining the bone trabeculae (5) in the marrow cavities (4) is a thin inner layer of cells called **endosteum (10)**. Cells in periosteum (2, 7) and in endosteum (10) give rise to bone-forming osteoblasts.

FIGURE 4.16 ■ Cancellous Bone: Sternum (Transverse Section, Decalcified)

This photomicrograph shows a section of cancellous bone from the sternum. Cancellous bone is composed of numerous **bony trabeculae (1)** separated by the **marrow cavity (5)** that contains **blood vessels (7)** and different types of **blood cells (8)**. Bony trabeculae (1) are lined by a thin inner layer of cells called the **endosteum (4, 6)**. Osteoprogenitor cells in endosteum (4, 6) give rise to osteoblasts. Formed bone matrix contains numerous **osteocytes in lacunae (2)**. The large, multinuclear **osteoclasts (3)** are eroding or remodeling the formed bone matrix. Osteoclasts (3) erode part of the bone through enzymatic action and lie in the eroded depressions called the Howship's lacunae.

FUNCTIONAL CORRELATIONS: Bone Characteristics

Bones are dynamic structures. They are continually renewed or remodeled in response to mineral needs of the body, mechanical stress, bone thinning as a result of age or disease, or fracture healing. Calcium and phosphate are either stored in the bone matrix or released into the blood to maintain proper levels. Maintenance of normal blood calcium levels is critical to life because calcium is essential for muscle contraction, blood coagulation, cell membrane permeability, transmission of nerve impulses, and other functions.

Hormones regulate calcium release into the blood and its deposition in bones. When the calcium level falls below normal, **parathyroid hormone,** released from the parathyroid glands, stimulates **osteoclasts** to resorb the bone matrix. This action releases more calcium into the blood. When the calcium level is above normal, a hormone called **calcitonin,** released by parafollicular cells in the thyroid gland, inhibits osteoclast activity and decreases bone resorption. These glands and hormones are discussed in more detail in Chapter 17, Endocrine System.

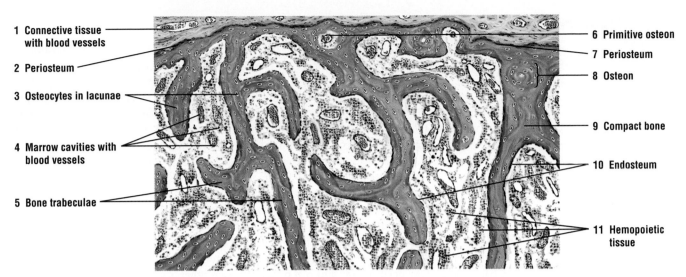

1 Connective tissue with blood vessels

2 Periosteum

3 Osteocytes in lacunae

4 Marrow cavities with blood vessels

5 Bone trabeculae

6 Primitive osteon

7 Periosteum

8 Osteon

9 Compact bone

10 Endosteum

11 Hemopoietic tissue

FIGURE 4.15 ■ Cancellous bone with trabeculae and bone marrow cavities: sternum (decalcified bone, transverse section). Stain: hematoxylin and eosin. Low magnification.

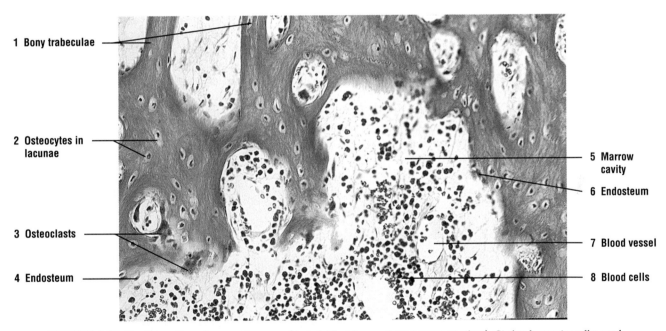

1 Bony trabeculae

2 Osteocytes in lacunae

3 Osteoclasts

4 Endosteum

5 Marrow cavity

6 Endosteum

7 Blood vessel

8 Blood cells

FIGURE 4.16 ■ Cancellous bone: sternum (decalcified bone, transverse section). Stain: hematoxylin and eosin. ×64.

FIGURE 4.17 ■ Compact Bone, Dried (Transverse Section)

This illustration depicts a transverse section of a dried compact bone. The bone was ground to a thin section to show empty canals for blood vessels, lacunae for osteocytes, and the connecting canaliculi.

The structural units of a compact bone matrix are the **osteons (Haversian systems) (3, 10).** Each osteon (3, 10) consists of layers of concentric **lamellae (3b)** arranged around a **central (Haversian) canal (3a).** Central canals are shown in cross section (3a) and in oblique section (10, middle leader). Lamellae are thin plates of bone that contain osteocytes in almond-shaped spaces called **lacunae (3c, 9).** Radiating from each lacuna in all directions are tiny canals, the **canaliculi (2).** Canaliculi (2) penetrate the lamellae (3b, 8), anastomose with canaliculi (2) from other lacunae (3c, 9), and form a network of communicating channels with other osteocytes. Some of the canaliculi (2) open directly into central (Haversian) canals (3a) of the osteon (3) and the marrow cavities of the bone. The small irregular areas of bone between osteons (3, 10) are the **interstitial lamellae (5, 12)** that represent the remnants of eroded or remodeled osteons.

External circumferential lamellae (7) form the external wall of a compact bone (beneath the connective tissue periosteum) and run parallel to each other and to the long axis of the bone. The internal wall of the bone (the endosteum along the marrow cavity) is lined by **internal circumferential lamellae (1).** Osteons (3, 10) are located between the internal circumferential lamellae (1) and external circumferential lamellae (7).

In a living bone, the lacunae of each osteon (3c, 9) house osteocytes. The central canals (3a) contain reticular connective tissue, blood vessels, and nerves. The boundary between each osteon (3, 10) is outlined by a refractile line of modified bone matrix called the **cement line (4, 11).** Anastomoses between central canals (3a) are called **perforating (Volkmann's) canals (6).**

FIGURE 4.18 ■ Compact Bone, Dried (Longitudinal Section)

This figure represents a small area of a dried compact bone, ground in a longitudinal plane. Because **central canals (1, 9)** course longitudinally, each central canal is seen as a vertical tube that shows branching. Central canals (1, 9) are surrounded by **lamellae (2, 6)** with **lacunae (4)** and radiating **canaliculi (5).** The lamellae (2, 6), lacunae (4), and the osteon boundaries, the **cement lines (3, 8),** course parallel to the central canals (1, 9).

Other canals that extend in either a transverse or oblique direction are called **perforating (Volkmann's) canals (7).** Perforating canals (7) join the central canals (1, 9) of osteons with the marrow cavity. The perforating canals (7) do not have concentric lamellae. Instead, they penetrate directly through the lamellae (2, 6).

1 Internal circumferential lamellae

6 Perforating (Volkmann's) canal

7 External circumferential lamellae

2 Canaliculi

3 Osteon
(Haversian
system)
  a. central
    (Haversian)
    canal
  b. lamellae
  c. lacunae

4 Cement line

5 Interstitial
  lamellae

8 Lamellae

9 Lacunae

10 Osteons
(Haversian
systems)

11 Cement line

12 Interstitial
   lamellae

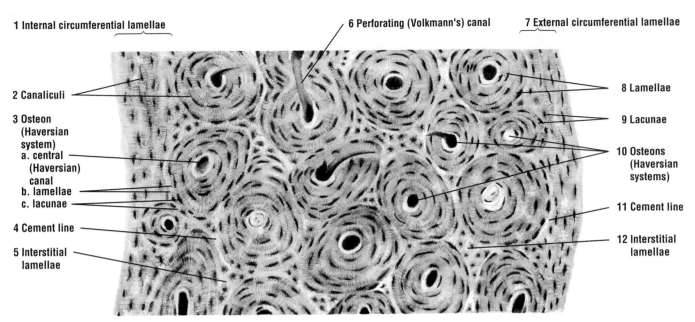

FIGURE 4.17 ■ Dry, compact bone: ground, transverse section. Low magnification.

1 Central
  (Haversian)
  canals

2 Lamellae

3 Cement line

4 Lacunae

5 Canaliculi

6 Lamellae

7 Perforating
(Volkmann's)
canal

8 Cement lines

9 Central
(Haversian)
canal

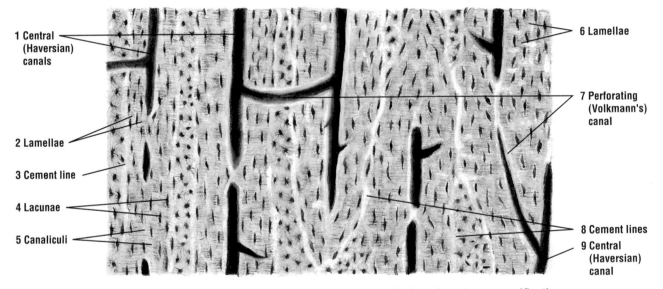

FIGURE 4.18 ■ Dry, compact bone: ground, longitudinal section. Low magnification.

FIGURE 4.19 ■ Compact Bone, Dried: Osteon (Transverse Section)

A higher magnification illustrates the details of one osteon and portions of adjacent osteons. Located in the center of the osteon is the dark-staining **central (Haversian) canal (3)** surronded by the concentric **lamellae (4)**. Between adjacent osteons are the **interstitial lamellae (5)**. The dark, almond-shaped structures between the lamellae (4) are the **lacunae (1, 7)** that house osteocytes in living bone.

Tiny **canaliculi (2)** radiate from individual lacuna (1, 7) to adjacent lacunae and form a system of communicating canaliculi (2) throughout the bony matrix and within the central canal (3). The canaliculi (2) contain tiny cytoplasmic extensions of the osteocytes. In this manner, osteocytes around the osteon communicate with each other and blood vessels in the central canals. The outer boundary of the osteon is separated by a **cement line (6)**.

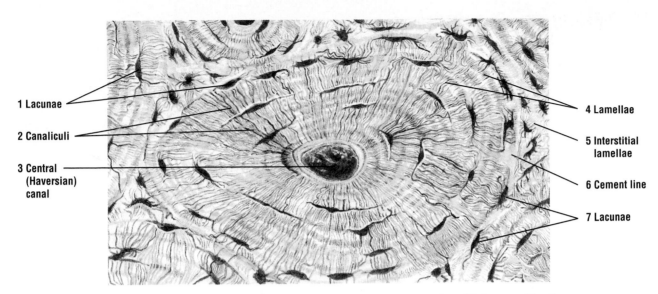

1 Lacunae

2 Canaliculi

3 Central (Haversian) canal

4 Lamellae

5 Interstitial lamellae

6 Cement line

7 Lacunae

FIGURE 4.19 ■ Dry, compact bone: an osteon, transverse section. High magnification.

CHAPTER 4 ■ Summary

Characteristics of Bone

- Consists of cells, fibers, and extracellular material
- Mineral deposits in bone matrix produce hard structure for protecting various organs
- Functions in hemopoiesis and as reservoir for calcium and minerals

Process of Bone Formation

Endochondral Ossification

- In endochondral ossification, hyaline cartilage model calcifies and cells die
- Mesenchyme cells in periosteum differentiate into osteoprogenitor cells and form osteoblasts
- Osteoblasts synthesize osteoid matrix, which calcifies and traps osteoblasts in lacunae as osteocytes
- Osteocytes establish cell-to-cell communication via canaliculi
- Primary ossification center forms in diaphysis and secondary center of ossification in epiphysis
- Epiphyseal plate between diaphysis and epiphysis allows for growth in bone length
- All cartilage is replaced except the articular cartilage

Intramembranous Ossification

- Bone develops directly from osteoblasts that produce the osteoid matrix
- Initially form spongy bone that consists of trabeculae
- Mandible, maxilla, clavicle, and flat skull bones are formed by this process
- Fontanelles in newborn skull represent areas where intramembranous ossification is occurring

Bone Types

- In long bones, outer part is compact bone and inner surface is cancellous bone
- Both bone types have the same microscopic appearance
- In compact bones, collagen fibers arranged in lamellae
- Lamellae deep to the periosteum are outer circumferential lamellae
- Lamellae surrounding the bone marrow are inner circumferential lamellae
- Lamellae surrounding the blood vessels, nerves, and loose connective tissue are osteons
- Within an osteon is the central canal, which is found in most compact bone

Bone Matrix

- Highly vascularized to aid diffusion in calcified matrix
- Organic components of bone resist tension, whereas mineral components resist compression
- Major component is coarse type I collagen fibers
- Glycoprotein components bind to calcium crystals during mineralization
- Hormones from parathyroid and thyroid glands responsible for proper mineral content of blood

Bone Cells

- Osteoprogenitor cells are located in the periosteum, endosteum, osteons, and perforating canals
- Osteoblasts are on the bone surfaces and synthesize osteoid matrix
- Osteocytes are mature osteoblasts, are branched, are located in lacunae, and use canaliculi for communication and exchange
- Osteocytes maintain homeostasis of bone and blood concentrations of calcium and phosphate

- Osteoclasts are multinucleated cells responsible for resorption, remodeling, and bone repair
- Osteoclasts belong to the mononuclear macrophage-monocyte cell line and are found in enzyme-eroded depressions (Howship's lacunae)

Bone Characteristics

- Continually remodeled in response to mineral needs, mechanical stress, thinning, or disease

- Maintain normal calcium levels in blood, critical to functions of numerous organs and life
- Parathyroid hormone stimulates osteoclasts to resorb bone and release calcium into blood
- Hormone from thyroid gland inhibits osteoclast action and decreases bone resorption

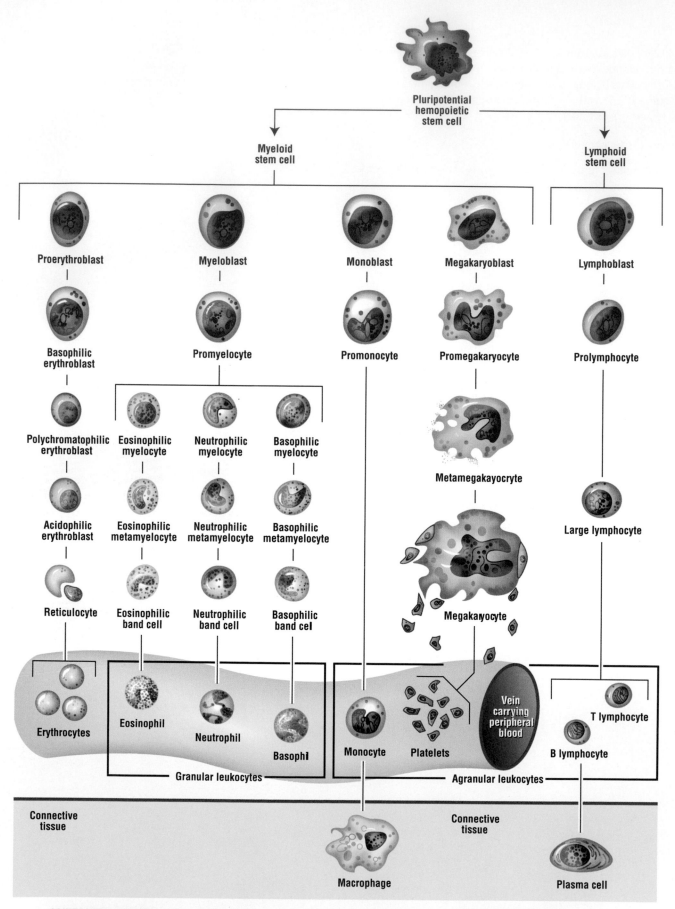

OVERVIEW FIGURE 5 ■ Differentiation of myeloid and lymphoid stem cells into their mature forms and their distribution in the blood and connective tissue.

Blood

Blood is a unique form of **connective tissue** that consists of three major cell types: erythrocytes (red blood cells), leukocytes (white blood cells), and platelets (thrombocytes). These cells, also called the **formed elements** of blood, are suspended in a liquid medium called **plasma.** Blood cells transport gases, nutrients, waste products, hormones, antibodies, various chemicals, ions, and other substances in the plasma to and from different cells in the body.

Hemopoiesis

Blood cells have a limited life span, and, as a result, they are continuously replaced in the body by a process called **hemopoiesis.** In this process, all blood cells are derived from a common stem cell in **red bone marrow.** Because the stem cell can produce all blood cell types, it is called the **pluripotential hemopoietic stem cell.** Pluripotential stem cells, in turn, produce two descendants that form pluripotential myeloid stem cells and pluripotential lymphoid stem cells. Before maturation and release into the bloodstream, the stem cells from each line undergo numerous divisions and intermediate stages of differentiation (Overview Figure 5).

Myeloid stem cells develop in red bone marrow and give rise to **erythrocytes, eosinophils, neutrophils, basophils, monocytes,** and **megakaryocytes. Lymphoid stem cells** also develop in red bone marrow. Some lymphoid cells remain in the bone marrow, proliferate, mature, and become **B lymphocytes.** Others leave the bone marrow and migrate via the bloodstream to **lymph nodes** and the **spleen,** where they proliferate and differentiate into B lymphocytes.

Other undifferentiated lymphoid cells migrate to the **thymus gland,** where they proliferate and differentiate into immunocompetent **T lymphocytes.** Afterward, T lymphocytes enter the bloodstream and migrate to specific regions of peripheral lymphoid organs. Both B and T lymphocytes reside in numerous peripheral lymphoid tissues, lymph nodes, and spleen. Here, they initiate immune responses when exposed to antigens.

Because all blood cells have a limited life span, the pluripotential hemopoietic stem cells continually divide and differentiate to produce new progeny. When the blood cells become worn out and die, they are destroyed in different lymphoid organs, such as the spleen (see Chapter 9).

Sites of Hemopoiesis

Hemopoiesis occurs in different organs of the body, depending on the stage of development. In the **embryo,** hemopoiesis initially occurs in the **yolk sac** and later in the liver, spleen, and lymph nodes. After birth, hemopoiesis continues almost exclusively in the red marrow of different bones (in the newborn, all bone marrow is red).

The red bone marrow is highly cellular and consists of hemopoietic stem cells and precursors of different blood cells. Red marrow also contains a loose arrangement of fine reticular fibers. In adults, red marrow is found primarily in the flat bones of the skull, sternum and ribs, vertebrae, and pelvic bones. The remaining bones, normally the long bones, gradually accumulate fat, their marrow becomes yellow, and they lose hemopoietic functions.

Major Blood Cell Types

Microscopic examination of a stained blood smear reveals the major blood cell types. **Erythrocytes** or red blood cells are nonnucleated cells and are the most numerous blood cells.

During the maturation process, the erythrocytes extrude their nuclei, and the mature blood cells enter the blood vessels without their nuclei. Erythrocytes remain in the blood and perform their major functions within the blood vessels.

In contrast, **leukocytes,** or white blood cells, are nucleated and subdivided into **granulocytes** and **agranulocytes,** depending on the presence or absence of granules in their cytoplasm. Granulocytes are the neutrophils, eosinophils, and basophils. Agranulocytes are the monocytes and lymphocytes. Leukocytes perform their major functions outside of the blood vessels. They migrate out of the blood vessels through capillary walls and enter the connective tissue, lymphatic tissue, and bone marrow.

The primary function of leukocytes is to defend the body against bacterial invasion or the presence of foreign material. Consequently, most leukocytes are concentrated in the connective tissue.

Platelets

Platelets or **thrombocytes** are not blood cells. Instead, they are the smallest, nonnucleated formed elements in the blood and appear in the blood of all mammals. Platelets are cytoplasmic fragments or remnants of **megakaryocytes,** the largest cells in the bone marrow. Platelets are produced when small, uneven portions of the cytoplasm separate or fragment from the peripheries of the megakaryocytes and are extruded into the bloodstream. Like the erythrocytes, platelets perform their major functions within the blood vessels. Their main function is to continually monitor the vascular system and to detect any damage to the endothelial lining of the vessels. If the endothelial lining breaks, the platelets adhere to the damaged site and initiate a highly complex chemical process that produces a blood clot.

FIGURE 5.1 ■ Human Blood Smear

A smear of human blood examined under lower magnification illustrates the formed elements. **Erythrocytes** or red blood cells (**1**) are the most abundant elements and the easiest to identify. Erythrocytes are enucleated (without nucleus) and stain pink with eosin. They are uniform in size and measure approximately 7.5 μm in diameter, which is the approximate size of capillaries. Erythrocytes can be used as a size reference for other cell types.

Several leukocytes or white blood cells are visible in the blood smear. Leukocytes are subdivided into categories according to the shape of their nuclei, the absence or presence of cytoplasmic granules, and the staining affinities of the granules. Two **neutrophils** (**2, 4**), one **eosinophil** (**7**) filled with red-pink granules, and one small **lymphocyte** (**5**) with a thin bluish cytoplasm are visible. Scattered among the blood cells are small, blue-staining fragments called **platelets** (**3, 6**).

FIGURE 5.2 ■ Human Blood Smear: Red Blood Cells, Neutrophils, Large Lymphocyte, and Platelets

A photomicrograph of a human blood smear shows different blood cell types. The most numerous blood cells are the **erythrocytes** (red blood cells) (**1**). Also visible are two **neutrophils** (**2, 4**), a **large lymphocyte** (**5**), and numerous **platelets** (**3**).

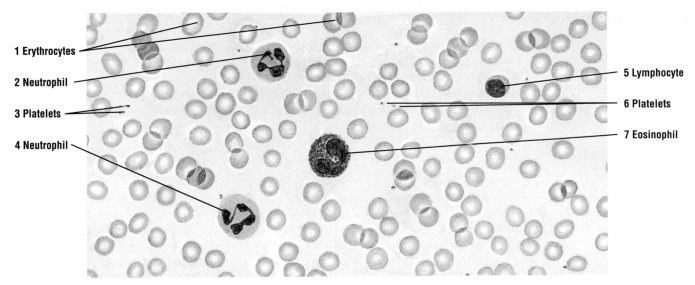

1 Erythrocytes
2 Neutrophil
3 Platelets
4 Neutrophil
5 Lymphocyte
6 Platelets
7 Eosinophil

FIGURE 5.1 ■ Human blood smear: erythrocytes, neutrophils, eosinophils, lymphocyte, and platelets. Stain: Wright's stain. High magnification.

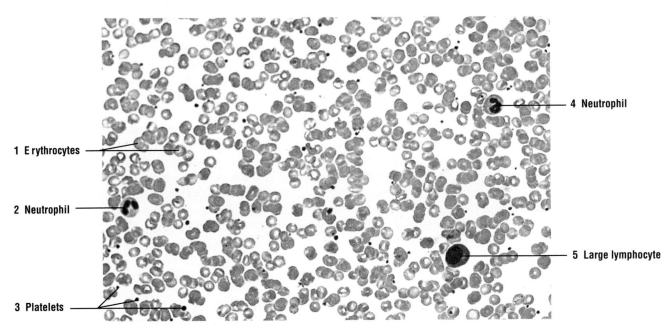

1 Erythrocytes
2 Neutrophil
3 Platelets
4 Neutrophil
5 Large lymphocyte

FIGURE 5.2 ■ Human blood smear: red blood cells, neutrophils, large lymphocytes, and platelets. Stain: Wright's stain. ×205.

FIGURE 5.3 ■ Erythrocytes and Platelets

This illustration shows numerous **erythrocytes** (1) and **platelets** (2) that are usually seen in a blood smear. Blood platelets (2) are the smallest of the formed elements; they are nonnucleated cytoplasmic remnants of large-cell megakaryocytes, which are found only in the red bone marrow. Platelets (2) appear as irregular masses of basophilic (blue) cytoplasm, and they tend to form clumps in blood smears. Each platelet exhibits a light blue peripheral zone and a dense central zone containing purple granules.

FIGURE 5.4 ■ Neutrophils

The leukocytes that contain cytoplasmic granules and lobulated nuclei are the polymorphonuclear granulocytes, of which the **neutrophils** (1) are the most abundant. The neutrophil cytoplasm (1) contains fine violet or pink granules that are difficult to see with a light microscope. As a result, the cytoplasm (1) appears clear or neutral. The nucleus (1) consists of several lobes connected by narrow chromatin strands. Immature neutrophils (1) contain fewer nuclear lobes.

The neutrophils (1) constitute approximately 60 to 70% of the blood leukocytes.

FUNCTIONAL CORRELATIONS OF FORMED ELEMENTS: Erythrocytes

Mature erythrocytes are specialized to transport **oxygen** and **carbon dioxide.** This specialization is attributable to the presence of the protein **hemoglobin** in their cytoplasm. Iron molecules in hemoglobin bind with oxygen molecules. As a result, most of the oxygen in the blood is carried in the combined form of **oxyhemoglobin,** which is responsible for the bright red color of arterial blood. Carbon dioxide diffuses from the cells and tissues into the blood vessels. It is carried to the lungs partly dissolved in the blood and partly in combination with hemoglobin in the erythrocytes as **carbaminohemoglobin,** which gives venous blood its bluish color.

During differentiation and maturation in the bone marrow, erythrocytes synthesize large amounts of hemoglobin. Before an erythrocyte is released into the systemic circulation, the nucleus is extruded from the cytoplasm, and the mature erythrocyte assumes a biconcave shape. This shape provides more surface area for carrying respiratory gases. Thus, mature mammalian erythrocytes in the circulation are **nonnucleated** biconcave disks that are surrounded by a membrane and filled with hemoglobin and some enzymes.

The life span of erythrocytes is approximately 120 days, after which the worn-out cells are removed from the blood and phagocytosed by macrophages in the **spleen, liver,** and **bone marrow.**

FUNCTIONAL CORRELATIONS OF FORMED ELEMENTS: Platelets

The main function of platelets is to promote **blood clotting.** When the wall and the endothelium of the blood vessel are damaged, platelets aggregate at the site and **adhere** to the damaged wall. The platelets are activated and form a plug to occlude the site of damage. The platelets in the plug release adhesive glycoproteins that increase the plug size, which is then reinforced by a polymer **fibrin** formed from numerous plasma proteins. Fibrin forms a mesh around the plug, trapping other platelets and blood cells to form a blood clot. After blood clot formation and cessation of bleeding, the aggregated platelets contribute to **clot retraction,** which is later removed through enzymatic action.

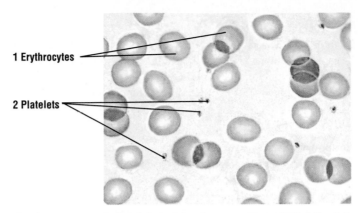

FIGURE 5.3 ■ Erythrocytes and platelets in blood smear. Stain: Wright's stain. Oil immersion.

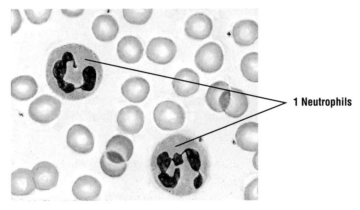

FIGURE 5.4 ■ Neutrophils and erythrocytes. Stain: Wright's stain. Oil immersion.

FIGURE 5.5 ■ Eosinophils

Eosinophils (1) are identified in a blood smear by their cytoplasm, which is filled with distinct, large, eosinophilic (bright pink) granules. The nucleus in eosinophils (1) typically is bilobed, but a small third lobe may be present.

Eosinophils (1) constitute approximately 2 to 4% of the blood leukocytes.

FIGURE 5.6 ■ Lymphocytes

Agranular leukocytes have few or no cytoplasmic granules and exhibit round to horseshoe-shaped nuclei. **Lymphocytes (1, 2)** vary in size from cells smaller than erythrocytes to cells almost twice as large. For size comparison among lymphocytes and erythrocytes, this illustration of a human blood smear depicts a **large lymphocyte (1)** and a **small lymphocyte (2)** surrounded by the red-staining erythrocytes. In small lymphocytes (2), the densely stained nucleus occupies most of the cytoplasm, which appears as a thin basophilic rim around the nucleus. The cytoplasm in lymphocytes is usually agranular but may sometimes contain a few granules. In large lymphocytes (1), basophilic cytoplasm is more abundant, and the larger and paler nucleus may contain one or two nucleoli.

Lymphocytes (1, 2) constitute approximately 20 to 30% of the blood leukocytes. Most of the lymphocytes in the blood, about 90%, are the small lymphocytes.

FIGURE 5.7 ■ Monocytes

Monocytes (1) are the largest agranular leukocytes. The nucleus (1) varies from round or oval to indented or horseshoe-shaped and stains lighter than the lymphocyte nucleus. The nuclear chromatin is finely dispersed in monocytes (1), and the abundant cytoplasm is lightly basophilic with few fine granules.

Monocytes (1) constitute approximately 3 to 8% of the blood leukocytes.

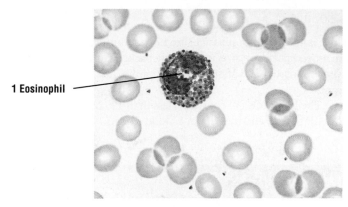

FIGURE 5.5 ■ Eosinophil. Stain: Wright's stain. Oil immersion.

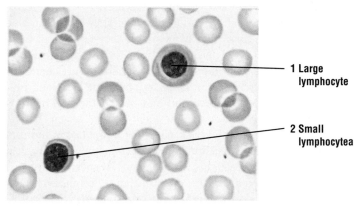

FIGURE 5.6 ■ Lymphocytes. Stain: Wright's stain. Oil immersion.

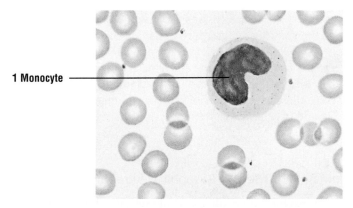

FIGURE 5.7 ■ Monocyte. Stain: Wright's stain. Oil immersion.

FIGURE 5.8 ■ Basophils

The granules in **basophils** (1) are not as numerous as in eosinophils (Figure 5.5); however, they are more variable in size, less densely packed, and stain dark blue or brown. Although the nucleus is not lobulated and stains pale basophilic, it is usually obscured by the density and number of granules.

The basophils (1) constitute less than 1% of the blood leukocytes and are therefore the most difficult to find and identify in a blood smear.

FUNCTIONAL CORRELATION OF FORMED ELEMENTS: Leukocytes

Neutrophils have a short life span. They circulate in blood for about 10 hours and then enter the connective tissue, where they survive for another 2 or 3 days. Neutrophils are active **phagocytes.** They are attracted by **chemotactic factors** (chemicals) released by damaged or dead cells, tissues, or microorganisms, especially bacterial, which they phagocytose (ingest) and quickly destroy with their lysosomal enzymes.

Eosinophils also have a short life span. They remain in blood for up to 10 hours and then migrate into the connective tissue, where they remain for up to 10 days. Eosinophils are also **phagocytic** cells with a particular affinity for **antigen–antibody complexes** that are formed in the tissues in allergic conditions. The cells also release chemicals that neutralize histamine and other mediators related to inflammatory allergic reactions. Eosinophils also increase in number during **parasitic infestation** and defend the organism against helminthic parasites by destroying them.

Lymphocytes have a variable life span, from days to months, and show size variability. The difference between small and large lymphocytes has a functional significance. Large lymphocytes represent the cells that were activated by specific antigens. Lymphocytes are essential for **immunologic defense** of the organism. Some lymphocytes (B lymphocytes), when stimulated by specific antigens, differentiate into **plasma cells** in the connective tissue and produce **antibodies** to counteract or destroy the invading organisms.

Monocytes can live in the blood for 2 to 3 days, after which they move into the connective tissue, where they may remain for a few months or longer. Blood monocytes are precursors of the mononuclear phagocyte system. After entering the connective tissue, monocytes become powerful **phagocytes.** At the site of infection, monocytes differentiate into **tissue macrophages** and then destroy bacteria, foreign matter, and cellular debris.

Basophils have a short life span and their function is similar to that of mast cells. Their granules contain **histamine** and **heparin.** Exposure to allergens results in release of histamine and other chemicals that mediate and intensify inflammatory responses. These reactions cause severe allergic reactions, vascular changes that lead to increased fluid leakage from blood vessels, and hypersensitivity responses and anaphylaxis.

FIGURE 5.9 ■ Human Blood Smear: Basophil, Neutrophil, Red Blood Cells, and Platelets

A high-magnification photomicrograph of a human blood smear shows **erythrocytes (3),** a **basophil (1),** a **neutrophil (5),** and **platelets (4).** The basophil (1) cytoplasm is filled with dense **basophilic granules (2)** that obscure the nucleus. In contrast, the neutrophil (5) cytoplasm does not show granules, and its **nucleus** is **multilobed (6).**

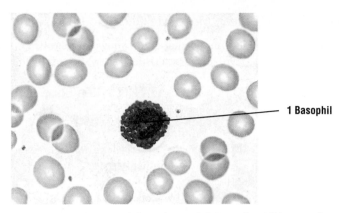

FIGURE 5.8 ■ Basophil. Stain: Wright's stain. Oil immersion.

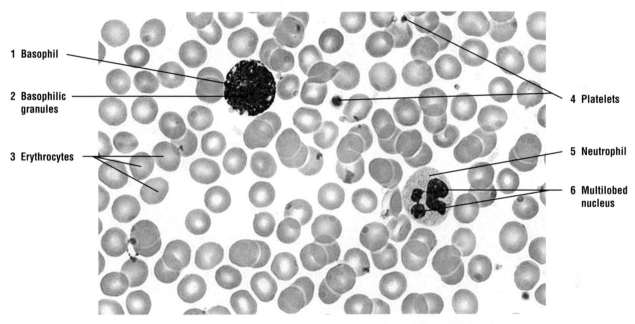

FIGURE 5.9 ■ Human blood smear: basophil, neutrophil, red blood cells, and platelets. Stain: Wright's stain. ×320.

FIGURE 5.10 ■ Human Blood Smear: Monocyte, Red Blood Cells, and Platelets

A high-magnification photomicrograph shows numerous **erythrocytes (1)**, **platelets (2)**, and a large **monocyte (3)** with a characteristic kidney-shaped nucleus and a nongranular cytoplasm.

FIGURE 5.11 ■ Development of Different Blood Cells in Red Bone Marrow (Decalcified Section)

In a section of red bone marrow, all types of developing blood cells are difficult to distinguish. The cells are densely packed, and different cell types are intermixed. During the maturation process, hemopoietic cells become smaller and their nuclear chromatin more condensed. As the blood cells pass through a series of developmental stages, they exhibit morphologic changes and become microscopically identifiable.

This section of bone marrow is stained with hematoxylin and eosin stain. At this magnification, little differentiation of cytoplasm is visible. In the erythrocytic line, early **basophilic erythroblasts (7, 21)** are recognized by a large but not very dense nucleus and basophilic cytoplasm. These cells give rise to the smaller **polychromatophilic erythroblasts (8, 22)** with a more condensed chromatin and a more variable color of the cytoplasm. The most recognizable cells of the erythrocytic line are **normoblasts (2, 23)**. They are characterized by small, dark-staining nuclei and a reddish or eosinophilic cytoplasm. Normoblasts (2, 23) exhibit **mitotic activity (6)** in the bone marrow. As normoblasts (2, 23) mature, they extrude their nuclei and become **erythrocytes (3)**. Cells of the erythrocytic lineage do not display any granules in their cytoplasm. Erythrocytes (3) are abundant in red bone marrow and are seen in the numerous **sinusoids (1, 12)**, **venule (14)**, and **arteriole (15)**.

The early granulocytes initially exhibit numerous primary or azurophilic granules in their cytoplasm. As a result, the immature forms of neutrophils, eosinophils, and basophils are morphologically indistinguishable and become recognizable only in the myelocyte stage, when specific granules appear in quantity in their cytoplasm. In neutrophilic cells, the specific granules are only faintly stained and the cytoplasm appears clear. In the eosinophilic line, the specific granules stain deep red or eosinophilic. Basophilic granulocytes are rarely observed in the bone marrow because of their small numbers. The cytoplasm of mature basophils exhibits a bilobed nucleus and dense blue or basophilic granules.

The granulocytic **myelocytes (13, 19)** exhibit a large spherical nucleus and a cytoplasm with many azurophilic granules. The myelocytes (13, 19) give rise to **metamyelocytes (4, 11, 20)** whose nuclei are bean or horseshoe shaped. The **neutrophilic metamyelocytes (17)** exhibit a deeply indented nuclei and cytoplasm with azurophilic granules and faintly stained specific granules. In contrast, a cell with bright-staining red or eosinophilic granules in the cytoplasm is an **eosinophilic myelocyte (18)**.

The stroma of the reticular connective tissue in the bone marrow is almost obscured by hemopoietic cells. In less dense areas, the reticular connective tissue with the elongated **reticular cells (16)** is visible. Also, numerous thin-walled sinusoids (1,12) and different types of blood vessels (14, 15) containing erythrocytes and leukocytes are present in the bone marrow. Conspicuous in the bone marrow are the large **adipose cells (5)**, each exhibiting a large vacuole (because of fat removal during section preparation) and a small, peripheral cytoplasm that surrounds the **nucleus (5)**. Other identifiable cells in the bone marrow are the very large **megakaryocytes (9, 10)** with varied nuclear lobulation. One of these megakaryocytes (10) is situated adjacent to a blood sinusoid, into which the fragments from its cytoplasmic extension can be discharged as platelets.

Selected blood cells from the red bone marrow are illustrated below at a higher magnification.

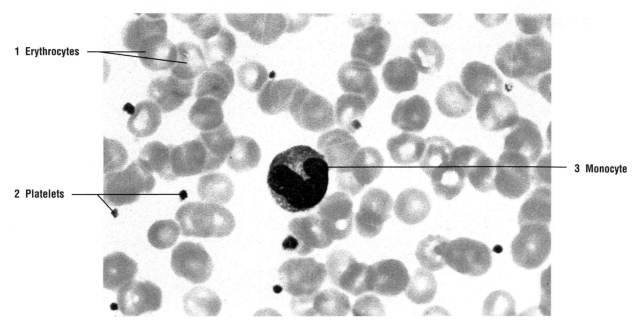

1 Erythrocytes

2 Platelets

3 Monocyte

FIGURE 5.10 ■ Human blood smear: monocyte, red blood cells, and platelets. Stain: Wright's stain. ×320.

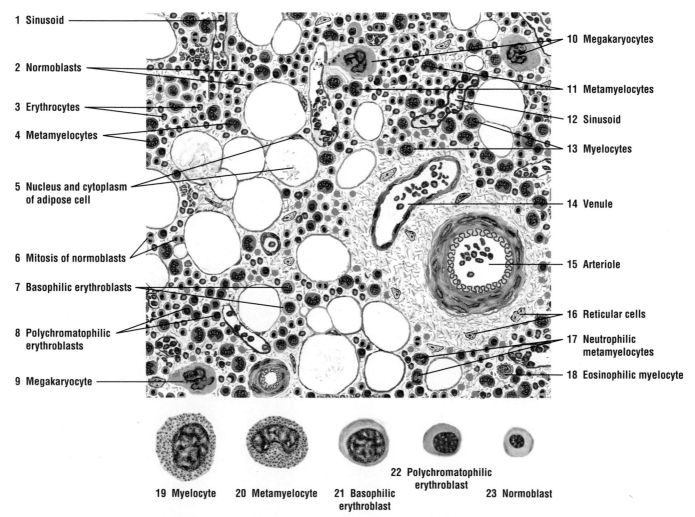

1 Sinusoid

2 Normoblasts

3 Erythrocytes

4 Metamyelocytes

5 Nucleus and cytoplasm of adipose cell

6 Mitosis of normoblasts

7 Basophilic erythroblasts

8 Polychromatophilic erythroblasts

9 Megakaryocyte

10 Megakaryocytes

11 Metamyelocytes

12 Sinusoid

13 Myelocytes

14 Venule

15 Arteriole

16 Reticular cells

17 Neutrophilic metamyelocytes

18 Eosinophilic myelocyte

19 Myelocyte   20 Metamyelocyte   21 Basophilic erythroblast   22 Polychromatophilic erythroblast   23 Normoblast

FIGURE 5.11 ■ Development of different blood cells in red bone marrow (decalcified). Stain: hematoxylin and eosin. Upper image: high magnification; lower image: oil immersion.

FIGURE 5.12 ■ Bone Marrow Smear: Development of Different Cell Types

A bone marrow smear shows a few typical blood cells in different stages of development. In the erythrocytic series, the precursor cell **proerythroblast (3)** exhibits a thin rim of basophilic cytoplasm and a large, oval nucleus that occupies most of the cell. The chromatin is dispersed uniformly, and two or more nuclei may be present. Azurophilic granules are absent from the cytoplasm in all cells of the erythrocytic series. The proerythroblasts (3) divide to form the smaller **basophilic erythroblasts (8, 16).**

Basophilic erythroblasts (8, 16) are characterized by a rim of basophilic cytoplasm and a decreased cell and nuclear size. The nuclear chromatin is coarse and exhibits the characteristic "checkerboard" pattern. Nucleoli are either inconspicuous or absent. Basophilic erythroblasts (8, 16) give rise to the **polychromatophilic erythroblasts (12),** which are similar in size to basophilic erythroblasts (8, 16). The cytoplasm of the polychromatophilic erythroblast (12) becomes progressively less basophilic and more acidophilic as a result of increased hemoglobin accumulation. The nuclei of polychromatophilic erythroblasts (12) are smaller and exhibit a coarse "checkerboard" pattern.

When the polychromatophilic cells (12) acquire a more acidophilic (pink) cytoplasm as a result of increased hemoglobin accumulation, their size decreases and they become **orthochromatophilic erythroblasts (normoblasts) (1).** These cells are capable of **mitosis (2).** Initially, the nucleus of orthochromatophilic erythroblasts (1) exhibits a concentrated "checkerboard" chromatin pattern. Eventually the nucleus decreases in size, becomes pyknotic, and is extruded from the cytoplasm, forming a biconcave-shaped cell with a bluish-pink cytoplasm called a reticulocyte or young erythrocyte. With special supravital staining, a delicate reticulum is seen in the reticulocyte cytoplasm because of the remaining polyribosomes (see Figure 5.13). After polyribosomes are lost from the cytoplasm, the cells become mature **erythrocytes (9).** Erythrocytes (9) are small cells with a homogeneous acidophilic or pink cytoplasm.

Also visible in the bone marrow smear are different types of myelocytes and metamyelocytes of the granulocytic cell line. Myelocytes exhibit an eccentric nucleus with condensed chromatin and a less basophilic cytoplasm with few azurophilic granules. Different types of myelocytes exhibit varying number of granules. More mature myelocytes, such as **neutrophilic myelocytes (14),** an **eosinophilic myelocyte (15),** and a rare **basophilic myelocyte (11),** show an abundance of specific granules in their slightly acidophilic cytoplasm. The myelocyte is the last cell of the granulocytic line capable of mitosis, after which they mature into metamyelocytes.

The shape of the nucleus in the neutrophilic line changes from oval to one with indentation, as seen in **neutrophilic metamyelocytes (4).** Before complete maturation and segmentation of the nucleus into distinct lobes, the neutrophils pass through a **band cell (10)** stage, in which the nucleus assumes a nearly uniform curved rod or band shape.

Mature neutrophils (13) with segmented nuclei are also present in the bone marrow smear, as well as a **mature eosinophil (7)** with specific pink granules filling its cytoplasm.

A section of a giant cell **megakaryocyte (17)** is visible. These cells measure approximately 80 to 100 µm in diameter and have a large, slightly acidophilic cytoplasm filled with fine azurophilic granules. Cytoplasmic fragments derived from megakaryocytes are shed as **platelets (18).**

1 Orthochromatophilic erythroblasts (normoblasts)

2 Mitosis of orthochromatophilic erythroblast (normoblast)

3 Proerythroblast

4 Neutrophilic metamyelocyte

5 Eosinophilic metamyelocyte

6 Platelets

7 Mature eosinophil

8 Basophilic erythroblast

9 Mature erythrocytes

10 Neutrophil (band cell)

11 Basophilic myelocyte

12 Polychromatophilic erythroblast

13 Mature neutrophils

14 Neutrophilic myelocytes

15 Eosinophilic myelocyte

16 Basophilic erythroblast

17 Megakaryocyte

18 Platelets derived from megakaryocyte

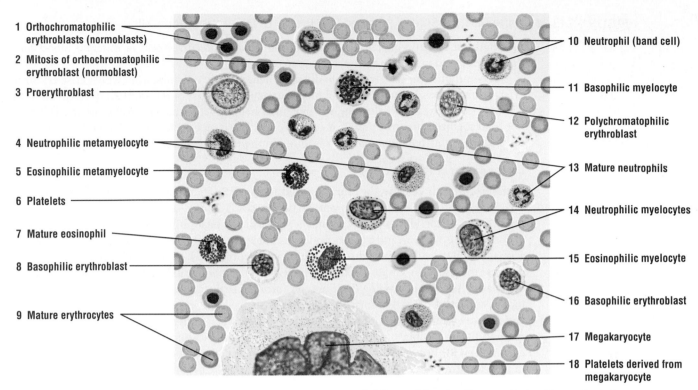

FIGURE 5.12 ■ Bone marrow smear: development of different blood cell types. Stain: Giemsa's stain. High magnification.

This figure shows at a higher magnification the selected precursor cells of different blood cells that develop and mature in the red bone marrow.

A common stem cell gives rise to different hemopoietic cell lines, from which arise erythrocytes, granulocytes, lymphocytes, and megakaryocytes. Because of its ability to differentiate into all blood cells, this cell is called the pluripotential hemopoietic stem cell. Although this cell cannot be recognized microscopically, it resembles a large lymphocyte. In adults, the greatest concentration of pluripotential stem cells is found in the red bone marrow.

Development of Erythrocytes

In the erythrocytic cell line, the **pluripotential stem cell** differentiates into a **proerythroblast (1)**, a large cell with loose chromatin, one or two nucleoli, and a basophilic cytoplasm. The proerythroblast (1) divides to produce a smaller cell called a **basophilic erythroblast (2)** with a rim of basophilic cytoplasm and a more condensed nucleus without visible nucleoli. In the next stage, a smaller cell called the **polychromatophilic erythroblast (3)** is produced. These cells show a decrease of basophilic ribosomes and an increase in the acidophilic hemoglobin content of their cytoplasm. As a result, staining these cells produces several colors in their cytoplasm. As differentiation continues, there is a further reduction of the cell size, condensation of nuclear material, and a more uniform eosinophilic cytoplasm. At this stage, the cell is called an **orthochromatophilic erythroblast (normoblast) (4)**. After extruding its nucleus, the orthochromatophilic erythroblast (4) becomes a **reticulocyte (5)** because a small number of ribosomes can be stained in its cytoplasm. After losing the ribosomes, the reticulocyte becomes a mature **erythrocyte (6)**.

Development of Granulocytes

The **myeloblast (7)** is the first recognizable precursor in the granulocytic cell line. The myeloblast (7) is a small cell with a large nucleus, dispersed chromatin, three or more nucleoli, and a basophilic cytoplasm rim that lacks specific granules. As development progresses, the cell enlarges, acquires azurophilic granules, and becomes a **promyelocyte (8, 9)**. The chromatin in the oval nucleus is dispersed, and multiple nucleoli are evident. In more advanced promyelocytes, the cells become smaller, the nucleoli become inconspicuous, the number of azurophilic granules increases, and specific granules with different staining properties begin to appear in the perinuclear region. Promyelocytes (8, 9) divide to form smaller **myelocytes (10, 13, 14)**. The cytoplasm of myelocytes (10, 13, 14) is less basophilic and contains many azurophilic granules. Myelocytes differentiate into three kinds of granulocytes, which can only be recognized by the increased accumulation and staining of the specific granules in their cytoplasm, as seen in the **eosinophilic myelocyte (13)** with red or eosinophilic granules and the rare **basophilic myelocyte (14)** with blue or basophilic granules. Myelocytes develop into metamyelocytes.

The cytoplasm of **neutrophilic metamyelocyte (11)** contains deep-staining azurophilic granules, lightly stained specific granules, and an indented, kidney-shaped nucleus. The **eosinophilic metamyelocytes (15)** are larger cells, and their specific cytoplasmic granules stain eosinophilic.

Megakaryoblasts (12) are large cells with a basophilic, homogeneous cytoplasm largely free of specific granules. The voluminous nucleus is ovoid or kidney shaped, contains numerous nucleoli, and exhibits a loose chromatin pattern. Platelets are not formed at this stage.

During differentiation, megakaryoblasts (12) become very large. Their nucleus becomes convoluted, with multiple, irregular lobes interconnected by constricted regions. The chromatin becomes condensed and coarse, and nucleoli are not visible. In mature **megakaryocytes (17)**, the plasma membrane invaginates the cytoplasm and forms demarcation membranes. This delimits the areas of the megakaryocyte cytoplasm that is then shed into the blood as small cell fragments in the form of **platelets (16)**.

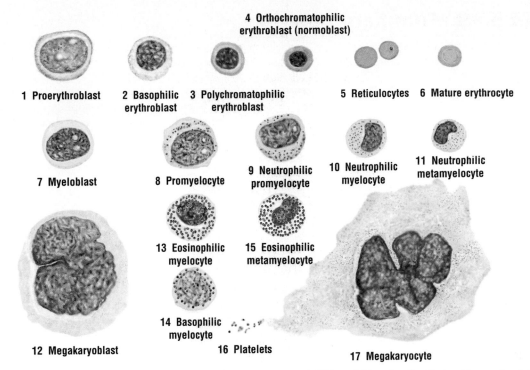

1 Proerythroblast

2 Basophilic erythroblast

3 Polychromatophilic erythroblast

4 Orthochromatophilic erythroblast (normoblast)

5 Reticulocytes

6 Mature erythrocyte

7 Myeloblast

8 Promyelocyte

9 Neutrophilic promyelocyte

10 Neutrophilic myelocyte

11 Neutrophilic metamyelocyte

13 Eosinophilic myelocyte

15 Eosinophilic metamyelocyte

14 Basophilic myelocyte

12 Megakaryoblast

16 Platelets

17 Megakaryocyte

FIGURE 5.13 ■ Bone marrow smear: selected precursors of different blood cells. Stain: Giemsa's stain. High magnification or oil immersion.

CHAPTER 5 ■ **Summary**

Blood

- Consists of formed elements, erythrocytes, leukocytes, and platelets suspended in plasma

Hemopoiesis

- Blood cells constantly replaced in red marrow because of limited life span
- Common pluripotential stem cell forms pluripotential myeloid and lymphoid stem cells
- Myeloid stem cells give rise to erythrocytes, eosinophils, neutrophils, basophils, monocytes, and megakaryocytes
- Lymphoid stem cells give rise to B lymphocytes and T lymphocytes
- B and T lymphocytes reside in peripheral lymphoid tissue, lymph nodes, and spleen

Sites of Hemopoiesis

- In embryo, hemopoiesis takes place in yolk sac, liver, spleen, and lymph nodes
- In adult, hemopoiesis is limited to red bone marrow (skull, sternum, ribs, vertebrae, pelvis)

Formed Elements: Major Blood Cell Types

Erythrocytes

- Most numerous cells in blood
- Erythrocytes are nonnucleated cells that remain in the blood
- Contain hemoglobin with iron molecules in cytoplasm
- Carry oxygen as oxyhemoglobin and carbon dioxide as carbaminohemoglobin
- Biconcave shape increases surface area to carry respiratory gases
- Life span is about 120 days, after which cells are phagocytosed in spleen, liver, and bone marrow

Platelets

- Are fragments of bone marrow megakaryocytes and not blood cells
- Function in blood vessels to promote blood clotting when blood vessel wall is damaged
- In damaged vessels form plug; increase plug size through adhesive glycoproteins and fibrin
- Fibrin traps platelets and blood cells, and forms blood clot
- Cause clot retraction and removal through enzymatic action

Leukocytes

- Granulocytes contain cytoplasmic granules; they are neutrophils, eosinophils, and basophils
- Agranulocytes are without cytoplasmic granules; they are monocytes and lymphocytes

Granulocytes

Neutrophils

- Cytoplasm appears clear under microscope
- Nucleus contains several lobes connected by thin chromatin strands
- Have a short life span in blood or connective tissue, from hours to days
- Are very active phagocytes that are attracted to foreign material by chemotactic factors
- Destroy phagocytosed (ingested) material with lysosomal enzymes
- Constitute about 60 to 70% of blood leukocytes

Eosinophils

- Cytoplasm filled with large pink or eosinophilic granules
- Nucleus typically bilobed
- Have a short life span, in blood or connective tissue
- Are phagocytic with affinity for antigen–antibody complexes
- Release chemical that neutralizes histamine and other mediators of inflammatory reactions
- Increase during parasitic infestation to destroy helminthic parasites
- Constitute about 2 to 4% of the blood leukocytes

Basophils

- Cytoplasm contains dark blue or brown granules
- Have a short life span
- Nucleus stains pale basophilic, but is normally obscured by dense cytoplasmic granules
- Granules contain histamine and heparin
- Exposure to allergens releases histamine that causes intense inflammatory response in severe allergic reactions
- Constitute less than 1% of blood leukocytes

Agranulocytes

Lymphocytes

- No granules in cytoplasm and vary in size from small to large
- Dense-staining nucleus surrounded by a narrow cytoplasmic rim

- Life span is from days to months
- Essential in immunologic defense of organism
- When exposed to specific antigens, B lymphocytes form plasma cells in connective tissue
- Plasma cells release antibodies to counteract or destroy invading organisms
- Constitute about 20 to 30% of blood leukocytes

Monocytes

- Largest agranular leukocyte characterized primarily by horseshoe-shaped nucleus
- Live in connective tissue for months where they become powerful phagocytes
- Are part of the mononuclear phagocyte system
- Constitute about 3 to 8% of blood leukocytes

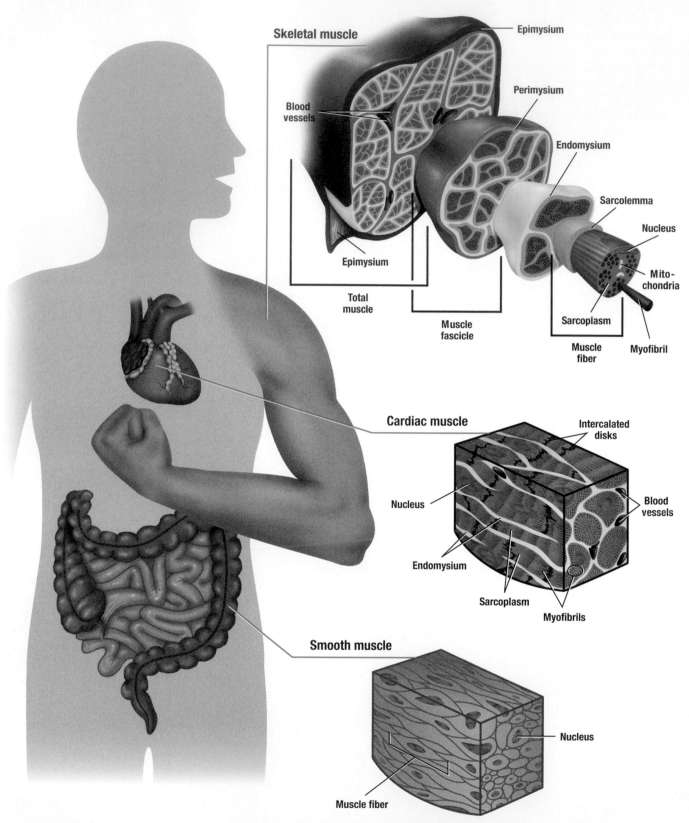

OVERVIEW FIGURE 6 ■ Diagrammatic representation of microscopic appearance of three muscle types: skeletal, cardiac, and smooth.

CHAPTER 6

Muscle Tissue

There are three types of muscle tissues in the body: **skeletal muscle, cardiac muscle,** and **smooth muscle.** Each muscle type has structural and functional similarities, as well as differences. All muscle tissues consist of elongated cells called **fibers.** The cytoplasm of muscle cells is called **sarcoplasm** and the surrounding cell membrane or plasmalemma is called **sarcolemma.** Each muscle fiber sarcoplasm contains numerous **myofibrils,** which contain two types of contractile protein filaments, **actin** and **myosin.**

Skeletal Muscle

Skeletal muscle fibers are long, cylindrical, **multinucleated cells,** with peripheral nuclei. The multiple nuclei in these muscles are owing to the fusion of muscle cell precursor **myoblasts** during the embryonic development. Each muscle fiber is composed of subunits called **myofibrils** that extend the length of the fiber. The myofibrils, in turn, are composed of **myofilaments** formed by the contractile thin proteins, **actin,** and thick proteins, **myosin.**

In the sarcoplasm, the arrangement of actin and myosin filaments is very regular, forming the distinct **cross-striation** patterns, which are seen under a light microscope as light **I bands** and dark **A bands** in each muscle fiber. Because of these cross-striations, skeletal muscle is also called **striated muscle.** Transmission electron microscopy illustrates the internal organization of the contractile proteins in each myofibril. These high-resolution images show that each light I band is bisected by a dense transverse **Z line** (disk or band). Between the two adjacent Z lines is found the smallest contractile unit of the muscle, the **sarcomere.** Sarcomeres are the repeating contractile units seen along the entire length of each myofibril and are characteristic features of the sarcoplasm of skeletal and cardiac muscle fibers.

Skeletal muscle is surrounded by a dense, irregular connective tissue layer called **epimysium.** From epimysium, a less dense irregular connective tissue layer, called **perimysium,** extends inward and divides the interior of the muscle into smaller bundles called **fascicles;** each fascicle is thus surrounded by perimysium. A thin layer of reticular connective tissue fibers, called **endomysium,** invests individual muscle fibers. Located in the different connective tissue sheaths are blood vessels, nerves, and lymphatics (see Overview Figure 6).

Sensitive stretch receptors called **neuromuscular spindles** are present within nearly all skeletal muscles. These spindles consist of a connective tissue **capsule,** in which are found modified muscle fibers called **intrafusal fibers** and numerous **nerve endings,** surrounded by a fluid-filled space. The neuromuscular spindles monitor the changes (distension) in the muscle lengths and activate complex reflexes to regulate muscle activity.

Cardiac Muscle

Cardiac muscle fibers are also cylindrical. They are primarily located in the walls and septa of the **heart** and in the walls of the large vessels attached to the heart (aorta and pulmonary trunk). Similar to skeletal muscle, cardiac muscle fibers exhibit distinct **cross-striations** as a result of the regular arrangements of actin and myosin filaments. Transmission electron microscopy reveals similar A bands, I bands, Z lines, and repeating sacromere units. In contrast to skeletal muscles, cardiac muscle fibers exhibit only one or two **central nuclei,** are shorter, and are **branched.**

The terminal ends of adjacent cardiac muscle fibers show characteristic and dense-staining, end-to-end junctional complexes called **intercalated disks.** These disks are special attachment sites that cross the cardiac cells at irregular intervals in steplike fashion. Located in the intercalated disks are the **gap junctions** that enable ionic communication and continuity between adjacent cardiac muscle fibers (see Overview Figure 6).

Smooth Muscle

Smooth muscle has a wide distribution and is found in numerous hollow organs. Smooth muscle fibers also contain contractile actin and myosin filaments; however, they are not arranged in the regular, cross-striated patterns that are visible in both the skeletal and cardiac muscle fibers. As a result, these muscle fibers appear **smooth** or **nonstriated.** Smooth muscle fibers are also **involuntary muscles** and are, therefore, under autonomic nervous system and hormonal control. The muscle fibers are small and spindle or fusiform in shape, and contain a single central **nucleus.**

Under a light microscope, smooth muscle appears as individual fibers or slender bundles called fascicles. Smooth muscles are predominantly found in the linings of **visceral hollow organs** and **blood vessels.** In digestive tract organs, uterus, ureters, and other hollow organs, smooth muscles occur in large sheets or layers. Connective tissue surrounds individual muscle fibers, as well as muscle layers. In the blood vessels, smooth muscle fibers are arranged in a circular pattern, where they control blood pressure by altering luminal diameters (see Overview Figure 6).

FIGURE 6.1 ■ Longitudinal and Transverse Sections of Skeletal (Striated) Muscles: Tongue

In the tongue, skeletal muscle fibers are arranged in bundles and course in different directions. This image illustrates the tongue muscle fibers in both the longitudinal (upper region) and transverse (lower region) sections.

Each skeletal **muscle fiber (9, transverse section; 11, longitudinal section)** is multinucleated. The **nuclei (1, 6)** are situated peripherally and immediately below the sarcolemma of each muscle fiber. (The sarcolemma is not visible in the figure.) Also, each skeletal muscle fiber shows **cross-striations (3),** which are visible as alternating dark or **A bands (3a)** and light or **I bands (3b).** With higher magnification and transmission electron microscopy, additional details of the cross-striations are visible (Figures 6.5–6.7).

Skeletal muscle fibers are aggregated into bundles or **fascicles (15),** surrounded by fibers of **connective tissue (5).** The connective tissue (5) sheath around each muscle fascicle (15) is called the **perimysium (12).** From each perimysium (12), thin partitions of connective tissue extend into each muscle fascicle (15) and invest individual muscle fibers (9, 11) with a connective tissue layer called the **endomysium (4, 7).** Small **blood vessels (8)** and **capillaries (2, 14)** are present in the connective tissue (5) around each muscle fiber (9, 11).

The skeletal muscle fibers that were sectioned longitudinally (11) show light and dark cross-striations (3a, 3b). The muscle fibers that were sectioned transversely (9) exhibit cross sections of **myofibrils (13)** and peripheral nuclei (6).

FIGURE 6.2 ■ Skeletal (Striated) Muscles: Tongue (Longitudinal Section)

A higher-magnification photomicrograph of the tongue illustrates individual **skeletal muscle fibers (1)** and their **cross-striations (2).** Note the peripheral **nuclei (3)** and the tiny **myofibrils (6).** Surrounding each skeletal muscle fiber (1) is the thin layer of connective tissue called **endomysium (5).** The thicker connective tissue layer called **perimysium (4)** invests aggregates of muscle fibers, or fascicles. Associated with the connective tissue perimysium (4) are the **adipose cells (7).**

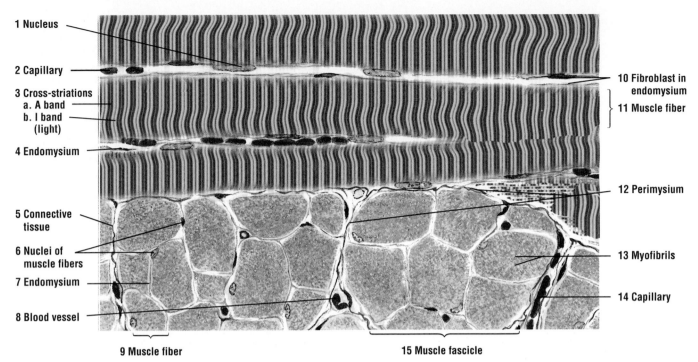

1 Nucleus
2 Capillary
3 Cross-striations
  a. A band
  b. I band
    (light)
4 Endomysium
5 Connective
  tissue
6 Nuclei of
  muscle fibers
7 Endomysium
8 Blood vessel

10 Fibroblast in
  endomysium
11 Muscle fiber
12 Perimysium
13 Myofibrils
14 Capillary

9 Muscle fiber   15 Muscle fascicle

FIGURE 6.1 ■ Longitudinal and transverse sections of skeletal (striated) muscles of the tongue. Stain: hematoxylin and eosin. High magnification.

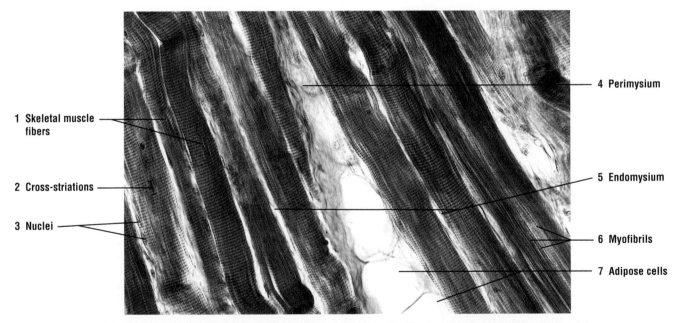

1 Skeletal muscle
  fibers

2 Cross-striations

3 Nuclei

4 Perimysium
5 Endomysium
6 Myofibrils
7 Adipose cells

FIGURE 6.2 ■ Skeletal (striated) muscles of the tongue (longitudinal section). Stain: Masson's trichrome. ×130.

FIGURE 6.3 ■ Skeletal Muscles, Nerves, and Motor End Plates

A group of **skeletal muscle fibers (6, 7)** have been teased apart and stained to illustrate nerve terminations or myoneural junctions on individual muscle fibers. Note the characteristic **cross-striations (2, 8)** of the skeletal muscle fibers (6, 7). The dark-stained, string-like structures between the separated muscle fibers (6, 7) are the myelinated motor **nerves (3)** and their branches, the **axons (1, 5, 10).** The motor nerve (3) courses within the muscle, branches, and distributes its axons (1, 5, 10) to the individual muscle fibers (6, 7). The axons (1, 5, 10) terminate on individual muscle fibers as specialized junctional regions called **motor end plates (4, 9).** The small, dark round structures seen in each motor end plate (4, 9) are the terminal expansion of the axons (1, 5, 10). Some axons (1) are also seen without motor end plates as a result of tissue preparation.

FUNCTIONAL CORRELATIONS: Skeletal Muscle and Motor End Plates

Skeletal muscles are **voluntary** because the stimulation for their contraction and relaxation is under conscious control. Large motor nerves or axons innervate skeletal muscles. Near the skeletal muscle, the motor nerve branches, and a smaller axon branch individually innervates a single muscle fiber. As a result, skeletal muscle fibers contract only when stimulated by an axon. Also, each skeletal muscle fiber exhibits a specialized site where the axon terminates. This **neuromuscular junction** or **motor end plate** is the site where the impulse from the axon is transmitted to the skeletal muscle fiber.

The terminal end of each efferent (motor) axon contains numerous small **vesicles** that contain the neurotransmitter **acetylcholine**. Arrival of a nerve impulse or **action potential** at the axon terminal causes the synaptic vesicles to fuse with the plasma membrane of the axon and release the acetylcholine into the **synaptic cleft,** a small gap between the axon terminal and cell membrane of the muscle fiber. The neurotransmitter then diffuses across the synaptic cleft, combines with **acetylcholine receptors** on the cell membrane of the muscle fiber, and stimulates the muscle to contract. An enzyme called **acetylcholinesterase,** located in the synaptic cleft near the surface of the muscle fiber cell membrane, inactivates or neutralizes the released acetylcholine. Inactivation of acetylcholine prevents further muscle stimulation and muscle contraction until the next impulse arrives at the axon terminal.

1 Axon terminals

2 Cross-striations

3 Myelinated
nerve

4 Motor end plates

5 Axons

6 Skeletal muscle
fibers

7 Skeletal muscle
fibers

8 Cross-striations

9 Motor end plates

10 Axons

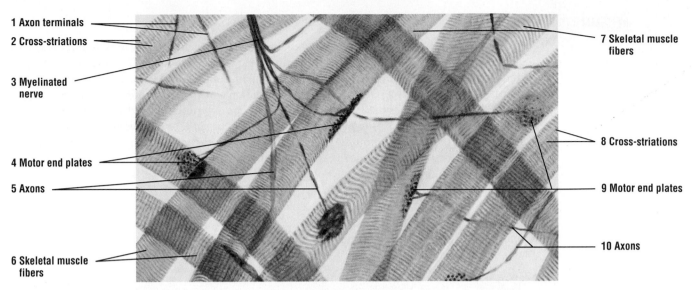

FIGURE 6.3 ■ Skeletal muscles, nerves, axons, and motor end plates. Stain: silver. High magnification.

FIGURE 6.4 ■ Skeletal Muscle With Muscle Spindle (Transverse Section)

A transverse section of an extraocular skeletal muscle shows individual **muscle fibers (2)** surrounded by connective tissue, the **endomysium (6)**. The muscle fibers (2) in turn are grouped into **fascicles (1)** and surrounded by interfascicular connective tissue called **perimysium (4)**. Located within the muscle fascicles (1) is a cross section of a **muscle spindle (3)**. Surrounding the muscle spindle (3) and the skeletal muscle fibers (2) are **arterioles (5)** in the perimysium (4).

The muscle spindle (3) is an encapsulated sensory organ. The connective tissue **capsule (8)** surrounding the muscle spindle (3) extends from the adjacent **perimysium (11)** and encloses several components of the spindle. The specialized muscle fibers located in the spindle and surrounded by the capsule (8) are called **intrafusal fibers (10)** [in contrast to the extrafusal **skeletal muscle fibers (7)** located outside of the spindle capsule (8)]. Small nerve fibers associated with the muscle spindles (3) are the myelinated and terminal unmyelinated **nerve fibers (axons) (9)** surrounded by the supportive Schwann cells. Small blood vessels and an **arteriole (12)** from the perimysium (11) are found in and around the capsule of the muscle spindle (3).

FUNCTIONAL CORRELATIONS: Muscle Spindles

Muscle spindles are highly specialized **stretch receptors** located parallel to muscle fibers in nearly all skeletal muscles. Their main function is to detect changes in the length of the muscle fibers. An increase in the length of muscle fibers stimulates the muscle spindle and sends **impulses** via the afferent (sensory) axons into the spinal cord. These impulses result in a **stretch reflex** that immediately causes **contraction** of the **extrafusal muscle fibers,** thereby shortening the stretched muscle and producing movement. A decrease in skeletal muscle length stops the stimulation of the muscle spindle fibers and the conduction of its impulses to the spinal cord.

The simple stretch **reflex arc** illustrates the function of these receptors. Gently tapping the patellar tendon on the knee with a rubber mallet stretches the skeletal muscle and stimulates the muscle spindle. This action results in rapid muscle contraction of the stretched muscle and produces an involuntary response, or stretch reflex.

FIGURE 6.5 ■ Skeletal Muscle Fibers (Longitudinal Section)

A higher-magnification illustration shows greater detail of individual skeletal muscle fibers. A cell membrane or **sarcolemma (4)** surrounds each skeletal **muscle fiber (2).** Note the peripheral location of the muscle fiber **nuclei (1, 15)** and their flattened appearance. Adjacent to the nuclei (1, 15) is the thin cytoplasm or **sarcoplasm (5)** with its organelles. Each muscle fiber (2) consists of **individual myofibrils (13)** that are arranged longitudinally. Myofibrils (13) are best seen in cross sections of the skeletal muscle fibers in Figure 6.3, label 13. Surrounding each skeletal muscle fiber (2) is a thin connective tissue **endomysium (14)** containing connective tissue cells called **fibrocytes (3, 11)**. Blood vessels and **capillaries (12)** with blood cells are found in the endomysium (14).

At higher magnification, the cross-striations of skeletal muscle fibers are recognized as the light-staining **I bands (6)** and dark-staining **A bands (7)**. Each A band (7) is bisected by the lighter H band and the darker **M line (8)**. Crossing the central region of each I band is a distinct, narrow **Z line (9)**. The cellular segments between the Z lines (9) represent a **sarcomere (10),** the structural and functional unit of striated muscles (skeletal and cardiac). When the myofibrils (13) are separated from the muscle fiber (2), the A, I, and Z lines remain visible. The close longitudinal arrangement of parallel myofibrils gives the skeletal muscle fibers their striated appearance.

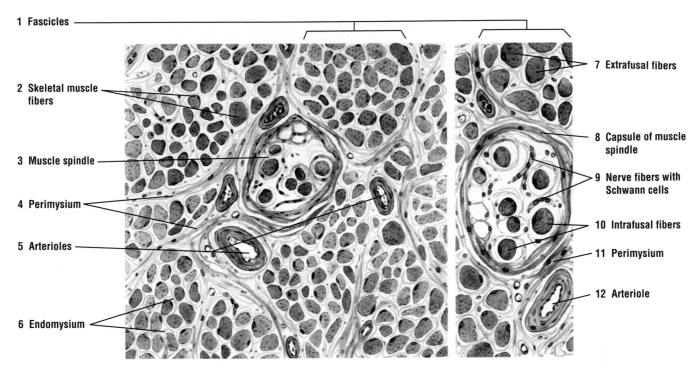

1 Fascicles
2 Skeletal muscle fibers
3 Muscle spindle
4 Perimysium
5 Arterioles
6 Endomysium
7 Extrafusal fibers
8 Capsule of muscle spindle
9 Nerve fibers with Schwann cells
10 Intrafusal fibers
11 Perimysium
12 Arteriole

FIGURE 6.4 ■ Skeletal muscle with muscle spindle (transverse section). Frozen section stained with modified Van Gieson method (hematoxylin, picric acid-ponceau stain). Left, medium magnification; right, high magnification. (Tissue samples provided by Dr. Mark De Santis, WWAMI Medical Program, University of Idaho, Moscow, Idaho.)

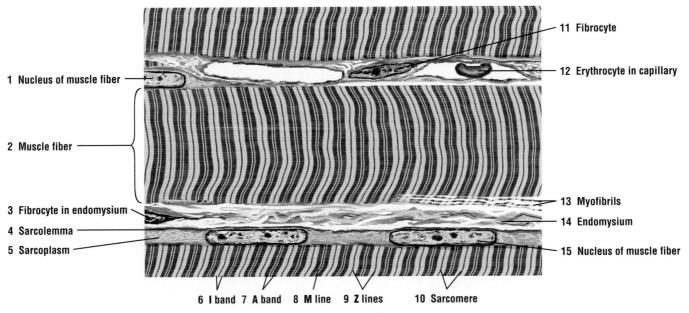

1 Nucleus of muscle fiber
2 Muscle fiber
3 Fibrocyte in endomysium
4 Sarcolemma
5 Sarcoplasm
11 Fibrocyte
12 Erythrocyte in capillary
13 Myofibrils
14 Endomysium
15 Nucleus of muscle fiber

6 I band   7 A band   8 M line   9 Z lines   10 Sarcomere

FIGURE 6.5 ■ Skeletal muscle fibers (longitudinal section). Stain: hematoxylin and eosin. Plastic section. High magnification.

FIGURE 6.6 ■ Ultrastructure of Myofibrils in Skeletal Muscle

A transmission electron micrograph illustrates the organization of myofibrils in a partially contracted skeletal muscle. Each myofibril consists of repeating units called sarcomeres, the contractile elements in striated muscles. A **sarcomere (9)** is located between two electron-dense **Z lines (8)**. Located in each sarcomere (9) are the thin actin and the thick myosin myofilaments. The thin actin filaments extend from the Z lines (8) and form the light-staining **I bands (2)**. In the center of each sarcomere (9) is the dark-staining **A band (5)**, which consists mainly of the thick myosin filaments overlapping the thin actin filaments. Each A band (5) is bisected by a denser **M band (7)** where the adjacent myosin filaments are linked. On each side of the M band (7) are small lighter **H bands (4, 6)** that consist only of myosin filaments. Surrounding each sarcomere in a repeating fashion are the tubules of **sacroplasmic reticulum (3)** and **mitochondria (1)**. During muscle contraction, the length of the thick and thin filaments remains unchanged, whereas the size of each sarcomere (9) decreases (see Figure 6.7).

FIGURE 6.7 ■ Ultrastructure of Sarcomeres, T tubules, and Triads in Skeletal Muscle

A higher magnification with the transmission electron micrograph illustrates the sarcomeres in a contracted skeletal muscle. Note that as the muscle contracts and the sarcomere shortens, the **Z lines (2. 6)** are drawn closer together and the thick and thin filaments slide past each other. This action narrows the **I bands (7)** and **H bands (8)**, whereas the **A band (1)** remains unchanged. Also visible in the middle of the sarcomere is the dense-staining **M band (4).** The tubules of the sarcoplasmic reticulum surround every sarcomere of every myofibril (see Figure 6.6). At the A band (1) and I band (7) junction (A-I junctions), the sarcoplasmic reticulum tubules expand into terminal cisternae. To allow synchronous stimulation and contraction of all sarcomeres, tiny tubular invaginations of the sarcolemma, called the **T tubules (3)**, penetrate every myofibril, and are located at the A-I junctions (1, 7). Here, one T tubule (3) is surrounded on each side by the expanded terminal cisternae of the sarcoplasmic reticulum and form **triads (5).** In mammalian skeletal muscles, the triads (5) are located at the A-I junctions. The stimulus for muscle contraction is then disseminated to each sarcomere through the T tubules (3) in the triads (5).

FUNCTIONAL CORRELATIONS: Contraction of Skeletal Muscles

Before the arrival of the nerve stimulus to the muscle, the muscle is relaxed and the calcium ions are stored in the cisternae of the sacroplasmic reticulum. After the arrival of the nerve stimulus and the release of the neurotransmitter at the motor end plates, the sarcolemma is depolarized or activated. The stimulus signal or action potential is propagated along the entire length of the sarcolemma and transmitted deep to every myofiber by the network of the T tubules. At each triad, the action potential is transmitted from the T tubules to the sarcoplasmic reticulum membrane. After its stimulation, cisternae of the sarcoplasmic reticulum release calcium ions into the individual sarcomeres and the overlapping thick and thin myofilaments of the myofiber. Calcium ions activate binding between actin and myosin that results in their sliding past each other and muscle contraction. When the stimulus subsides and the membrane is no longer stimulated, calcium ions are actively transported back into and stored in the cisternae of the sarcoplasmic reticulum, causing muscle relaxation.

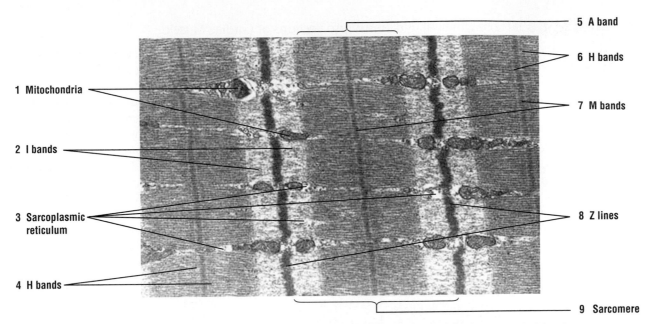

1 Mitochondria

2 I bands

3 Sarcoplasmic reticulum

4 H bands

5 A band

6 H bands

7 M bands

8 Z lines

9 Sarcomere

FIGURE 6.6 ■ Ultrastructure of myofibrils in skeletal muscle. ×33,500. Image provided by Carter Rowley, Fort Collins, CO.

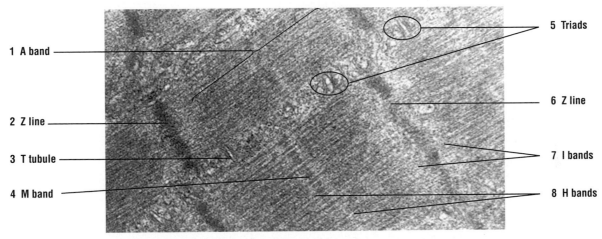

1 A band

2 Z line

3 T tubule

4 M band

5 Triads

6 Z line

7 I bands

8 H bands

FIGURE 6.7 ■ Ultrastructure of sarcomeres, T tubules, and triads in skeletal muscle. ×50,000. Image provided by Carter Rowley, Fort Collins, CO.

FIGURE 6.8 ■ Longitudinal and Transverse Sections of Cardiac Muscle

Cardiac muscle fibers exhibit some of the features that are seen in skeletal muscle fibers. This figure illustrates a section of a cardiac muscle cut in both longitudinal (upper portion) and transverse (lower portion) planes. The **cross-striations (2)** in cardiac muscle fibers closely resemble those seen in skeletal muscles. In contrast, the cardiac muscle fibers show **branching (5, 10)** without much change in their diameters. Also, each cardiac muscle fiber is shorter than a skeletal muscle fiber and contains a single, centrally located **nucleus (3, 7). Binucleate (two nuclei) muscle fibers (8)** are also occasionally seen. The nuclei (7) are clearly visible in the center of each muscle fiber when they are cut in a transverse section. Around these nuclei (3, 7, 8) are the clear zones of nonfibrillar **perinuclear sarcoplasm (1, 13).** In transverse sections, the perinuclear sarcoplasm (13) appears as a clear space if the section is not through the nucleus. Also visible in transverse sections are **myofibrils (14)** of individual cardiac muscle cells.

A distinguishing and characteristic feature of cardiac muscle fibers are the **intercalated disks (4, 9).** These dark-staining structures are found at irregular intervals in the cardiac muscle and represent the specialized junctional complexes between cardiac muscle fibers.

The cardiac muscle has a vast blood supply. Numerous small blood vessels and **capillaries (6)** are found in the **connective tissue (11)** septa and the delicate **endomysium (12)** between individual muscle fibers.

Other examples of cardiac muscles are seen in Chapter 8, Circulatory System.

FIGURE 6.9 ■ Cardiac Muscle (Longitudinal Section)

A high-magnification photomicrograph illustrates a section of the cardiac muscle cut in a longitudinal plane. The **cardiac muscle fibers (2)** exhibit **cross-striations (4), branching (3),** and a single central **nucleus (5).** The dark-staining **intercalated disks (1)** connect individual cardiac muscle fibers (2). Small **myofibrils (6)** are visible within each cardiac muscle fiber. Delicate strands of **connective tissue fibers (7)** surround the individual cardiac muscle fibers.

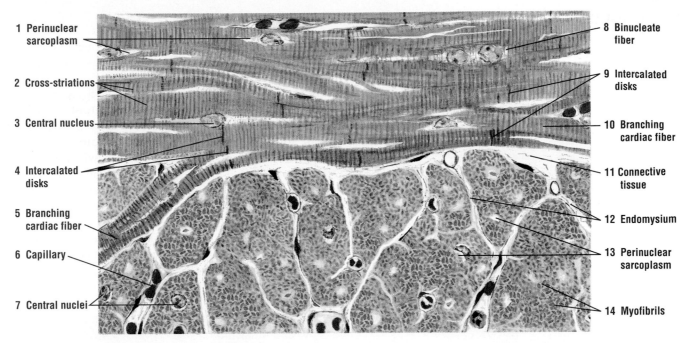

1 Perinuclear sarcoplasm

2 Cross-striations

3 Central nucleus

4 Intercalated disks

5 Branching cardiac fiber

6 Capillary

7 Central nuclei

8 Binucleate fiber

9 Intercalated disks

10 Branching cardiac fiber

11 Connective tissue

12 Endomysium

13 Perinuclear sarcoplasm

14 Myofibrils

FIGURE 6.8 ■ Longitudinal and transverse sections of cardiac muscle. Stain: hematoxylin and eosin. High magnification.

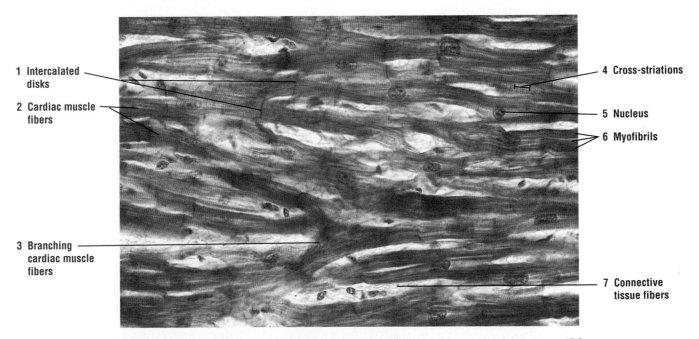

1 Intercalated disks

2 Cardiac muscle fibers

3 Branching cardiac muscle fibers

4 Cross-striations

5 Nucleus

6 Myofibrils

7 Connective tissue fibers

FIGURE 6.9 ■ Cardiac muscle (longitudinal section). Stain: Masson's trichrome. ×130.

FIGURE 6.10 ■ Cardiac Muscle in Longitudinal Section

Comparison of cardiac muscle fibers with skeletal muscles at higher magnification and with the same stain (Figure 6.5) illustrates the similarities and differences between the two types of muscle tissue.

The **cross-striations (1)** are similar in both the skeletal and cardiac muscle types but are less prominent in cardiac muscle fibers. The branching **cardiac fibers (9)** are in contrast to the individual, elongated fibers of the skeletal muscle. The characteristic **intercalated disks (5, 7)** of cardiac muscle fibers and their irregular structure are more prominent at higher magnification. The intercalated disks (5, 7) appear as either straight bands (5) or staggered (7) across individual fibers.

The large, oval **nuclei (3),** usually one per cell, occupy the central position of the cardiac fibers, in contrast to the numerous flattened and peripheral nuclei in each skeletal muscle fiber. Surrounding the nucleus of a cardiac muscle fiber is a prominent **perinuclear sarcoplasm (2, 10)** that is devoid of cross-striations and myofibrils.

The connective tissue **fibrocytes (6, 8)** and fine connective tissue fibers of **endomysium (4)** surround the cardiac muscle fibers. **Capillaries** with **erythrocytes (11)** are normally seen in the endomysium (4, 6, 8).

FUNCTIONAL CORRELATIONS: Cardiac Muscle

Although the organization of the contractile proteins in the cardiac myofibers and sarcomeres is essentially the same as in the skeletal muscles, there are important differences. The T tubules are located at the Z lines, are larger than in skeletal muscles, and the sarcoplasmic reticulum is less well developed. Also, the mitochondria are more abundant in the cardiac cells, which reflects on the increased metabolic demands on the cardiac muscle fibers for continuous action.

The cardiac cells are joined end to end by specialized, interdigitating junctional complexes called **intercalated disks.** Besides fascia adherens and desmosomes, these disks contain **gap junctions** that functionally couple all cardiac muscle fibers to rapidly spread the stimuli for contraction of the heart muscle. Conduction of excitatory impulses to the cardiac sarcomeres is through the T tubules and the sacroplasmic reticulum. Diffusion of ions through the pores in gap junctions between individual cardiac muscle fibers coordinates heart functions and allows the cardiac muscle to act as a **functional syncytium,** allowing the stimuli for contraction to pass through the entire cardiac muscle.

Cardiac muscle fibers exhibit **autorhythmicity,** an ability to spontaneously generate stimuli. Both the **parasympathetic** and **sympathetic divisions** of the autonomic nervous system innervate the heart. Nerve fibers from the parasympathetic division, by way of the vagus nerve, slow the heart and decrease blood pressure. Nerve fibers from the sympathetic division produce the opposite effect and increase heart rate and blood pressure.

Additional information on cardiac muscle histology, heart pacemaker, Purkinje fibers, and heart hormones is presented in more detail in Chapter 8, Circulatory System.

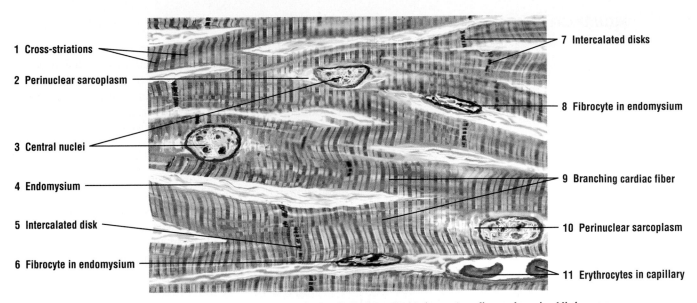

1 Cross-striations

2 Perinuclear sarcoplasm

3 Central nuclei

4 Endomysium

5 Intercalated disk

6 Fibrocyte in endomysium

7 Intercalated disks

8 Fibrocyte in endomysium

9 Branching cardiac fiber

10 Perinuclear sarcoplasm

11 Erythrocytes in capillary

FIGURE 6.10 ■ Cardiac muscle in longitudinal section. Stain: hematoxylin and eosin. High magnification.

FIGURE 6.11 ■ Longitudinal and Transverse Sections of Smooth Muscle: Wall of Small Intestine

In the muscular region of the small intestine, smooth muscle fibers are arranged in two concentric layers: an inner circular layer and an outer longitudinal layer. Here, the muscle fibers are tightly packed and the muscle fibers of one layer are arranged at right angles to the fibers of the adjacent layer.

The upper region of the illustration shows the smooth muscle fibers of the inner circular layer cut in longitudinal section. **Smooth muscle fibers (1)** are spindle-shaped cells with tapered ends. The cytoplasm (sarcoplasm) of each muscle fiber stains dark. An elongated or ovoid **nucleus (7)** is present in the center of each smooth muscle fiber.

The lower region of the figure shows the muscles of the adjacent longitudinal layer cut in transverse section. Because the spindle-shaped cells are sectioned at different places along their length, the cells with their nuclei exhibit different shapes and sizes. Large **nuclei (5)** are seen only in those **smooth muscle fibers (5)** that have been sectioned through their center. Muscle fibers that were not sectioned through the center appear only as deeply stained areas of clear **cytoplasm (sarcoplasm) (3, lower leader; 9, lower leader)** or exhibit only a small portion of their nuclei.

In the small intestine, the smooth muscle layers are close to each other with only a minimal amount of **connective tissue fibers** and **fibroblasts (2, 4, 8, 10)** present between the two layers. Smooth muscle also has a rich blood supply, evidenced by the numerous **capillaries (6, 11)** between individual fibers and layers.

FIGURE 6.12 ■ Smooth Muscle: Wall of the Small Intestine (Transverse and Longitudinal Sections)

A photomicrograph of the small intestine illustrates its muscular outer wall. The smooth muscle fibers are arranged in two layers: an **inner circular layer (7)** and an **outer longitudinal layer (8).** In the inner circular layer (7), a single **nucleus (1)** is visible in the center of the **cytoplasm (2)** of different fibers. In the outer longitudinal layer (8), cut in transverse section, the **cytoplasm (5)** appears empty, and single **nuclei (6)** of individual muscle fibers are visible if the plane of section passes through them. Located between the two smooth muscle layers is a group of autonomic **neurons** of the **myenteric nerve plexus (3)**. Small **blood vessels (4)** are seen between individual muscle fibers and muscle layers.

FUNCTIONAL CORRELATIONS: Smooth Muscle

In smooth muscle, the actin and myosin myofilaments do not show the regular arrangement seen in striated muscles. Instead, intermediate myofilaments, myosin, and actin form a lattice network in the sarcoplasm. Both thin and intermediate filaments insert into **dense bodies** in the sarcoplasm that correspond to the Z lines of the striated muscles. In response to a stimulus, the increased presence of calcium causes smooth muscle contraction. Actin and intermediate filaments insert into the dense bodies. Both actin and myosin contract by a sliding filament mechanism that is similar to that in skeletal muscles. When the actin-myosin complex contracts, the attachment of the filaments to the dense bodies produces cell shortening.

Smooth muscle usually exhibits spontaneous wavelike activity that passes in a slow, sustained contraction throughout the entire muscle. In this manner, smooth muscle produces a continuous contraction of low force and maintains **tonus** in hollow structures. In ureters, uterine tubes, and digestive organs, contraction of smooth muscle produces **peristaltic contractions,** which propel the contents along the lengths of these organs. In arteries and other blood vessels, smooth muscles regulate the luminal diameters.

Smooth muscle fibers also make close contacts with each other via specialized **gap junctions.** These gap junctions allow for rapid ionic communications between the smooth muscle fibers, resulting in coordinated activity in smooth muscle sheets or layers. Smooth muscles are **involuntary** muscles. They are innervated and regulated by nerves from postganglionic neurons whose cell bodies are located in the **sympathetic** and **parasympathetic divisions** of the **autonomic nervous system.** These innervations influence the rate and force of contractility. In addition, smooth muscle fibers contract and relax in response to nonneural stimulation, such as **stretching** or exposure to different **hormones.**

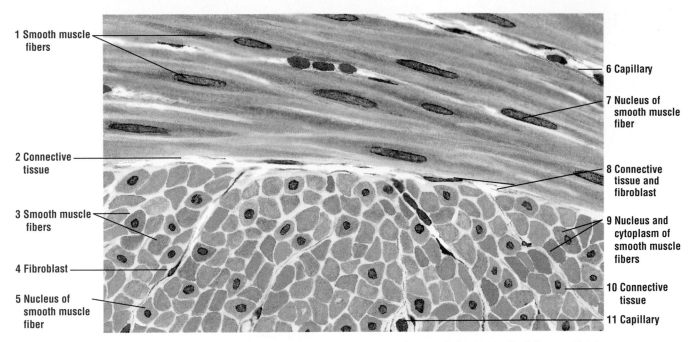

1 Smooth muscle fibers

2 Connective tissue

3 Smooth muscle fibers

4 Fibroblast

5 Nucleus of smooth muscle fiber

6 Capillary

7 Nucleus of smooth muscle fiber

8 Connective tissue and fibroblast

9 Nucleus and cytoplasm of smooth muscle fibers

10 Connective tissue

11 Capillary

FIGURE 6.11 ■ Longitudinal and transverse sections of smooth muscle in the wall of the small intestine. Stain: hematoxylin and eosin. High magnification.

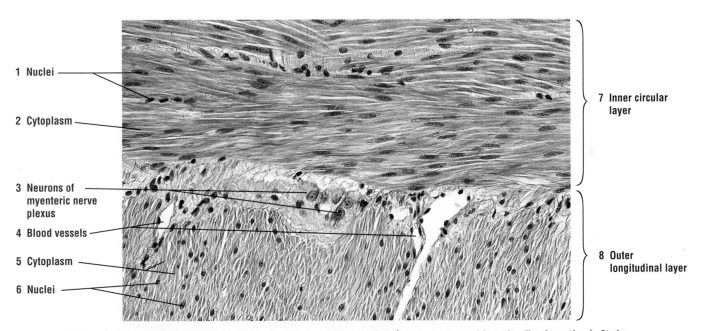

1 Nuclei

2 Cytoplasm

3 Neurons of myenteric nerve plexus

4 Blood vessels

5 Cytoplasm

6 Nuclei

7 Inner circular layer

8 Outer longitudinal layer

FIGURE 6.12 ■ Smooth muscle: wall of the small intestine (transverse and longitudinal section). Stain: hematoxylin and eosin. ×80.

Muscle Tissue

- Three muscle types: skeletal muscle, cardiac muscle, and smooth muscle
- All muscles composed of elongated cells called fibers
- Muscle cytoplasm is sarcoplasm and muscle cell membrane is sarcolemma
- Muscle fibers contain myofibrils, made of contractile proteins actin and myosin

Skeletal Muscle

- Fibers are multinucleated with peripheral nuclei
- Actin and myosin filaments form distinct cross-striation patterns
- Muscle is surrounded by connective tissue epimysium
- Muscle fascicles surrounded by connective tissue perimysium
- Each muscle fiber surrounded by connective tissue endomysium
- Voluntary muscles under conscious control
- Motor end plates the site of nerve innervation and transmission of stimuli to muscle
- Axon terminals contain neurotransmitter acetylcholine
- Action potential releases acetylcholine into synaptic cleft
- Acetylcholine combines with its receptors on muscle membrane
- Acetylcholinesterase in synaptic cleft neutralizes acetylcholine and prevents further contraction
- Neuromuscular spindles are specialized stretch receptors in almost all skeletal muscles
- Stretching of muscle produces a stretch reflex and movement to shorten muscle

Transmission Electron Microscopy of Skeletal Muscle

- Light bands are I bands and are formed by thin actin filaments
- I bands are crossed by dense Z lines
- Between Z lines is the smallest contractile unit of muscle, the sarcomere
- Dark bands are A bands and are located in the middle of sarcomere
- A bands are formed by overlapping actin and myosin filaments
- M bands in the middle of A bands represent linkage of myosin filaments
- H bands on each side of M bands contain only myosin filaments
- Sarcoplasmic reticulum and mitochondria surround each sarcomere
- When muscle contracts, I and H bands shorten, while A bands stay same
- Sarcolemma invaginations into each myofiber form T tubules
- Expanded terminal cisternae of sarcoplasmic reticulum and T tubules form triads
- Triads are located at A-I junctions in mammalian skeletal muscles
- Stimulus for muscle contraction carried by T tubules to every myofiber
- After stimulation, sarcoplasmic reticulum releases calcium ions into sarcomeres
- Calcium activates the binding of actin and myosin, causing muscle contraction
- After end of contraction, calcium actively transported and stored in sarcoplasmic reticulum

Cardiac Muscle

- Located in heart and large vessels attached to heart
- Cross-striations of actin and myosin form similar I bands, A bands, and Z lines as in skeletal muscle
- Contains one or two central nuclei; fibers are branched
- Characterized by dense junctional complexes called intercalated disks that contain gap junctions
- T tubules located at Z lines; larger than in skeletal muscle
- Sarcoplasmic reticulum less well developed
- Gap junctions couple all fibers for rhythmic contraction
- Exhibit autorhythmicity and spontaneously generate stimuli
- Autonomic nervous system innervates heart and influences heart rate and blood pressure

Smooth Muscle

- Found in hollow organs and blood vessels
- Contain actin and myosin filaments without cross-striation patterns
- Fibers are fusiform in shape and contain single nuclei
- In intestines, muscles arranged in concentric layers
- Actin and myosin filaments do not show regular arrangement and there are not striations
- Actin and myosin form lattice network and insert into dense bodies in the sarcoplasm
- Actin and myosin contract and shorten muscle by sliding mechanism similar to skeletal muscle
- Exhibit spontaneous activity and maintain tonus in hollow organs
- Peristaltic contractions propel contents in the organs
- Gap junctions couple muscle and allow ionic communication between all fibers
- Involuntary muscles regulated by autonomic nervous system, hormones, and stretching

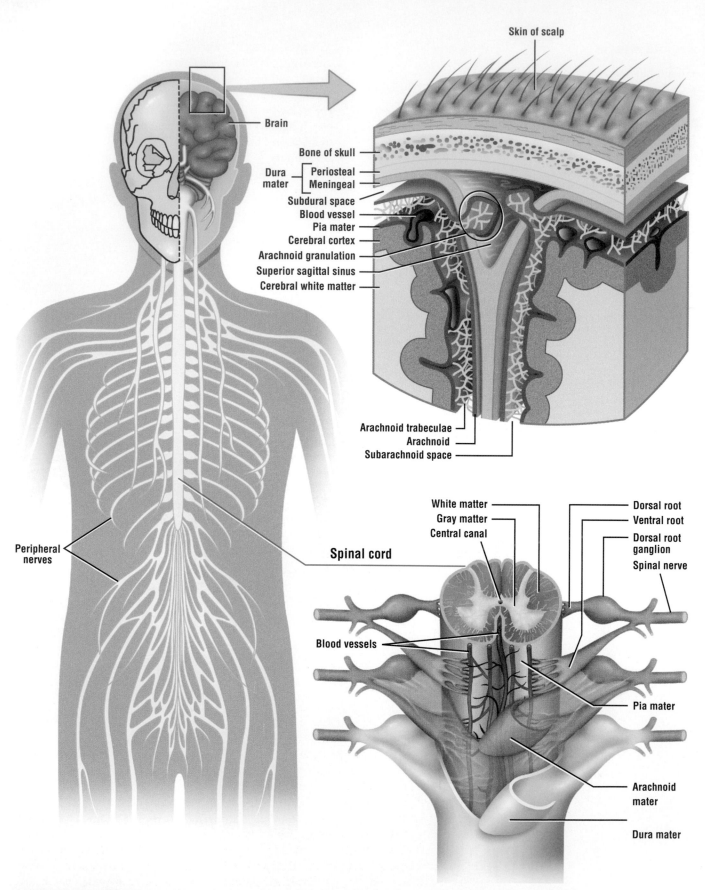

OVERVIEW FIGURE 7.1 ■ Central nervous system. The central nervous system is composed of the brain and spinal cord. A section of the brain and spinal cord is illustrated with their protective connective tissue layers called meninges (dura mater, arachnoid mater, and pia mater).

Nervous Tissue

SECTION 1 ■ The Central Nervous System: Brain and Spinal Cord

Introduction

The mammalian nervous system is divided into two major parts, the **central nervous system (CNS)** and the **peripheral nervous system (PNS).** The CNS consists of the **brain** and **spinal cord.** The components of the PNS—the cranial and spinal nerves—are located outside the CNS.

The Protective Layers of the Central Nervous System (CNS)

Because the nervous tissue is very delicate, bones, connective tissue layers, and a watery cerebrospinal fluid (CSF) surround and protect the brain and the spinal cord. Deep to the cranial bones in the skull and the vertebral foramen are the meninges, a connective tissue that consists of three layers: the dura mater, arachnoid mater, and pia mater (Overview Figure 7.1 Central Nervous System).

The outermost meningeal layer is the **dura mater,** a tough, strong, and thick layer of dense connective tissue fibers. Deep to the dura mater is a more delicate connective tissue, the **arachnoid mater.** The dura mater and arachnoid mater surround the brain and spinal cord on their external surfaces. The innermost meningeal layer is the delicate connective tissue **pia mater.** This layer contains numerous blood vessels and adheres directly to the surfaces of the brain and spinal cord.

Between the arachnoid mater and the pia mater is the **subarachnoid space.** Delicate, weblike strands of collagen and elastic fibers attach the arachnoid mater to the pia mater. Circulating in the subarachnoid space is the cerebrospinal fluid (CSF) that bathes and protects both the brain and spinal cord.

The Cerebrospinal Fluid

The **cerebrospinal fluid (CSF)** is a clear, colorless fluid that cushions the brain and spinal cord, and gives them buoyancy as a means of protection from physical injuries. The CSF is continually produced by the **choroid plexuses** in the lateral, third, and fourth ventricles, or cavities, of the brain. Choroid plexuses are small, vascular extensions of dilated and fenestrated capillaries that penetrate the interior of brain ventricles. CSF circulates through the ventricles and around the outer surfaces of the brain and spinal cord in the subarachnoid space. CSF also fills the central canal of the spinal cord.

CSF is important for homeostasis and brain metabolism. It brings nutrients to nourish brain cells, removes metabolites that enter the CSF from the brain cells, and provides an optimal chemical environment for neuronal functions and impulse conduction. After circulation, CSF is reabsorbed from the arachnoid space via the **arachnoid villi** into venous blood, mainly at the superior sagittal sinus that drains the brain. Arachnoid villi are small, thin-walled arachnoid extensions that project into the venous sinuses located between the periosteal and meningeal layers of dura mater.

Morphology of a Typical Neuron

The nervous system is composed of highly complex intercommunicating networks of nerve cells that receive and conduct **impulses** along their neural pathways or axons to the CNS for analysis, integration, interpretation, and response. Ultimately, the appropriate response to a given stimulus from the neurons of the CNS is the activation of muscles (skeletal, smooth, or cardiac) or glands (endocrine or exocrine).

The structural and functional cells of the nervous tissue are the **neurons.** (A general structure of a neuron and examples of different types of neurons are shown in the Overview Figure 7.2, Section 2: Peripheral Nervous System.) Although neurons vary in size and shape, a general structure of these cells can be described. Each neuron consists of **soma** or **cell body,** numerous **dendrites,** and a single **axon.** The cell body or soma contains the nucleus, nucleolus, numerous different organelles, and the surrounding cytoplasm or perikaryon. Projecting from the cell body are numerous cytoplasmic extensions called dendrites that form a dendritic tree.

Surrounding the neurons are the smaller and more numerous supportive cells collectively called **neuroglia.** These cells form the nonneural components of the CNS.

Types of Neurons in the CNS

The three major types of neurons in the nervous system are multipolar, bipolar, and unipolar. This anatomic classification is based on the number of dendrites and axons that originate from the cell body.

Multipolar neurons. These are the most common type in the CNS and include all **motor neurons** and **interneurons** of the brain, cerebellum, and spinal cord. Projecting from the cell body of a multipolar neuron are numerous branched dendrites. On the opposite side of the multipolar neuron is a single axon.

Bipolar neurons. These are not as common and are purely **sensory neurons.** In bipolar neurons, a single dendrite and a single axon are associated with the cell body. Bipolar neurons are found in the retina of the eye, in the organs of hearing and equilibrium in the inner ear, and in the olfactory epithelium in the upper region of the nose (the latter two are found in the PNS).

Unipolar neurons. Most neurons in the adult organism that exhibit only one process leaving the cell body were initially bipolar during embryonic development. The two neuronal processes fuse during later development and form one process. The unipolar neurons (formerly called **pseudounipolar neurons**) are also **sensory.** Unipolar neurons are found in numerous sensory ganglia of cranial and spinal nerves.

Myelin Sheath and Myelination of Axons

Highly specialized cells present in both the CNS and the PNS wrap around the axon numerous times to build up successive layers of modified cell membrane and form a lipid-rich, insulating sheath around the axon called the **myelin sheath.** The sheath extends from the initial segments of the axon to the terminal branches. Interspersed along the length of a myelinated axon are small gaps or spaces in the myelin sheath between individual cells that myelinated the axons. These gaps are called **nodes of Ranvier.** Axons in both the CNS and the PNS can be either myelinated or remain unmyelinated.

In the PNS, all axons are surrounded by specialized **Schwann cells** that either myelinate the axons or envelope the unmyelinated axons. Schwann cells myelinate individual peripheral axons and extend along their length, from their origin to their termination in the muscle or gland. In contrast, each Schwann cell can envelope numerous unmyelinated axons; unmyelinated axons do not show nodes of Ranvier because the Schwann cells form a continuous sheath. Smaller axons in the peripheral nerves, such as those in the autonomic nervous system (ANS), are unmyelinated and surrounded only by the Schwann cell cytoplasm.

There are no Schwann cells in the CNS. Instead, neuroglial cells called **oligodendrocytes** myelinate the axons in the CNS. Oligodendrocytes differ from Schwann cells in that the cytoplasmic extensions of one oligodendrocyte envelopes and myelinates numerous axons.

White and Gray Matter

The brain and the spinal cord contain gray matter and white matter. The **gray matter** of the CNS consists of neurons, their dendrites, and the supportive cells called **neuroglia.** This region represents the site of connections or **synapses** between a multitude of neurons and dendrites. Gray matter covers the surface of the brain (cerebrum) and cerebellum. The size, shape, and mode of branching of these neurons are highly variable and depend on which region of the CNS is examined.

White matter in the CNS is devoid of neuronal cell bodies and consists primarily of myelinated axons, some unmyelinated axons, and the supportive neuroglial oligodendrocytes. The myelin sheaths around the axons impart a white color to this region of the CNS.

Supporting Cells in the CNS: Neuroglia

Neuroglia are the highly branched, supportive, nonneuronal cells in the CNS that surround the neurons, their axons, and dendrites. These cells do not become stimulated or conduct impulses, but are morphologically and functionally different from the neurons. Neuroglial cells can be distinguished by their much smaller size and dark-staining nuclei. The CNS contains approximately tenfold more neuroglial cells than neurons. The four types of neuroglia cells are **astrocytes, oligodendrocytes, microglia,** and **ependymal cells.**

FIGURE 7.1 ■ Spinal Cord: Midthoracic Region (Transverse Section)

A transverse section of a spinal cord cut in the midthoracic region and stained with hematoxylin and eosin is illustrated. Although a basic structural pattern is seen throughout the spinal cord, the shape and structure of the cord vary at different levels (cervical, thoracic, lumbar, and sacral).

The thoracic region of the spinal cord differs from the cervical region illustrated in Figure 7.3. The thoracic spinal cord exhibits slender **posterior gray horns (6)** and smaller **anterior gray horns (10, 20)** with fewer **motor neurons (10, 20)**. The **lateral gray horns (8, 19)**, on the other hand, are well developed in the thoracic region of the spinal cord. These contain the **motor neurons (8, 19)** of the sympathetic division of the autonomic nervous system.

The remaining structures in the midthoracic region of the spinal cord closely correspond to the structures illustrated in the cervical cord region in Figure 7.3. These are the **posterior median sulcus (15), anterior median fissure (22), fasciculus gracilis (16)** and **fasciculus cuneatus (17)** (seen in the mid to upper thoracic region of the spinal cord) of the **posterior white column (16, 17), lateral white column (7), central canal (9)**, and the **gray commissure (18)**. Associated with the posterior gray horns (6) are axons of the **posterior roots (5)**, and leaving the anterior gray horns (10, 20) are the **axons (11, 21)** of the **anterior roots (11)**.

Surrounding the spinal cord are the connective tissue layers of the meninges. These are the thick and fibrous outer **dura mater (2)**, the thinner and middle **arachnoid mater (3)**, and the delicate inner **pia mater (4)**, which closely adheres to the surface of the spinal cord. Located in the pia mater (4) are numerous anterior and posterior **spinal blood vessels (1, 12)** of various sizes. Between the arachnoid (3) and the pia mater (4) is the **subarachnoid space (14)**. Fine trabeculae located in the subarachnoid space (14) connect the pia mater (4) with the arachnoid mater (3). In life, the subarachnoid space (14) is filled with circulating CSF. Between the arachnoid mater (3) and the dura mater (2) is the **subdural space (13)**. In this preparation, the subdural space (13) appears unusually large because of the artifactual retraction of the arachnoid during the specimen preparation.

FIGURE 7.2 ■ Spinal Cord: Anterior Gray Horn, Motor Neurons, and Adjacent Anterior White Matter

A higher magnification of a small section of the spinal cord illustrates the appearance of gray matter, white matter, neurons, neuroglia, and axons stained with hematoxylin and eosin. The cells in the anterior gray horn of the thoracic region of the spinal cord are **multipolar motor neurons (2, 6)**. Their cytoplasm is characterized by a prominent vesicular **nucleus (7)**, a distinct **nucleolus (7)**, and coarse clumps of basophilic material called the **Nissl substance (3)**. The Nissl substance extends into the **dendrites (5)** but not into the axons. One such neuron exhibits the root of an axon and the **axon hillock (4)**, which is devoid of the Nissl substance and characterizes the axon hillock.

The nonneural **neuroglia (8)**, seen here only as basophilic nuclei, are small in comparison to the prominent multipolar neurons (2, 4). The neuroglia (8) occupy the spaces between the neurons. The anterior white matter of the spinal cord contains myelinated axons of various sizes. Because of the chemicals used in histologic preparation of this section, the myelin sheaths appear as clear spaces around the dark-staining **axons (1)**.

In certain neurons (2), the plane of section did not include the nucleus, and the cytoplasm appears enucleated (without nucleus).

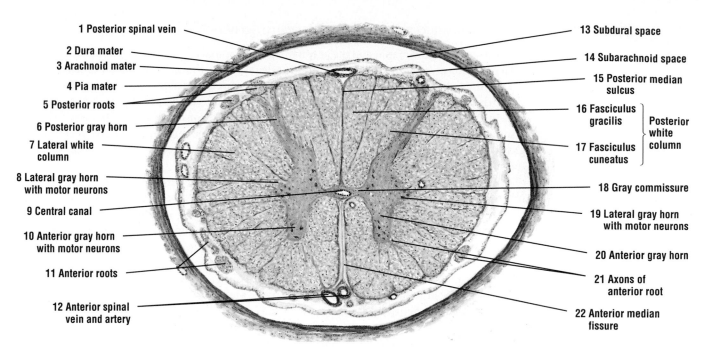

1 Posterior spinal vein

2 Dura mater

3 Arachnoid mater

4 Pia mater

5 Posterior roots

6 Posterior gray horn

7 Lateral white column

8 Lateral gray horn with motor neurons

9 Central canal

10 Anterior gray horn with motor neurons

11 Anterior roots

12 Anterior spinal vein and artery

13 Subdural space

14 Subarachnoid space

15 Posterior median sulcus

16 Fasciculus gracilis \
17 Fasciculus cuneatus — Posterior white column

18 Gray commissure

19 Lateral gray horn with motor neurons

20 Anterior gray horn

21 Axons of anterior root

22 Anterior median fissure

FIGURE 7.1 ■ Spinal cord: midthoracic region (transverse section). Stain: hematoxylin and eosin. Low magnification.

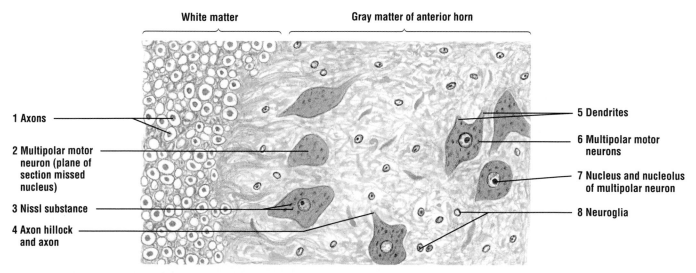

White matter

Gray matter of anterior horn

1 Axons

2 Multipolar motor neuron (plane of section missed nucleus)

3 Nissl substance

4 Axon hillock and axon

5 Dendrites

6 Multipolar motor neurons

7 Nucleus and nucleolus of multipolar neuron

8 Neuroglia

FIGURE 7.2 ■ Spinal cord: anterior gray horn, motor neuron, and adjacent white matter. Stain: hematoxylin and eosin. Medium magnification.

FIGURE 7.3 ■ Spinal Cord: Midcervical Region (Transverse Section)

To illustrate the white matter and the gray matter of the spinal cord, a cross section of the cord was prepared with silver impregnation technique. After staining, the dark brown, outer **white matter** (3) and the light-staining, inner **gray matter** (4, 14) are clearly visible. The white matter (3) consists primarily of ascending and descending myelinated nerve fibers or axons. By contrast, the gray matter contains the cell bodies of neurons and interneurons. The gray matter also exhibits a symmetrical H-shape, with the two sides connected across the midline of the spinal cord by the **gray commissure** (15). The center of the gray commissure is located at the **central canal** (16) of the spinal cord.

The **anterior horns** (6) of the gray matter extend toward the front of the cord and are more prominent than the **posterior horns** (2, 13). The anterior horns contain the cell bodies of the large **motor neurons** (7, 17). Some **axons** (8, 20) from the motor neurons of the anterior horns cross the white matter and exit from the spinal cord as components of the **anterior roots** (9, 21) of the peripheral nerves. The posterior horns (2, 13) are the sensory areas and contain cell bodies of smaller neurons.

The spinal cord is surrounded by connective tissue meninges, consisting of an outer dura mater, a middle **arachnoid mater** (5), and an inner **pia mater** (18). The spinal cord is also partially divided into right and left halves by a narrow, posterior (dorsal) groove, the **posterior median sulcus** (10), and a deep, anterior (ventral) cleft, the **anterior median fissure** (19). In this illustration, pia mater (18) is best seen in the **anterior median fissure** (19).

Between the posterior median sulcus (10) and the posterior horns (2, 13) of the gray matter are the prominent posterior columns of the white matter. In this midcervical region of the spinal cord, each dorsal column is subdivided into two fascicles, the posteromedial column, the **fasciculus gracilis** (11), and the posterolateral column, the **fasciculus cuneatus** (1, 12).

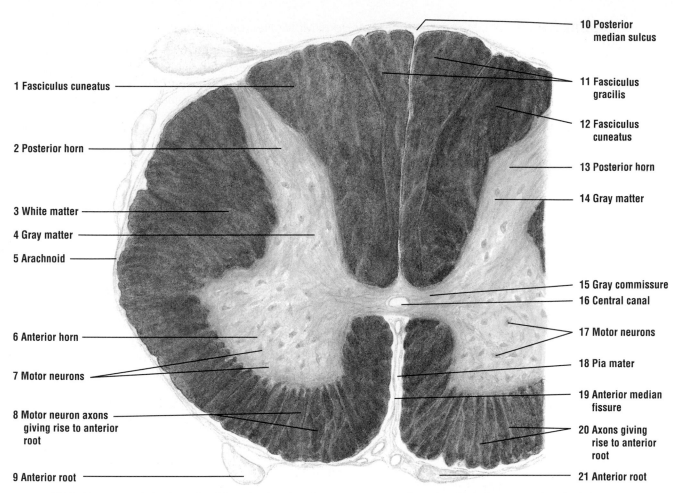

1 Fasciculus cuneatus

2 Posterior horn

3 White matter

4 Gray matter

5 Arachnoid

6 Anterior horn

7 Motor neurons

8 Motor neuron axons giving rise to anterior root

9 Anterior root

10 Posterior median sulcus

11 Fasciculus gracilis

12 Fasciculus cuneatus

13 Posterior horn

14 Gray matter

15 Gray commissure

16 Central canal

17 Motor neurons

18 Pia mater

19 Anterior median fissure

20 Axons giving rise to anterior root

21 Anterior root

FIGURE 7.3 ■ Spinal cord: midcervical region (transverse section). Stain: silver impregnation (Cajal's method). Low magnification.

FIGURE 7.4 ■ Spinal Cord: Anterior Gray Horn, Motor Neurons, and Adjacent Anterior White Matter

A small section of the white matter and the gray matter of the anterior horn of the spinal cord are illustrated at a higher magnification. The gray matter of the anterior horn contains large, **multipolar motor neurons (2, 3).** These are characterized by numerous **dendrites (5, 6)** that extend in different directions from the perikaryon (cell bodies). In some sections of the neurons, the **nucleus (8)** is visible with its prominent **nucleolus (8).** In other neurons, the plane of section has missed the nucleus and the perikaryon appears empty (2). Located in the vicinity of the motor neurons are the small, light-staining, supportive cells, the **neuroglia (7).**

The white matter contains closely packed groups of myelinated axons. In cross sections, the **axons (1)** appear dark-stained and surrounded by clear spaces, which are the remnants of the myelin sheaths. The axons of the white matter represent the ascending and descending tracts of the spinal cord. On the other hand, the **axons (4)** of the anterior horn motor neurons aggregate into groups, pass through the white matter, and exit from the spinal cord as the anterior (ventral) root fibers (see Figure 7.3).

FUNCTIONAL CORRELATIONS: Neurons, Interneurons, Axons, and Dendrites

Functionally, neurons are classified as **afferent** (sensory), **efferent** (motor), or **interneurons.** Sensory or afferent neurons conduct impulses from receptors in the internal organs or from the external environment to the CNS. Motor or efferent neurons convey impulses from the CNS to the effector muscles or glands in the periphery. Interneurons constitute the majority of the neurons in the CNS. They serve as intermediaries or integrators of nerve impulses and connect neuronal circuits between sensory neurons, motor neurons, and other interneurons in the CNS.

Neurons are highly specialized for **irritability, conductivity,** and **synthesis** of neuroactive substances such as **neurotransmitters** and **neurohormones.** After a mechanical or chemical stimulus, these neurons react (irritability) to the stimulus and transmit (conductivity) the information via axons to other neurons in different regions of the nervous system. Strong stimuli create a wave of excitation, or nerve impulse (action potential), that is then propagated along the entire length of the axon (nerve fiber).

Axons arise from the funnel-shaped region of the cell body called the axon hillock. The **initial segmen**t of the axon is located between the axon hillock and where myelination starts. It is at the initial segment that the stimuli, whether inhibitory or stimulatory, are summated and the resulting nerve stimuli generated. The rate of conduction of the stimulus is dependent on the size of the axon and myelination. Myelinated axons conduct impulses at a much faster rate (velocity) than the unmyelinated axons of the same size. In addition to conducting impulses, axons also transport chemical substances or neurotransmitters. These are first synthesized in the cell body and transported in small tubules called microtubules to the region where the axon terminates or **synapses** with other dendrites, a cell body, or other axons. Neurotransmitters are released during a nerve stimulus.

The surface of the dendrites is covered by **dendritic spines** that connect (synapse) with axon terminals from other neurons. The surface membrane of the soma and the dendrites are specialized to receive and to integrate information from other dendrites, neurons, or axons. The axons, in turn, conduct the received information away from the neuron to an interneuron, another neuron, or to an effector organ such as a muscle or gland.

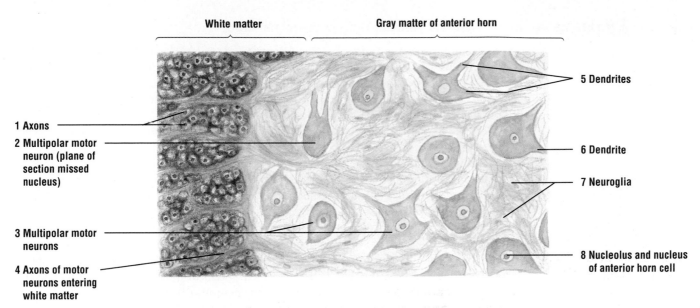

White matter   **Gray matter of anterior horn**

1 Axons

2 Multipolar motor
  neuron (plane of
  section missed
  nucleus)

3 Multipolar motor
  neurons

4 Axons of motor
  neurons entering
  white matter

5 Dendrites

6 Dendrite

7 Neuroglia

8 Nucleolus and nucleus
  of anterior horn cell

FIGURE 7.4 ■ Spinal cord: anterior gray horn, motor neurons, and adjacent anterior white matter. Stain: silver impregnation (Cajal's method). Medium magnification.

FIGURE 7.5 ■ Motor Neurons: Anterior Horn of the Spinal Cord

The large, multipolar **motor neurons (7)** of the CNS have a large central **nucleus (11)**, a prominent **nucleolus (12)**, and several radiating cell processes, the **dendrites (10, 16)**. A single, thin **axon (5, 14)** arises from a cone-shaped, clear area of the neuron; this is the **axon hillock (6, 13)**. The axons (5, 14) that leave the motor neurons (7) are thinner and much longer than the thicker but shorter dendrites (10, 16).

The cytoplasm or perikaryon of the neuron is characterized by numerous clumps of coarse granules (basophilic masses). These are the **Nissl bodies (4, 8),** and they represent the granular endoplasmic reticulum of the neuron. When the plane of section misses the nucleus (4), only the dark-staining Nissl bodies (4) are seen in the perikaryon of the neuron. The Nissl bodies (4, 8) extend into the dendrites (10, 16) but not into the axon hillock (6, 13) or into the axon (5, 14). This feature distinguishes the axons (5, 14) from the dendrites (10, 16). The nucleus of the neuron (11) is outlined distinctly and stains light because of the uniform dispersion of the chromatin. The nucleolus (12), on the other hand, is prominent, dense, and stains dark. The **nuclei (2, 9)** of the surrounding **neuroglia (2, 9)** are stained prominently, whereas their small cytoplasm remains unstained. The neuroglia (2, 9) are nonneural cells of the central nervous system; they provide the structural and metabolic support for the neurons (7).

Surrounding the neurons (7) and the neuroglia (2, 9) are numerous blood vessels (**1, 3, 15**) of various sizes.

FIGURE 7.6 ■ Neurofibrils and Motor Neurons in the Gray Matter of the Anterior Horn of the Spinal Cord

This section of the anterior horn of the spinal cord was prepared by silver impregnation (Cajal's method) to demonstrate the distribution of neurofibrils in both the gray matter and motor neurons. Fine **neurofibrils (2, 4)** are distributed throughout the **cytoplasm (perikaryon) (4)** and **dendrites (2, 9)** of the **motor neurons (1, 10, 11)**.

Because of the silver impregnation technique, axons and additional details of the motor neurons are not visible. The nuclei of the **motor neurons (1, 11)** appear yellow stained and their **nucleoli (5, 10)** dark stained. Not all motor neurons were sectioned through the middle. As a result, some motor neurons show only a **nucleus (1)** without a nucleolus, whereas others only show **peripheral cytoplasm (8)** without a nucleus.

There are also many **neurofibrils** in the **gray matter (3)**. Some of these neurofibrils (3) belong to the axons of anterior horn neurons (1, 11) or the adjacent **neuroglia (7)**, whose **nuclei (7)** are visible throughout the gray matter (3) (see also Figure 7.7).

The clear spaces around the neurons and their processes are artifacts that were caused by the chemical preparations of the nervous tissue.

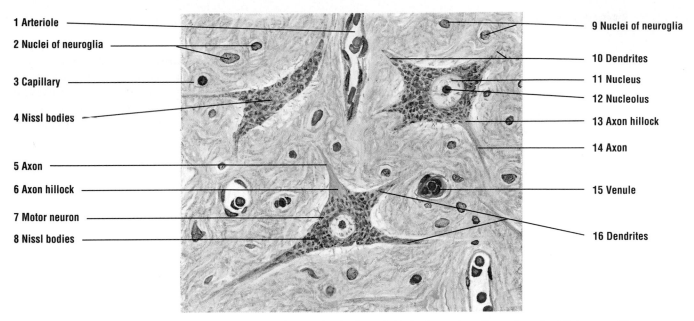

1 Arteriole
2 Nuclei of neuroglia
3 Capillary
4 Nissl bodies
5 Axon
6 Axon hillock
7 Motor neuron
8 Nissl bodies
9 Nuclei of neuroglia
10 Dendrites
11 Nucleus
12 Nucleolus
13 Axon hillock
14 Axon
15 Venule
16 Dendrites

FIGURE 7.5 ■ Motor neurons: anterior horn of spinal cord. Stain: hematoxylin and eosin. High magnification.

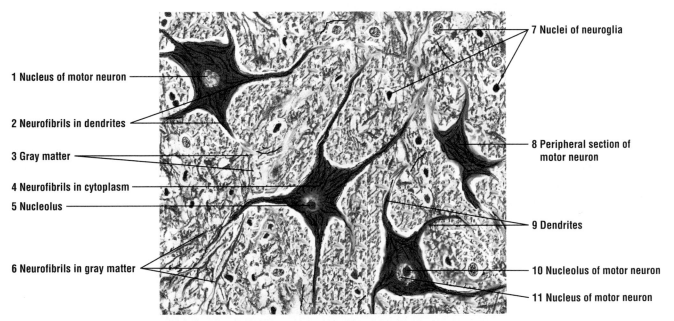

1 Nucleus of motor neuron
2 Neurofibrils in dendrites
3 Gray matter
4 Neurofibrils in cytoplasm
5 Nucleolus
6 Neurofibrils in gray matter
7 Nuclei of neuroglia
8 Peripheral section of motor neuron
9 Dendrites
10 Nucleolus of motor neuron
11 Nucleus of motor neuron

FIGURE 7.6 ■ Neurofibrils and motor neurons in the gray matter of the anterior horn of the spinal cord. Stain: silver impregnation (Cajal's method). High magnification.

FIGURE 7.7 ■ Anterior Gray Horn of Spinal Cord: Multipolar Motor Neurons, Axons, and Neuroglial Cells

This medium-magnification photomicrograph of the anterior horn of the spinal cord was prepared with silver stain to show the morphology of neurons and axons of the central nervous system. The large multipolar **motor neurons (1)** of the gray horn exhibit numerous **dendrites (4).** Each motor neuron (1) contains a distinct **nucleus (5)** and a prominent **nucleolus (6).** Within the cytoplasm of the motor neurons (1) is the cytoskeleton, which consists of numerous **neurofibrils (3)** that course through the cell body and extend into the dendrites (4) and **axons (8).** Coursing past the motor neurons (1) are numerous axons of different size (8) from other nerve cells in the spinal cord. Surrounding the motor neurons (1) are numerous **nuclei** of **neuroglial cells (2)** and a **blood vessel (7)** with blood cells.

Similar to Figure 7.6, the clear spaces around the neurons and their processes are artifacts caused by tissue shrinkage during the preparation of the spinal cord.

FIGURE 7.8 ■ Cerebral Cortex: Gray Matter

The different cell types that constitute the gray matter of the cerebral cortex are distributed in six layers, with one or more cell types predominant in each layer. Although there are variations in the arrangement of cells in different parts of the cerebral cortex, distinct layers are recognized in most regions. Horizontal and radial axons associated with neuronal cells in different layers give the cerebral cortex a laminated appearance. The different layers are labeled with Roman numerals on the right side of the figure.

The most superficial is the **molecular layer (I).** Overlying and covering the molecular cell layer (I) is the delicate connective tissue of the brain, the **pia mater (1).** The peripheral portion of molecular layer (I) is composed predominantly of **neuroglial cells (2)** and horizontal cells of Cajal. Their axons contribute to the horizontal fibers that are seen in the molecular layer (I).

The **external granular layer (II)** contains mainly different types of neuroglial cells and **small pyramidal cells (3).** Note that the pyramidal cells get progressively larger in successively deeper layers of the cortex. The **apical dendrites** of the **pyramidal cells (4, 7)** are directed toward the periphery of the cortex, whereas their axons extend from the cell bases [see Figure 7.9 (4, 10) below]. In the **external pyramidal layer (III), medium-sized pyramidal cells (5)** predominate. The **internal granular layer (IV)** is a thin layer and contains mainly small **granule cells (6),** some pyramidal cells, and different neuroglia that form numerous complex connections with the pyramidal cells. The **internal pyramidal layer (V)** contains numerous neuroglial cells and the largest **pyramidal cells (8),** especially in the motor area of the cerebral cortex. The deepest layer is the **multiform layer (VI).** This layer is adjacent to the **white matter (10)** of the cerebral cortex. The multiform layer (VI) contains intermixed cells of varying shapes and sizes, such as the fusiform cells, granule cells, stellate cells, and cells of Martinotti. **Bundles of axons (9)** enter and leave the white matter (10).

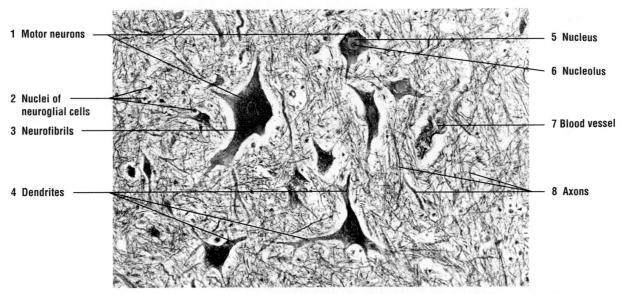

1 Motor neurons
2 Nuclei of neuroglial cells
3 Neurofibrils
4 Dendrites
5 Nucleus
6 Nucleolus
7 Blood vessel
8 Axons

FIGURE 7.7 ■ Anterior gray horn of the spinal cord: multipolar neurons, axons, and neuroglial cells. Stain: silver impregnation (Cajal's method). ×80.

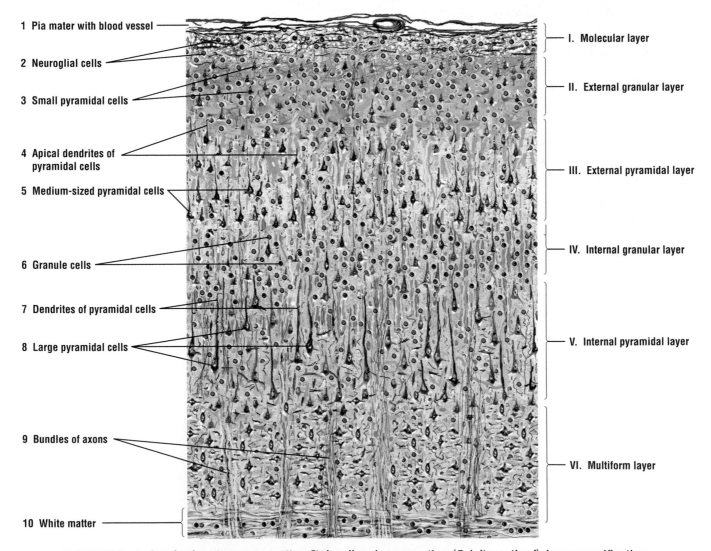

1 Pia mater with blood vessel
2 Neuroglial cells
3 Small pyramidal cells
4 Apical dendrites of pyramidal cells
5 Medium-sized pyramidal cells
6 Granule cells
7 Dendrites of pyramidal cells
8 Large pyramidal cells
9 Bundles of axons
10 White matter

I. Molecular layer
II. External granular layer
III. External pyramidal layer
IV. Internal granular layer
V. Internal pyramidal layer
VI. Multiform layer

FIGURE 7.8 ■ Cerebral cortex: gray matter: Stain: silver impregnation (Cajal's method). Low magnification.

FIGURE 7.9 ■ Layer V of the Cerebral Cortex

A higher magnification of layer V of the cerebral cortex illustrates the large **pyramidal cells (3)**. Note the typical large vesicular **nucleus (3)** with its prominent **nucleolus (3)**. The silver stain also shows the presence of numerous **neurofibrils (9)** in the pyramidal cells (3). The most prominent cell processes are the **apical dendrites (1, 7)** of the pyramidal cells (3), which are directed toward the surface of the cortex. The **axons (4, 10)** of the pyramidal cells (3) arise from the base of the cell body and pass into the white matter [see Figure 7.8 (10) above].

The intercellular area is occupied by **neuroglial cells (2, 8)** in the cortex, small astrocytes, and blood vessels, **venule (5)** and **capillary (6)**.

FIGURE 7.10 ■ Cerebellum (Transverse Section)

The **cerebellar cortex (1, 10)** exhibits numerous deeply convoluted folds called **cerebellar folia (6)** (singular, folium) separated by **sulci (9)**. The cerebellar folia (6) are covered by the thin connective tissue, the **pia mater (7)**, that follows the surface of each folium (6) into the adjacent sulci (9). The detachment of the pia mater (7) from the cerebellar cortex (1, 10) is an artifact caused by tissue fixation and preparation.

The cerebellum (1, 10) consists of an outer **gray matter or cortex (1, 10)** and an inner **white matter (5, 8)**. Three distinct cell layers can be distinguished in the cerebellar cortex (1, 10): an outer **molecular layer (2)** with relatively fewer and smaller neuronal cell bodies and many fibers that extend parallel to the length of the folium; a central or middle **Purkinje cell layer (3);** and an inner **granular layer (4)** with numerous small neurons that exhibit intensely stained nuclei. The Purkinje cells (3) are pyriform or pyramidal in shape with ramified dendrites that extend into the molecular layer (2).

The white matter (5, 8) forms the core of each cerebellar folium (6) and consists of myelinated nerve fibers or axons. The nerve axons are the afferent and efferent fibers of the cerebellar cortex.

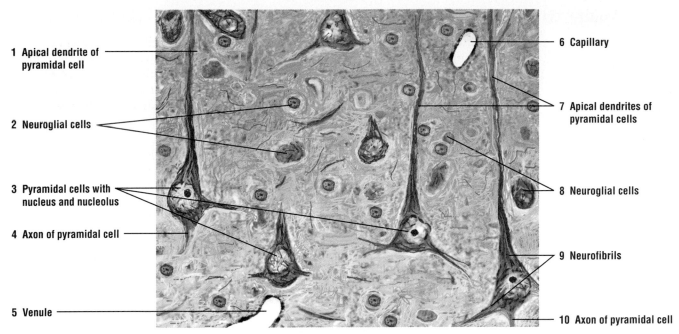

1 Apical dendrite of pyramidal cell

2 Neuroglial cells

3 Pyramidal cells with nucleus and nucleolus

4 Axon of pyramidal cell

5 Venule

6 Capillary

7 Apical dendrites of pyramidal cells

8 Neuroglial cells

9 Neurofibrils

10 Axon of pyramidal cell

FIGURE 7.9 ■ Layer V of the cerebral cortex. Stain: silver impregnation (Cajal's method). High magnification.

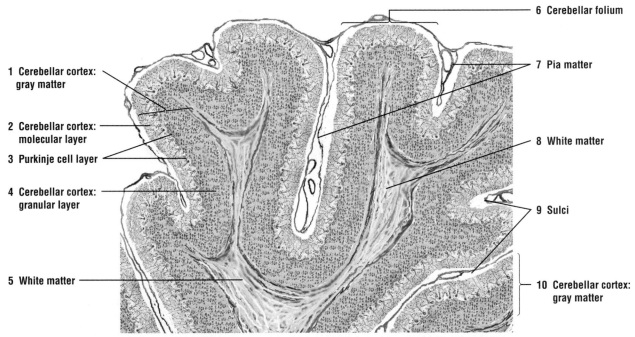

1 Cerebellar cortex: gray matter

2 Cerebellar cortex: molecular layer

3 Purkinje cell layer

4 Cerebellar cortex: granular layer

5 White matter

6 Cerebellar folium

7 Pia matter

8 White matter

9 Sulci

10 Cerebellar cortex: gray matter

FIGURE 7.10 ■ Cerebellum (transverse section). Stain: silver impregnation (Cajal's method). Low magnification.

FIGURE 7.11 ■ Cerebellar Cortex: Molecular Layer, Purkinje Cell Layer, and Granular Cell Layer

This illustration shows a small section of cerebellar cortex above the white matter at a higher magnification. The **Purkinje cells (3)** comprising the **Purkinje cell layer (7)**, with their prominent nuclei and nucleoli, are arranged in a single row between the **molecular cell layer (6)** and the **granular cell layer (4)**. The large "flask-shaped" bodies of the Purkinje cells (3, 7) give off thick **dendrites (2)** that branch extensively throughout the molecular cell layer (6) to the cerebellar surface. Thin axons (not shown) leave the base of the Purkinje cells, pass through the granular cell layer (4), become myelinated, and enter the **white matter (5, 11)**.

The molecular cell layer (6) contains scattered **basket cells (1)** whose unmyelinated axons normally course horizontally. Descending collaterals of more deeply placed basket cells (1) arborize around the Purkinje cells (3, 7). Axons of the **granule cells (9)** in the granular cell layer (4) extend into the molecular layer (6) and also course horizontally as unmyelinated axons.

In the granular cell layer (4) are numerous small granule cells (9) with dark-staining nuclei and a small amount of cytoplasm. Also scattered in the granular cell layer (4) are larger **Golgi type II cells (8)** with typical vesicular nuclei and more cytoplasm. Throughout the granular layer are small, irregularly dispersed, clear spaces called the **glomeruli (10).** These regions contain only synaptic complexes.

FIGURE 7.12 ■ Fibrous Astrocytes of the Brain

A section of the brain was prepared by Cajal's method to demonstrate the supportive neuroglial cells called astrocytes. The **fibrous astrocytes (2, 5)** exhibit a small **cell body (5)**, a large oval **nucleus (5)**, and a **dark-stained nucleolus (5).** Extending from the cell body are long, thin, and smooth radiating **processes (4, 6)** that are found between the neurons and blood vessels. A **perivascular fibrous astrocyte (2)** surrounds a **capillary (8)** with red blood cells (erythrocytes). From other fibrous astrocytes (2, 5), the long processes (4, 6) extend to and terminate on the capillary (8) as **perivascular end feet (3, 7).**

Also seen in the illustration are nuclei of different **neuroglial (1)** cells of the brain.

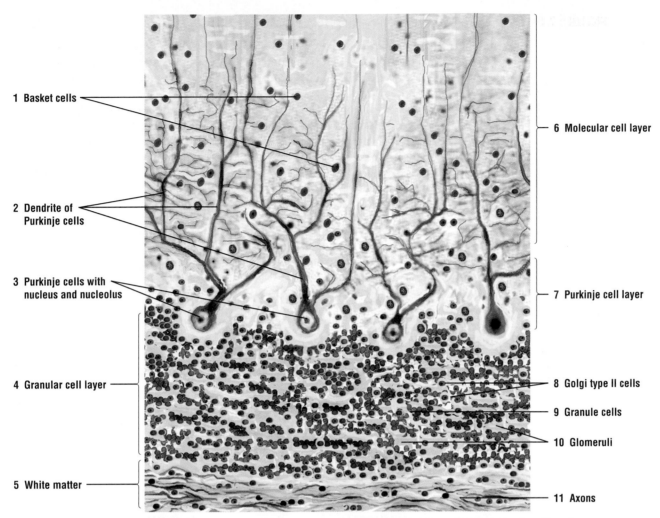

1 Basket cells

2 Dendrite of Purkinje cells

3 Purkinje cells with nucleus and nucleolus

4 Granular cell layer

5 White matter

6 Molecular cell layer

7 Purkinje cell layer

8 Golgi type II cells

9 Granule cells

10 Glomeruli

11 Axons

FIGURE 7.11 ■ Cerebellar cortex: molecular, Purkinje cell, and granular cell layers. Stain: silver impregnation (Cajal's method). High magnification.

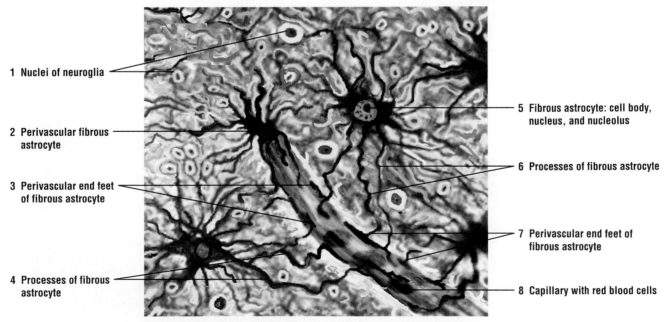

1 Nuclei of neuroglia

2 Perivascular fibrous astrocyte

3 Perivascular end feet of fibrous astrocyte

4 Processes of fibrous astrocyte

5 Fibrous astrocyte: cell body, nucleus, and nucleolus

6 Processes of fibrous astrocyte

7 Perivascular end feet of fibrous astrocyte

8 Capillary with red blood cells

FIGURE 7.12 ■ Fibrous astrocytes and capillary in the brain. Stain: silver impregnation (Cajal's method). Medium magnification.

FIGURE 7.13 ■ Oligodendrocytes of the Brain

This section of the brain was also prepared with Cajal's method to show the supportive neuroglial cells called **oligodendrocytes (1, 4, 7).** In comparison to a **fibrous astrocyte (3),** the oligodendrocytes (1, 4, 7) are smaller and exhibit few, thin, short processes without excessive branching.

The oligodendrocytes (1, 4, 7) are found in both the gray and white matter of the CNS. In the white matter, the oligodendrocytes form myelin sheaths around numerous axons and are analogous to the Schwann cells that myelinate individual axons in the nerves of the PNS.

Two **neurons (2, 6)** are also illustrated to contrast their size with those of fibrous astrocyte (3) and the oligodendrocytes (1, 4, 7). A **capillary (5)** passes between the different cells.

FIGURE 7.14 ■ Microglia of the Brain

This section of the brain was prepared with Hortega's method to show the smallest neuroglial cells called **microglia (2, 3).** The microglia (2, 3) vary in shape and often exhibit irregular contours, and the small, deeply stained nucleus almost fills the entire cell. The cell processes of the microglia (2, 3) are few, short, and slender. Both the cell body and the processes of microglia (2, 3) are covered with small spines. Two **neurons (1)** and a **capillary** with **red blood cells (erythrocytes) (4)** provide a size comparison with the microglia (2, 3).

Microglia are found in both the white and gray matter of the CNS, and are the main phagocytes of the CNS.

FUNCTIONAL CORRELATIONS: Neuroglia

There are four types of neuroglial cells recognized in the CNS: astrocytes, oligodendrocytes, microglia, and ependymal cells.

Astrocytes are the largest and most abundant neuroglia cells in the gray matter and consist of two types: fibrous astrocytes and protoplasmic astrocytes. In the CNS, both types of astrocytes abut the surface **capillaries** and **neurons.** The perivascular feet of astrocytes cover the capillary basement membrane and form part of the **blood-brain barrier,** which restricts the movement of molecules from the blood into the interstitium of the CNS. The processes of astrocytes also extend to the basal lamina of the pia mater to form an impermeable barrier, the **glia limitans** or glial limiting membrane, that surrounds the brain and spinal cord. They also support **metabolic exchange** between neurons and the capillaries of the CNS. In addition, the astrocytes control the **chemical environment** around neurons by clearing intercellular spaces of increased **potassium ions** and released **neurotransmitters,** such as **glutamate,** at active synaptic sites to maintain a proper ionic environment for their function. If these metabolic chemicals are not quickly removed from these sites, they can interfere with neuronal functions. Astrocytes remove glutamate and convert it to glutamine, which is then returned to the neurons. Astrocytes also contain reserves of glycogen, from which they release as glucose, and in this manner, they contribute to the energy metabolism of the CNS.

Oligodendrocytes are smaller than astrocytes with fewer cytoplasmic processes. Oligodendrocytes **myelinate** the axons in the CNS. Because oligodendrocytes have numerous processes, a single oligodendrocyte can surround and myelinate several axons. In the PNS, a different type of supporting cell, called the **Schwann cell,** myelinates the axons. In contrast to oligodendrocytes, a Schwann cell only forms a myelin sheath around the internode of a single myelinated axon.

Microglia are the smallest neuroglial cells. The dark-staining microglia are believed to be part of the **mononuclear phagocyte system** of the CNS that originates from precursor cells in the bone marrow. Microglia are found throughout the CNS, and their main function is similar to that of the **macrophages** of the connective tissue. When nervous tissue is injured or damaged, microglia migrate to the region, proliferate, become phagocytic, and remove dead or foreign tissue.

Ependymal cells are simple cuboidal or low columnar epithelial cells that line the ventricles of the brain and the central canal in the spinal cord. Their apices contain cilia and microvilli. Cilia facilitate the movement of the cerebrospinal fluid through the central canal of the spinal cord, whereas microvilli may have some absorptive functions.

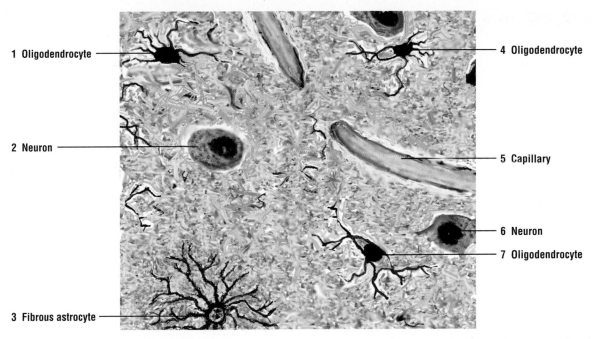

1 Oligodendrocyte

2 Neuron

3 Fibrous astrocyte

4 Oligodendrocyte

5 Capillary

6 Neuron

7 Oligodendrocyte

FIGURE 7.13 ■ Oligodendrocytes of the brain. Stain: silver impregnation (Cajal's method). Medium magnification.

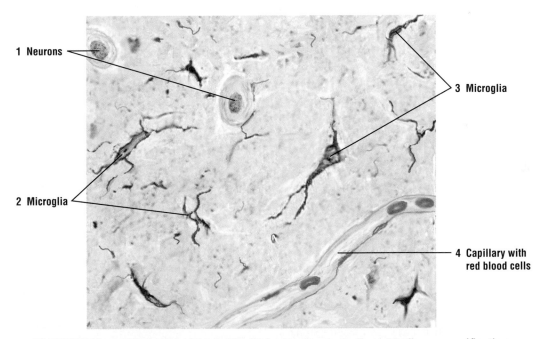

1 Neurons

2 Microglia

3 Microglia

4 Capillary with red blood cells

FIGURE 7.14 ■ Microglia of the brain. Stain: Hortega's method. Medium magnification.

CHAPTER 7 ■ Summary

SECTION 1 ■ The Central Nervous System: Brain and Spinal Cord

The Mammalian Nervous System

- Central nervous system (CNS) consists of the brain and spinal cord
- Peripheral nervous system (PNS) consists of cranial and spinal nerves

Central Nervous System

- Surrounded by bones and cerebrospinal fluid
- Dura mater is the tough outermost connective tissue layer around the CNS
- Delicate arachnoid mater and dura cover CNS on external surfaces
- Pia mater adheres to surface of brain and spinal cord
- Between pia mater and arachnoid mater is subarachnoid space
- Cerebrospinal fluid circulates in subarachnoid space

Cerebrospinal Fluid

- Clear, colorless fluid cushions and protects brain and spinal cord
- Continually produced by choroid plexuses in brain ventricles
- Important for homeostasis and brain metabolism
- Reabsorbed into venous blood (superior sagittal sinus) via arachnoid villi

Morphology and Types of Neurons in CNS

- Structural and functional units of CNS
- Consist of soma or cell body, dendrites, and axon
- Three main types are multipolar, bipolar, and unipolar
- Multipolar are most common and include all motor neurons and interneurons
- Multipolar neurons contain numerous dendrites and a single axon
- Bipolar neurons are sensory and found in eyes, nose, and ears
- Bipolar neurons contain single dendrite and single axon
- Unipolar neurons are found in sensory ganglia and spinal nerves
- Unipolar neurons contain one process from the cell body and are sensory
- Interneurons found in CNS integrate and coordinate stimuli between sensory, motor, and other interneurons

Myelin Sheath and Myelination of Axons

- Specialized cells wrap around axons to form lipid-rich, insulating myelin sheath
- Myelin sheath extends along length of axon to its terminal branches
- Gaps between myelin sheath are nodes of Ranvier
- In PNS, Schwann cells myelinate axons and envelope unmyelinated axons
- Unmyelinated axons do not show nodes of Ranvier
- In CNS, neuroglial oligodendrocyte cells myelinate numerous axons

White and Gray Matter

- Gray matter contains neurons, dendrites, and neuroglia
- Site of synapse between neurons and dendrites in gray matter
- Posterior horns of spinal cord associated with axons of posterior roots
- Anterior horns of spinal cord associated with axons of anterior roots
- White matter contains only myelinated axons, unmyelinated axons, and neuroglia

Spinal Cord

- Thoracic region of spinal cord contains anterior, posterior, and lateral gray horns
- Lateral horns contain motor neurons of sympathetic division of autonomic nervous system
- Anterior horns of gray matter contain motor neurons
- Axons from anterior horns form anterior roots of spinal nerves
- White matter contains closely packed ascending and descending axons
- Posterior columns of white matter contain fasciculus gracilis and fasciculus cuneatus
- Gray matter inside the spinal cord is H-shaped and contains neurons and interneurons
- Gray commissure connects two sides of the gray matter and contains the central canal

Neurons, Axons, and Dendrites

- Classified as afferent (sensory), efferent (motor), or interneurons
- Neuron cell body and dendrites contain Nissl substance (granular endoplasmic reticulum)
- Neurofibrils in neuron cell body extend into dendrites and axons
- Axons arise from funnel-shaped region called axon hillock
- Axon and axon hillock are devoid of Nissl substance
- Afferent neurons conduct impulses via axons from internal or external receptor into the CNS
- Efferent neurons conduct impulses via axons from CNS to muscles or glands
- Neurons synthesize neurotransmitters in cell body
- Axons transport neurotransmitters in microtubules to synapses

- Stimuli cause conduction of nerve impulse (action potential) along the axons
- Initial segment of axon is site where stimuli are summated and nerve impulse generated
- Rate of impulse conduction dependent on axon size and myelination
- Dendrites are covered with dendritic spines for connections (synapses) with other neurons
- Dendrites receive and integrate information from dendrites, neurons, or axons

Supportive Cells in the CNS: Neuroglia

- Supportive, nonneural cells that surround neurons, axons, and dendrites
- Small cells that do not conduct impulses
- Ten times more numerous than neurons
- Four types: astrocytes, oligodendrocytes, microglia, and ependymal cells

Astrocytes

- Are the largest and most numerous in gray matter
- Consist of two types, fibrous astrocytes and protoplasmic astrocytes
- Both types abut on capillaries and neurons, and form blood-brain barrier
- Form glial limiting membrane that surrounds the brain and spinal cord
- Support metabolic exchange and contribute to energy metabolism of CNS
- Control chemical environment around neurons by clearing neurotransmitters

Oligodendrocytes

- Surround and myelinate numerous axons at one time, in contrast to Schwann cells

Microglia

- Part of the mononuclear phagocyte system and found throughout CNS
- Phagocytic cells in the CNS, similar to connective tissue macrophages

Ependymal Cells

- Line the ventricles in the brain and central canal of the spinal cord
- Ciliated cells move the CSF through the central canal of spinal cord

Cerebral Cortex: Gray Matter (Layers I to IV)

- Molecular layer (I): most superficial and covered by pia mater; contains neuroglial cells and horizontal cells of Cajal
- External granular layer (II): contains neuroglial cells and small pyramidal cells
- External pyramidal layer (III): medium-sized pyramidal cells predominant type
- Internal granular layer (IV): thin layer with small granule, pyramidal cells, and neuroglia
- Internal pyramidal layer (V): contains neuroglial cells and largest pyramidal cells
- Multiform layer (VI): deepest layer, adjacent to white matter with various cell types

Cerebellar Cortex

- Deep folds in cortex called cerebellar folia separated by sulci
- Outer molecular layer contains small neurons and fibers
- Middle Purkinje layer contains large Purkinje cells whose dendrites branch in molecular layer
- Granule cell layer contains small granule cells, Golgi type II cells, and empty spaces called glomeruli

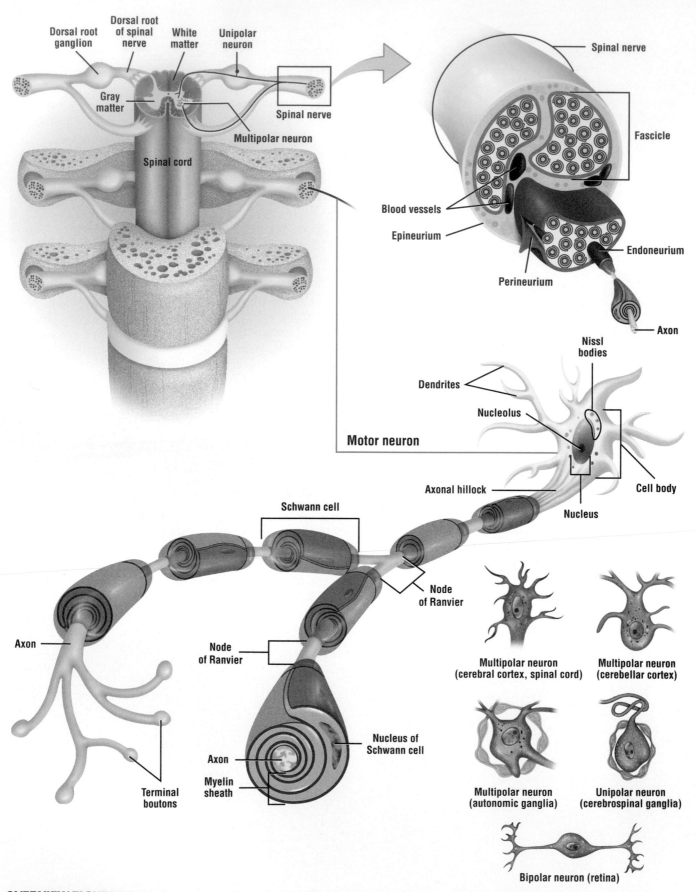

OVERVIEW FIGURE 7.2 ■ Peripheral nervous system. The peripheral nervous system is composed of the cranial and spinal nerves. A cross section of the spinal cord is illustrated with the characteristic features of the motor neuron and a cross section of a peripheral nerve. Also illustrated are types of neurons located in different ganglia and organs outside of the central nervous system.

SECTION 2 ■ The Peripheral Nervous System

The **peripheral nervous system (PNS)** consists of neurons, supportive cells, nerves, and axons that are located outside of the central nervous system (CNS). These include **cranial nerves** from the brain and **spinal nerves** from the spinal cord along with their associated ganglia. Ganglia (singular, ganglion) are small accumulations of neurons and supportive glial cells surrounded by a connective tissue capsule. The nerves of the PNS contain both sensory and motor axons. These axons transmit information between the peripheral organs and the CNS. The neurons of the peripheral nerves are located either within the CNS or outside of the CNS in different ganglia.

Connective Tissue Layers in the PNS

A peripheral nerve is composed of numerous axons of various sizes that are surrounded by several layers of connective tissue, which partition the nerve into several nerve (axon) bundles or **fascicles.** The outermost connective tissue layer is the strong sheath **epineurium** that binds all fascicles together. It consists of dense irregular connective tissue that completely surrounds the peripheral nerve. A thinner connective tissue layer called the **perineurium** extends into the nerve and surrounds one or more individual nerve fascicles. Within each fascicle are individual axons and their supporting cells, the **Schwann cells.** Each myelinated axon or a cluster of unmyelinated axons associated with a Schwann cell is surrounded by a loose vascular connective tissue layer of thin reticular fibers, called the **endoneurium.**

FIGURE 7.15 ■   Peripheral Nerves and Blood Vessels (Transverse Section)

Several bundles of nerve axons (fibers) or **nerve fascicles (1)** and accompanying blood vessels have been sectioned in the transverse plane. Each nerve fascicle (1) is surrounded by a sheath of connective tissue **perineurium (5)** that merges with surrounding **interfascicular connective tissue (9).** Delicate connective tissue strands from the perineurium (5) surround individual nerve axons (fibers) in a fascicle and form the innermost layer endoneurium (not visible in this figure and at this magnification).

Numerous nuclei are seen between individual nerve axons (fibers) in the nerve fascicles (1). Most of these are the **nuclei** of **Schwann cells (2).** Schwann cells (2) surround and myelinate the axons. The myelin sheaths that surrounded the tiny **axons (3)** are seen as empty spaces because of the chemicals used in preparation of the tissue. Other nuclei in the nerve fascicles (1) are the **fibrocytes (4)** of the endoneurium (see Figure 7.18).

The arterial blood vessels in the interfascicular connective tissue (9) send branches into each nerve fascicle (1) where they branch into capillaries in the endoneurium. Different size **arterioles (7, 12)** and **venules (11)** are found in the interfascicular connective tissue (9) that surrounds the nerve fascicles (1). In the larger arteriole (7) are visible blood cells, an **internal elastic membrane (8),** and a muscular **tunica media (6).** Different size **adipose cells (10)** are also present in the interfascicular connective tissue (9).

1 **Nerve fascicles**

2 **Nuclei of Schwann cells**

3 **Myelinated axons**

4 **Fibrocytes**

5 **Perineurium with fibrocytes**

6 **Tunica media of arteriole**

7 **Arteriole**

8 **Internal elastic membrane**

9 **Interfascicular connective tissue**

10 **Adipose cells**

11 **Venules**

12 **Arteriole**

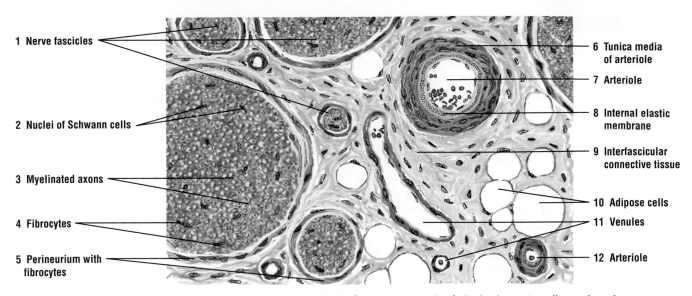

FIGURE 7.15 ■ Peripheral nerves and blood vessels (transverse section). Stain: hematoxylin and eosin. Medium magnification.

FIGURE 7.16 ■ Myelinated Nerve Fibers

Schwann cells surround the axons in peripheral nerves and form a myelin sheath. To illustrate the myelin sheath, nerve fibers are fixed with osmic acid; this preparation stains the lipid in the myelin sheath black. In this illustration, a portion of the peripheral nerve has been prepared in a longitudinal section (upper figure) and in a cross section (lower figure).

In the longitudinal section, the **myelin sheath (1)** appears as a thick, black band surrounding a lighter, central **axon (2)**. At intervals of a few millimeters, the myelin sheath exhibits discontinuity between adjacent Schwann cells. These regions of discontinuity represent the **nodes of Ranvier (4)**.

A group of nerve fibers or fascicle is also illustrated. Each fascicle is surrounded by a light-appearing connective tissue layer, called the **perineurium (3, 5, 8)**. In turn, each individual nerve fiber or axon is surrounded by a thin layer of connective tissue, called the **endoneurium (7, 10)**. In the transverse plane (lower figure), different diameters of myelinated axons are seen. The **myelin sheath (9)** appears as a thick, black ring around the light, unstained **axon (12)**, which in most fibers is seen in the center.

The connective tissue surrounding individual nerve fibers or the fascicle exhibits a rich supply of **blood vessels (6, 11)** of different sizes.

FUNCTIONAL CORRELATIONS: Axon Myelination and Supporting Cells in the PNS

The supportive cells in the PNS are the **Schwann cells.** Their main function is to encircle and form the insulating, lipid-rich **myelin sheaths** around the larger axons. Each Schwann cell myelinates a single axon. Also, a single Schwann cell can enclose several unmyelinated axons. The function of Schwann cells in the PNS is similar to that of the **oligodendrocytes** in the **CNS**, except that processes from a single oligodendrocyte can form myelin sheaths around numerous axons. Myelin sheaths are not continuous, solid sheets along the axon; rather, they are punctuated by gaps called **nodes of Ranvier.** These nodes significantly accelerate the conduction of **nerve impulses** (action potentials) along the axons. In large, myelinated axons, the nerve impulse or action potential jumps from node to node, resulting in a more efficient and faster conduction of the impulse. This type of impulse propagation in myelinated axons is called **saltatory conduction.**

Small unmyelinated axons conduct nerve impulses at a much slower rate than larger, myelinated axons. In unmyelinated axons, even though they are surrounded by the cytoplasm of the Schwann cell, the impulse travels along the entire length of the axon; as a result, conduction efficiency of the impulse and velocity is reduced. Thus, the larger, myelinated axons have the highest velocity of impulse conduction. Also, the rate of impulse conduction depends directly on the axon size and the myelin sheath.

The **satellite cells** are small, flat cells that surround the neurons of PNS ganglia. Ganglia are collections of neurons that are located outside of the CNS. Peripheral ganglia are located parallel to the vertebral column near the junction of the dorsal and ventral roots of the spinal nerves and near various visceral organs. Satellite cells provide **structural support** for the neuronal bodies, insulate them, and regulate the exchange of different metabolic substances between the neurons and the interstitial fluid.

1 Myelin sheath

2 Axons

3 Perineurium

4 Nodes of Ranvier

5 Perineurium

6 Blood vessels

7 Endoneurium

8 Perineurium

9 Myelin sheath

10 Endoneurium

11 Blood vessel

12 Axons

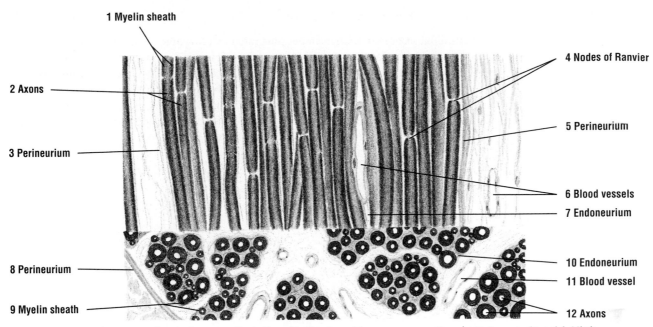

FIGURE 7.16 ■ Myelinated nerve fibers (longitudinal and transverse sections). Stain: osmic acid. High magnification.

FIGURE 7.17 ■ Sciatic Nerve (Longitudinal Section)

A longitudinal section of sciatic nerve is illustrated at a low magnification. A small portion of the outer layer of dense connective tissue **epineurium (1)** that surrounds the entire nerve is visible. The deeper layer of the epineurium (1) contains numerous **blood vessels (5)** and **adipose cells (6).**

The connective tissue sheath directly inferior to the epineurium (1) that surrounds bundles of nerve fibers or **nerve fascicles (3)** is **the perineurium (2).** Extensions of the epineurium (1) with **blood vessels (4)** between the nerve fascicles (3) form the **interfascicular connective tissue (7).**

In a longitudinal section, the individual axons usually follow a characteristic wavy pattern. Located among the wavy axons in the nerve fascicle (3) are numerous **nuclei (8)** of the Schwann cells and fibrocytes of the endoneurium connective tissue. Schwann cells and fibrocytes cannot be differentiated at this magnification.

FIGURE 7.18 ■ Sciatic Nerve (Longitudinal Section)

A small portion of the sciatic nerve, illustrated in Figure 7.17, is presented at a higher magnification. The central **axons (1)** appear as slender threads stained lightly with hematoxylin and eosin. The surrounding myelin sheath has been dissolved by chemicals during histologic preparation, leaving a **neurokeratin network (6)** of protein. The sheath or cell membrane of the **Schwann cells (4)** is not always distinguishable from the connective tissue **endoneurium (5)** that surrounds each axon. At the **node of Ranvier (2)**, the Schwann cell membrane (4) is seen as a thin, peripheral boundary that descends toward the axon.

Two **Schwann cell nuclei (4)**, cut in different planes, are shown around the periphery of the myelinated axons (1). The **fibrocytes** of the connective tissue **endoneurium (3a)** and **perineurium (3b)** are also seen in the illustration. The fibrocyte of the endoneurium (3a) is outside of the myelin sheath, in contrast to the Schwann cells (4) that myelinate or surround the axons (1). However, it is often difficult to distinguish between the nuclei of Schwann cells (4) and the fibrocytes (3) of the endoneurium.

FIGURE 7.19 ■ Sciatic Nerve (Transverse Section)

A higher magnification of a transverse section of the sciatic nerve illustrated in Figure 7.17 shows the myelinated nerve fibers. The **axons (5)** appear as thin, dark central structures, surrounded by the dissolved remnants of myelin, the **neurokeratin network (2)** of protein with peripheral radial lines. The nuclei and cell membranes of the **Schwann cells (1)** are peripheral to the myelinated axon (5). The crescent shape of the Schwann cells (1), as they appear to encircle the axons, allows their identification.

The collagen fibers of the connective tissue endoneurium are faintly distinguishable, whereas the **fibrocytes (3a)** in the connective tissue of endoneurium and **perineurium (3b, 6)** are clearly seen. Located in the **interfascicular connective tissue (4)** and draining the nerve fascicles is a small **venule (7).**

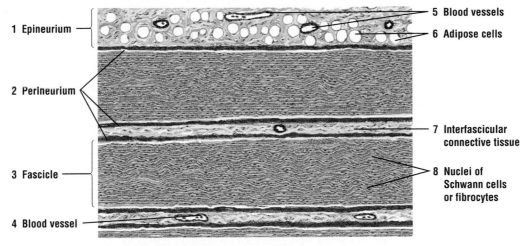

1 Epineurium
2 Perineurium
3 Fascicle
4 Blood vessel
5 Blood vessels
6 Adipose cells
7 Interfascicular connective tissue
8 Nuclei of Schwann cells or fibrocytes

FIGURE 7.17 ■ Sciatic nerve (longitudinal section). Stain: hematoxylin and eosin. Low magnification.

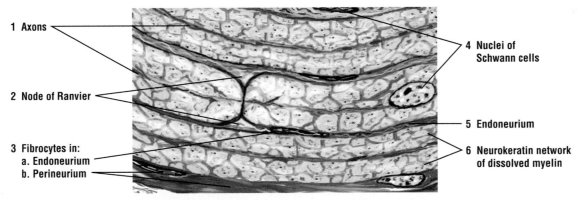

1 Axons
2 Node of Ranvier
3 Fibrocytes in:
 a. Endoneurium
 b. Perineurium
4 Nuclei of Schwann cells
5 Endoneurium
6 Neurokeratin network of dissolved myelin

FIGURE 7.18 ■ Sciatic nerve (longitudinal section). Stain: hematoxylin and eosin. High magnification (oil immersion).

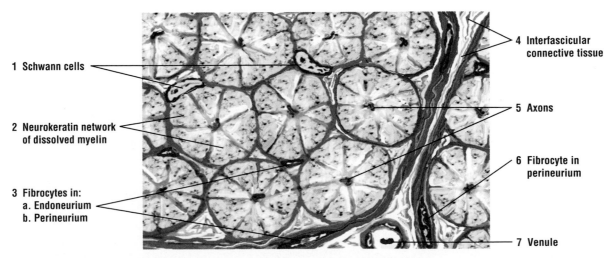

1 Schwann cells
2 Neurokeratin network of dissolved myelin
3 Fibrocytes in:
 a. Endoneurium
 b. Perineurium
4 Interfascicular connective tissue
5 Axons
6 Fibrocyte in perineurium
7 Venule

FIGURE 7.19 ■ Sciatic nerve (transverse section). Stain: hematoxylin and eosin. High magnification (oil immersion).

FIGURE 7.20 ■ Peripheral Nerve: Nodes of Ranvier and Axons

A medium magnification photomicrograph of a peripheral nerve sectioned in a longitudinal plane is shown. The myelin sheaths that normally surround the axons have been washed out in this preparation and only **myelin spaces (7)** are seen. A centrally located **axon (2, 8)** can be seen in some of the nerve fibers that exhibited myelin sheaths. At regular intervals along the axon are seen indentations in the myelin sheaths. These represent the **nodes of Ranvier (1, 9)**, which indicate the edges of two different myelin sheaths that enclose the axon. A possible **Schwann cell nucleus (3)** is seen associated with one of the axons (2, 8) and a thin, blue connective tissue layer **endoneurium (6)** that surrounds some of the axons (2, 8). Outside of the axons (2, 8) are seen a **capillary (4)** with blood cells and **fibrocytes (5)** of the surrounding connective tissue layers.

FIGURE 7.21 ■ Dorsal Root Ganglion With Dorsal and Ventral Roots, and Spinal Nerve (Longitudinal Section)

The dorsal root ganglia are aggregations of neuron cell bodies that are located outside of the CNS. The **dorsal (posterior) root ganglion (7)** is situated on the **dorsal (posterior) nerve root (9),** which joins the spinal cord. Numerous round (pseudo) **unipolar neurons (2)** or sensory neurons constitute the majority of the ganglion. Numerous fascicles of **nerve fibers (3)** pass between the unipolar neurons (2) and course either in the dorsal nerve root (9) or the **spinal nerve (5).** The nerve fibers (3) represent the peripheral processes that are formed by the bifurcation of a single axon that emerges from each unipolar neuron (2).

Each dorsal root ganglion (7) is enclosed by an irregular **connective tissue layer (1)** that contains adipose cells, **nerves (6),** and **blood vessels (6).** The connective tissue (1, 6) around the ganglion (7) merges with the connective tissue **epineurium (4)** of the peripheral spinal nerve (5). The nerve fibers in the **ventral (anterior) root (11)** join the nerve fibers that emerge from the ganglion (7) to form the spinal nerve (5). The spinal nerve (5) is formed when the dorsal nerve root (9) and the ventral (anterior) root (11) unite.

On emerging from the spinal cord, the dorsal (9) and ventral roots (11) are surrounded by pia mater and an **arachnoid sheath (8, 10).** These become continuous with the epineurium (4) of the spinal nerve (5). The connective tissue perineurium around the nerve fascicles (3) and the endoneurium around individual nerve fibers in the spinal nerve (5) or in the ganglion (7) are not distinguishable at this magnification.

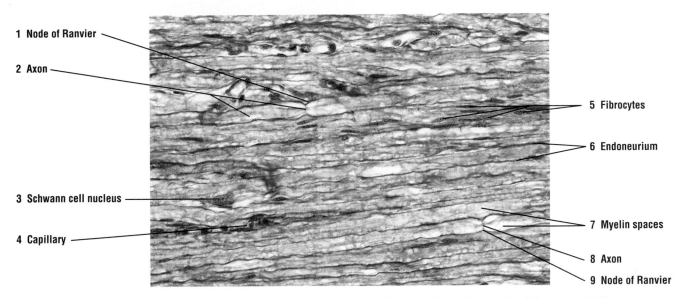

1 Node of Ranvier

2 Axon

3 Schwann cell nucleus

4 Capillary

5 Fibrocytes

6 Endoneurium

7 Myelin spaces

8 Axon

9 Node of Ranvier

FIGURE 7.20 ■ Peripheral nerve: nodes of Ranvier and axons. Stain: Masson's trichrome. ×100.

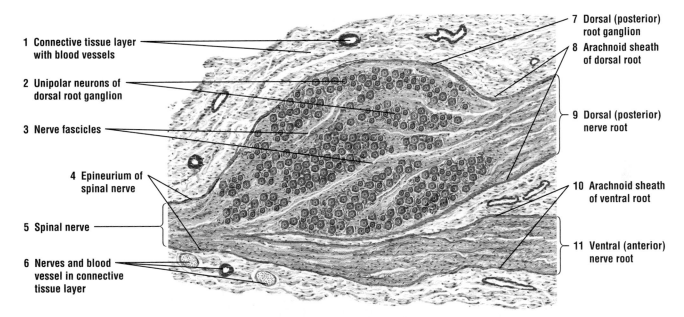

1 Connective tissue layer
  with blood vessels

2 Unipolar neurons of
  dorsal root ganglion

3 Nerve fascicles

4 Epineurium of
  spinal nerve

5 Spinal nerve

6 Nerves and blood
  vessel in connective
  tissue layer

7 Dorsal (posterior)
  root ganglion

8 Arachnoid sheath
  of dorsal root

9 Dorsal (posterior)
  nerve root

10 Arachnoid sheath
   of ventral root

11 Ventral (anterior)
   nerve root

FIGURE 7.21 ■ Dorsal root ganglion, with dorsal and ventral roots, spinal nerve (longitudinal section. Stain: hematoxylin and eosin. Low magnification.

FIGURE 7.22 ■ Cells and Unipolar Neurons of a Dorsal Root Ganglion

The **unipolar neurons (1, 6)** of a dorsal (posterior) root ganglion are illustrated at higher magnification. When the plane of section passes through the middle of a neuron (1, 6), a pink-staining **cytoplasm (1b, 4)** and a round **nucleus (1a)** is visible with its characteristic, dark-staining **nucleolus (1b)**. Some of the unipolar neurons (1, 6) contain small clumps of brownish **lipofuscin pigment (9)** in their cytoplasm (Also Fig. 7).

The cell body of each unipolar neuron (1, 6) is surrounded by two cellular capsules. The inner cell layer is within the perineuronal space and closely surrounds the unipolar neurons (1, 6). These are the smaller, flat epithelium-like **satellite cells (3, 8)**. The satellite cells (3, 8) have spherical nuclei, are of neuroectodermal origin, and are continuous with similar **Schwann cells (11)** that surround the unmyelinated and **myelinated axons (5, 10)**. The satellite cells (3, 8) are surrounded by an outer layer of **capsule cells (7)** of the connective tissue. Between the unipolar neurons (1, 6) are numerous **fibrocytes (2)** that are randomly arranged in the surrounding connective tissue and continue into the endoneurium between the axons (5).

With hematoxylin and eosin stain, small axons and individual connective tissue fibers are not clearly defined. Large myelinated axons (5) are recognizable when sectioned longitudinally.

FIGURE 7.23 ■ Multipolar Neurons, Surrounding Cells, and Nerve Fibers of a Sympathetic Ganglion

In contrast to the neurons of the dorsal root ganglion (Figure 7.22), the **neurons (3, 9)** of the sympathetic trunk are multipolar, smaller, and more uniform in size. As a result, the outlines of the neurons (3, 9) and their **dendritic processes (2, 11)** appear often irregular. Also, if the plane of section does not pass through the middle of the cell, only the **cytoplasm** of the **neuron (1, 10)** is visible. The sympathetic neurons (3, 9) also often exhibit **eccentric nuclei (9)**, and binucleated cells are not uncommon. In older individuals, a brownish **lipofuscin pigment (12)** accumulates in the cytoplasm of numerous neurons (3, 9).

The **satellite cells (8)** surround the multipolar neurons (3, 9), but are usually less numerous than around the cells in the dorsal root ganglion. Also, the connective tissue capsule with its capsule cells may not be well defined. Surrounding the neurons (3, 9) are **fibrocytes (5)** of the intercellular connective tissue and different size blood vessels, such as a **venule** with **blood cells (6)**. Unmyelinated and myelinated nerve **axons (4, 7)** aggregate into bundles and course through the sympathetic ganglion. The flattened nuclei on the peripheries of the myelinated axons (4, 7) are the **Schwann cells (4, 7)**. These nerve fibers represent the preganglionic axons, postganglionic visceral efferent axons, and visceral afferent axons.

FIGURE 7.24 ■ Dorsal Root Ganglion: Unipolar Neurons and Surrounding Cells

A medium-magnification photomicrograph of the dorsal root ganglion illustrates the spherical shape of the sensory **unipolar neurons (2)**. The cytoplasm of these neurons contains a central **nucleus (6)** and a prominent dense **nucleolus (5)**. Surrounding the unipolar neurons (2) are the smaller **satellite cells (1)**. Other cells outside of the satellite cells are the connective tissue **fibrocytes (3)**. Coursing through the dorsal root ganglion between the unipolar neurons (2) are numerous **bundles of sensory axons (4)** from the periphery.

The clear space around the neurons and the surrounding cells is an artifact caused by the tissue shrinkage during chemical preparation of the dorsal root ganglion.

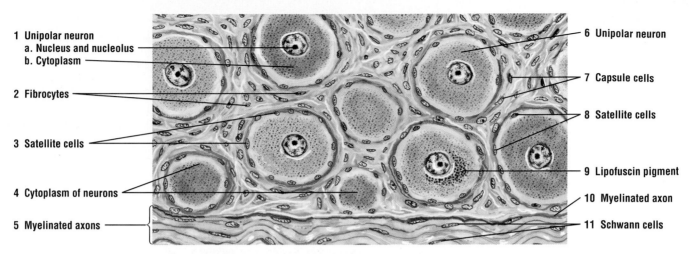

1 **Unipolar neuron**
  a. **Nucleus and nucleolus**
  b. **Cytoplasm**

2 **Fibrocytes**

3 **Satellite cells**

4 **Cytoplasm of neurons**

5 **Myelinated axons**

6 **Unipolar neuron**

7 **Capsule cells**

8 **Satellite cells**

9 **Lipofuscin pigment**

10 **Myelinated axon**

11 **Schwann cells**

FIGURE 7.22 ■ Cells and unipolar neurons of a dorsal root ganglion. Stain: hematoxylin and eosin. High magnification.

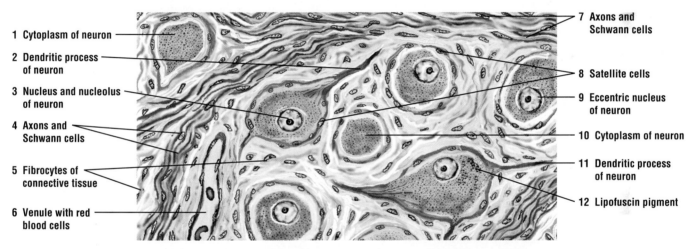

1 **Cytoplasm of neuron**

2 **Dendritic process of neuron**

3 **Nucleus and nucleolus of neuron**

4 **Axons and Schwann cells**

5 **Fibrocytes of connective tissue**

6 **Venule with red blood cells**

7 **Axons and Schwann cells**

8 **Satellite cells**

9 **Eccentric nucleus of neuron**

10 **Cytoplasm of neuron**

11 **Dendritic process of neuron**

12 **Lipofuscin pigment**

FIGURE 7.23 ■ Multipolar neurons, surrounding cells, and nerve fibers of the sympathetic ganglion. Stain: hematoxylin and eosin. High magnification.

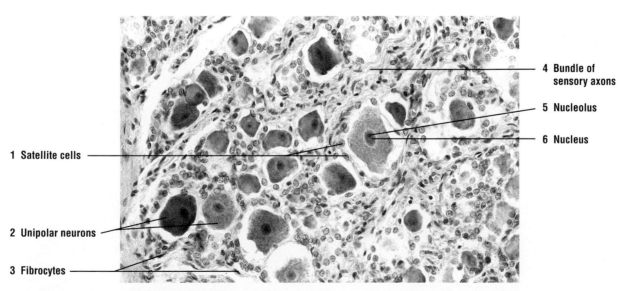

1 **Satellite cells**

2 **Unipolar neurons**

3 **Fibrocytes**

4 **Bundle of sensory axons**

5 **Nucleolus**

6 **Nucleus**

FIGURE 7.24 ■ Dorsal root ganglion: unipolar neurons and surrounding cells. Stain: hematoxylin and eosin. ×100.

CHAPTER 7 ■ Summary

Peripheral Nervous System

- Consists of neurons, neuroglia, nerves, and axons outside of the CNS
- Cranial nerves arise from brain and spinal nerves from spinal cord
- Ganglia are accumulations of neurons and ganglia covered by connective tissue
- Contains both sensory and motor nerves
- Neurons of peripheral nerves can be located in CNS or in ganglia

Connective Tissue Layers in Peripheral Nerves

- Peripheral nerves are partitioned by layers of connective tissue into fascicles
- Outermost connective tissue around the nerve is epineurium
- Connective tissue perineurium surrounds one or more nerve fascicles
- Vascular connective tissue layer endoneurium surrounds individual axons

Peripheral Nerves

- Nuclei seen between individual axons are Schwann cells and fibrocytes
- Schwann cells myelinate and surround individual axons, or enclose unmyelinated axons
- Between individual Schwann cells in myelinated axons are the nodes of Ranvier
- Conduction along myelinated axon is called saltatory conduction
- Small satellite cells surround neurons of PNS ganglia
- Satellite cells provide structural support, insulate, and regulate metabolic exchanges

Dorsal Root Ganglia and Unipolar Neurons of PNS

- Situated on dorsal nerve roots that join the spinal cord
- Sensory or round unipolar neurons constitute the ganglia
- Bundles of sensory nerve fibers or axons pass between the unipolar neurons
- Connective tissue capsule encloses the ganglia and merges with epineurium of peripheral nerve
- Unipolar neurons are surrounded by satellite cells, which are enclosed by connective tissue capsule cells

PART II

ORGANS

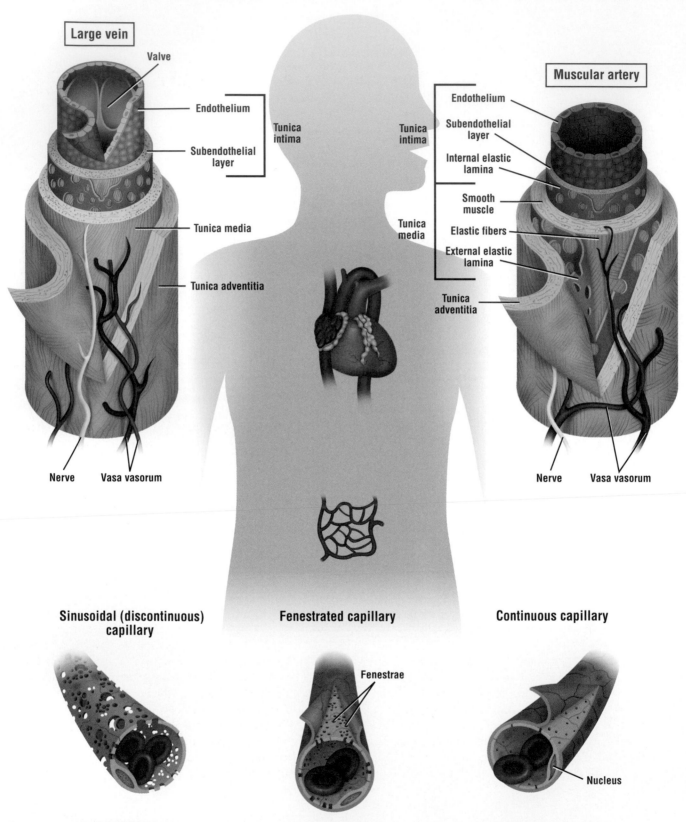

Large vein

Valve

Endothelium

Subendothelial layer

Tunica intima

Tunica media

Tunica adventitia

Nerve　　Vasa vasorum

Muscular artery

Endothelium

Subendothelial layer

Internal elastic lamina

Smooth muscle

Elastic fibers

External elastic lamina

Tunica intima

Tunica media

Tunica adventitia

Nerve　　Vasa vasorum

Sinusoidal (discontinuous) capillary

Fenestrated capillary

Fenestrae

Continuous capillary

Nucleus

OVERVIEW FIGURE 8 ■ Comparison of a muscular artery, a large vein, and the three types of capillaries (transverse sections).

Circulatory System

The Blood Vascular System

The mammalian **blood vascular system** consists of the heart, major arteries, arterioles, capillaries, venules, and veins. The main function of this system is to deliver oxygenated blood to cells and tissues and to return venous blood to the lungs for gaseous exchange. The histology of the heart muscle has been described in detail in Chapter 6 as one of the four main tissues. In this chapter, heart histology is illustrated only as part of the cardiovascular system.

Types of Arteries

There are three types of arteries in the body: elastic arteries, muscular arteries, and arterioles. Arteries that leave the heart to distribute the oxygenated blood exhibit progressive branching. With each branching, the luminal diameters of the arteries gradually decrease, until the smallest vessel, the capillary, is formed.

Elastic arteries are the largest blood vessels in the body and include the **pulmonary trunk** and **aorta** with their major branches, the brachiocephalic, common carotid, subclavian, vertebral, pulmonary, and common iliac arteries. The walls of these vessels are primarily composed of elastic connective tissue fibers. These fibers provide great resilience and flexibility during blood flow. The large elastic arteries branch and become medium-sized **muscular arteries,** the most numerous vessels in the body. In contrast to the walls of elastic arteries, those of muscular arteries contain greater amounts of **smooth muscle fibers. Arterioles** are the smallest branches of the arterial system. Their walls consist of one to five layers of smooth muscle fibers. Arterioles deliver blood to the smallest blood vessels, the capillaries. Capillaries connect arterioles with the smallest veins or venules.

Structural Plan of Arteries

The wall of a typical artery contains three concentric layers or **tunics.** The innermost layer is the **tunica intima.** This layer consists of a simple squamous epithelium, called **endothelium** in the vascular system, and the underlying **subendothelial connective tissue.** The middle layer is the **tunica media,** composed primarily of smooth muscle fibers. Interspersed among the smooth muscle cells are variable amounts of elastic and reticular fibers. In these arteries, smooth muscles produce the extracellular matrix. The outermost layer is the **tunica adventitia,** composed primarily of collagen and elastic connective tissue fibers; adventitia consists primarily of collagen type I.

The walls of some muscular arteries also exhibit two thin, wavy bands of elastic fibers. The **internal elastic lamina** is located between the tunica intima and the tunica media; this layer is not seen in smaller arteries. The **external elastic lamina** is located on the periphery of the muscular tunica media and is primarily seen in large muscular arteries.

Structural Plan of Veins

Capillaries unite to form larger blood vessels called **venules;** venules usually accompany arterioles. The venous blood initially flows into smaller **postcapillary venules** and then into veins of increasing size. The veins are arbitrarily classified as small, medium, and large. Compared with arteries, veins typically are more numerous and have thinner walls, larger diameters, and greater structural variation.

Small-sized and medium-sized veins, particularly in the extremities, have **valves.** Because of the low blood pressure in the veins, blood flow to the heart in the veins is slow and can even back up. The presence of valves in veins assists venous blood flow by preventing backflow. When blood flows toward the heart, pressure in the veins forces the valves to open. As the blood begins to flow backward, the valve flaps close the lumen and prevent backflow of blood. Venous blood between the valves in the extremities flows toward the heart as a result of contraction of muscles that surround the veins. Valves are absent in veins of the central nervous system, the inferior and superior venae cavae, and viscera.

The walls of the veins, like the arteries, also exhibit three layers or tunics. However, the muscular layer is much less prominent. The **tunica intima** in large veins exhibits a prominent endothelium and subendothelial connective tissue. In large veins, the muscular **tunica media** is thin, and the smooth muscles intermix with connective tissue fibers. In large veins, the **tunica adventitia** is the thickest and best-developed layer of the three tunics. Longitudinal bundles of smooth muscle fibers are common in the connective tissue of this layer (see Overview Figure 8).

Vasa Vasorum

The walls of larger arteries and veins are too thick to receive nourishment by direct diffusion from their lumina. As a result, these walls are supplied by their own small blood vessels called the **vasa vasorum** (vessels of the vessel). The vasa vasorum allows for exchange of nutrients and metabolites with cells in the tunica adventitia and tunica media.

Types of Capillaries

Capillaries are the smallest blood vessels. Their average diameter is about **8 μm,** which is about the size of an **erythrocyte** (red blood cell). There are three types of capillaries: continuous capillaries, fenestrated capillaries, and sinusoids. These structural variations in capillaries allow for different types of metabolic exchange between blood and the surrounding tissues.

Continuous capillaries are the most common. They are found in muscle, connective tissue, nervous tissue, skin, respiratory organs, and exocrine glands. In these capillaries, the **endothelial cells** are joined and form an uninterrupted, solid endothelial lining.

Fenestrated capillaries are characterized by large openings or **fenestrations** (pores) in the cytoplasm of endothelial cells designed for a rapid exchange of molecules between blood and tissues. Fenestrated capillaries are found in endocrine tissues and glands, small intestine, and kidney glomeruli.

Sinusoidal (discontinuous) capillaries are blood vessels that exhibit irregular, tortuous paths. Their much wider diameters slow down the flow of blood. Endothelial cell junctions are rare in sinusoidal capillaries, and wide gaps exist between individual endothelial cells. Also, because a **basement membrane** underlying the endothelium is either incomplete or absent, a direct exchange of molecules occurs between blood contents and cells. Sinusoidal capillaries are found in the liver, spleen, and bone marrow (see Overview Figure 8).

The Lymph Vascular System

The **lymphatic system** consists of lymph capillaries and lymph vessels. This system starts as blind-ending tubules or lymphatic capillaries in the connective tissue of different organs. These vessels collect the excess **interstitial fluid (lymph)** from the tissues and return it to the venous blood via the large **lymph vessels,** the thoracic duct and right lymphatic duct. Also, to allow greater permeability, the **endothelium** in lymph capillaries and vessels is extremely thin. The structure of larger lymph vessels is similar to that of veins except that their walls are much thinner.

Lymph movement in the lymphatic vessels is similar to that of blood movement; that is, the contractions of surrounding skeletal muscles forces the lymph to move forward. Also, the lymph vessels contain more **valves** to prevent a backflow of collected lymph. Lymph vessels are found in all tissues except the central nervous system, cartilage, bone and bone marrow, thymus, placenta, and teeth.

FIGURE 8.1   ■Different Blood and Lymphatic Vessels in the Connective Tissue

This composite figure illustrates a section of irregular connective tissue with nerve fibers, blood and lymphatic vessels, and adipose tissue. To illustrate structural differences, the vessels have been sectioned in transverse, longitudinal, or oblique planes.

A **small artery (3)** with its wall structure is shown in the lower left corner of the illustration. In contrast to **veins (11),** an artery has a relatively thick wall and a small lumen. In cross section, the wall of a small artery (3) exhibits the following layers:

a. **Tunica intima (4)** is the innermost layer. It is composed of **endothelium (4a),** a **subendothelial (4b)** layer of connective tissue, and an **internal elastic lamina (membrane) (4c),** which separates the tunica intima (4) from the next layer, the tunica media.
b. **Tunica media (5)** is composed predominantly of circular smooth muscle fibers. A loose network of fine elastic fibers is interspersed among the smooth muscle cells.
c. **Tunica adventitia (6)** is the connective tissue layer that surrounds the vessel. This layer contains small nerves and blood vessels. In tunica adventitia (6), the blood vessels are collectively called **vasa vasorum (7)** or blood vessels of the blood vessel.

When arteries acquire about 25 or more layers of smooth muscle fibers in the tunica media, they are called muscular or distributing arteries. Elastic fibers become more numerous in the tunica media but are still present as thin fibers and networks.

A **venule (9)** and small vein (11) are also illustrated. Note the relatively thin wall and a large lumen. The thin wall, however, appears to have many cell layers when the vein is sectioned in an **oblique plane (9).** In cross section, the wall of the vein exhibits the following layers:

a. Tunica intima is composed of **endothelium (11a)** and an extremely thin layer of fine collagen and elastic fibers, which blend with the connective tissue of the tunica media.
b. **Tunica media (11b)** consists of a thin layer of circularly arranged smooth muscle loosely embedded in connective tissue. Tunica media (11b) is much thinner in veins than tunica media in arteries (5).
c. **Tunica adventitia (11c)** contains a wide layer of connective tissue. In veins, the tunica adventitia (11c) layer is thicker than the tunica media (11b).

Two arterioles, cut in different planes, are also illustrated. The **arterioles (2, 8)** have a thin internal elastic lamina and a layer of smooth muscle fibers in the tunica media. One **arteriole (8)** is shown cut in longitudinal plane with a branching **capillary (10).** When an arteriole (8) is cut at an oblique angle, only the circular smooth muscle layer of tunica media is seen. Also visible in the illustration are capillaries (10) sectioned in longitudinal and oblique planes, and small **nerves (1)** in transverse planes.

The **lymphatic vessels (12, 13)** are recognized by having the thinnest walls. When the lymphatic vessel is cut in a longitudinal plane, the flaps of a **valve (13)** are seen in its lumen. Many veins in the arms and legs have similar valves in their lumina.

Numerous **adipose cells (14)** are found in the surrounding connective tissue.

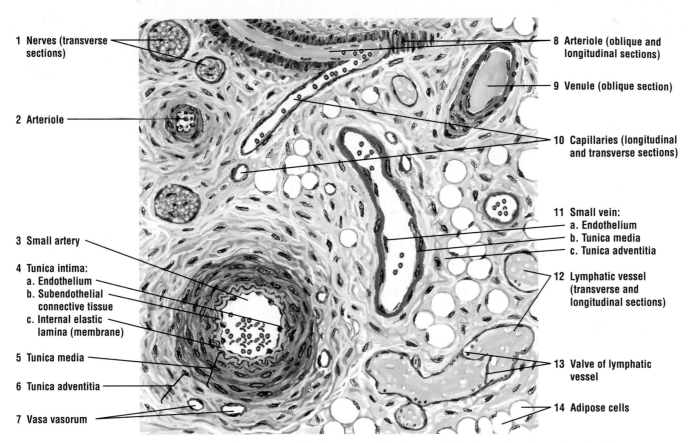

1 Nerves (transverse sections)

2 Arteriole

3 Small artery

4 Tunica intima:
   a. Endothelium
   b. Subendothelial connective tissue
   c. Internal elastic lamina (membrane)

5 Tunica media

6 Tunica adventitia

7 Vasa vasorum

8 Arteriole (oblique and longitudinal sections)

9 Venule (oblique section)

10 Capillaries (longitudinal and transverse sections)

11 Small vein:
    a. Endothelium
    b. Tunica media
    c. Tunica adventitia

12 Lymphatic vessel (transverse and longitudinal sections)

13 Valve of lymphatic vessel

14 Adipose cells

FIGURE 8.1 ■ Blood and lymphatic vessels in the connective tissue. Stain: hematoxylin and eosin. Low magnification.

FIGURE 8.2 ■ Muscular Artery and Vein (Transverse Section)

The walls of blood vessels contain elastic tissue that allows them to expand and contract. In this illustration, a muscular **artery (1)** and **vein (4)** have been cut in transverse plane and prepared with a plastic stain to illustrate the distribution of elastic fibers in their walls. The elastic fibers stain black, and the collagen fibers stain light yellow.

The wall of the artery (1) is much thicker and contains more smooth muscle fibers than the wall of the vein (4). The innermost layer tunica intima of the artery (1) is stained dark because of the thick **internal elastic lamina (1a)**. The thick middle layer of the muscular artery, the **tunica media (1b)**, contains several layers of smooth muscle fibers, arranged in a circular pattern, and thin dark strands of **elastic fibers (1b)**. On the periphery of the tunica media (1b) is the less conspicuous **external elastic lamina (1c)**. Surrounding the artery is the connective tissue **tunica adventitia (1d)**, which contains both the light-staining **collagen fibers (2)** and the dark-staining **elastic fibers (3)**.

The wall of the vein (4) also contains the layers **tunica intima (4a), tunica media (4b)**, and **tunica adventitia (4c)**. However, these three layers in the vein (4) are not as thick as those in the wall of the artery (1).

Surrounding both vessels are **capillary (5), arteriole (7), venule (6)**, and cells of the **adipose tissue (8)**. Present in the lumina of both vessels (1, 4) are numerous erythrocytes and leukocytes.

FIGURE 8.3 ■ Artery and Vein in Connective Tissue of Vas Deferens

This photomicrograph illustrates the structural differences between a **small artery (1)** and a small **vein (6)** in a dense irregular **connective tissue (5)**. The small artery (1) has a relatively thick muscular wall and a small lumen. The arterial wall consists of the **tunica intima (2)**, composed of an inner layer of **endothelium (2a)**, a **subendothelial (2b)** layer of connective tissue, and an **internal elastic lamina (membrane) (2c)**. This membrane (2c) separates the tunica intima (2) from the **tunica media (3)**, which consists predominantly of circular smooth muscle fibers. Surrounding the tunica media (3) is the connective tissue layer **tunica adventitia (4)**.

Adjacent to the small artery (1) is a small vein (6) with a much larger lumen that is filled with blood cells. The wall of the vein (6) is much thinner in comparison to that of the artery (1) but also consists of **tunica intima (7)** composed of **endothelium (7a)**, a thin layer of circular smooth muscle **tunica media (8)**, and the layer of connective tissue **tunica adventitia (9)**.

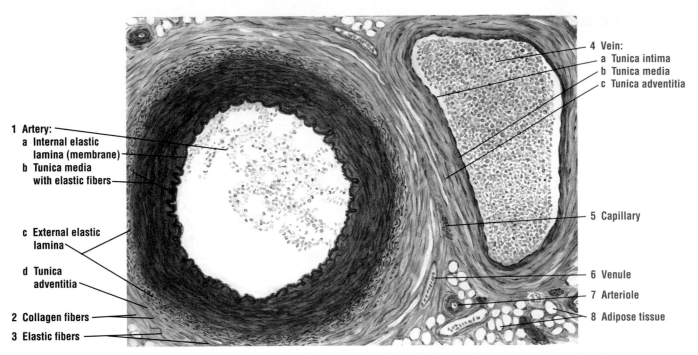

1 **Artery:**
  **a Internal elastic
    lamina (membrane)**
  **b Tunica media
    with elastic fibers**

  **c External elastic
    lamina**

  **d Tunica
    adventitia**

2 **Collagen fibers**
3 **Elastic fibers**

4 Vein:
  a Tunica intima
  b Tunica media
  c Tunica adventitia

5 Capillary

6 Venule
7 Arteriole
8 Adipose tissue

FIGURE 8.2 ■ Muscular artery and vein (transverse section). Stain: elastic stain. Low magnification.

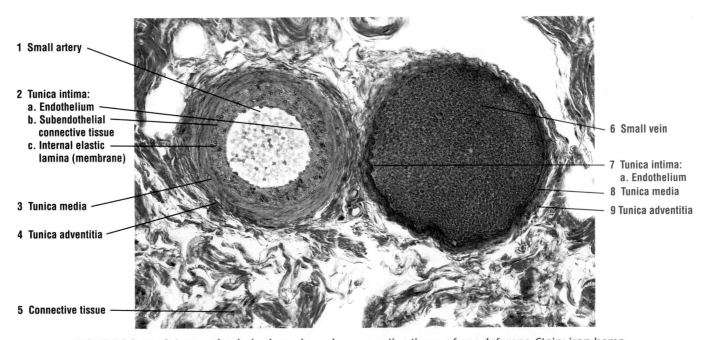

1 **Small artery**

2 **Tunica intima:**
  a. Endothelium
  **b. Subendothelial
    connective tissue**
  **c. Internal elastic
    lamina (membrane)**

3 **Tunica media**

4 **Tunica adventitia**

5 **Connective tissue**

6 Small vein

7 Tunica intima:
    a. Endothelium
8 Tunica media
9 Tunica adventitia

FIGURE 8.3 ■ Artery and vein in dense irregular connective tissue of vas deferens. Stain: iron hematoxylin and Alcian blue. ×64.

FIGURE 8.4 ■ Wall of an Elastic Artery: Aorta (Transverse Section)

The wall of the aorta is similar in morphology to that of the artery illustrated in Figure 8.3. Instead of smooth muscle fibers, the **elastic fibers (4)** constitute the bulk of the **tunica media (6),** with **smooth muscle fibers (10)** less abundant than in the muscular arteries. The size and arrangement of the elastic fibers (4) in the tunica media (6) are demonstrated with the elastic stain. Other tissues in the wall of the aorta, such as fine elastic fibers and smooth muscle fibers (10) are either lightly stained or remain colorless.

The simple squamous **endothelium (1)** and the **subendothelial connective tissue (2)** in the **tunica intima (5)** are indicated but remain unstained. The first visible elastic membrane is the **internal elastic lamina (membrane) (3).**

The **tunica adventitia (7),** somewhat less stained with elastic stain, is a narrow, peripheral zone of connective tissue. A **venule (9a)** and an **arteriole (9b)** of the **vasa vasorum (9)** supply the tunica adventitia (7). In such large blood vessels as the aorta and the pulmonary arteries, tunica media (6) occupies most of the vessel wall, whereas tunica adventitia (7) is reduced to a proportionately smaller area, as illustrated in the figure.

FIGURE 8.5 ■ Wall of a Large Vein: Portal Vein (Transverse Section)

In contrast to the wall of a large artery (above, Figure 8.4), the wall of a large vein is characterized by thick, muscular **tunica adventitia (6)** in which the **smooth muscle fibers (7)** show a longitudinal orientation. In the transverse section of the portal vein, the smooth muscle fibers (7) are segregated into bundles and are seen mainly in cross section, surrounded by the connective tissue of the tunica adventitia (6). An **arteriole (8a),** two **venules (8b),** and a **capillary (8c)** in longitudinal section of **vasa vasorum (8)** are visible in the connective tissue of the tunica adventitia (6).

In contrast to the thick tunica adventitia (6), the **tunica media (5)** is thinner. The **smooth muscle fibers (3)** exhibit a circular orientation. In other large veins, the tunica media (5) may be extremely thin and compact.

The **tunica intima (4)** is part of the **endothelium (1)** and is supported by a small amount of **subendothelial connective tissue (2).** In addition, large veins may also exhibit an internal elastic lamina that is not as well developed as in the arteries.

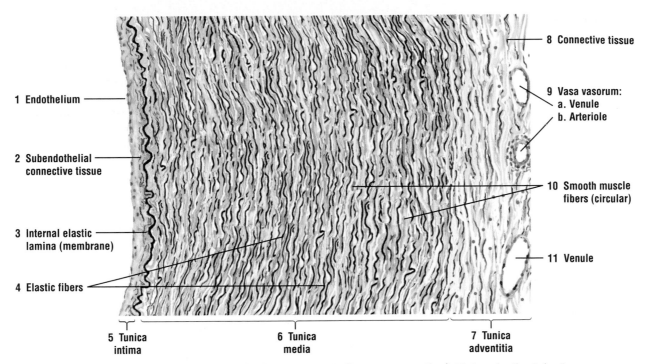

1 Endothelium

2 Subendothelial connective tissue

3 Internal elastic lamina (membrane)

4 Elastic fibers

8 Connective tissue

9 Vasa vasorum:
a. Venule
b. Arteriole

10 Smooth muscle fibers (circular)

11 Venule

5 Tunica intima   6 Tunica media   7 Tunica adventitia

FIGURE 8.4 ■ Wall of a large elastic artery: aorta (transverse section). Stain: elastic stain. Low magnification.

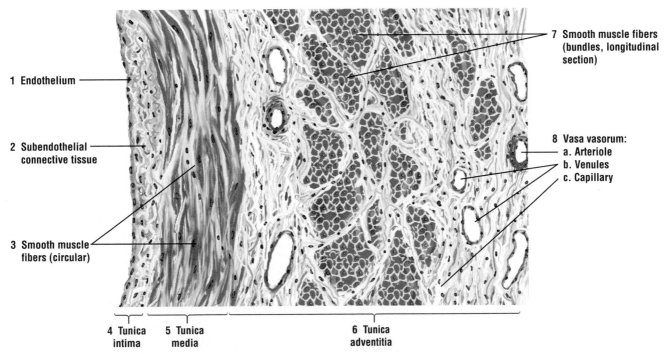

1 Endothelium

2 Subendothelial connective tissue

3 Smooth muscle fibers (circular)

7 Smooth muscle fibers (bundles, longitudinal section)

8 Vasa vasorum:
a. Arteriole
b. Venules
c. Capillary

4 Tunica intima   5 Tunica media   6 Tunica adventitia

FIGURE 8.5 ■ Wall of a large vein: portal vein (transverse section). Stain: hematoxylin and eosin. Low magnification.

FIGURE 8.6 ◼ Heart: Left Atrium, Atrioventricular Valve, and Left Ventricle (Longitudinal Section)

The wall of the heart consists of three layers: an inner endocardium, a middle myocardium, and an outer epicardium. The endocardium consists of a simple squamous endothelium and a thin subendothelial connective tissue. Deeper to the endocardium is the subendocardial layer of connective tissue. Here are found small blood vessels and Purkinje fibers. The subendocardial layer attaches to the endomysium of the cardiac muscle fibers. The myocardium is the thickest layer and consists of cardiac muscle fibers. The epicardium consists of a simple squamous mesothelium and an underlying subepicardial layer of connective tissue. The subepicardial layer contains coronary blood vessels, nerves, and adipose tissue.

A longitudinal section through the left side of the heart illustrates a portion of the **atrium (1)**, the **cusps** of the **atrioventricular (mitral) valve (5)**, and a section of the **ventricle (19)**. The **endocardium (1, 9)** lines the cavities of the atrium and ventricle. Below the endocardium (1, 9) is the **subendocardial connective tissue (2)**. The **myocardium (3, 19)** in both the atrium (3) and ventricle (19) consists of cardiac muscle fibers.

The outer **epicardium (13, 16)** of the atrium (13) and ventricle (16) is continuous and covers the heart externally with mesothelium. A **subepicardial layer (17)** contains connective tissue, **adipose tissue (15)**, and numerous **coronary blood vessels (15)**, which vary in amount in different regions of the heart. The epicardium (13, 16) also extends into the coronary (atrioventricular) sulcus and interventricular sulcus of the heart.

Between the atrium (1) and ventricle (19) is a layer of dense fibrous connective tissue called the **annulus fibrosus (4)**. A bicuspid (mitral) atrioventricular valve separates the atrium (1) from the ventricle (19). The cusps of the atrioventricular (mitral) valve (5) are formed by a double membrane of the **endocardium (6)** and a dense **connective tissue core (7)** that is continuous with the annulus fibrosus (4). On the ventral surface of each cusp (5) are the insertions of the connective tissue cords, the **chorda tendineae (8),** which extend from the cusps of the valve (5) and attach to the **papillary muscles (11),** which project from the ventricle wall. The inner surface of the ventricle also contains prominent muscular (myocardial) ridges called **trabeculae carneae (10)** that give rise to the papillary muscles (11). The papillary muscles (11) via the chorda tendineae (8) hold and stabilize the cusps in the atrioventricular valves of the right and left ventricles during ventricular contractions.

The **Purkinje fibers (18),** or impulse-conducting fibers, are located in the subendocardial connective tissue (2). They are distinguished by their larger size and lighter-staining properties. The Purkinje fibers are illustrated in greater detail and higher magnification in Figures 8.8 and 8.9.

A large blood vessel of the heart, the **coronary artery (12),** is found in the subepicardial connective tissue (17). Below the coronary artery is the **coronary sinus (14)**, a blood vessel that drains the heart. Entering the coronary sinus (14) is a **coronary vein (14)** with its valve. Smaller coronary blood vessels (15) are seen in the subepicardial connective tissue (17) and in the connective tissue septa that are found in the myocardium (19).

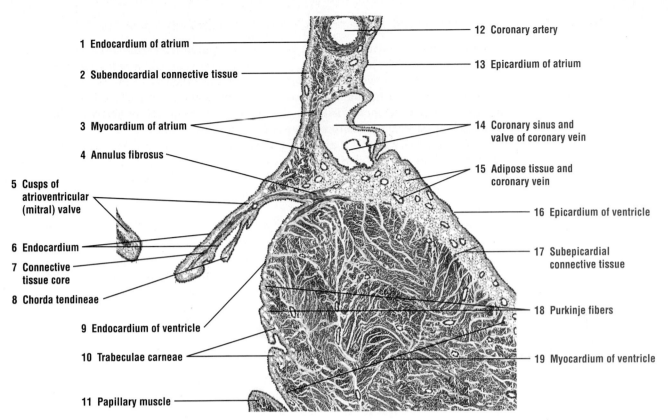

1 Endocardium of atrium

2 Subendocardial connective tissue

3 Myocardium of atrium

4 Annulus fibrosus

5 Cusps of atrioventricular (mitral) valve

6 Endocardium

7 Connective tissue core

8 Chorda tendineae

9 Endocardium of ventricle

10 Trabeculae carneae

11 Papillary muscle

12 Coronary artery

13 Epicardium of atrium

14 Coronary sinus and valve of coronary vein

15 Adipose tissue and coronary vein

16 Epicardium of ventricle

17 Subepicardial connective tissue

18 Purkinje fibers

19 Myocardium of ventricle

FIGURE 8.6 ■ Heart: a section of the left atrium, atrioventricular valve, and left ventricle (longitudinal section). Stain: hematoxylin and eosin. Low magnification.

FIGURE 8.7 ■ Heart: Right Ventricle, Pulmonary Trunk, and Pulmonary Valve (Longitudinal Section)

A section of the right ventricle and a lower portion of **pulmonary trunk (5)** are illustrated. As in other blood vessels, the pulmonary trunk (5) is lined by endothelium of the **tunica intima (5a)**. The **tunica media (5b)** constitutes the thickest portion of the wall of the pulmonary trunk (5); however, its thick, elastic laminae are not seen at this magnification. The thin connective tissue **tunica adventitia (5c)** merges with the surrounding **subepicardial connective tissue (2)**, which contains adipose tissue and **coronary arterioles and venules (2, 3)**.

The pulmonary trunk (5) arises from the **annulus fibrosus (8)**. One cusp of its **semilunar (pulmonary) valve (6)** is illustrated. Similar to the atrioventricular valve (see Figure 8.6), the semilunar valve (6) of the pulmonary trunk (5) is covered with **endocardium (6)**. A **connective tissue core (7)** from the annulus fibrosus (8) extends into the base of the semilunar valve (6) and forms its central core.

The thick **myocardium (4)** of the right ventricle is lined internally by **endocardium (9)**. The endocardium (9) extends over the pulmonary valve (6) and the annulus fibrosus (8), and blends in with the tunica intima (5a) of the pulmonary trunk (5).

The pulmonary trunk (6) is lined by the **subepicardial connective tissue** and **adipose tissue (2)**, which, in turn, is covered by **epicardium (1)**. Both of these layers cover the external surface of the right ventricle. Coronary arterioles and venules (3) are seen in the subepicardial connective tissue (2).

FIGURE 8.8 ■ Heart: Contracting Cardiac Muscle Fibers and Impulse-Conducting Purkinje Fibers

This figure illustrates a section of the heart stained with Mallory-Azan stain. With this preparation, the blue-stained collagen fibers accentuate the **subendocardial connective tissue (9)** that surrounds the **Purkinje fibers (6, 10)**. The characteristic features of Purkinje fibers (6, 10) are demonstrated in both longitudinal and transverse planes of section. In transverse plane (6), the Purkinje fibers exhibit fewer myofibrils that are distributed peripherally, leaving a perinuclear zone of comparatively clear sarcoplasm. A nucleus is seen in some transverse sections; in others, a central area of clear sarcoplasm is seen, with the plane of section bypassing the nucleus.

The Purkinje fibers (6, 10) are located under the **endocardium (7)**, which represents the endothelium of the heart cavities. The Purkinje fibers (6, 10) are different from typical **cardiac muscle fibers (1, 3)**. In contrast to cardiac muscle fibers (1, 3), the Purkinje fibers (6, 10) are larger in size and show less intense staining.

The cardiac muscle fibers (1, 3) are connected to each other via the prominent **intercalated disks (4)**. The intercalated disks (4) are not observed in the Purkinje fibers (6, 10). Instead, the Purkinje fibers (6, 10) are connected to each other via desmosomes and gap junctions, and eventually merge with cardiac muscle fibers (1, 3).

The heart musculature has a rich blood supply. Seen in this illustration are a **capillary (8)**, **arteriole (5)**, and **venule (2)**.

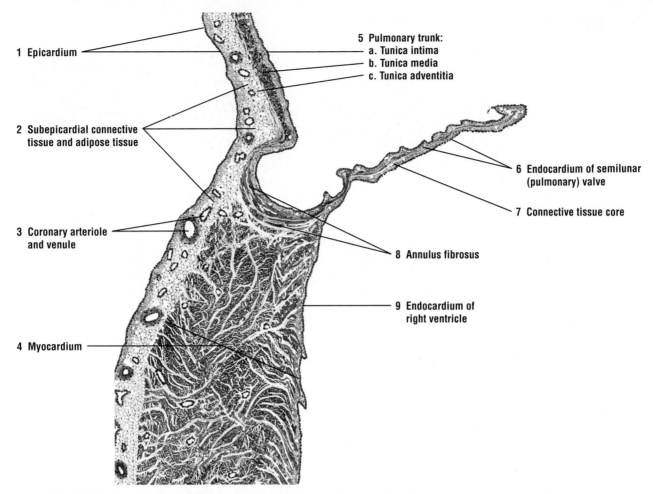

1 Epicardium

5 Pulmonary trunk:
  a. Tunica intima
  b. Tunica media
  c. Tunica adventitia

2 Subepicardial connective tissue and adipose tissue

6 Endocardium of semilunar (pulmonary) valve

7 Connective tissue core

3 Coronary arteriole and venule

8 Annulus fibrosus

9 Endocardium of right ventricle

4 Myocardium

FIGURE 8.7 ■ Heart: a section of right ventricle, pulmonary trunk, and pulmonary valve (longitudinal section). Stain: hematoxylin and eosin. Low magnification.

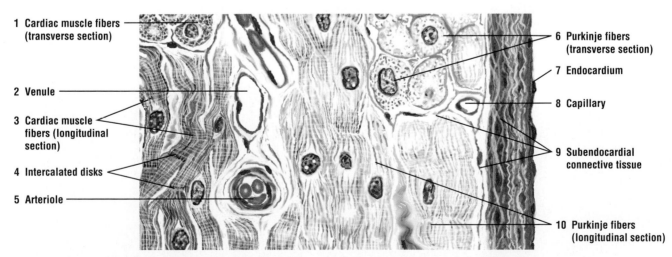

1 Cardiac muscle fibers (transverse section)

2 Venule

3 Cardiac muscle fibers (longitudinal section)

4 Intercalated disks

5 Arteriole

6 Purkinje fibers (transverse section)

7 Endocardium

8 Capillary

9 Subendocardial connective tissue

10 Purkinje fibers (longitudinal section)

FIGURE 8.8 ■ Heart: contracting cardiac muscle fibers and impulse-conducting Purkinje fibers. Stain: Mallory-azan. High magnification.

FIGURE 8.9 ■ Heart Wall: Purkinje Fibers

A photomicrograph of the ventricular heart wall illustrates the **endocardium** (3) of the heart chamber, **subendocardial connective tissue** (4), and the underlying **Purkinje fibers** (5). In comparison with the adjacent, red-stained **cardiac muscle fibers (1),** the Purkinje fibers (5) are larger in size and exhibit less intense staining. Also, the Purkinje fibers (5) exhibit fewer myofibrils, which are peripherally distributed and which leave a perinuclear zone of clear sarcoplasm. Purkinje fibers (5) gradually merge with the cardiac muscle fibers (1). Surrounding both the Purkinje fibers (5) and the cardiac muscle fibers (1) are bundles of **connective tissue fibers (2).**

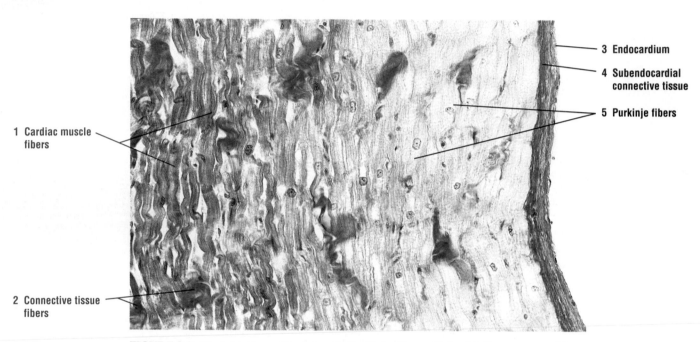

FIGURE 8.9 ■ A section of heart wall: Purkinje fibers. Stain: Mallory-azan. ×64.

FUNCTIONAL CORRELATIONS OF THE CIRCULATORY SYSTEM

Blood Vessels

The **elastic arteries** transport blood from the heart and move it along the systemic vascular path. The presence of an increased number of **elastic fibers** in their walls allows the elastic arteries to greatly expand in diameter during **systole** (heart contraction), when a large volume of blood is forcefully ejected from the ventricles into their lumina. During **diastole** (heart relaxation), the expanded elastic walls recoil upon the volume of blood in their lumina and force the blood to move forward through the vascular channels. As a result, a less variable systemic blood pressure is maintained, and blood flows more evenly through the body during heart beats.

In contrast, the **muscular arteries** control blood flow and blood pressure through **vasoconstriction** or **vasodilation** of their lumina. Vasoconstriction and vasodilation, owing to a high proportion of **smooth muscle fibers** in the artery walls, are controlled by unmyelinated axons of the **sympathetic division** of the **autonomic nervous system.** Similarly, by autonomic constriction or dilation of their lumina, the smooth muscle fibers in smaller muscular arteries or arterioles regulate blood flow into the capillary beds.

Terminal arterioles give rise to the smallest blood vessels, called **capillaries.** Because of their very thin walls, capillaries are major sites for exchange of gases, metabolites, nutrients, and waste products between blood and interstitial tissues.

In **veins,** blood pressure is lower than in the arteries. As a result, venous blood flow is **passive.** Venous blood flow in the head and trunk is primarily owing to negative pressures in the thorax and abdominal cavities resulting from respiratory movements. Venous blood return from the extremities is aided by surrounding **muscle contractions** and prevented from flowing back by numerous valves in the large veins of the extremities.

The Endothelium

The endothelium lining the lumina of blood vessels performs important functions in blood homeostasis. The endothelial cells form a **permeability barrier** between blood and the interstitial tissue. Also, the endothelium provides a smooth surface that allows blood cells and platelets to flow through the vessels without damage. The smooth lining of the blood vessels and the secretion of **anticoagulants** by the endothelial cells prevents blood clotting. Endothelium also produces vasoactive chemicals that stimulate the **dilation** or **constriction** of the blood vessels. When endothelium is damaged, platelets adhere at the site and form a blood clot. During inflammation of tissues around the vessel, the endothelium produces **cell adhesion molecules** that induce leukocytes to adhere and congregate at the site where their defensive actions can be used. Other functions of the endothelium include the conversion of **angiotensin I** to **angiotensin II,** which is a powerful vasoconstrictor that results in increased blood pressure. Endothelium also converts such compounds as prostaglandins, bradykinin, serotonin, and other substances to biologically inactive compounds, degrades lipoproteins, and produces growth factors for fibroblasts, blood cell colonies, and platelets, as well as having other functions.

Lymphatic Vessels

The main function of the **lymph vascular system** is to passively collect excess tissue fluid and proteins, called **lymph,** from the intercellular spaces of the connective tissue and return it into the venous portion of the blood vascular system. Lymph is a clear fluid and an **ultrafiltrate** of the blood plasma. Numerous lymph nodes are located along the route of the lymph vessels. In the maze of lymph node channels, the collected lymph is filtered of cells and particulate matter. Lymph that flows through the lymph nodes is also exposed to the numerous macrophages that reside here. These engulf any foreign microorganisms, as well as other suspended matter. The lymph vessels also bring to the systemic bloodstream **lymphocytes, fatty acids** absorbed through the capillary lymph vessels called **lacteals** in the small intestine, and **immunoglobulins** (antibodies) produced in the lymph nodes. Thus, the lymphatic vessels are an integral part of the immune system of the body.

The Heart Wall

Pacemaker of the Heart

Cardiac muscle is **involuntary** and contracts rhythmically and automatically. The **impulse-generating** and **impulse-conducting** portions of the heart are specialized or modified cardiac muscle fibers located in the **sinoatrial (SA) node** and the **atrioventricular (AV) node** in the wall of the **right atrium** of the heart. The modified cardiac muscle fibers in these nodes exhibit spontaneous rhythmic depolarization or impulse conduction, which sends a wave of stimulation throughout the myocardium of the heart. Because the fibers in the SA node depolarize and repolarize faster than those in the AV node, the SA node sets the pace for the heartbeat, and is, therefore, the **pacemaker.**

Intercalated disks bind all cardiac muscle fibers as stimulatory impulses from the SA node are conducted via **gap junctions** to the atrial musculature, causing rapid spread of stimuli and their contraction. Impulses from the SA node travel through the heart musculature via **internodal pathways** to stimulate the AV node that lies in the interatrial septum. From the AV node, the impulses spread along a bundle of specialized conducting cardiac fibers, called the **atrioventricular bundle (of His),** located in the interventricular septum. The atrioventricular bundle divides into right and left bundle branches. Approximately halfway down the interventricular septum, the atrioventricular bundle branches become the **Purkinje fibers,** which branch and transmit stimulation throughout the ventricles.

The pacemaker activities of the heart are influenced by the axons from the **autonomic nervous system** and by certain **hormones.** Axons from both the parasympathetic and sympathetic division innervate the heart and form a wide plexus at its base. Although these axons innervate the heart myocardium, they do not affect the initiation of rhythmic activity of the nodes. Instead, they affect the heart rate. Stimulation by the sympathetic nerves accelerates the heart rate, whereas stimulation by the parasympathetic nerves produces the opposite effect and decreases the heart rate.

Purkinje Fibers

Purkinje fibers are thicker and larger than cardiac muscle fibers and contain a greater amount of **glycogen.** They also contain fewer contractile filaments. Purkinje fibers are part of the conduction system of the heart. These fibers are located beneath the **endocardium** on either side of the interventricular septum and are recognized as separate tracts. Because Purkinje fibers branch throughout the myocardium, they deliver continuous waves of stimulation from the atrial nodes to the rest of the heart musculature via the **gap junctions.** This produces ventricular contractions (systole) and ejection of blood from both ventricular chambers.

Atrial Natriuretic Hormone

Certain cardiac muscle fibers in the atria exhibit dense granules in their cytoplasm. These granules contain **atrial natriuretic hormone,** a chemical that is released in response to atrial distension or stretching. The main function of this hormone is to decrease blood pressure by regulating blood volume. This action is accomplished by inhibiting the release of **renin** by the specialized cells in the kidney and **aldosterone** from the adrenal gland cortex. This induces the kidney to lose more sodium and water (diuresis). As a result, the blood volume and blood pressure are reduced, and the distension of the atrial wall is relieved.

CHAPTER 8 ■ Summary

Blood Vascular System

- Consists of heart, major arteries, arterioles, capillaries, veins, and venules

Type of Arteries

Elastic Arteries

- Are the largest vessels in the body
- Include aorta, pulmonary trunk, and their major branches
- Wall primarily composed of elastic connective tissue
- Exhibit resilience and flexibility during blood flow
- Walls greatly expand during systole (heart contraction)
- During diastole (heart relaxation), walls recoil and force blood forward

Muscular Arteries, Arterioles, and Capillaries

- Wall contains much smooth muscle
- Control of blood flow through vasoconstriction or vasodilation of lumina
- Smooth muscles in arterial walls controlled by autonomic nervous system
- Arterioles are the small blood vessels with one to five layers of smooth muscle
- Terminal arterioles deliver blood to smallest blood vessels, the capillaries
- Capillaries are sites of metabolic exchanges between blood and tissues
- Capillaries connect arterioles with venules

Structural Plan of Arteries

- Wall consists of three layers: inner tunica intima, middle tunica media, and outer tunica adventitia
- Tunica intima consists of endothelium and subendothelial connective tissue
- Tunica media is composed mainly of smooth muscle fibers
- Tunica adventitia contains primarily collagen and elastic fibers
- Smooth muscles produce the extracellular matrix
- Internal elastic lamina separates tunica intima from tunica media
- External elastic lamina separates tunica media from tunica adventitia

Structural Plan of Veins

- Capillaries unite to form larger vessels called venules and postcapillary venules
- Thinner walls, larger diameters, and more structural variation than arteries
- In veins of extremities, valves present to prevent backflow of blood
- Blood flows toward heart owing to muscular contractions around veins
- Wall consists of three layers: inner tunica intima, middle tunica media, and outer tunica adventitia
- Tunica intima consists of endothelium and subendothelial connective tissue
- Tunica media is thin, and smooth muscle intermixes with connective tissue fibers
- Tunica adventitia is the thickest layer with longitudinal smooth muscle fibers

Vasa Vasorum

- Found in walls of large arteries and veins
- Small blood vessels supply tunica media and tunica adventitia

Types of Capillaries

- Average diameter is about the size of red blood cell
- Continuous capillaries are most common; endothelium forms solid lining
- Continuous capillaries found in most organs
- Fenestrated capillaries contain pores or fenestrations in endothelium
- Fenestrated capillaries found in endocrine glands, small intestine, and kidney glomeruli
- Sinusoidal capillaries exhibit wide diameters with wide gaps between endothelial cells
- Basement membrane incomplete or absent in sinusoidal capillaries
- Sinusoidal capillaries found in liver, spleen, and bone marrow

Lymph Vascular System

- Consists of lymph capillaries and vessels
- Starts as blind lymphatic capillaries
- Collects excess interstitial fluid lymph and returns it to venous blood
- Vessels very thin for greater permeability
- Lymph vessels contain valves
- Lymph flows through lymph nodes and is exposed to macrophages
- Lymph contains lymphocytes, fatty acids, and immunoglobulins (antibodies)

Endothelium

- Forms a permeability barrier between blood and interstitial tissue
- Provides smooth surface for blood flow and produces anticoagulants to prevent blood clotting
- Dilates and constricts blood vessels

- Produces cell adhesion molecules to induce leukocyte adhesion and accumulation
- Converts angiotensin I to angiotensin II to increase blood pressure
- Converts certain chemicals to inactive compounds, degrades lipoproteins, and produces growth factors

Heart Wall – Endocardium, Myocardium, and Epicardium

Pacemaker

- Impulse conduction by specialized cardiac cells located in SA and AV nodes
- SA and AV nodes located in the wall of the right atrium
- SA node sets the pace for the heart and is the pacemaker of the heart
- Impulse from SA node conducted via gap junctions to all heart musculature
- Atrioventricular bundles located on right and left sides of the interventricular septum
- Atrioventricular bundles become Purkinje fibers
- Pacemaker activities influenced by autonomic nervous system and hormones

Purkinje Fibers

- Larger than cardiac fibers with more glycogen and lighter staining
- Part of the conduction system of the heart
- Located beneath the endocardium on either side of the interventricular septum
- Branch throughout the myocardium and deliver stimuli via gap junctions to rest of heart

Atrial Natriuretic Hormone

- Certain atrial cells contain granules of atrial natriuretic hormone
- Released when atrial wall is stretched
- Decreases blood pressure by inhibiting renin and aldosterone release
- Kidney loses more sodium and water, which decreases blood volume and pressure

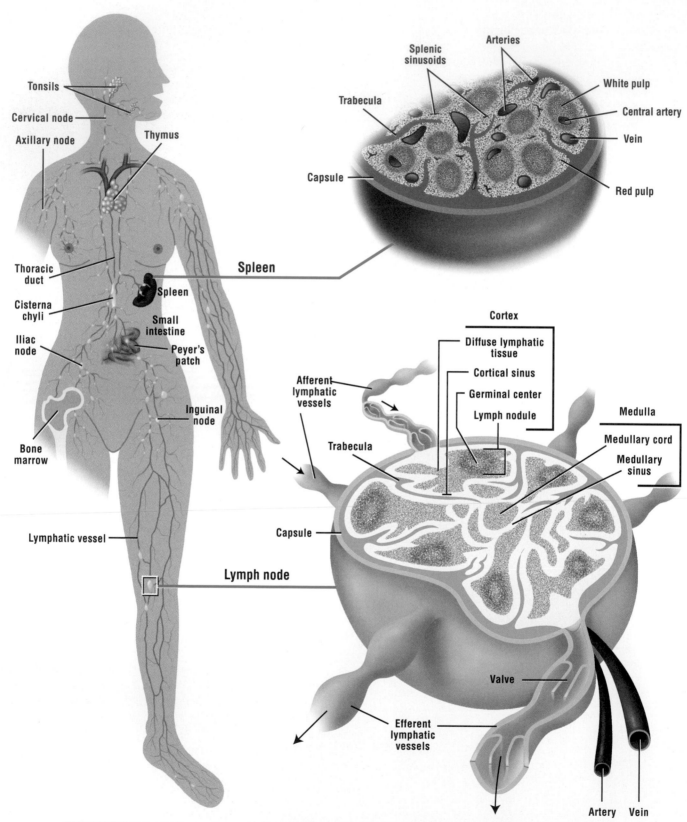

Tonsils

Cervical node

Axillary node

Thymus

Thoracic duct

Spleen

Cisterna chyli

Small intestine

Iliac node

Peyer's patch

Bone marrow

Inguinal node

Lymphatic vessel

Spleen

Splenic sinusoids

Arteries

Trabecula

White pulp

Central artery

Vein

Capsule

Red pulp

Cortex

Diffuse lymphatic tissue

Cortical sinus

Germinal center

Lymph nodule

Medulla

Medullary cord

Medullary sinus

Afferent lymphatic vessels

Trabecula

Capsule

Valve

Lymph node

Efferent lymphatic vessels

Artery   Vein

OVERVIEW FIGURE 9 ■ Location and distribution of the lymphoid organs and lymphatic channels in the body. Internal contents of the lymph node and spleen are illustrated in greater detail.

Lymphoid System

The **lymphoid system** collects excess interstitial fluid into lymphatic capillaries, transports absorbed lipids from the small intestine, and responds immunologically to invading foreign substances. The main function of the lymphoid organs is to protect the organism against invading pathogens or antigens (bacteria, parasites, and viruses). The immune response occurs when the organism detects the pathogens, which can enter the organism at any point. For this reason, lymphatic cells, tissues, and organs have wide distribution in the body.

The lymphoid system includes all cells, tissues, and organs in the body that contain aggregates of immune cells called **lymphocytes.** Cells of the immune system, especially lymphocytes, are distributed throughout the body either as single cells, as isolated accumulations of cells, as distinct nonencapsulated lymphatic nodules in the loose connective tissue of **digestive, respiratory, and reproductive systems,** or as encapsulated individual lymphoid organs. The major lymphoid organs are the lymph nodes, tonsils, thymus, and spleen. Because bone marrow produces lymphocytes, it is considered a lymphoid organ and part of the lymphoid system.

Lymphoid Organs: Lymph Nodes, Spleen, and Thymus

The overview figure illustrates the distribution of the lymphoid system in the body and the general structures of two encapsulated lymphoid organs, the **lymph node** and **spleen.** A connective tissue **capsule** surrounds the lymph node and sends its **trabeculae** into its interior. Each lymph node contains an outer **cortex** and an inner **medulla.** A network of reticular fibers and spherical, nonencapsulated aggregations of lymphocytes called **lymphoid nodules** characterize the cortex. Some lymphoid nodules exhibit lighter-staining central areas called **germinal centers.** The medulla consists of **medullary cords** and **medullary sinuses.** Medullary cords are networks of reticular fibers filled with plasma cells, macrophages, and lymphocytes separated by capillary-like channels called medullary sinuses. Lymph enters the lymph node via **afferent lymphatic vessels** that penetrate the capsule on the convex surface. Lymph flows through the medullary sinuses and exits the lymph node on the opposite side via the **efferent lymphatic vessels** (see Overview Figure 9).

The spleen is a large lymphoid organ with a rich blood supply. A connective tissue capsule surrounds the spleen and divides its interior into incomplete compartments called the **splenic pulp. White pulp** consists of dark-staining lymphoid aggregations or **lymphatic nodules** that surround a blood vessel called the **central artery.** White pulp is located within the blood-rich red pulp. **Red pulp,** in turn, consists of **splenic cords** and **splenic (blood) sinusoids.** Splenic cords contain networks of reticular fibers in which are found macrophages, lymphocytes, plasma cells, and different blood cells. Splenic sinuses are interconnected blood channels that drain splenic blood into larger sinuses that eventually leave the spleen via the splenic vein (see Overview Figure 9).

The **thymus gland** is a soft, lobulated lymphoepithelial organ located in the upper anterior mediastinum and lower part of the neck. The gland is most active during childhood, after which it undergoes slow involution; in adults, it is filled with adipose tissue. The thymus gland is surrounded by a connective tissue capsule, under which is a dark-staining **cortex** with an extensive network of interconnecting spaces. These spaces become colonized by **immature lymphocytes** that migrate here from hemopoietic tissues in the developing individual to undergo maturation and differentiation. The epithelial cells of the thymus gland provide structural support for the increased lymphocyte population. In the lighter-staining **medulla,** the epithelial cells form a coarser framework that contains fewer lymphocytes and whorls of epithelial cells that combine to form **thymic (Hassall's) corpuscles.**

Lymphoid Cells: T Lymphocytes and B Lymphocytes

All components of the lymphoid system are an essential part of the **immune system.** Lymphocytes are the cells that carry out immune responses. Different types of lymphocytes are present in various organs of the body. Morphologically, all types of lymphocytes appear very similar, but functionally, they are very different. When lymphocytes are properly stimulated, **B lymphocytes** or **B cells** and **T lymphocytes** or **T cells** are produced. These two subclasses of lymphocytes are distinguished on the basis of where they differentiate and mature into immunocompetent cells, and on the types of surface receptors present on their cell membranes. These two functionally distinct types of lymphocytes are found in blood, lymph, lymphoid tissues, and lymphoid organs. Like all blood cells, both types of lymphocytes originate from precursor **hemopoietic stem cells** in the **bone marrow** and then enter the bloodstream.

T cells arise from lymphocytes that are carried from the bone marrow to the **thymus gland.** Here, they mature, differentiate, and acquire surface receptors and **immunocompetence** before migrating to peripheral lymphoid tissues and organs. The thymus gland produces mature T cells early in life. After their stay in the thymus gland, T cells are distributed throughout the body in blood and populate lymph nodes, the spleen, and lymphoid aggregates or nodules in connective tissue. In these regions, the T cells carry out immune responses when stimulated. On encountering an antigen, T cells destroy the antigen either by cytotoxic action or by activating B cells. There are four main types of differentiated T cells: **helper T cells, cytotoxic T cells, memory T cells,** and **suppressor T cells.**

When encountering an antigen, **helper T cells** assist other lymphocytes by secreting immune chemicals called **cytokines,** also called **interleukins.** Cytokines are protein hormones that stimulate proliferation, secretion, differentiation, and maturation of B cells into **plasma cells,** which then produce immune proteins called **antibodies,** also called **immunoglobulins.**

Cytotoxic T cells specifically recognize antigenically different cells such as virus-infected cells, foreign cells, or malignant cells and destroy them. These lymphocytes become activated when they combine with antigens that react with their receptors.

Memory T cells are the long-living progeny of T cells. They respond rapidly to the same antigens in the body and stimulate immediate production of cytotoxic T cells. Memory T cells are the counterparts of memory B cells.

Suppressor T cells may decrease or inhibit the functions of helper T cells and cytotoxic T cells, and thus modulate the immune response.

B cells mature and become immunocompetent in bone marrow. After maturation, blood carries B cells to the nonthymic lymphoid tissues such as lymph nodes, spleen, and connective tissue. B cells are able to recognize a particular type of antigen owing to the presence of **antigen receptors** on the surface of their cell membrane. Immunocompetent B cells become activated when they encounter a specific antigen and it binds to the surface antigen receptor of the B lymphocyte. The response of B cells to an antigen, however, is more intense when antigen-presenting cells, such as **helper T cells,** present the antigen to the B cells. Helper T cells secrete a cytokine (**interleukin 2**) that induces increased proliferation and differentiation of antigen-activated B cells. Numerous progeny of activated B cells enlarge, divide, proliferate, and differentiate into **plasma cells.** Plasma cells then secrete large amounts of antibodies specific to the antigen that triggered plasma cell formation. Antibodies react with the antigens and initiate a complex process that eventually destroys the foreign substance that activated the immune response. Other activated B cells do not become plasma cells. Instead, they persist in lymphoid organs as **memory B cells.** These memory cells produce a more rapid immunologic response should the same antigen reappear.

In addition to T cells and B cells, cells called macrophages, natural killer cells, and antigen-presenting cells perform important functions in immune responses. **Natural killer cells** attack virally infected cells and cancer cells. **Antigen-presenting cells** are found in most tissues. These cells phagocytose and process antigens, and then present the antigen to T cells, inducing their activation. Most antigen-presenting cells belong to the mononuclear phagocytic system. Included in this group are the connective tissue **macrophages, perisinusoidal macrophages** in the liver (Kupffer cells), **Langerhans cells** in the skin, and macrophages within lymphoid organs.

Basic Types of Immune Responses

The presence of foreign cells or antigens in the body stimulates a highly complex series of reactions. These result in either production of antibodies, which bind to the antigens, or stimulation of cells that destroy foreign cells. B cells and T cells respond to antigens by different means. Two types of closely related immune responses take place in the body, both of which are triggered by antigens.

In the **cell-mediated immune response,** T cells are stimulated by the presence of antigens on the surface of antigen-presenting cells. The T cells proliferate and secrete cytokines. These chemical signals stimulate other T cells, B cells, and cytotoxic T cells. On activation and binding to target cells, cytoxic T cells produce protein molecules called **perforin,** which perforate or puncture the target cell membranes, causing cell death. Cytotoxic T cells also destroy foreign cells by attaching to them and inducing **apoptosis** or programmed cell death. The activated lymphocytes then destroy foreign microorganisms, parasites, tumor cells, or virus-infected cells. T cells may also attack indirectly by activating B cells or **macrophages** of the immune system. T cells provide specific immune protection without secreting antibodies.

In the **humoral immune response,** exposure of **B cells** to an antigen induces proliferation and transformation of some of the B cells into **plasma cells.** These, in turn, secrete specific **antibodies** into blood and lymph that bind to, inactivate, and destroy the specific foreign substance or antigens. The activation and proliferation of B cells against most antigens require the cooperation of helper T cells that respond to the same antigen and the production of certain cytokines. The presence of the B cells, plasma cells, and antibodies in the blood and lymph are the basis of the humoral immune response.

FIGURE 9.1 ■ Lymph Node (Panoramic View)

The lymph node consists of dense masses of lymphocyte aggregations intermixed with dilated lymphatic sinuses that contain lymph and are supported by a framework of fine reticular fibers. A lymph node has been sectioned in half to show the outer dark-staining **cortex (4)** and the inner light-staining **medulla (10).** The lymph node is surrounded by a **pericapsular adipose tissue (1)** that contains numerous blood vessels, shown here as an **arteriole** and **venule (9).** A dense connective tissue **capsule (2)** surrounds the lymph node. From the capsule (2), **connective tissue trabeculae (6)** extend into the node, initially between the lymphatic nodules, and then ramifying throughout the medulla (10) for a variable distance. The trabecular connective tissue (6) also contains the major **blood vessels (5, 8)** of the lymph node.

Afferent lymphatic vessels with **valves (7)** course in the connective tissue capsule (2) of the lymph node and, at intervals, penetrate the capsule to enter a narrow space called the **subcapsular sinus (3, 15).** From here, the sinuses (cortical sinuses) extend along the trabeculae (6) to pass into the **medullary sinuses (11).**

The cortex (4) of the lymph node contains numerous lymphocyte aggregations called **lymphatic nodules (16).** When the lymphatic nodules (16) are sectioned through the center, lighter-stained areas become visible. These lighter areas are the **germinal centers (17)** of the lymphatic nodules (16) and represent the active sites of lymphocyte proliferation.

In the medulla (10) of the lymph node, the lymphocytes are arranged as irregular cords of lymphatic tissue called **medullary cords (14).** Medullary cords (14) contain macrophages, plasma cells, and small lymphocytes. The dilated medullary sinuses (11) drain the lymph from the cortical region of the lymph node and course between the medullary cords (14) toward the hilus of the organ.

The concavity of the lymph node represents the **hilus (12).** Nerves, blood vessels, and veins that supply and drain the lymph node are located in the hilus (12). **Efferent lymphatic vessels (13)** drain the lymph from the medullary sinuses (11) and exit the lymph node in the hilus (12).

1 Pericapsular adipose
  tissue

2 Capsule

3 Subcapsular sinus

4 Cortex

5 Trabecular blood
  vessels

6 Connective tissue
  trabeculae

7 Afferent lymphatic
  vessels with valves

8 Trabecular blood
  vessels

9 Arteriole and venule

10 Medulla

11 Medullary sinuses

12 Hilus

13 Efferent lymphatic
   vessels

14 Medullary cords

15 Subcapsular sinus

16 Lymphatic nodules

17 Germinal centers of
   lymphatic nodules

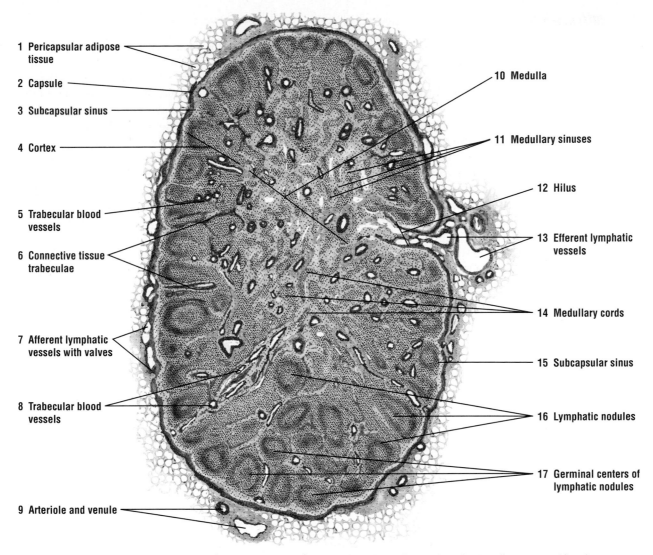

FIGURE 9.1 ■ Lymph node (panoramic view). Stain: hematoxylin and eosin. Medium magnification.

FIGURE 9.2 ■ Lymph Node Capsule, Cortex, and Medulla (Sectional View)

A small section of a cortical region of the lymph node is illustrated at a higher magnification.

A layer of **connective tissue (1)** with a **venule** and **arteriole (11)** surrounds the lymph node **capsule (3).** Visible in the connective tissue (1) is an afferent **lymphatic vessel (2)** lined with endothelium and containing a **valve (2).** Arising from the inner surface of the capsule (3), the connective tissue **trabeculae (5, 14)** extend through the cortex and medulla. Associated with the connective tissue trabeculae (5, 14) are numerous **trabecular blood vessels (16).**

The cortex of the lymph node is separated from the connective tissue capsule (3) by the **subcapsular (marginal) sinus (4, 12).** The cortex consists of **lymphatic nodules (13)** situated adjacent to each other but incompletely separated by internodular connective tissue trabeculae (5, 14) and **trabecular (cortical) sinuses (6).** In this illustration, two complete lymphatic nodules (13) are illustrated. When sectioned through the middle, the lymphatic nodules exhibit a central, light-staining **germinal center (7, 15)** surrounded by a deeper-staining peripheral portion of the nodule (13). In the germinal centers (7, 15) of the lymphatic nodules (13), the cells are more loosely aggregated and the developing lymphocytes have larger and lighter-staining nuclei with more cytoplasm.

The deeper portion of the lymph node cortex is the **paracortex (8, 17).** This area is the thymus-dependent zone and is primarily occupied by T cells. This is also a transition area from the lymphatic nodules (7, 13) to the **medullary cords (9, 19)** of the lymph node medulla. The medulla consists of anastomosing cords of lymphatic tissue, the medullary cords (9, 19), interspersed with **medullary sinuses (10, 18)** that drain the lymph from the node into the efferent lymphatic vessels that are located at the hilus (see Figure 9.1).

Fine reticular connective tissue provides the main structural support for the lymph node and forms the core of the lymphatic nodules (13) in the cortex, the medullary cords (9, 19), and all medullary sinuses (10, 18) in the medulla. Relatively few lymphocytes are seen in the medullary sinuses (10, 18); thus, it is possible to distinguish the reticular framework of the node in the lymphatic nodules (13) and the medullary cords (9, 19). The lymphocytes are so abundant that the fine reticulum is obscured, unless it is specifically stained, as shown in Figure 9.5. Most of the lymphocytes are small with large, deep-staining nuclei and condensed chromatin, and exhibit either a small amount of cytoplasm or none at all.

FUNCTIONAL CORRELATIONS: Lymph Nodes

Lymph nodes are important components of the defense mechanism. They are distributed throughout the body along the paths of **lymphatic vessels** and are most prominent in the **inguinal** and **axillary regions.** Their major functions are **lymph filtration** and **phagocytosis** of bacteria or foreign substances from the lymph, preventing them from reaching the general circulation. Trapped within the reticular fiber network of each node are fixed or free macrophages that destroy any foreign substances. Thus, as lymph is filtered, the nodes participate in localizing and preventing the spread of infection into the general circulation and other organs.

Lymph nodes also produce, store, and recirculate **B cells** and **T cells.** Here the lymphocytes can proliferate and the B cells can transform into plasma cells. As a result, lymph that leaves the lymph nodes may contain increased amounts of antibodies that can then be distributed to the entire body. B cells congregate in the **lymphatic nodules** of lymph nodes, whereas T cells are concentrated below the nodules in the deep **cortical** or **paracortical regions.** Lymph nodes are also the sites of **antigenic recognition** and **antigenic activation** of B cells, which give rise to **plasma cells** and **memory B cells.**

All of the lymph that is formed in the body eventually reaches the blood, and lymphocytes that leave the lymph nodes via the efferent lymph vessels also return to the bloodstream. The arteries that supply the lymph nodes and branch into capillaries in the cortical and paracortical regions also provide an entryway for lymphocytes into the lymph nodes. Most of the lymphocytes enter the lymph nodes through the postcapillary venules located deep in the cortex. Here, the postcapillary venules exhibit tall cuboidal or columnar endothelium containing specialized **lymphocyte-homing receptors.** Because these venules are lined by taller endothelium, they are called **high endothelial venules.** The circulating lymphocytes recognize the receptors in the endothelial cells and leave the bloodstream to enter the lymph node. Both B and T cells leave the bloodstream via the high endothelial venules. These specialized venules are also present in other lymphoid organs, such as Peyer's patches in the small intestine, tonsils, appendix, and cortex of the thymus; high endothelial venules are absent from the spleen.

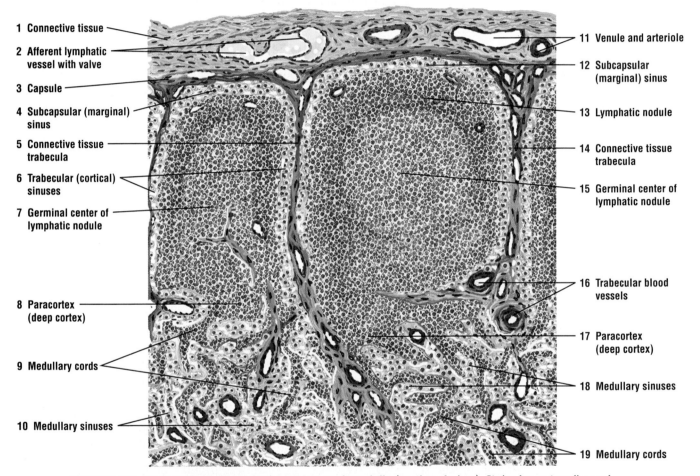

1 Connective tissue
2 Afferent lymphatic vessel with valve
3 Capsule
4 Subcapsular (marginal) sinus
5 Connective tissue trabecula
6 Trabecular (cortical) sinuses
7 Germinal center of lymphatic nodule
8 Paracortex (deep cortex)
9 Medullary cords
10 Medullary sinuses

11 Venule and arteriole
12 Subcapsular (marginal) sinus
13 Lymphatic nodule
14 Connective tissue trabecula
15 Germinal center of lymphatic nodule
16 Trabecular blood vessels
17 Paracortex (deep cortex)
18 Medullary sinuses
19 Medullary cords

FIGURE 9.2 ■ Lymph node: capsule, cortex, and medulla (sectional view). Stain: hematoxylin and eosin. Medium magnification.

FIGURE 9.3 ■ Cortex and Medulla of a Lymph Node

This low-power photomicrograph illustrates the cortex and medulla of the lymph node. A loose connective tissue **capsule (4)** with blood vessels and **adipose cells (7)** covers the lymph node. Inferior to the capsule (4) is the **subcapsular (marginal) sinus (5),** which overlies the darker-staining and peripheral lymph node **cortex (3).** In the cortex (3) are found numerous **lymphatic nodules (1, 6),** some of which contain a lighter-staining **germinal center (2).**

The central region of the lymph node is the lighter-staining **medulla (9).** This region is characterized by the dark-staining **medullary cords (12)** and the light-staining lymphatic channels, the **medullary sinuses (11).** The medullary sinuses (11) drain the lymph that enters the lymph node through the afferent lymphatic vessels in the capsule (see Figure 9.2) and converges toward the hilum of the lymph node (see Figure 9.1). In the hilum are found numerous **arteries (8)** and veins. The lymph leaves the lymph node via the **efferent lymphatic vessels** with **valves (10)** at the hilum.

FIGURE 9.4 ■ Lymph Node: Subcortical Sinus and Lymphatic Nodule

This figure illustrates, at a higher magnification and in greater detail, a portion of the lymph node with the connective tissue **capsule (3), trabecula (4),** and **subcapsular sinus (1)** that continue on both sides of the trabecula (4) as **trabecular sinuses (12)** into the interior of the lymph node.

The reticular connective tissue of the lymph node, the **reticular cells (8, 11),** is seen in different regions of the node. Reticular cells (8, 11) are visible in the subcapsular sinus (1), trabecular sinuses (12), and the **germinal center (9)** of the **lymphatic nodule (14).** Numerous free **macrophages (2, 6, 16)** are also seen in the subcapsular sinus (1), trabecular sinuses (12), and the germinal center (9) of the lymphatic nodule (14).

A lymphatic nodule with a small section of its **peripheral zone (14)** and a germinal center (9) with developing lymphocytes are also visible. **Endothelial cells (5, 13)** line the sinuses (1, 12) and form an incomplete cover over the surface of the lymphatic nodules (14).

The peripheral zone of the lymphatic nodule (14) stains dense because of the accumulation of **small lymphocytes (7).** The small lymphocytes (7) are characterized by dark-staining nuclei, condensed chromatin, and little or no cytoplasm. Small lymphocytes (7) are also present in the subcapsular sinus (1) and trabecular sinuses (12).

The germinal center (9) of the lymphatic nodule (14) contains **medium-sized lymphocytes (10).** These cells are characterized by larger, lighter nuclei and more cytoplasm than is seen in the small lymphocytes (7). The nuclei of medium-sized lymphocytes (10) exhibit variations in size and density of chromatin. The largest cells, with less condensed chromatin, are derived from **lymphoblasts (17).** The lymphoblasts (17) are visible in small numbers in the germinal center (9) of the lymphatic nodules (14) as large, round cells with a broad band of cytoplasm and a large vesicular nucleus with one or more nucleoli. **Lymphoblasts** undergoing mitosis (15) produce other lymphoblasts and medium-sized lymphocytes (10). With successive mitotic divisions of lymphoblasts (15), the chromatin condenses and the cells decrease in size, resulting in the formation of small lymphocytes (7).

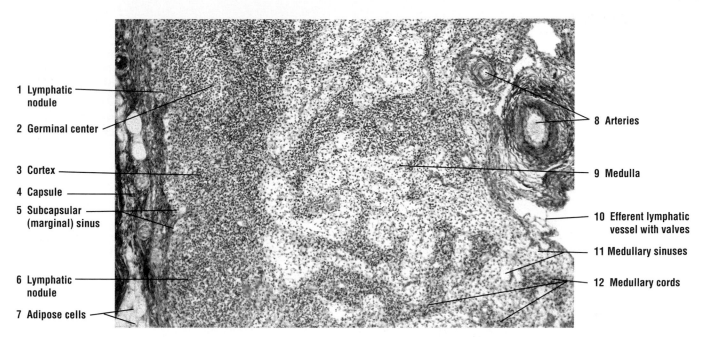

1 Lymphatic nodule

2 Germinal center

3 Cortex

4 Capsule

5 Subcapsular (marginal) sinus

6 Lymphatic nodule

7 Adipose cells

8 Arteries

9 Medulla

10 Efferent lymphatic vessel with valves

11 Medullary sinuses

12 Medullary cords

FIGURE 9.3 ■ Cortex and medulla of a lymph node. Stain: Mallory-azan. ×25.

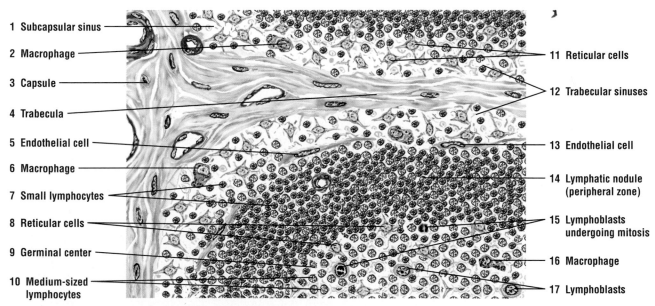

1 Subcapsular sinus

2 Macrophage

3 Capsule

4 Trabecula

5 Endothelial cell

6 Macrophage

7 Small lymphocytes

8 Reticular cells

9 Germinal center

10 Medium-sized lymphocytes

11 Reticular cells

12 Trabecular sinuses

13 Endothelial cell

14 Lymphatic nodule (peripheral zone)

15 Lymphoblasts undergoing mitosis

16 Macrophage

17 Lymphoblasts

FIGURE 9.4 ■ Lymph node: subcortical sinus, trabecular sinus, reticular cells, and lymphatic nodule. Stain: hematoxylin and eosin. High magnification.

FIGURE 9.5 ■ Lymph Node: High Endothelial Venule in Paracortex (Deep Cortex) of a Lymph Node

The paracortex region of lymph nodes contains postcapillary venules. These venules have an unusual morphology to facilitate the migration of lymphocytes from the blood into the lymph node. This image shows a **high endothelial venule** (2) that is lined by tall cuboidal endothelium, instead of the usual squamous endothelium. Several **migrating lymphocytes** (3) are seen moving through the venule wall between the high endothelium (2) into the paracortex of the lymph node. Surrounding the high endothelial venule (2) are **lymphocytes** in the **paracortex** (5), a **medullary sinus** (1), and a **venule** (4) with blood cells.

FIGURE 9.6 ■ Lymph Node: Subcapsular Sinus, Trabecular Sinus, and Supporting Reticular Fibers

A section of a lymph node has been stained with the silver method to illustrate the intricate arrangement of the supporting **reticular fibers** (6, 9) of a lymph node. The thicker and denser collagen fibers in the connective tissue **capsule** (3) stain pink. Both the capsule and the rest of the lymph node are supported by delicate reticular fibers (6, 9) that stain black and form a fine meshwork throughout the organ.

The various zones that are illustrated in Figure 9.2 with hematoxylin and eosin stain are readily recognizable with the silver stain. A connective tissue **trabecula** (4) from the capsule (3) penetrates the interior of the lymph node between two **lymphatic nodules** (8, 12). Inferior to the capsule (3) are **subcapsular (marginal) sinuses** (1, 7) that continue on each side of the trabecula (4) as **trabecular sinuses** (2, 5) into the medulla of the node and eventually exit through the efferent lymph vessels in the hilum. Also observed are **medullary cords** (10) and **medullary sinuses** (11).

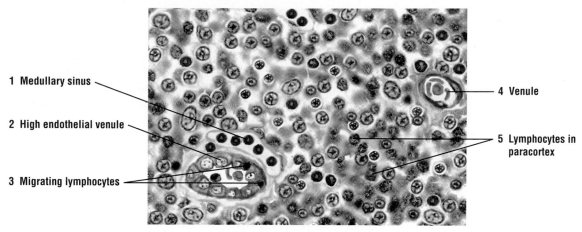

1 Medullary sinus

2 High endothelial venule

3 Migrating lymphocytes

4 Venule

5 Lymphocytes in paracortex

FIGURE 9.5 ■ Lymph node: high endothelial venule in the paracortex (deep cortex) of a lymph node. Stain: hematoxylin and eosin. High magnification.

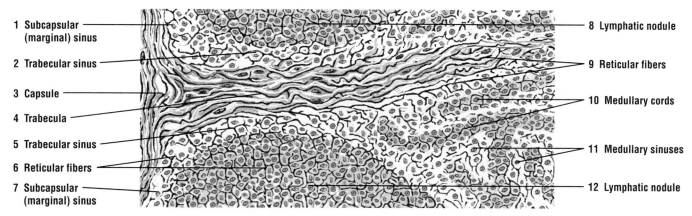

1 Subcapsular (marginal) sinus

2 Trabecular sinus

3 Capsule

4 Trabecula

5 Trabecular sinus

6 Reticular fibers

7 Subcapsular (marginal) sinus

8 Lymphatic nodule

9 Reticular fibers

10 Medullary cords

11 Medullary sinuses

12 Lymphatic nodule

FIGURE 9.6 ■ Lymph node: subcapsular sinus, trabecular sinus, and supporting reticular fibers. Stain: Silver stain. Medium magnification.

FIGURE 9.7 ■ Thymus Gland (Panoramic View)

The thymus gland is a lobulated lymphoid organ enclosed by a connective tissue **capsule (1)** from which arise connective tissue **trabeculae (2, 10).** The trabeculae (2, 10) extend into the interior of the organ and subdivide the thymus gland into numerous incomplete **lobules (8).** Each lobule consists of a dark-staining outer **cortex (3, 13)** and a light-staining inner **medulla (4, 12).** Because the lobules are incomplete, the medulla shows continuity between the neighboring lobules (4, 12). **Blood vessels (5, 14)** pass into the thymus gland via the connective tissue capsule (1) and the trabeculae (2, 10).

The cortex (3, 13) of each lobule contains densely packed lymphocytes that do not form lymphatic nodules. In contrast, the medulla (4, 12) contains fewer lymphocytes but more epithelial reticular cells (see Figure 9.7). The medulla also contains numerous **thymic (Hassall's) corpuscles (6, 9)** that characterize the thymus gland.

The histology of the thymus gland varies with the age of the individual. The thymus gland attains its greatest development shortly after birth. By the time of puberty, thymus glands begin to involute or show signs of gradual regression and degeneration. As a consequence, lymphocyte production declines, and the thymic (Hassall's) corpuscles (6, 9) become more prominent. In addition, the parenchyma or cellular portion of the gland is gradually replaced by loose **connective tissue (10)** and **adipose cells (7, 11).** The thymus gland depicted in this illustration exhibits adipose tissue accumulation and initial signs of involution associated with increasing age.

FIGURE 9.8 ■ Thymus Gland (Sectional View)

A small section of the cortex and medulla of a thymus gland lobule is illustrated at a higher magnification. The thymic lymphocytes in the **cortex (1, 5)** form dense aggregations. In contrast, the **medulla (3)** contains only a few lymphocytes but more **epithelial reticular cells (7, 10).**

The **thymic (Hassall's) corpuscles (8, 9)** are oval structures consisting of round or spherical aggregations (whorls) of flattened epithelial cells. The thymic corpuscles also exhibit calcification or **degeneration centers (9)** that stain pink or eosinophilic. The functional significance of these corpuscles remains unknown.

Blood vessels (6) and **adipose cells (4)** are present in both the thymic lobules and in a connective tissue **trabecula (2).**

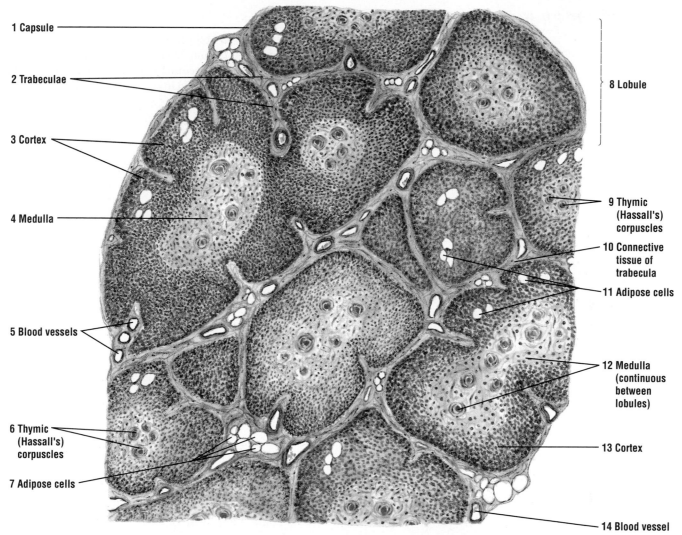

1 Capsule

2 Trabeculae

3 Cortex

4 Medulla

5 Blood vessels

6 Thymic (Hassall's) corpuscles

7 Adipose cells

8 Lobule

9 Thymic (Hassall's) corpuscles

10 Connective tissue of trabecula

11 Adipose cells

12 Medulla (continuous between lobules)

13 Cortex

14 Blood vessel

FIGURE 9.7 ■ Thymus gland (panoramic view). Stain: hematoxylin and eosin. Low magnification.

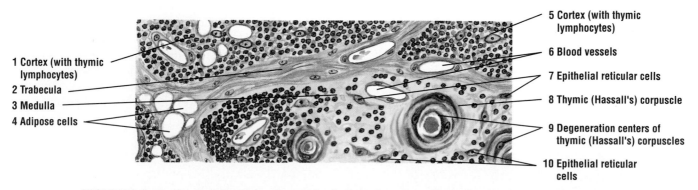

1 Cortex (with thymic lymphocytes)

2 Trabecula

3 Medulla

4 Adipose cells

5 Cortex (with thymic lymphocytes)

6 Blood vessels

7 Epithelial reticular cells

8 Thymic (Hassall's) corpuscle

9 Degeneration centers of thymic (Hassall's) corpuscles

10 Epithelial reticular cells

FIGURE 9.8 ■ Thymus gland (sectional view). Stain: hematoxylin and eosin. High magnification.

FIGURE 9.9 ■ Cortex and Medulla of a Thymus Gland

A low-magnification photomicrograph shows a portion of the lobule of the thymus gland. A **connective tissue trabecula (1)** subdivides the gland into incomplete lobules. Each lobule consists of the darker-staining **cortex (2)** and the lighter-staining **medulla (3)**. A characteristic **thymic (Hassall's) corpuscle (4)** is present in the center of the medulla in one of the lobules.

FUNCTIONAL CORRELATIONS: Thymus Gland

The **thymus gland** performs an important role early in childhood in **immune system development.** Undifferentiated **lymphocytes** are carried from bone marrow by the bloodstream to the thymus gland. In much of the thymic cortex, the **epithelial reticular cells,** also called **thymic nurse cells,** surround the lymphocytes and promote their differentiation, proliferation, and maturation. Here, the lymphocytes mature into **immunocompetent T cells, helper T cells,** and **cytotoxic T cells,** whereby they acquire their surface receptors for recognition of antigens. Furthermore, the developing lymphocytes are prevented from exposure to blood-borne antigens by a physical **blood-thymus barrier,** formed by endothelial cells, epithelial reticular cells, and macrophages. Macrophages outside of the capillaries ensure that substances transported in the blood vessels do not interact with the developing T cells in the cortex and induce an autoimmune response against the body's own cells or tissues. After maturation, the T cells leave the thymus gland via the bloodstream and populate the **lymph nodes, spleen,** and other thymus-dependent **lymphatic tissues** in the organism.

The maturation and selection of T cells within the thymus gland is a very complicated process that includes **positive** and **negative** selection of T cells. Only a small fraction of lymphocytes generated in the thymus gland reach maturity. As maturation progresses in the cortex, the cells are presented by antigen-presenting cells with self and foreign antigens. Lymphocytes that are unable to recognize or that recognize self-antigens die and are eliminated by macrophages (negative selection), which is about 95% of the total. Those lymphocytes that recognize the foreign antigens (positive selection) reach maturity, enter the medulla from the cortex, and are then distributed in the bloodstream.

In addition to forming the blood-thymus barrier, the epithelial reticular cells secrete hormones that are necessary for the proliferation, differentiation, and maturation of T cells and expression of their surface markers. The hormones are **thymulin, thymopoietin, thymosin, thymic humoral factor, interleukins,** and **interferon.** The epithelial reticular cells also form distinctive whorls called **thymic (Hassall's) corpuscles** in the medulla of the gland, which are characteristic features in identifying the thymus gland.

The thymus gland involutes after puberty, becomes filled with adipose tissue, and the production of T cells decreases. However, because T lymphocyte progeny has been established, immunity is maintained without the need for new T cell production. If the thymus gland is removed from a newborn, the lymphoid organs will not receive the immunocompetent T cells and the individual will not acquire the immunologic competence to fight pathogens. Death may occur early in life as a result of complications of an infection and the lack of a functional immune system.

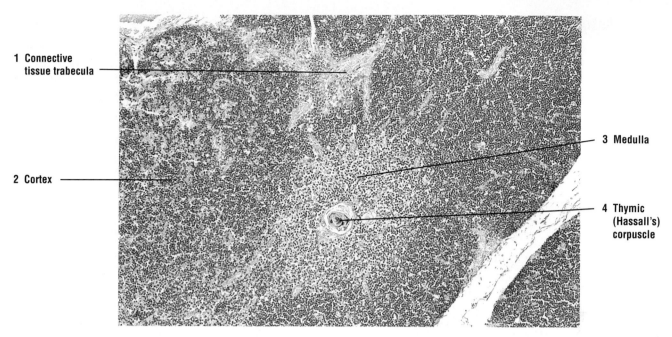

1 Connective
tissue trabecula

2 Cortex

3 Medulla

4 Thymic
(Hassall's)
corpuscle

FIGURE 9.9 ■ Cortex and medulla of a thymus gland. Stain: hematoxylin and eosin. ×30.

FIGURE 9.10 ■ Spleen (Panoramic View)

The spleen is surrounded by a dense connective tissue **capsule (1),** from which arise connective tissue **trabeculae (3, 5, 11)** that extend deep into the spleen's interior. The main trabeculae enter the spleen at the hilus and extend throughout the organ. Located within the trabeculae (3, 5, 11) are **trabecular arteries (5b)** and **trabecular veins (5a).** Trabeculae that are cut in transverse section (11) appear round or nodular and may contain blood vessels.

The spleen is characterized by numerous aggregations of **lymphatic nodules (4, 6).** These nodules constitute the **white pulp (4, 6)** of the organ. The lymphatic nodules (4, 6) also contain **germinal centers (8, 9)** that decrease in number with age. Passing through each lymphatic nodule (4, 6) is a blood vessel called a **central artery (2, 7, 10)** that is located in the periphery of the lymphatic nodules (4, 6). Central arteries (2, 7, 10) are branches of trabecular arteries (5b) that become ensheathed with lymphatic tissue as they leave the connective tissue trabeculae (3, 5, 11). This periarterial lymphatic sheath also forms the lymphatic nodules (4, 6) that constitute the white pulp (4, 6) of the spleen.

Surrounding the lymphatic nodules (4, 6) and intermeshed with the connective tissue trabeculae (3, 5, 11) is a diffuse cellular meshwork that makes up the bulk of the organ. This meshwork collectively forms the **red** or **splenic pulp (12, 13).** In fresh preparations, red pulp is red because of its extensive vascular tissue. The red pulp (12, 13) also contains **pulp arteries (14), venous sinuses (13),** and **splenic cords** (of Billroth) **(12).** The splenic cords (12) appear as diffuse strands of lymphatic tissue between the venous sinuses (13) and form a spongy meshwork of reticular connective tissue, usually obscured by the density of other tissue.

The spleen does not exhibit a distinct cortex and a medulla, as seen in lymph nodes. However, lymphatic nodules (4, 6) are found throughout the spleen. In addition, the spleen contains venous sinuses (13), in contrast to lymphatic sinuses that are found in the lymph nodes. The spleen also does not exhibit subcapsular or trabecular sinuses. The capsule (1) and trabeculae (3, 5, 11) in the spleen are thicker than those around the lymph nodes and contain some smooth muscle cells.

FIGURE 9.11 ■ Spleen: Red and White Pulp

A higher magnification of a section of the spleen illustrates the red and white pulp and associated connective tissue trabeculae, blood vessels, venous sinuses, and splenic cords.

The large **lymphatic nodule (3)** represents the white pulp of the spleen. Each nodule normally exhibits a peripheral zone, the periarterial lymphatic sheath, with densely packed small lymphocytes. The **central artery (4)** in the lymphatic nodule (3) has a peripheral or an eccentric position. Because the artery occupies the center of the periarterial lymphatic sheath, it is called the central artery. The cells found in the periarterial lymphatic sheath are mainly T cells. A **germinal center (5)** may not always be present. In the more lightly stained germinal center (5) are found B cells, many medium-sized lymphocytes, some small lymphocytes, and lymphoblasts.

The red pulp contains the **splenic cords** (of Billroth) **(1, 8)** and **venous sinuses (2, 9)** that course between the cords. The splenic cords (1, 8) are thin aggregations of lymphatic tissue containing small lymphocytes, associated cells, and various blood cells. Venous sinuses (2, 9) are dilated vessels lined with modified endothelium of elongated cells that appear cuboidal in transverse sections.

Also present in the red pulp are the **pulp arteries (10).** These represent the branches of the central artery (4) after it leaves the lymphatic nodule (3). Capillaries and pulp veins (venules) are also present.

Connective tissue trabeculae with a **trabecular artery (6)** and **trabecular vein (7)** are evident. These vessels have endothelial tunica intima and muscular tunica media. The tunica adventitia is not apparent because the connective tissue of the trabeculae surrounds the tunica media.

1 Capsule

2 Central artery

3 Trabeculae

4 Lymphatic nodule
(white pulp)

5 Trabecular:
  a. Vein
  b. Artery

6 Lymphatic nodule
(white pulp)

7 Central artery

8 Germinal center

9 Germinal center

10 Central artery

11 Trabeculae

12 Splenic cords
(in red pulp)

13 Venous sinuses
(in red pulp)

14 Pulp arteries

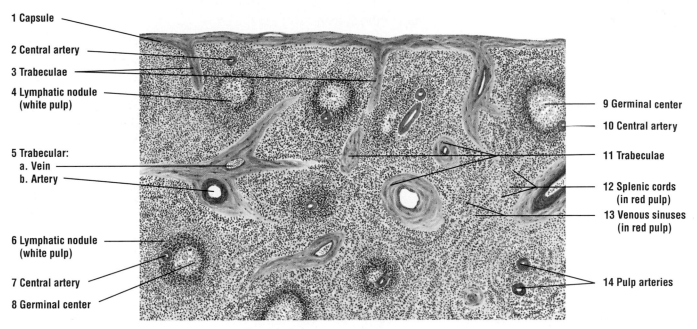

FIGURE 9.10 ■ Spleen (panoramic view). Stain: hematoxylin and eosin. Low magnification.

1 Splenic cord

2 Venous sinus

3 Lymphatic nodule

4 Central artery

5 Germinal center

6 Trabecular artery

7 Trabecular vein

8 Splenic cords

9 Venous sinuses

10 Pulp arteries

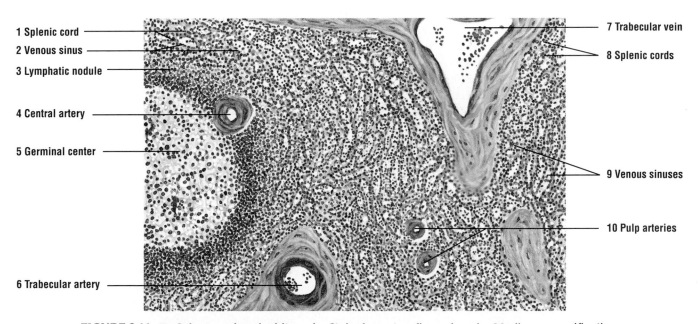

FIGURE 9.11 ■ Spleen: red and white pulp. Stain: hematoxylin and eosin. Medium magnification.

FIGURE 9.12 ■ Red and White Pulp of the Spleen

A low-magnification photomicrograph illustrates a section of the spleen. A dense irregular **connective tissue capsule (1)** covers the organ. From the capsule (1), **connective tissue trabeculae (3)** with blood vessels extend into the interior of the organ. The spleen is composed of white pulp and red pulp. **White pulp (2)** consists of lymphocytes and aggregations of **lymphatic nodules (2a).** Within the lymphatic nodule (2a) are found the **germinal center (2b)** and a **central artery (2c)** that is located off-center. Surrounding the white pulp lymphatic nodules (2) is the **red pulp (4).** It is primarily composed of **venous sinuses (4a)** and **splenic cords (4b).**

FUNCTIONAL CORRELATIONS: The Spleen

The **spleen** is the largest lymphoid organ with an extensive blood supply. It filters blood and is the site of immune responses to bloodborne antigens. The spleen consists of red pulp and white pulp. **Red pulp** consists of a dense network of reticular fibers that contains numerous erythrocytes, lymphocytes, plasma cells, macrophages, and other granulocytes. The main function of the red pulp is to filter the blood. It removes antigens, microorganisms, platelets, and aged or abnormal erythrocytes from the blood.

The **white pulp** is the immune component of the spleen and consists mainly of **lymphatic tissue.** Lymphatic cells that surround the **central arteries** of the white pulp are primarily **T cells,** whereas the lymphatic nodules contain mainly **B cells. Antigen-presenting cells** and **macrophages** reside within the white pulp. These cells detect trapped bacteria and antigens and initiate immune responses against them. As a result, T cells and B cells interact, become activated, proliferate, and perform their immune response.

Macrophages in the spleen also break down **hemoglobin** of worn-out **erythrocytes.** Iron from hemoglobin is recycled and returned to the **bone marrow,** where it is reused during the synthesis of new hemoglobin by developing erythrocytes. The **heme** from the hemoglobin is further degraded and excreted into **bile** by the liver cells.

During fetal life, the spleen is a **hemopoietic organ,** producing **granulocytes** and **erythrocytes.** This hemopoietic capability, however, ceases after birth. The spleen also serves as an important **reservoir** for blood. Because it has a spongelike microstructure, much blood can be stored in its interior. When needed, the stored blood is returned from the spleen to the general circulation. Although the spleen performs various important functions in the body, it is not an essential organ for life.

FIGURE 9.13 ■ Palatine Tonsil

The paired palatine tonsils consist of aggregates of lymphatic nodules located in the oral cavity. The palatine tonsils are not surrounded by a connective tissue capsule. As a result, the surface of the palatine tonsil is covered by a protective **stratified squamous nonkeratinized epithelium (1, 6)** that covers the rest of the oral cavity. Each tonsil is invaginated by deep grooves called **tonsillar crypts (3, 9)** that are also lined by stratified squamous nonkeratinized epithelium (1, 6).

Below the epithelium (1, 6) in the underlying connective tissue are numerous **lymphatic nodules (2)** that are distributed along the lengths of the tonsillar crypts (3, 9). The lymphatic nodules (2) frequently merge with each other and usually exhibit lighter-staining **germinal centers (7).**

A dense connective tissue underlies the palatine tonsil and forms its **capsule (4, 10).** The connective tissue **trabeculae,** some with **blood vessels (8),** arise from the capsule (4, 10) and pass toward the surface of the tonsil between the lymphatic nodules (2).

Below the connective tissue capsule (10) are sections of **skeletal muscle (5)** fibers.

1 **Connective tissue capsule**

2 **White pulp:**
   a. Lymphatic nodule

   b. Germinal center

   c. Central artery

3 **Connective tissue trabeculae**

4 **Red pulp:**
   a. Venous sinuses

   b. Splenic cords

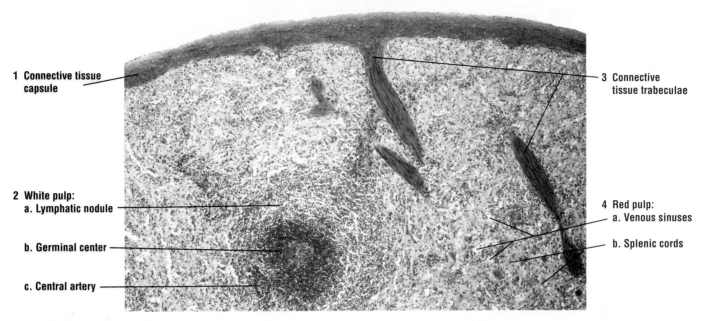

FIGURE 9.12 ■ Red and white pulp of the spleen. Stain: Mallory-azan. ×21.

1 **Stratified squamous nonkeratinized epithelium**

2 **Lymphatic nodules**

3 **Tonsillar crypts**

4 **Capsule**

5 **Skeletal muscle**

6 **Stratified squamous nonkeratinized epithelium**

7 **Germinal centers**

8 **Trabeculae with blood vessels**

9 **Tonsillar crypts**

10 **Capsule**

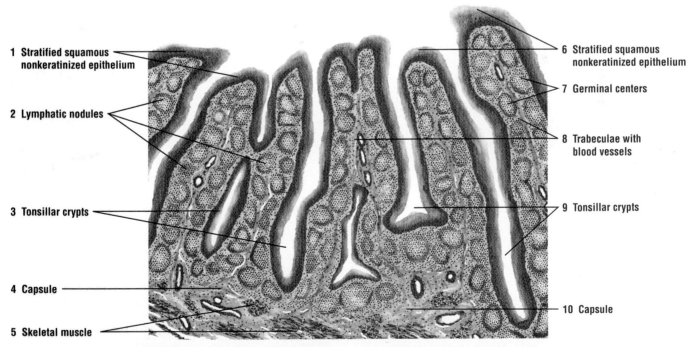

FIGURE 9.13 ■ Palatine tonsil. Stain: hematoxylin and eosin. Low magnification.

CHAPTER 9 ■ **Summary**

Lymphoid System

- Collects excess interstitial fluid
- Protects organism against invading pathogens or antigens by producing immune responses
- Includes all cells, tissues, and organs that contain lymphocytes
- Major organs are lymph nodes, spleen, thymus, and tonsils

Lymphoid Organs

Lymph Nodes

- Distributed along the paths of lymphatic vessels
- Most prominent in inguinal and axillary regions
- Surrounded by connective tissue capsule that sends trabeculae into interior
- Afferent lymph vessels with valves penetrate the capsule and enter subcapsular sinus
- Major blood vessels present in connective tissue trabeculae
- Exhibit an outer dark-staining cortex and an inner light-staining medulla
- Medullary cords in the medulla contain plasma cells, macrophages, and lymphocytes
- Medullary sinuses are capillary channels that drain lymph from cortical regions
- Efferent lymphatic vessels drain lymph from medullary sinuses to exit at the hilus
- Deeper region of the cortex is the paracortex, occupied by T cells
- Major function is lymph filtration and phagocytosis of foreign material from lymph
- Produce, store, and recirculate B and T cells
- B cells accumulate in lymphatic nodules
- T cells concentrate in deep cortical or paracortex regions
- Activate B cells to give rise to plasma cells and memory B cells
- B and T cells enter lymph nodes through postcapillary venules
- Postcapillary venules contain lymphocyte-homing receptors and high endothelium

Lymphatic Nodules

- Contain nonencapsulated lymphocytes collected in the cortex
- Peripheral zone stains dense owing to accumulation of small lymphocyte
- A lighter central region is the germinal center with medium-sized lymphocytes

Lymphoid Cells

- Originate from hemopoietic stem cells in bone marrow

T Lymphocytes (T Cells)

- Stimulated lymphocytes produce B cells and T cells

- T cells arise from lymphocytes that left bone marrow and matured in thymus gland
- After maturation, T cells are distributed to all lymph tissues and organs
- On encountering antigens, T cells destroy them by cytotoxic action or activating B cells
- Four types of differentiated T cells: helper T cells, cytotoxic T cells, memory T cells, and suppressor T cells
- Helper T cells secrete cytokines or interleukins when encounter antigens
- Cytokines stimulate B cells to differentiate into plasma cells and to secrete antibodies
- Cytotoxic T cells attack and destroy virus-infected, foreign, or malignant cells
- Memory T cells are long-living progeny of T cells and respond to same antigens
- Suppressor T cells inhibit the functions of helper T cells
- Maturation of T cells a very complicated process, involving positive and negative selection
- Most T cells recognize self-antigens and die (negative selection)
- T cells that recognize foreign antigens reach maturity and enter bloodstream (positive selection)

B Lymphocytes (B Cells)

- B cells remain and mature in bone marrow, then move to lymphoid tissues and organs
- Recognize antigens as a result of antigen receptors on cell membranes and become activated
- Response more intense when helper T cells present antigens to B cells
- Cytokines secreted by helper T cells increase proliferation of activated B cells
- B cells secrete antibodies and destroy foreign substance
- Other activated B cells remain as memory B cells for future defense against same antigens

Other Cells in Immune Responses

- Natural killer cells attack virally infected cells and cancer cells
- Antigen-presenting cells phagocytose and present antigens to T cells for immune response
- Connective tissue macrophages such as perisinusoidal cells in liver, Langerhans cells in skin, and other lymphoid organs

Types of Immune Responses

Cell-Mediated Immune Response

- T cells stimulated by antigens secrete cytokines that stimulate other lymphocytes
- Cytotoxic T cells produce protein perforin to puncture target cells or induce apoptosis

Humoral Immune Response

- Exposure of B cells to antigen induces proliferation and plasma cell formation
- Plasma cells produce antibodies to destroy specific foreign substance
- Helper T cells cooperate and produce cytokines

Spleen

- Largest lymphoid organ with extensive blood supply; filters blood and serves as blood reservoir
- Surrounded by connective tissue capsule that divides it into compartments called splenic pulp
- White pulp consists of lymphatic nodules with germinal center around a central artery
- Red pulp consists of splenic cords and splenic (blood) sinusoids
- Splenic cords contain macrophages, lymphocytes, plasma cells, and different blood cells
- Does not exhibit cortex and medulla, but contains lymphatic nodules
- White pulp is the site of immune response to bloodborne antigens
- T cells surround the central arteries, whereas B cells are mainly in the lymphatic nodules
- Antigen-presenting cells and macrophages are found in white pulp

- Breaks down hemoglobin from worn-out erythrocytes and recycles iron to bone marrow
- Degrades heme from hemoglobin, which is then excreted in the bile
- During fetal life is an important hemopoietic organ

Thymus Gland

- Lobulated lymphoepithelial organ with dark-staining cortex and light-staining medulla
- Most active in childhood and has an important role early in life in immune system development
- Site where immature lymphocytes from bone marrow mature into T cells, helper T cells, and cytotoxic T cells
- Thymic nurse cells promote lymphocyte differentiation, proliferation, and maturation
- Blood-thymus barrier prevents developing lymphocytes contacting bloodborne antigens
- Sends mature T cells to populate lymph nodes, spleen, and lymphatic tissues
- Epithelial reticular cells secrete hormones needed for lymphocyte maturation
- Epithelial reticular cells form thymic (Hassall's) corpuscles in medulla
- Involutes and becomes filled with adipose tissues as individual ages
- Removal early in life results in loss of immunologic competence

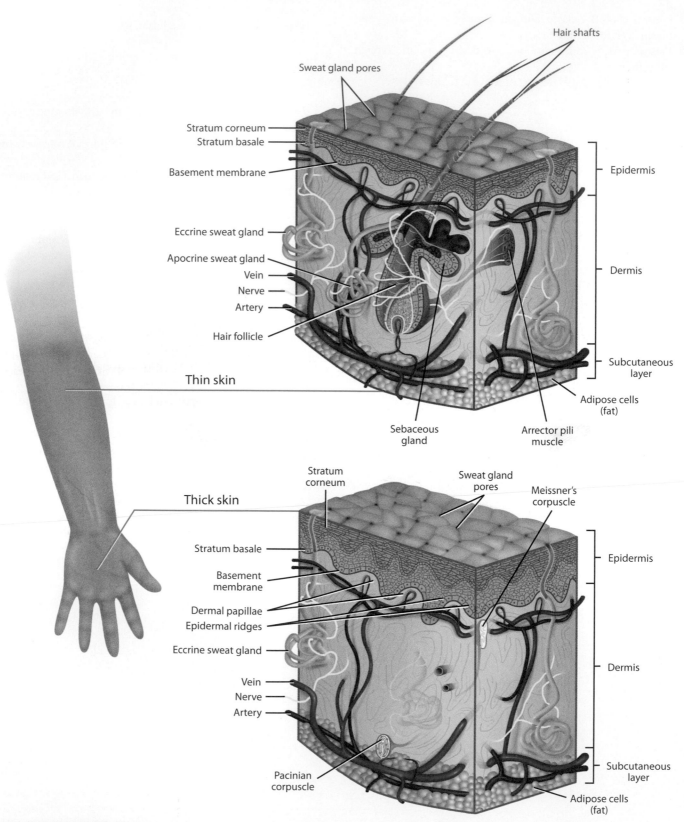

OVERVIEW FIGURE 10 ■ Comparison between thin skin in the arm and thick skin in the palm, including the contents of the connective tissue dermis.

CHAPTER 10

Integumentary System

Skin and its derivatives and appendages form the **integumentary system.** In humans, skin derivatives include nails, hair, and several types of sweat and sebaceous glands. Skin, or **integument,** consists of two distinct regions, the superficial epidermis and a deep dermis. The superficial **epidermis** is nonvascular and lined by **keratinized stratified squamous epithelium** with distinct cell types and cell layers. Inferior to the epidermis is the vascular **dermis,** characterized by dense irregular connective tissue. Beneath the dermis is **hypodermis** or a **subcutaneous layer** of connective tissue and adipose tissue that forms the superficial fascia seen in gross anatomy.

Epidermis: Thick Versus Thin Skin

The basic histology of skin is similar in different regions of the body, except in the thickness of the epidermis. **Palms** and **soles** are constantly exposed to increased wear, tear, and abrasion. As a result, the epidermis in these regions is thick, especially the outermost stratified keratinized layer. The skin in these regions is called **thick skin.** Thick skin also contains numerous **sweat glands,** but lacks hair follicles, sebaceous glands, and smooth muscle fibers.

The remainder of the body is covered by **thin skin.** In these regions, the epidermis is thinner and its cellular composition simpler than that of thick skin. Present in thin skin are **hair follicles, sebaceous glands,** and **sweat glands.** Attached to the connective tissue sheath of hair follicles and the connective tissue of the dermis are smooth muscle fibers, called **arrector pili.** Also associated with the hair follicles are numerous sebaceous glands (Overview Figure 10).

In addition to the keratinocytes that become keratinized in the epithelium, the epidermis also contains three less abundant types of cells. These are **melanocytes, Langerhans cells,** and **Merkel's cells.**

Dermis: Papillary and Reticular Layers

Dermis is the connective tissue layer that binds to epidermis. A distinct **basement membrane** separates the epidermis from the dermis. In addition, dermis also contains epidermal derivatives such as the sweat glands, sebaceous glands, and hair follicles.

The junction of the dermis with the epidermis is irregular. The superficial layer of the dermis forms numerous raised projections called **dermal papillae,** which interdigitate with evaginations of epidermis, called **epidermal ridges.** This region of skin is the **papillary layer** of the dermis. This layer is filled with loose irregular connective tissue fibers, capillaries, blood vessels, fibroblasts, macrophages, and other loose connective tissue cells.

The deeper layer of dermis is called the **reticular layer.** This layer is thicker and is characterized by dense irregular connective tissue fibers (mainly type I collagen), and is less cellular than the papillary layer. There is no distinct boundary between the two dermal layers, and the papillary layer blends with the reticular layer. Also, dermis blends inferiorly with the **hypodermis** or the **subcutaneous layer,** which contains the superficial fascia and adipose tissue.

The connective tissue of the dermis is highly vascular and contains numerous blood vessels, lymph vessels, and nerves. Certain regions of skin exhibit **arteriovenous anastomoses** used for temperature regulation. Here, blood passes directly from arteries into veins. In addition, the dermis contains numerous sensory receptors. **Meissner's corpuscles** are located closer to the surface of the skin in dermal papillae, whereas **Pacinian corpuscles** are found deeper in the connective tissue of the dermis (Overview Figure 10).

FUNCTIONAL CORRELATIONS

Epidermal Cells

There are four cell types in the epidermis of skin, with the **keratinocytes** being the dominant cells. Keratinocytes divide, grow, migrate up, and undergo **keratinization or cornification**, and form the protective epidermal layer for the skin. The epidermis is composed of stratified keratinized squamous epithelium. There are other less abundant cell types in the epidermis. These are the melanocytes, Langerhans cells, and Merkel's cells, which are interspersed among the keratinocytes in the epidermis. In thick skin, five distinct and recognizable cell layers can be identified.

The Epidermal Cell Layers

Stratum Basale (Germinativum)

The **stratum basale** is the deepest, or basal layer, in the epidermis. It consists of a single layer of columnar to cuboidal cells that rest on a **basement membrane** separating the dermis from the epidermis. The cells are attached to one another by cell junctions, called **desmosomes,** and to the underlying basement membrane by **hemidesmosomes.** Cells in the stratum basale serve as **stem cells** for the epidermis; thus, much increased mitotic activity is seen in this layer. The cells divide and mature as they migrate up toward the superficial layers. All cells in the stratum basale produce and contain **intermediate keratin filaments** that increase in number as the cells move superficially.

Stratum Spinosum

As the keratinocytes move upward in the epidermis, a second cell layer, or **stratum spinosum,** forms. This layer consists of four to six rows of cells. In routine histologic preparations, cells in this layer shrink. As a result, the developed intercellular spaces between cells appear to form numerous cytoplasmic extensions, or spines, that project from their surfaces. The spines represent the sites where desmosomes are anchored to bundles of intermediate keratin filaments, or tonofilaments, and to neighboring cells. The synthesis of keratin filaments continues in this layer that become assembled into bundles of **tonofilaments.** Tonofilaments maintain cohesion among cells and provide resistance to abrasion of the epidermis.

Stratum Granulosum

Cells above the stratum spinosum become filled with dense basophilic **keratohyalin granules** and form the third layer, the **stratum granulosum.** Three to five layers of flattened cells form this layer. The granules are not surrounded by a membrane and are associated with bundles of keratin tonofilaments. The combination of keratin tonofilaments with keratohyalin granules in these cells produces **keratin.** The keratin formed by this process is the soft keratin of skin. In addition, the cytoplasm of these cells contains membrane-bound **lamellar granules** formed by lipid bilayers. The lamellar granules are discharged into the intercellular spaces of stratum granulosum as layers of **lipid** and seal the skin. This process renders the skin relatively impermeable to water.

Stratum Lucidum

In thick skin only, the **stratum lucidum** is translucent and barely visible; it lies just superior to the stratum granulosum and inferior to the stratum corneum. The tightly packed cells lack nuclei or organelles and are dead. The flattened cells contain densely packed keratin filaments.

Stratum Corneum

The **stratum corneum** is the fifth and most superficial layer of skin. All nuclei and organelles have disappeared from the cells. Stratum corneum primarily consists of flattened, dead cells filled with soft **keratin filaments.** The keratinized, superficial cells from this layer are continually shed or **desquamated** and are replaced by new cells arising from the deep stratum basale. During the keratinization process, the hydrolytic enzymes disrupt the nucleus and cytoplasmic organelles, which disappear as the cells fill with keratin.

Other Skin Cells

In addition to keratinocytes, the epidermis contains three other cell types: melanocytes, Langerhans cells, and Merkel's cells. Unless skin is prepared with special stains, these cells are normally not distinguishable with hematoxylin and eosin preparations.

Melanocytes are derived from the neural crest cells. They have long irregular cytoplasmic extensions that branch into the epidermis. Melanocytes are located between the stratum basale and the stratum spinosum of the epidermis and synthesize the dark brown pigment **melanin.** Melanin is synthesized from the amino acid tyrosine by the melanocytes. The melanin granules in the melanocytes migrate to their cytoplasmic extensions, from which they are transferred to keratinocytes in the basal cell layers of the epidermis. Melanin imparts a dark color to the skin, and exposure of the skin to sunlight promotes increased synthesis of melanin. The function of melanin is to protect the skin from the damaging effects of ultraviolet radiation.

Langerhans cells are found mainly in the stratum spinosum. They participate in the body's immune responses. Langerhans cells recognize, phagocytose, and process foreign **antigens,** and then present them to T lymphocytes for an immune response. Thus, these cells function as **antigen-presenting** cells of the skin.

Merkel's cells are found in the basal layer of the epidermis and are most abundant in the fingertips. Because these cells are closely associated with afferent (sensory) **unmyelinated axons,** it is believed that they function as **mechanoreceptors** to detect pressure.

Major Skin Functions

The skin comes in direct contact with the external environment. As a result, skin performs numerous important functions, most of which are protective.

Protection

The **keratinized stratified epithelium** of the epidermis protects the body surfaces from mechanical abrasion and forms a physical barrier to pathogens or foreign microorganisms. Because a **glycolipid layer** is present between the cells of the stratum granulosum, the epidermis is also **impermeable** to water. This layer also prevents the loss of body fluids through dehydration. Increased synthesis of the pigment melanin protects the skin against ultraviolet radiation.

Temperature Regulation

Physical exercise or a warm environment increases **sweating.** Sweating reduces the body temperature after **evaporation** of sweat from skin surfaces. In addition to sweating, temperature regulation also involves increased **dilation** of blood vessels for maximum blood flow to the skin. This function also increases heat loss. Conversely, in cold temperatures, body heat is conserved by **constriction** of blood vessels and decreased blood flow to the skin.

Sensory Perception

The skin is a large **sensory organ** of the external environment. Numerous encapsulated and free **sensory nerve endings** within the skin respond to stimuli for temperature (heat and cold), touch, pain, and pressure.

Excretion

Through production of sweat by the **sweat glands,** water, sodium salts, urea, and nitrogenous wastes are excreted to the surface of skin.

Formation of Vitamin D

Vitamin D is formed from precursor molecules synthesized in the epidermis during exposure of the skin to **ultraviolet** rays from the sun. Vitamin D is essential for **calcium absorption** from the intestinal mucosa and for proper mineral metabolism.

FIGURE 10.1 ■ Thin Skin

This illustration depicts a section of thin skin from the general body surface, where wear and tear are minimal. To differentiate between the cellular and connective tissue components of the skin, a special stain was used. With this stain, the collagen fibers of the connective tissue components stain blue and the cellular components stain bright red.

Skin consists of two principal layers: **epidermis (10)** and **dermis (14).** The epidermis (10) is the superficial cellular layer with different cell types. The dermis (14), located directly below the epidermis (10), contains connective tissue fibers and cellular components of epidermal origin.

In thin skin, the epidermis (10) exhibits a stratified squamous epithelium and a thin layer of keratinized cells called the **stratum corneum (1).** The most superficial cells in the stratum corneum (1) are constantly shed or desquamate from the surface. Also, the stratum corneum (1) of thin skin is much thinner in contrast to that of thick skin, in which the stratum corneum is much thicker. In this illustration, a few rows of polygonal-shaped cells are visible in the epidermis (10). These cells form the layer **stratum spinosum (2).**

The narrow zone of irregular, lighter-staining connective tissue directly below the epidermis (10) is the **papillary layer (11)** of the dermis (14). The papillary layer (11) indents the base of the epidermis to form the **dermal papillae (3).** The deeper **reticular layer (12)** comprises the bulk of the dermis (14) and consists of dense irregular connective tissue. A small portion of **hypodermis (13),** the superficial region of the underlying subcutaneous **adipose tissue (9),** is also illustrated.

Skin appendages, such as the **sweat gland (7)** and **hair follicles (8),** develop from the epidermis (10) and are located in the dermis (14). The sweat gland is illustrated in greater detail in Figure 10.3. The expanded terminal portion of the hair follicle (8) observed in longitudinal section is the **hair bulb (8a).** The base of the hair bulb (8a) is indented by the connective tissue to form a **dermal papilla (8b).** Within each dermal papilla (8b) is a capillary network vital for sustaining the hair follicle. Attached to hair follicles (8) are thin strips of smooth muscle called the **arrector pili muscles (5).** Associated also with hair follicles (8) are numerous **sebaceous glands (6).**

In the reticular layer of the dermis (14) are found examples of the cross sections of a coiled portion of the sweat gland (7). The elongated portions of the sweat gland (7) that continue to the surface of skin are the excretory **ductal portions** of the **sweat glands (4, 7a).** The more circular and deeper-lying parts of the sweat gland are the **secretory (7b)** portions of the sweat gland.

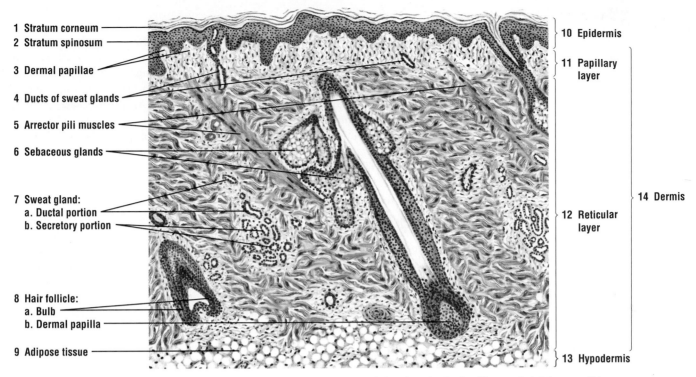

1 Stratum corneum
2 Stratum spinosum

3 Dermal papillae

4 Ducts of sweat glands

5 Arrector pili muscles

6 Sebaceous glands

7 Sweat gland:
   a. Ductal portion
   b. Secretory portion

8 Hair follicle:
   a. Bulb
   b. Dermal papilla

9 Adipose tissue

10 Epidermis

11 Papillary
    layer

12 Reticular
    layer

13 Hypodermis

14 Dermis

FIGURE 10.1 ■ Thin skin: epidermis and the contents of the dermis. Stain: Masson's trichrome (blue stain). Low magnification.

FIGURE 10.2 ■ Skin: Scalp

This low-magnification section of the thin skin of the scalp is prepared with routine histologic stain. It illustrates both the epidermis and dermis, and some of the skin derivatives in the deeper connective tissue layers. The epidermis stains darker than the underlying connective tissue of the dermis. In the epidermis are visible the cell layers **stratum corneum (1)**, with desquamating superficial cells; **stratum spinosum (2)**; and the basal cell layer, the **stratum basale (3)**, with brown **melanin (pigment) granules (3)**.

The connective tissue **dermal papillae (4)** indent the underside of the epidermis. The thin connective tissue papillary layer of the dermis is located immediately under the epidermis. The thicker connective tissue **reticular layer (12)** of the dermis extends from just below the epidermis to the **subcutaneous layer (8)** with **adipose tissue (8)**. Located inferior to the subcutaneous layer (8) are **skeletal muscle fibers (9)**, sectioned in transverse and longitudinal planes.

Hair follicles (13) in the skin of the scalp are numerous, closely packed, and oriented at an angle to the surface. A complete hair follicle in longitudinal section is illustrated in the figure. Parts of other hair follicles, sectioned in different planes, are also visible (13). When the hair follicle (13) is cut in a transverse plane, the following structures are visible: cuticle, **internal root sheath (13a), external root sheath (13b), connective tissue sheath (13c), hair bulb (13d)**, and connective tissue dermal **papilla (13e)**. The hair passes upward through the follicle (13) to the skin surface. Numerous **sebaceous glands (11)** surround each hair follicle (13). The sebaceous glands are aggregates of clear cells that are connected to a duct that opens into the hair follicle (see Figure 10.5).

The **arrector pili muscles (5, 10)** are smooth muscles aligned at an oblique angle to the hair follicles (13). The arrector pili muscles (5, 10) attach to the papillary layer of the dermis and to the connective tissue sheath (13c) of the hair follicle (13). The contraction of arrector pili muscles (5, 10) causes the hair shaft to move into a more vertical position.

Deep in the dermis or subcutaneous layer (8) are the basal portions of the highly coiled **sweat glands (6)**. Sections of the sweat gland (6) that exhibit lightly stained columnar epithelium are the **secretory portions (6b)** of the gland. These are distinct from the **excretory ducts (6a)** of the sweat glands (6), which are lined by stratified cuboidal epithelium of smaller, darker-stained cells. Each sweat gland duct (6a) is coiled deep in the dermis but straightens out in the upper dermis, and follows a spiral course through the epidermis to the surface of the skin (see Figure 10.3).

The skin contains many **blood vessels (14)** and has a rich sensory innervation. The sensory receptors for pressure and vibration are the **Pacinian corpuscles (7)**, located in the subcutaneous tissue (8). The Pacinian corpuscles (7) are illustrated in greater detail and higher magnification in Figure 10.10.

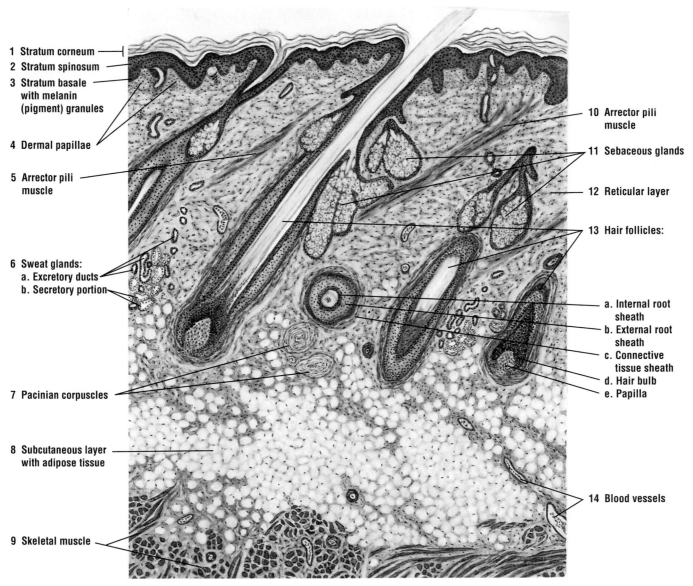

1 **Stratum corneum**
2 **Stratum spinosum**
3 **Stratum basale with melanin (pigment) granules**
4 **Dermal papillae**
5 **Arrector pili muscle**
6 **Sweat glands:**
   a. **Excretory ducts**
   b. **Secretory portion**
7 **Pacinian corpuscles**
8 **Subcutaneous layer with adipose tissue**
9 **Skeletal muscle**

10 **Arrector pili muscle**
11 **Sebaceous glands**
12 **Reticular layer**
13 **Hair follicles:**
    a. **Internal root sheath**
    b. **External root sheath**
    c. **Connective tissue sheath**
    d. **Hair bulb**
    e. **Papilla**
14 **Blood vessels**

FIGURE 10.2 ■ Skin: epidermis, dermis, and hypodermis in the scalp. Stain: hematoxylin and eosin. Low magnification.

FIGURE 10.3 ■   Hairy Thin Skin of the Scalp: Hair Follicles and Surrounding Structures

This low-power photomicrograph illustrates a section of the thin skin of the scalp. In the **epidermis (1)** of the thin skin, the **stratum corneum (1a), stratum granulosum (1b),** and **stratum spinosum (1c)** layers are thinner than the same layers in the thick skin. In the dense irregular connective tissue of the **dermis (4)** are **hair follicles (3)** and associated **sebaceous glands (2, 5).** An **arrector pili muscle (6)** extends from the deep connective tissue around the hair follicle (3) to the connective tissue of the papillary layer of the dermis (4).

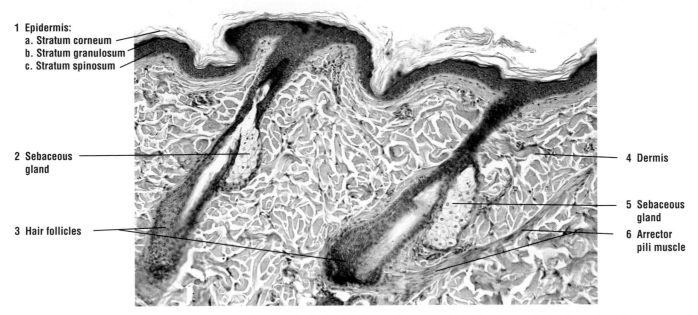

1 Epidermis:
   a. Stratum corneum
   b. Stratum granulosum
   c. Stratum spinosum

2 Sebaceous
   gland

3 Hair follicles

4 Dermis

5 Sebaceous
   gland

6 Arrector
   pili muscle

FIGURE 10.3 ■ Hairy thin skin of the scalp: hair follicles and surrounding structures. Stain: hematoxylin and eosin. ×40.

FIGURE 10.4 ■ Section of a Hair Follicle With the Surrounding Structures

This figure illustrates a longitudinal section of a hair follicle and surrounding glands and structures. The different layers of the hair follicle are identified in the right side. The hair follicle is surrounded by an outer **connective tissue sheath** (15) of the **dermis** (7). Under the connective tissue sheath (15) is an **external root sheath** (14) composed of several cell layers. These cell layers are continuous with the epithelial layer of the epidermis. The **internal root sheath** (13) is composed of a thin, pale epithelial stratum (Henle's layer) and a thin, granular epithelial stratum (Huxley's layer). These two cell layers become indistinguishable as their cells merge with the cells in the expanded part of the hair follicle called the **hair bulb** (21). Internal to the cell layers of the internal root sheath (13) are cells that produce the **cuticle** (12) of the hair and the keratinized **cortex** (11) of the hair follicle, which appears as a pale yellow layer. The **hair root** (16) and the **dermal papilla** (18) form the hair bulb (21). In the hair bulb (21), the external root sheath (14) and internal root sheath (13) merge into an undifferentiated group of cells called the **hair matrix** (17), which is situated above the dermal papilla (18). Cell mitoses and **melanin pigment** (19) can be seen in the matrix cells (17). Numerous **capillaries** (20) supply the connective tissue of the dermal papilla (18).

In the connective tissue of the dermis (7) and adjacent to the hair follicle are visible transverse sections of the basal portion of a coiled **sweat gland** (8, 9). The **secretory cells** (9) of the sweat gland are tall and stain light. Along the bases of the secretory cells (9) are flattened nuclei of the contractile **myoepithelial cells** (10). The **excretory ducts** (8) of the sweat gland are smaller in diameter, are lined with a stratified cuboidal epithelium, and stain darker than the secretory cells (9).

A **sebaceous gland** (4) that is connected to the hair follicle is sectioned through the middle. The sebaceous gland (4) is lined with a stratified epithelium that has continuity with the external root sheath (14) of the hair follicle. The epithelium of the sebaceous gland is modified, and along its base is a row of columnar or cuboidal cells, the **basal cells** (3), whose nuclei may be flattened. These cells rest on a basement membrane, which is surrounded by the connective tissue of the dermis (7). The basal cells (3) of the sebaceous gland divide and fill the acinus of the gland with larger, polyhedral **secretory cells** (5) that enlarge, accumulate secretory material, and become round. The secretory cells (5) in the interior of the acinus undergo **degeneration** (2), a process in which the cells become the oily secretory product of the gland called sebum. Sebum passes through the short **duct** of the **sebaceous gland** (1) into the lumen of the hair follicle.

Each hair follicle is surrounded by numerous sebaceous glands (4). The sebaceous glands lie in the connective tissue of the dermis (7) and in the angle between the hair follicle and the smooth muscle strip called the **arrector pili muscle** (6). When the arrector pili muscle contracts, the hair stands up, forming a dimple or a goose bump on the skin and forcing the sebum out of the sebaceous gland into the lumen of the hair follicle.

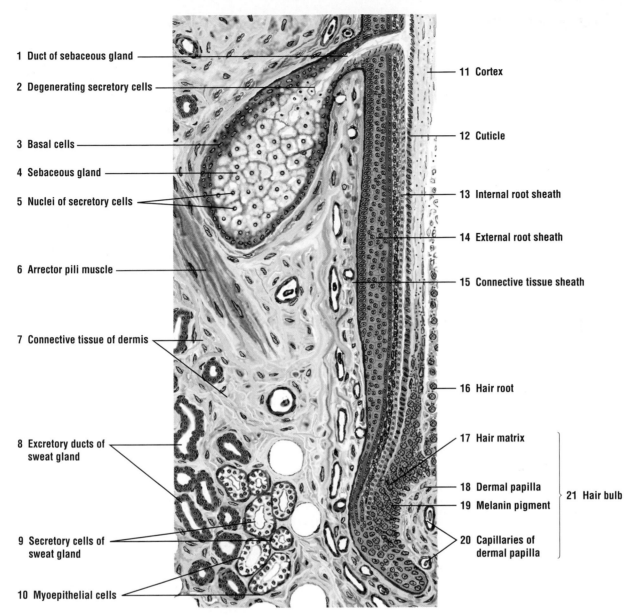

1 Duct of sebaceous gland

2 Degenerating secretory cells

3 Basal cells

4 Sebaceous gland

5 Nuclei of secretory cells

6 Arrector pili muscle

7 Connective tissue of dermis

8 Excretory ducts of sweat gland

9 Secretory cells of sweat gland

10 Myoepithelial cells

11 Cortex

12 Cuticle

13 Internal root sheath

14 External root sheath

15 Connective tissue sheath

16 Hair root

17 Hair matrix

18 Dermal papilla

19 Melanin pigment

20 Capillaries of dermal papilla

21 Hair bulb

FIGURE 10.4 ■ Hair follicle: bulb of the hair follicle, sweat gland, sebaceous gland, and arrector pili muscle. Stain: hematoxylin and eosin. Medium magnification.

FIGURE 10.5 ■ Thick Skin of the Palm, Superficial Cell Layers, and Melanin Pigment

Thick skin is best illustrated by examining a section from the palm. The epidermis of thick skin exhibits five distinct cell layers and is much thicker than that of the thin skin (Figures 10.1–10.3). The different cell layers of the epidermis are illustrated in greater detail and at higher magnification on the left.

The outermost layer of thick skin is the **stratum corneum (1, 9),** a wide layer of flattened, dead or keratinized cells that are constantly shed or **desquamated (8)** from the skin surface. Inferior to the stratum corneum (1, 9) is a narrow, lightly stained **stratum lucidum (2).** This thin layer is difficult to see in most slide preparations. At higher magnification, the outlines of flattened cells and eleidin droplets in this layer are occasionally seen.

Located below the stratum lucidum (2) is the **stratum granulosum (3, 11),** whose cells are filled with dark-staining **keratohyalin granules (3).** Directly under the stratum granulosum (3, 11) is the thick **stratum spinosum (4, 12)** composed of several layers of polyhedral-shaped cells. These cells are connected to each other by spinous processes or intercellular bridges that represent the attachment sites of desmosomes (macula adherens).

The deepest cell layer in the skin is the columnar **stratum basale (5, 13)** that rests on the connective tissue **basement membrane (6, 15).** Mitotic activity and the brown melanin pigment (5, 13) are normally seen in the deeper layers of stratum spinosum (4, 12) and stratum basale (5, 13).

The **excretory duct** of a **sweat gland (10)** located deep in the dermis penetrates the epidermis, loses its epithelial wall, and spirals through the epidermal cell layers (1–5) to the skin surface as small channels with a thin lining.

Dermal papillae (7) are prominent in thick skin. Some dermal papillae may contain tactile or sensory **Meissner's corpuscles (14)** and **capillary loops (16).**

FIGURE 10.6 ■ Thick Skin: Epidermis and Superficial Cell Layers

A higher-magnification photomicrograph shows a clear distinction between the different cell layers in the **epidermis (1)** of the thick skin of the palm. The outermost and the thickest layer is the **stratum corneum (1a).** Inferior to the stratum corneum (1a) are two to three layers of dark cells filled with granules. This is the **stratum granulosum (1b).** Below the stratum granulosum (1b) is the **stratum spinosum (1c),** a thicker layer of polyhedral cells. The deepest cell layer in the epidermis (1) is the **stratum basale (1d).** The cells in this layer contain brown **melanin granules (6).** The stratum basale (1d) is attached to a thin connective tissue **basement membrane (4)** that separates the epidermis (1) from the **dermis (2).** The connective tissue of the dermis (2) indents the epidermis (1) to form **dermal papillae (5).** Passing through the dermis (2) and the cell layers of the epidermis (1) is the **excretory duct (3)** of a sweat gland that is located deep in the dermis.

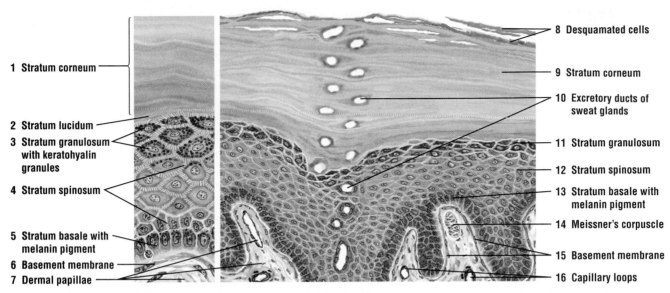

1 Stratum corneum

2 Stratum lucidum
3 Stratum granulosum with keratohyalin granules
4 Stratum spinosum

5 Stratum basale with melanin pigment
6 Basement membrane
7 Dermal papillae

8 Desquamated cells

9 Stratum corneum

10 Excretory ducts of sweat glands

11 Stratum granulosum

12 Stratum spinosum

13 Stratum basale with melanin pigment

14 Meissner's corpuscle

15 Basement membrane

16 Capillary loops

FIGURE 10.5 ■ Thick skin of the palm, superficial cell layers, and melanin pigment. Stain: hematoxylin and eosin. Medium magnification.

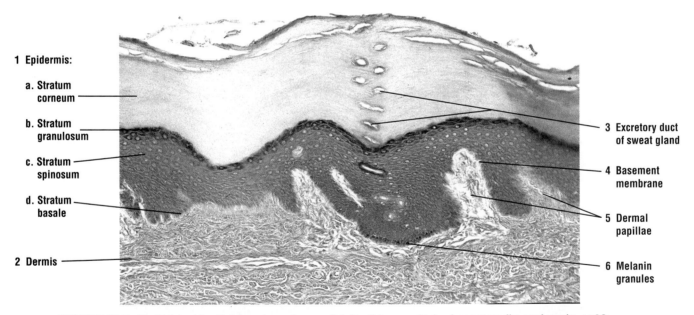

1 Epidermis:

a. Stratum corneum

b. Stratum granulosum

c. Stratum spinosum

d. Stratum basale

2 Dermis

3 Excretory duct of sweat gland

4 Basement membrane

5 Dermal papillae

6 Melanin granules

FIGURE 10.6 ■ Thick skin: Epidermis and superficial cell layers. Stain: hematoxylin and eosin. ×40.

FIGURE 10.7 ■ Thick Skin: Epidermis, Dermis, and Hypodermis of the Palm

A low-power photomicrograph illustrates the superficial and deep structures in the thick skin of the palm. The following cell layers are recognized in the **epidermis (6): stratum corneum (7), stratum granulosum (8),** and **stratum basale (9).** Inferior to the epidermis (6) is the dense irregular connective tissue **dermis (5). Dermal papillae (11)** from the dermis (5) indent the base of the epidermis (6). Deep in the dermis (5) and the **hypodermis (4)** are cross sections of the coiled simple tubular **sweat glands (3)** and the **excretory ducts of the sweat glands (10).** A thick layer of **adipose tissue (1)** deep to the dermis (5) is the hypodermis (4) or the superficial fascia. Hypodermis (4) is not part of the integument. Two sensory receptors called the **Pacinian corpuscles (2)** are seen inferior to the adipose tissue (1) of the hypodermis (4).

FIGURE 10.8 ■ Apocrine Sweat Glands

The apocrine glands are large, coiled sweat glands that deliver their secretions into the adjacent **hair follicle (7).** This illustration shows numerous cross sections of an apocrine sweat gland and a few secretory units of an eccrine sweat gland for comparison. The **secretory portion** of the **apocrine sweat gland (3)** consists of wide and dilated lumina. The gland is embedded deep in the **connective tissue** of the **dermis (5)** or hypodermis with **adipose cells (4)** and numerous **blood vessels (8).** In comparison, the **secretory portion** of an **eccrine sweat gland (6)** is smaller and exhibits much smaller lumina. The cuboidal secretory cells of the apocrine sweat gland (3) are surrounded by numerous **myoepithelial cells (2)** that are located at the base of the secretory cells. When cut at an oblique angle, the myoepithelial cells (2) loop over the secretory cells to surround them. The **excretory portion** of the **sweat gland (1)** is lined by a double layer of dark-staining cuboidal cells, which is similar to the excretory duct of the eccrine sweat gland.

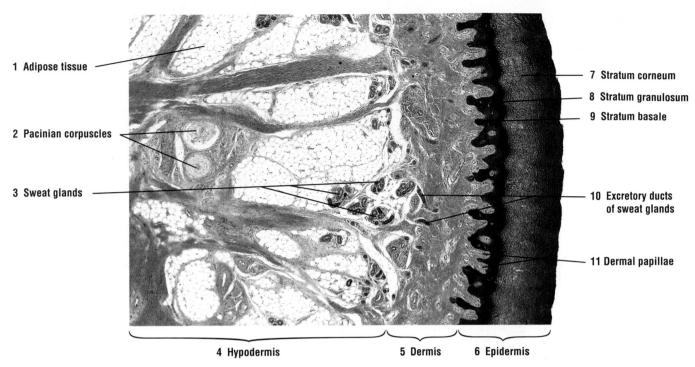

1 Adipose tissue

2 Pacinian corpuscles

3 Sweat glands

7 Stratum corneum

8 Stratum granulosum

9 Stratum basale

10 Excretory ducts
    of sweat glands

11 Dermal papillae

4 Hypodermis   5 Dermis   6 Epidermis

FIGURE 10.7 ■ Thick skin: epidermis, dermis, and hypodermis of the palm. Stain: hematoxylin and eosin. ×17.

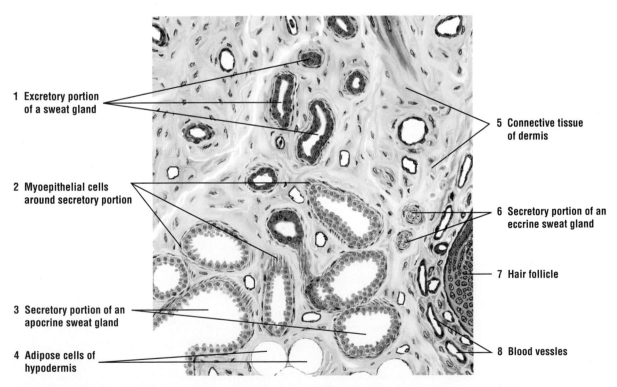

1 Excretory portion
   of a sweat gland

2 Myoepithelial cells
   around secretory portion

3 Secretory portion of an
   apocrine sweat gland

4 Adipose cells of
   hypodermis

5 Connective tissue
   of dermis

6 Secretory portion of an
   eccrine sweat gland

7 Hair follicle

8 Blood vessels

FIGURE 10.8 ■ Apocrine sweat gland: secretory and excretory potions of the sweat gland. Stain: hematoxylin and eosin. Medium magnification.

FIGURE 10.9 ■ Eccrine Sweat Glands

The eccrine sweat gland is a simple, highly coiled tubular gland that extends deep into the dermis or the upper hypodermis. To illustrate this extension, the sweat gland is shown in both cross-sectional (left side) and three-dimensional views (right side).

The coiled portion of the sweat gland in the dermis is the **secretory (8)** region. The **secretory cells (3, 4)** are large and columnar, and stain lightly eosinophilic. Surrounding the secretory cells (3, 4) are thin, spindle-shaped **myoepithelial cells (5)** that are located between the base of the secretory cells (3, 4) and the basement membrane (not illustrated) that surrounds the cells.

A thinner, darker-staining **excretory duct (2, 7)** leaves the secretory region of the sweat gland. The cells of the excretory duct are smaller than the secretory cells (3, 4). Also, the excretory duct (2, 7) is smaller in diameter and is lined by deep-staining, stratified cuboidal cells. There are no myoepithelial cells around the excretory duct. As the excretory duct ascends, it straightens out and penetrates the cell layers of the **epidermis (1, 6)**, where it loses its epithelial wall. In the epidermis (1, 6), the duct follows a spiral course through the cells to the surface of the skin.

FUNCTIONAL CORRELATIONS: Skin Derivatives or Appendages

Nails, hairs, and **sweat glands** are derivatives of skin that develop directly from the surface epithelium of the epidermis. During development, these appendages grow into and reside deep within the connective tissue of the **dermis.** Sweat glands may also extend deeper into the **subcutaneous layer** or **hypodermis.**

Hairs are the hard, cornified, cylindrical structures that arise from **hair follicles** in the skin. One portion of the hair projects through the epithelium of the skin to the exterior surface; the other portion remains embedded in the dermis. Hair grows in the expanded portion at the base of the hair follicle called the **hair bulb.** The base of the hair bulb is indented by a **connective tissue papilla,** a highly vascularized region that brings essential nutrients to hair follicle cells. Here, the hair cells divide, grow, cornify, and form the hairs.

Associated with each hair follicle are one or more **sebaceous glands** that produce an oily secretion called **sebum.** Sebum forms when cells die in sebaceous glands. Also, extending from the connective tissue around the hair follicle to the **papillary layer** of the **dermis** are bundles of smooth muscle called **arrector pili.** The sebaceous glands are located between the arrector pili muscle and the hair follicle. Arrector pili muscles are controlled by the **autonomic nervous system** and contract during strong emotions, fear, and cold. Contraction of the arrector pili muscle erects the hair shaft, depresses the skin where it inserts, and produces a small bump on the surface of skin, often called a goose bump. In addition, this contraction forces the sebum from sebaceous glands onto the hair follicle and skin. Sebum oils and keeps the skin smooth, waterproofs it, prevents it from drying, and gives it some antibacterial protection.

Sweat glands are widely distributed in skin, and are of two types, eccrine and apocrine. **Eccrine** sweat glands are simple, coiled tubular glands. Their **secretory portion** is found deep in the dermis, from which a coiled **excretory duct** leads to the skin surface. The eccrine sweat glands contain two cell types: **clear cells** without secretory granules and **dark cells** with secretory granules. Secretion from the dark cells is primarily mucous, whereas secretion from clear cells is watery. Surrounding the basal region of the secretory portion of each sweat gland are **myoepithelial cells,** whose contraction expels the secretion (sweat) from sweat glands. Eccrine sweat glands are most numerous in the skin of the palms and soles. The eccrine sweat glands assist in temperature regulation. Sweat glands also excrete water, sodium salts, ammonia, uric acid, and urea.

Apocrine sweat glands are also found in the dermis and are primarily limited to the axilla, anus, and areolar regions of the breast. These sweat glands are larger than eccrine sweat glands, and their ducts open into the **hair follicle.** The secretory portion of the gland is coiled and tubular. In contrast to eccrine sweat glands, the lumina of the secretory portion of the gland are wide and dilated, and the secretory cells are low cuboidal. Similar to eccrine sweat glands, the secretory portion of the apocrine glands is surrounded by contractile **myoepithelial cells.** The apocrine sweat glands become functional at puberty, when the **sex hormones** are produced. The glands produce a **viscous secretion**, which acquires a distinct and unpleasant odor after bacterial decomposition.

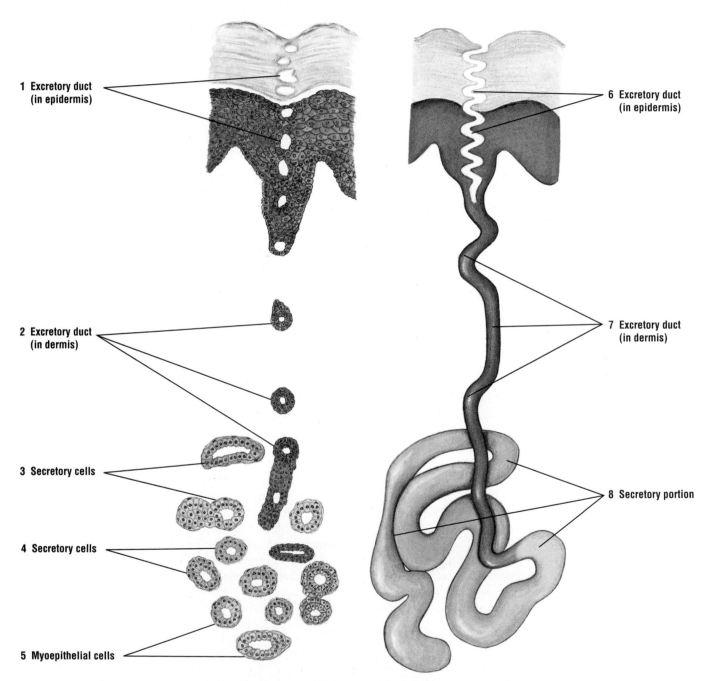

1 **Excretory duct**
   (in epidermis)

2 **Excretory duct**
   (in dermis)

3 **Secretory cells**

4 **Secretory cells**

5 **Myoepithelial cells**

6 **Excretory duct**
   (in epidermis)

7 **Excretory duct**
   (in dermis)

8 **Secretory portion**

FIGURE 10.9 ■ Cross section and three-dimensional appearance of an eccrine sweat gland. Stain: hematoxylin and eosin. Low magnification.

FIGURE 10.10 ■ Glomus in the Dermis of Thick Skin

Arteriovenous anastomoses are numerous in the thick skin of the fingers and toes. In some arteriovenous anastomoses, there is a direct connection between the artery and vein. In others, the arterial portion of the anastomosis forms a specialized thick-walled structure called the **glomus (2)**. The blood vessel in the glomus (2) is highly coiled or convoluted and, as a result, more than one lumen of the coiled vessel may be seen in a transverse section of the glomus (2).

The smooth muscle cells in the tunica media of the glomus artery (2) have enlarged and become **epithelioid cells (6)**. The tunica media of the glomus artery (2) becomes thin again before it empties into a venule at the **arteriovenous junction (5)**.

All arteriovenous anastomoses are richly innervated and supplied by blood vessels. A **connective tissue sheath (7)** encloses the glomus (2). The **dermis (4)** that surrounds the glomus (2) contains numerous **blood vessels (8)**, peripheral **nerves (1)**, and excretory **ducts** of **sweat glands (3)**.

FUNCTIONAL CORRELATIONS: Arteriovenous Anastomoses and Glomus

In numerous tissues, direct communications between arteries and veins called **arteriovenous anastomoses** bypass the capillaries. Their main functions are regulation of blood pressure, blood flow, and temperature, and conservation of body heat. A more complex structure that also forms shunts is called a **glomus.** A glomus consists of a highly coiled arteriovenous shunt that is surrounded by collagenous connective tissue. The function of the glomus is also to regulate blood flow and conserve body heat. These structures are found in the fingertips, external ear, and other peripheral areas that are exposed to excessive cold temperatures and where arteriovenous shunts are needed.

FIGURE 10.11 ■ Pacinian Corpuscles in the Dermis of Thick Skin
(Transverse and Longitudinal Sections)

Located deep in the **dermis (3)** of the thick skin and subcutaneous tissue are the **Pacinian corpuscles (2, 9)**. One Pacinian corpuscle is illustrated in a longitudinal section (2) and the other in transverse section (9).

Each Pacinian corpuscle (2, 9) is an ovoid structure with an elongated central myelinated **axon (2b, 9b)**. The axon (2b, 9b) in the corpuscle is surrounded by **concentric lamellae (2a, 9a)** of compact collagenous fibers that become denser in the periphery to form the **connective tissue capsule (2c, 9c)**. Between the connective tissue lamellae (2c, 9c) is a small amount of lymphlike fluid. In a transverse section, the layers of connective tissue lamellae (9a) surrounding the central axon (9b) of the Pacinian corpuscle (9) resemble a sliced onion.

In the connective tissue of the dermis (3) and surrounding the Pacinian corpuscles (2, 9) are numerous **adipose cells (5)**, blood vessels such as a **venule (10)**, peripheral **nerves (4, 6)**, and cross sections of an **excretory duct (1)** and the **secretory portion** of the **sweat gland (8)**. The contractile **myoepithelial cells (7)** surround the secretory portion of the sweat gland (8).

The Pacinian (2, 9) corpuscles are important sensory receptors for pressure, vibration, and touch.

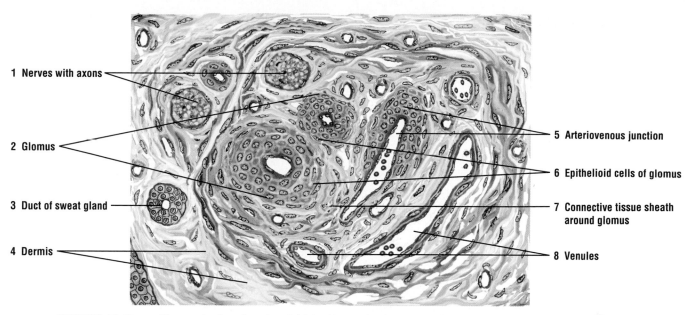

1 Nerves with axons

2 Glomus

3 Duct of sweat gland

4 Dermis

5 Arteriovenous junction

6 Epithelioid cells of glomus

7 Connective tissue sheath around glomus

8 Venules

FIGURE 10.10 ■ Glomus in the dermis of thick skin. Stain: hematoxylin and eosin. High magnification.

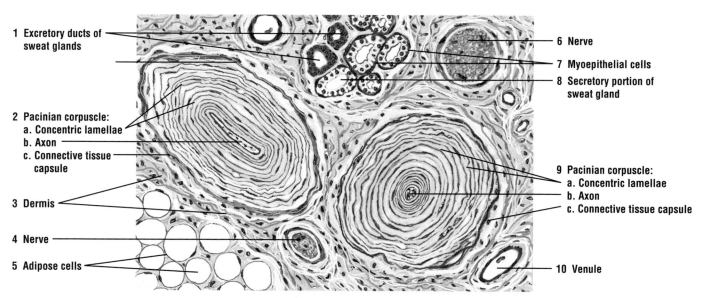

1 Excretory ducts of sweat glands

2 Pacinian corpuscle:
  a. Concentric lamellae
  b. Axon
  c. Connective tissue capsule

3 Dermis

4 Nerve

5 Adipose cells

6 Nerve

7 Myoepithelial cells

8 Secretory portion of sweat gland

9 Pacinian corpuscle:
  a. Concentric lamellae
  b. Axon
  c. Connective tissue capsule

10 Venule

FIGURE 10.11 ■ Pacinian corpuscles in the dermis of thick skin (transverse and longitudinal sections). Stain: hematoxylin and eosin. High magnification.

Integumentary System

- Skin and derivatives form the integumentary system
- Consists of superficial epidermis and deeper dermis
- Nonvascular epidermis is covered by keratinized stratified squamous epithelium
- Vascular dermis consists of irregular connective tissue

Epidermis: Thick Versus Thin Skin

- Palms and soles, because of wear and tear, are covered by thick skin
- Thick skin contains sweat glands, but lacks hair, sebaceous glands, and smooth muscle
- Thin skin contains sebaceous glands, hair, sweat glands, and arrector pili smooth muscle
- Keratinocytes are predominant cell type in the epidermis
- Less numerous epidermal cells are the melanocytes, Langerhans cells, and Merkel's cells
- Basement membrane separates dermis from epidermis

Dermis

Papillary Layer

- Is the superficial layer in dermis and contains loose irregular connective tissue
- Dermal papillae and epidermal ridges form evaginations and interdigitations
- Connective tissue filled with fibers, cells, and blood vessels
- Sensory receptors Meissner's corpuscles are present in dermal papillae

Reticular Layer

- Is the deeper and thicker layer in dermis, filled with dense irregular connective tissue
- Few cells present and collagen is type I
- No distinct boundary between papillary and reticular layers
- Blends inferiorly with hypodermis or subcutaneous layer (hypodermis) of superficial fascia
- Contains arteriovenous anastomoses and sensory receptors Pacinian corpuscles
- Concentric lamellae of collagen fibers surround myelinated axons in Pacinian corpuscles

Epidermal Cell Layers

Stratum Basale (Germinativum)

- Deepest or basal single layer of cells that rests on the basement membrane
- Cells attached by desmosomes and by hemidesmosomes to basement membrane

- Cells serve as stem cells for epidermis and show increased mitosis
- Cells migrate upward in epidermis and produce intermediate keratin filaments

Stratum Spinosum

- Is the second layer above stratum basale that consists of four to six rows of cells
- During histologic preparation, cells shrink and intercellular spaces appear as spines
- Cells synthesize keratin filaments that become assembled into tonofilaments
- Spines represent sites of desmosome attachments to keratin tonofilaments

Stratum Granulosum

- Cells are above stratum spinosum and consists of three to five cell layers of flattened cells
- Cells filled with dense keratohyalin granules and membrane-bound lamellar granules
- Keratohyalin granules associate with keratin tonofilaments to produce soft keratin
- Lamellar granules discharge lipid material between cells and waterproof the skin

Stratum Lucidum

- Lies superior to stratum granulosum, found in thick skin only, translucent and barely visible
- Cells lack nuclei or organelles and are packed with keratin filaments

Stratum Corneum

- Most superficial layer and consists of flat, dead cells filled with soft keratin
- Keratinized cells continually shed or desquamated and replaced by new cells
- During keratinization, hydrolytic enzymes eliminate nucleus and organelles

Other Skin Cells

Melanocytes

- Arise from neural crest cells and are located between stratum basale and stratum spinosum
- Long irregular cytoplasmic extensions branch into epidermis
- Synthesize from amino acid tyrosine a dark brown pigment, melanin
- Melanin transferred to keratinocytes in basal cell layers
- Melanin darkens skin color and protect it from ultraviolet radiation

Langerhans Cells

- Found mainly in stratum spinosum; part of immune system of body
- Are antigen-presenting cells of the skin

Merkel's Cells

- Present in the basal layer of epidermis and function as mechanoreceptors for pressure

Major Skin Functions

- Protection through keratinized epidermis from abrasion and entrance of pathogens
- Impermeable to water owing to lipid layer in epidermis
- Body temperature regulation as a result of sweating and changes in vessel diameters
- Sensory perception of touch, pain, pressure, and temperature changes because of nerve endings
- Excretions through sweat of water, sodium salts, urea, and nitrogenous waste
- Formation of vitamin D from precursor molecules produced in epidermis when exposed to sun

Skin Derivatives

Hairs

- Develop from surface epithelium of the epidermis and reside deep in the dermis
- Are hard cylindrical structures that arise from hair follicles
- Surrounded by external and internal root sheaths
- Grow from expanded hair bulb of the hair follicle
- Hair bulb indented by connective tissue (dermal) papilla that is highly vascularized
- Hair matrix situated above papilla contain mitotic cells and melanocytes

Sebaceous Glands

- Numerous sebaceous glands associated with each hair follicle
- Cells in sebaceous glands grow, accumulate secretions, die, and become oily secretion sebum

- Smooth muscles arrector pili attach to papillary layer of dermis and to sheath of hair follicle
- Contraction of arrector pili muscle stands hair up and forces sebum into lumen of hair follicle

Sweat Glands

- Widely distributed in skin and are of two types: eccrine and apocrine
- Assist in temperature regulation and excretion of water, salts, and some nitrogenous waste

Eccrine Sweat Glands

- Are simple coiled glands located deep in dermis in skin of palms and soles
- Consist of clear and dark secretory cells, and excretory duct
- Clear cells secrete watery product, whereas dark cells secrete mainly mucus
- Contractile myoepithelial cells surround only the secretory cells
- Excretory duct is thin, dark-staining, and lined by stratified cuboidal cells
- Excretory duct ascends, straightens, and penetrates epidermis to reach surface of skin

Apocrine Sweat Glands

- Found coiled in deep dermis of axilla, anus, and areolar regions of the breast
- Ducts of glands open into hair follicles
- Lumina wide and dilated, with low cuboidal epithelium
- Contractile myoepithelial cells surround secretory portion of glands
- Become functional at puberty, when sex hormones are present
- Secretion has unpleasant odor after bacterial decomposition

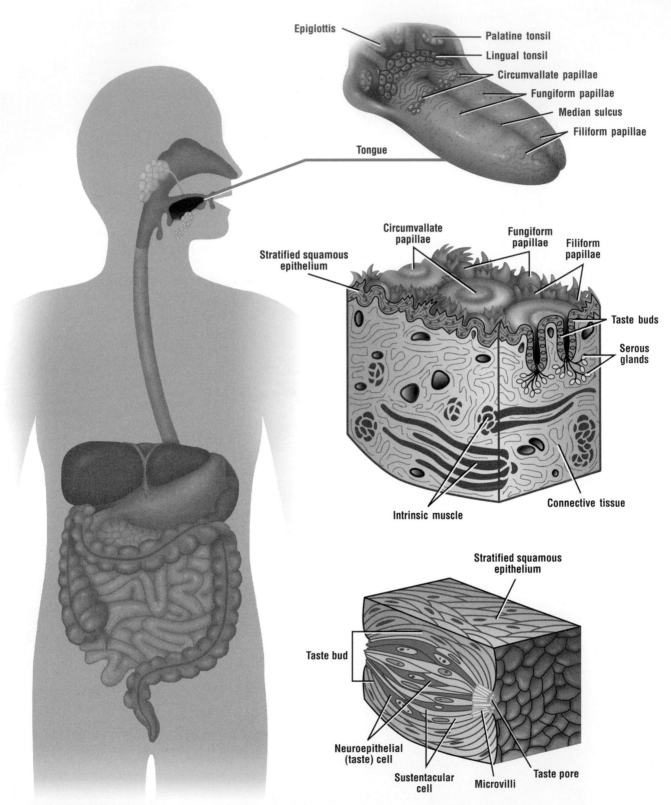

OVERVIEW FIGURE 11.1 ■ Oral cavity. The salivary glands and their connections to the oral cavity, morphology of the tongue in cross section, and added detail of a taste bud are illustrated.

CHAPTER 11

Digestive System: Oral Cavity and Salivary Glands

The digestive system is a long **hollow tube** or tract that starts at the oral cavity and terminates at the anus. The system consists of the **oral cavity, esophagus, stomach, small intestine, large intestine, rectum,** and **anal canal.** Associated with the digestive tract are the accessory digestive organs, the **salivary glands, liver,** and **pancreas.** The accessory organs are located outside of digestive tract. Their secretory products are delivered to the digestive tract through excretory ducts that penetrate the digestive tract wall (Overview Figure 11.1: Oral Cavity).

The Oral Cavity

In the oral cavity, food is ingested, masticated (chewed), and lubricated by saliva for swallowing. Because food is physically broken down in the oral cavity, this region is lined by a protective, nonkeratinized, **stratified squamous epithelium,** which also lines the inner or labial surface of the lips.

The Lips

The oral cavity is formed, in part, by the lips and cheeks. The lips are lined by a very thin skin covered by a stratified squamous keratinized epithelium. Blood vessels are close to the lip surface, imparting a red color to the lips. The outer surface of the lip contains hair follicles, sebaceous glands, and sweat glands. The lips also contain skeletal muscle called **orbicularis oris.** Inside the free margin of the lip, the outer lining changes to a thicker, stratified squamous nonkeratinized oral epithelium. Beneath the oral epithelium are found mucus-secreting **labial glands.**

The Tongue

The **tongue** is a muscular organ located in the oral cavity. The core of the tongue consists of **connective tissue** and interlacing bundles of **skeletal muscle fibers.** The distribution and random orientation of individual skeletal muscle fibers in the tongue allows for increased movement during chewing, swallowing, and speaking.

Papillae

The epithelium on the dorsal surface of the tongue is irregular or rough owing to numerous elevations or projections called **papillae.** These are indented by the underlying connective tissue called **lamina propria.** All papillae on the tongue are covered by **stratified squamous epithelium** that shows partial or incomplete **keratinization.** In contrast, the epithelium on the ventral surface of the tongue is smooth.

There are four types of papillae on the tongue: filiform, fungiform, circumvallate, and foliate.

Filiform Papillae

The most numerous and smallest papillae on the surface of the tongue are the narrow, conical-shaped **filiform papillae.** They cover the entire dorsal surface of the tongue.

Fungiform Papillae

Less numerous but larger, broader, and taller than the filiform papillae are the **fungiform papillae.** These papillae exhibit a mushroom-like shape and are more prevalent in the anterior region of the tongue. Fungiform papillae are interspersed among the filiform papillae.

Circumvallate Papillae

Circumvallate papillae are much larger than the fungiform or filiform papillae. Eight to 12 circumvallate papillae are located in the posterior region of the tongue. These papillae are characterized by deep moats or **furrows** that completely encircle them. Numerous excretory ducts from underlying **serous (von Ebner's) glands,** located in the connective tissue, empty into the base of the furrows.

Foliate Papillae

Foliate papillae are well developed in some animals but are rudimentary or poorly developed in humans.

Taste Buds

Located in the epithelium of the foliate and fungiform papillae, and on the lateral sides of the circumvallate papillae, are barrel-shaped structures called the **taste buds.** In addition, taste buds are found in the epithelium of the soft palate, pharynx, and epiglottis. The free surface of each taste bud contains an opening called the **taste pore.** Each taste bud occupies the full thickness of the epithelium.

Located within each taste bud are elongated **neuroepithelial (taste) cells** that extend from the base of the taste bud to the taste pore. The apices of each taste cell exhibit numerous **microvilli** that protrude through the taste pore. The cells that are receptors for taste are closely associated with small afferent nerve fibers. Also present within the confines of the taste buds are elongated supporting **sustentacular cells.** These cells are not sensory. At the base of each taste bud are **basal cells.** These cells are undifferentiated and are believed to serve as **stem cells** for the specialized cells in taste buds (Overview Figure 11.1, Oral Cavity).

Lymphoid Aggregations: Tonsils (Palatine, Pharyngeal, and Lingual)

The tonsils are aggregates of diffuse lymphoid tissue and lymphoid nodules that are located in the oral pharynx. The **palatine tonsils** are located on the lateral walls of the oral part of the pharynx. These tonsils are lined with stratified squamous nonkeratinized epithelium and exhibit numerous **crypts.** A connective tissue capsule separates the tonsils from adjacent tissue. The **pharyngeal tonsil** is a single structure situated in the superior and posterior portion of the pharynx. It is covered by pseudostratified ciliated epithelium. The **lingual tonsils** are located on the dorsal surface of the posterior one third of the tongue. They are several in number and are seen as small bulges composed of masses of lymphoid aggregations. The lingual tonsils are lined by stratified squamous nonkeratinized epithelium. Each lingual tonsil is invaginated by the covering epithelium to form numerous crypts, around which are found aggregations of lymphatic nodules.

FIGURE 11.1 ■ Lip (Longitudinal Section)

Thin skin or thin **epidermis (11)** lines the external surface of the lip. The epidermis (11) is composed of stratified squamous keratinized epithelium with **desquamating surface cells (10).** Beneath the epidermis (11) is the **dermis (14)** with **sebaceous glands (2, 12)** that are associated with **hair follicles (4, 15),** and the simple tubular **sweat glands (16)** located deeper in the dermis (14). The dermis (14) also contains the **arrector pili muscles (3, 13),** smooth muscles that attach to the hair follicles (4, 15). Also visible in the lip periphery are blood vessels, an **artery (6a)** and **venule (6b).** The core of the lip contains a layer of striated muscles, the **orbicularis oris (5, 17).**

The **transition zone (1)** of the skin epidermis **(11)** to oral epithelium illustrates a mucocutaneous junction. The internal or oral surface of the lip is lined with a moist, stratified, squamous nonkeratinized **oral epithelium (8)** that is thicker than the epithelium of the epidermis (11). The surface cells of the oral epithelium (8), without becoming cornified, are sloughed off (desquamated) into the fluids of the **mouth (10).** In the deeper connective tissue of the lip are found tubuloacinar, mucus-secreting **labial glands (9, 18).** The secretions from these glands moisten the oral mucosa. The small excretory ducts of the labial glands (9, 18) open into the oral cavity.

In the underlying connective tissue of the lip are also numerous **adipose cells (7),** blood vessels (6), and numerous capillaries. Because the blood vessels (6) are very close to the surface, the color of the blood shows through the overlying thin epithelium, giving the lips a characteristic red color.

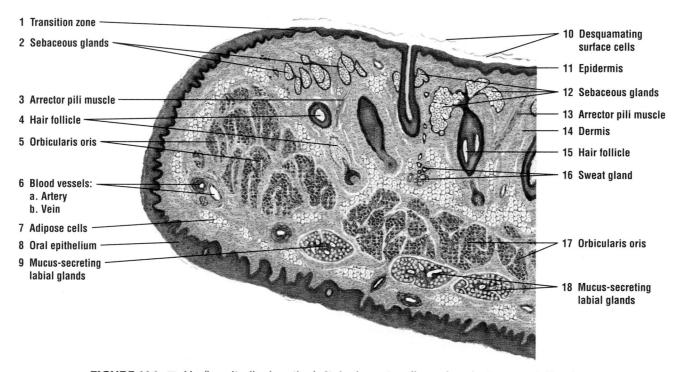

1 Transition zone
2 Sebaceous glands
3 Arrector pili muscle
4 Hair follicle
5 Orbicularis oris
6 Blood vessels:
   a. Artery
   b. Vein
7 Adipose cells
8 Oral epithelium
9 Mucus-secreting
   labial glands

10 Desquamating
   surface cells
11 Epidermis
12 Sebaceous glands
13 Arrector pili muscle
14 Dermis
15 Hair follicle
16 Sweat gland
17 Orbicularis oris
18 Mucus-secreting
   labial glands

FIGURE 11.1 ■ Lip (longitudinal section). Stain: hematoxylin and eosin. Low magnification.

FIGURE 11.2 ■ Anterior Region of the Tongue: Apex (Longitudinal Section)

This illustration shows a longitudinal section of an anterior portion of the tongue. The oral cavity is lined by a protective **mucosa (5)** that consists of an outer epithelial layer (**epithelium**) **(5a)** and an underlying connective tissue layer called the **lamina propria (5b).**

The dorsal surface of the tongue is rough and characterized by numerous mucosal projections called **papillae (1, 2, 6).** In contrast, the mucosa (5) of the ventral surface of the tongue is smooth. The slender, conical-shaped **filiform papillae (2, 6)** are the most numerous papillae and cover the entire dorsal surface of the tongue. The tips of the filiform papillae (2, 6) show partial keratinization.

Less numerous are the **fungiform papillae (1)** with a broad, round surface of noncornified epithelium and a prominent core of **lamina propria (5b).**

The core of the tongue consists of crisscrossing bundles of **skeletal muscle (3, 7).** As a result, the skeletal muscles of the tongue are typically seen in longitudinal, transverse, or oblique planes of section. In the **connective tissue (9)** around the muscle bundles may be seen **blood vessels (4, 8),** such as an **artery (4a, 8a)** and **vein (4b, 8b),** and **nerve fibers (11).**

In the lower half of the tongue and surrounded by skeletal muscle fibers (3, 7) is a portion of the **anterior lingual gland (10).** This gland is of a mixed type and contains both **mucous acini (10b)** and **serous acini (10c),** as well as mixed acini. The **interlobular ducts (10a)** from the anterior lingual gland (10) pass into the larger **excretory duct** of the **lingual gland (12)** that opens into the oral cavity on the ventral surface of the tongue.

FIGURE 11.3 ■ Tongue: Circumvallate Papilla (Cross Section)

A cross section of a circumvallate papilla of the tongue is illustrated. The **lingual epithelium (2)** of the tongue that covers the circumvallate papilla is **stratified squamous epithelium (1).** The underlying connective tissue, the **lamina propria (3),** exhibits numerous **secondary papillae (7)** that project into the overlying stratified squamous epithelium (1, 2) of the papilla. A deep trench or **furrow (5, 10)** surrounds the base of each circumvallate papilla.

The oval **taste buds (4, 9)** are located in the epithelium of the lateral surfaces of the circumvallate papilla and in the epithelium on the outer wall of the furrow (5, 10). (Figure 11.4 illustrates the taste buds (4, 9) in greater detail with higher magnification.)

Located deep in the lamina propria (3) and core of the tongue are numerous, tubuloacinar **serous** (von Ebner's) **glands (6, 11),** whose **excretory ducts (6a, 11a)** open at the base of the circular furrows (5, 10) in the circumvallate papilla. The secretory product from the **serous secretory acini (6b, 11b)** acts as a solvent for taste-inducing substances.

Most of the core of the tongue consists of interlacing bundles of **skeletal muscles (12).** Examples of skeletal muscle fibers sectioned in **longitudinal (12a)** and **transverse planes (12b)** are abundant. This interlacing arrangement of skeletal muscles (12) gives the tongue the necessary mobility for phonating and chewing and swallowing of food. The lamina propria (3) surrounding the serous glands (6, 11) and muscles (12) also contains an abundance of **blood vessels (8).**

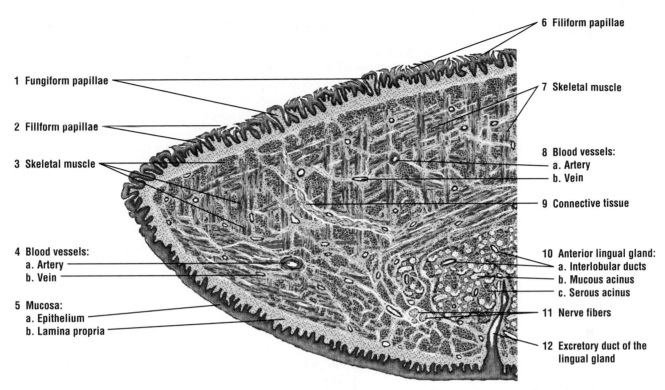

1 Fungiform papillae

2 Fillform papillae

3 Skeletal muscle

4 Blood vessels:
   a. Artery
   b. Vein

5 Mucosa:
   a. Epithelium
   b. Lamina propria

6 Filiform papillae

7 Skeletal muscle

8 Blood vessels:
   a. Artery
   b. Vein

9 Connective tissue

10 Anterior lingual gland:
   a. Interlobular ducts
   b. Mucous acinus
   c. Serous acinus

11 Nerve fibers

12 Excretory duct of the lingual gland

FIGURE 11.2 ■ Anterior region of the tongue (longitudinal section). Stain: hematoxylin and eosin. Low magnification.

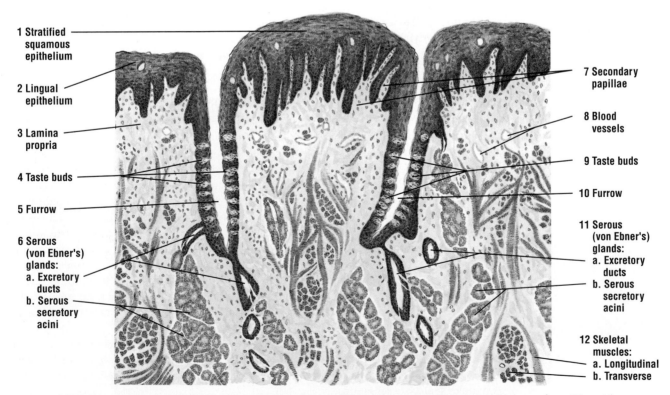

1 Stratified squamous epithelium

2 Lingual epithelium

3 Lamina propria

4 Taste buds

5 Furrow

6 Serous (von Ebner's) glands:
  a. Excretory ducts
  b. Serous secretory acini

7 Secondary papillae

8 Blood vessels

9 Taste buds

10 Furrow

11 Serous (von Ebner's) glands:
   a. Excretory ducts
   b. Serous secretory acini

12 Skeletal muscles:
   a. Longitudinal
   b. Transverse

FIGURE 11.3 ■ Posterior tongue: circumvallate papilla, surrounding furrow, and serous (von Ebner's) glands (cross section). Stain: hematoxylin and eosin. Medium magnification.

FIGURE 11.4 ■ Tongue: Filiform and Fungiform Papillae

A low-power photomicrograph shows a section of the dorsal surface of the tongue. In the center is a large **fungiform papilla (2)**. The surface of the fungiform papilla (2) is covered by **stratified squamous epithelium (3)** that is not cornified or keratinized. The fungiform papilla (2) also exhibits numerous **taste buds (4)** that are located in the epithelium on the apical surface of the papilla, in contrast to the circumvallate papillae, in which the taste buds are located in the peripheral epithelium (see Figure 11.3 above).

The underlying connective tissue core, the **lamina propria (5)**, projects into the surface epithelium of the fungiform papilla (2) to form numerous indentations. Surrounding the fungiform papilla (2) are the slender **filiform papillae (1)**, whose conical tips are covered by stratified squamous epithelium that exhibits partial keratinization.

FIGURE 11.5 ■ Tongue: Taste Buds

The **taste buds (5, 12)** at the bottom of a **furrow (14)** of the circumvallate papilla are illustrated in greater detail. The taste buds (5, 12) are embedded within and extend the full thickness of the stratified **lingual epithelium (1)** of the circumvallate papilla. The taste buds (5, 12) are distinguished from the surrounding stratified epithelium (1) by their oval shapes and elongated cells (modified columnar) that are arranged perpendicular to the epithelium (1).

Several types of cells are found in the taste buds (5, 12). Three different types of cells can be identified in this illustration. The supporting or **sustentacular cells (3, 8)** are elongated and exhibit a darker cytoplasm and a slender, dark nucleus. The **taste** or **gustatory cells (7, 11)** exhibit a lighter cytoplasm and a more oval, lighter nucleus. The **basal cells (13)** are located at the periphery of the taste bud (5, 12) near the basement membrane.

Because unmyelinated nerve fibers are associated with both sustentacular cells (3, 8) and gustatory cells (7, 11), both types may be responsible for taste functions. The basal cells (13) give rise to both the sustentacular cells (3, 8) and gustatory cells (7, 11).

Each taste bud (5, 12) exhibits a small opening onto the epithelial surface called the **taste pore (9)**. The apical surfaces of both the sustentacular cells (3, 8) and gustatory cells (7, 11) exhibit long **microvilli (taste hairs) (4)** that extend into and protrude through the taste pore (9) into the furrow (14) that surrounds the circumvallate papilla.

The underlying **lamina propria (2)** adjacent to the epithelium and the taste buds (5, 12) consists of loose connective tissue with numerous **blood vessels (6, 10)** and nerve fibers.

FUNCTIONAL CORRELATIONS: Tongue and Taste Buds

The main functions of the tongue during food processing are to perceive **taste** and to assist with mastication (chewing) and swallowing of the food mass, called a **bolus.** In the oral cavity, taste sensations are detected by receptor taste cells located in the **taste buds** of the **fungiform** and **circumvallate papillae** of the tongue. In addition to the tongue, where taste buds are most numerous, taste buds are also found in the mucous membrane of the **soft palate, pharynx,** and **epiglottis.**

Substances to be tasted are first dissolved in **saliva** that is present in the oral cavity during food intake. The dissolved substance then contacts the taste cells through the taste pore. In addition to saliva, taste buds located in the epithelium of circumvallate papillae are continuously washed by watery secretions produced by the underlying **serous (von Ebner's) glands.** This secretion enters the **furrow** at the base of the papillae and continues to dissolve different substances, which then enter the **taste pores** in taste buds. The receptor taste cells are then stimulated by coming in direct contact with the dissolved substances and conduct an impulse over the afferent nerve fibers.

There are four basic taste sensations: **sour, salt, bitter,** and **sweet.** All remaining taste sensations are various combinations of the basic four tastes. The tip of the tongue is most sensitive to sweet and salt, the posterior portion of the tongue to bitter, and the lateral edges of the tongue to sour taste sensations.

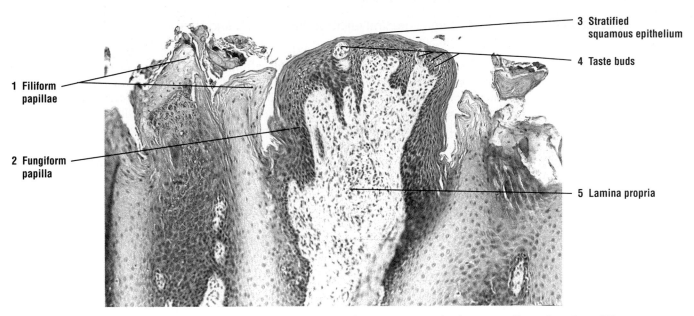

FIGURE 11.4 ■ Filiform and fungiform papillae of the tongue. Stain: hematoxylin and eosin. ×25.

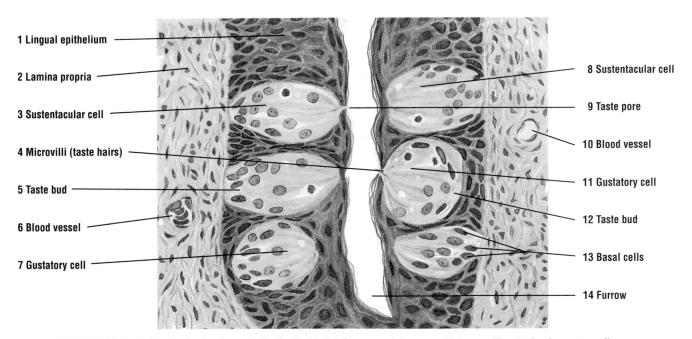

FIGURE 11.5 ■ Posterior tongue: taste buds in the furrow of circumvallate papilla. Stain: hematoxylin and eosin. High magnification.

FIGURE 11.6 ■ Posterior Tongue: Behind Circumvallate Papilla and Near Lingual Tonsil (Longitudinal Section)

The anterior two thirds of the tongue is separated from the posterior one third of the tongue by a depression or a sulcus terminalis. The posterior region of the tongue is located behind the circumvallate papillae and near the lingual tonsils. The dorsal surface of the posterior region typically exhibits large **mucosal ridges (1)** and elevations or **folds (7)** that resemble the large fungiform papillae of the anterior tongue. A **stratified squamous epithelium (6)** without keratinization covers the mucosal ridges (1) and the folds (7). The filiform and fungiform papillae that are normally seen in the anterior region of the tongue are absent from the posterior tongue. Lymphatic nodules of the lingual tonsils can be seen in these folds (7).

The **lamina propria (7)** of the mucosa is wider but similar to that in the anterior two thirds of the tongue. Under the stratified squamous epithelium (6) are seen aggregations of diffuse **lymphatic tissue (2)**, accumulations of **adipose tissue (4)**, **nerve fibers (3)** (in longitudinal section), and blood vessels, an **artery (8)** and **vein (9)**.

Deep in the connective tissue of the lamina propria (7) and between the interlacing **skeletal muscle fibers (5)** are found the mucous acini of the **posterior lingual glands (11)**. The **excretory ducts (10)** of the posterior lingual glands (11) open onto the dorsal surface of the tongue, usually between bases of the mucosal ridges and folds (1, 7). The posterior lingual glands (11) come in contact with the serous glands (von Ebner's) of the circumvallate papilla in the anterior region of the tongue. In the posterior region of the tongue, the posterior lingual glands (11) extend through the root of the tongue.

FIGURE 11.7 ■ Lingual Tonsils (Transverse Section)

The lingual tonsils are aggregations of small, individual tonsils, each with its own **tonsillar crypt (2, 8)**. Lingual tonsils are situated on the dorsal surface of the posterior region or the root of the tongue. A nonkeratinized **stratified squamous epithelium (1)** lines the tonsils and their crypts (2, 8). The tonsillar crypts (2, 8) form deep invaginations on the surface of the tongue and may extend deep into the **lamina propria (5)**.

Numerous **lymphatic nodules (3, 9)**, some exhibiting **germinal centers (3, 9)**, are located in the lamina propria (5) below the stratified squamous surface epithelium (1). Dense **lymphatic infiltration (4, 10)** surrounds the individual lymphatic nodules (3, 9) of the tonsils.

Located deep in the lamina propria (5) are fat cells of the **adipose tissue (7)** and the secretory **mucous acini** of the **posterior lingual glands (11)**. Small excretory ducts from the lingual glands (11) unite to form larger **excretory ducts (6)**. Most of the excretory ducts (6) open into the tonsillar crypts (2, 8), although some may open directly on the lingual surface. Interspersed among the connective tissue of the lamina propria (5), adipose tissue (7), and the secretory mucous acini of the posterior lingual glands (11) are fibers of the **skeletal muscles (12)** of the tongue.

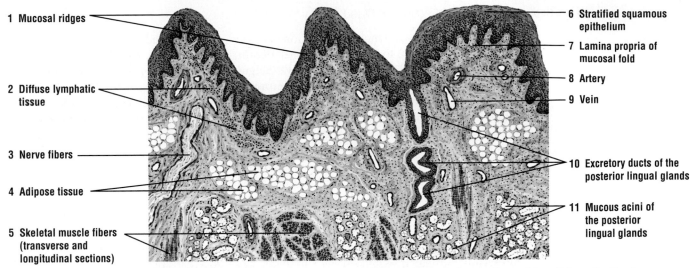

1 Mucosal ridges

2 Diffuse lymphatic tissue

3 Nerve fibers

4 Adipose tissue

5 Skeletal muscle fibers (transverse and longitudinal sections)

6 Stratified squamous epithelium

7 Lamina propria of mucosal fold

8 Artery

9 Vein

10 Excretory ducts of the posterior lingual glands

11 Mucous acini of the posterior lingual glands

FIGURE 11.6 ■ Posterior tongue: posterior to circumvallate papillae and near lingual tonsil (longitudinal section). Stain: hematoxylin and eosin. Low magnification.

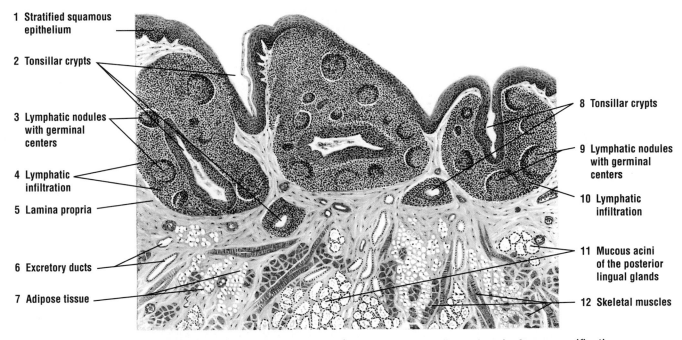

1 Stratified squamous epithelium

2 Tonsillar crypts

3 Lymphatic nodules with germinal centers

4 Lymphatic infiltration

5 Lamina propria

6 Excretory ducts

7 Adipose tissue

8 Tonsillar crypts

9 Lymphatic nodules with germinal centers

10 Lymphatic infiltration

11 Mucous acini of the posterior lingual glands

12 Skeletal muscles

FIGURE 11.7 ■ Lingual tonsils (transverse section). Stain: hematoxylin and eosin. Low magnification.

FIGURE 11.8 ■ Longitudinal Section of Dried Tooth

This illustration shows a longitudinal section of a dried, nondecalcified, and unstained tooth. The mineralized parts of a tooth are the enamel, dentin, and cementum. **Dentin (3)** is covered by **enamel (1)** in the region that projects above the gum. Enamel is not present at the root of the tooth, and here the dentin is covered by **cementum (6).** Cementum (6) contains lacunae with the cementum-producing cells called cementocytes and their connecting canaliculi. Dentin (3) surrounds both the **pulp cavity (5)** and its extension into the root of the tooth as the **root canal (11).** In living persons, the pulp cavity and root canal are filled with fine connective tissue, fibroblasts, histiocytes, and dentin-forming cells, the odontoblasts. Blood capillaries and nerves enter the pulp cavity (5) through an **apical foramen (13)** at the tip of each root.

Dentin (3) exhibits wavy, parallel dentinal tubules. The earlier or primary dentin is located at the periphery of the tooth. The later or secondary dentin lies along the pulp cavity, where it is formed throughout life by odontoblasts. In the crown of a dried tooth at **the dentinoenamel junction (2)** are numerous irregular, air-filled spaces that appear black in the section. These **interglobular spaces (4, 10)** are filled with incompletely calcified dentin (interglobular dentin) in living persons. Similar areas, but smaller and spaced closer together, are present in the root, close to the dentinal-cementum junction, where they form the **granular layer (of Tomes) (12).**

The dentin in the crown of the tooth is covered with a thicker layer of enamel (1), composed of enamel rods or prisms held together by an interprismatic cementing substance. The **lines of Retzius (7)** represent the variations in the rate of enamel deposition. Light rays passing through a dried section of the tooth are refracted by twists that occur in the enamel rods as they course toward the surface of the tooth. These are the light **lines of Schreger (8).** Poor calcification of enamel rods during enamel formation can produce **enamel tufts (9)** that extend from the dentinoenamel junction into the enamel (see Figure 11.9).

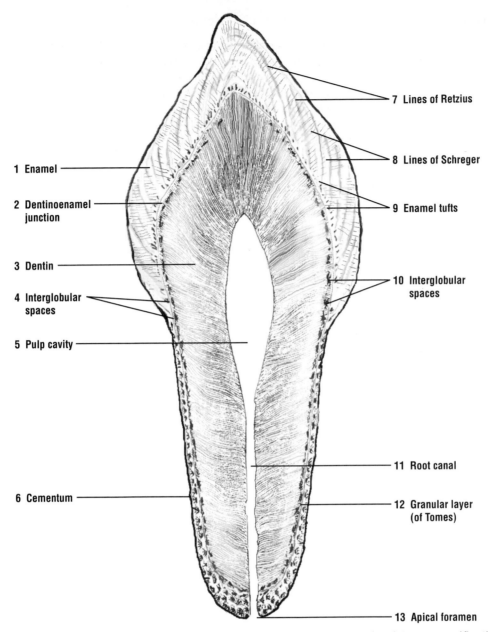

1 Enamel

2 Dentinoenamel junction

3 Dentin

4 Interglobular spaces

5 Pulp cavity

6 Cementum

7 Lines of Retzius

8 Lines of Schreger

9 Enamel tufts

10 Interglobular spaces

11 Root canal

12 Granular layer (of Tomes)

13 Apical foramen

FIGURE 11.8 ■ Longitudinal section of dry tooth. Ground and unstained. Low magnification.

FIGURE 11.9 ■ Dried Tooth: Dentinoenamel Junction

A section of the **dentin matrix (4)** and **enamel (5)** at the **dentinoenamel junction (1)** is illustrated at a higher magnification. The enamel is produced by cells called ameloblasts as successive segments that form elongated **enamel rods** or **prisms (7)**. The **enamel tufts (6),** which are the poorly calcified, twisted enamel rods or prisms, extend from the dentinoenamel junction (1) into the enamel (5). Dentin matrix (4) is produced by cells called odontoblasts. The odontoblastic processes of the odontoblasts occupy tunnel-like spaces in the dentin, forming the clearly visible **dentin tubules (3)** and black, air-filled **interglobular spaces (2).**

FIGURE 11.10 ■ Dried Tooth: Cementum and Dentin Junction

The junction between the **dentin matrix (5)** and **cementum (2)** is illustrated at a higher magnification at the root of the tooth. At the junction of the cementum (2) with the dentin matrix (5) is a layer of small interglobular spaces, the **granular layer of Tomes (7).** Internal to this layer in the dentin matrix (5) are the large, irregular **interglobular spaces (4, 8)** that are commonly seen in the crown of the tooth, but may also be present in the root of the tooth.

Cementum (2) is a thin layer of bony material secreted by cells called cementoblasts (mature forms, cementocytes). The bonelike cementum exhibits **lacunae (1)** that house the cementocytes and numerous **canaliculi (3)** for the cytoplasmic processes of cementocytes.

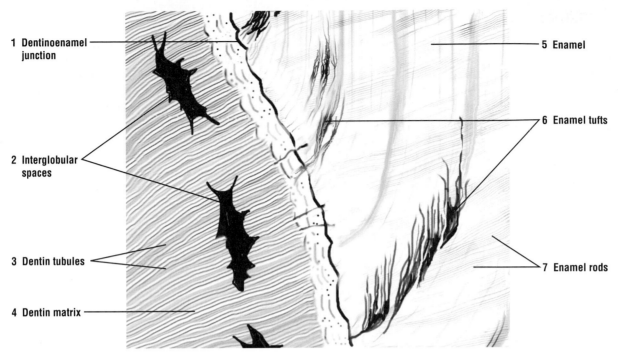

1 Dentinoenamel junction

2 Interglobular spaces

3 Dentin tubules

4 Dentin matrix

5 Enamel

6 Enamel tufts

7 Enamel rods

FIGURE 11.9 ■ Dried tooth. Dentinoenamel junction. Ground and unstained. Medium magnification.

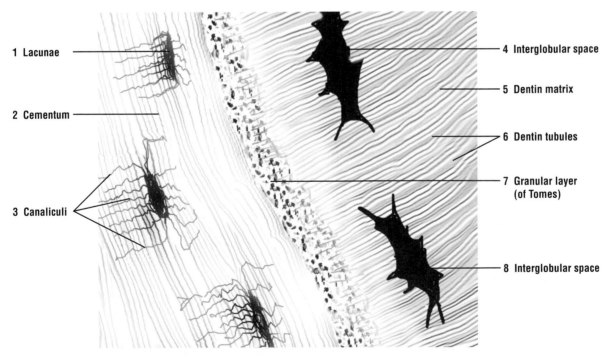

1 Lacunae

2 Cementum

3 Canaliculi

4 Interglobular space

5 Dentin matrix

6 Dentin tubules

7 Granular layer (of Tomes)

8 Interglobular space

FIGURE 11.10 ■ Dried tooth. Cementum and dentin junction. Ground and unstained. Medium magnification.

FIGURE 11.11 ■ Developing Tooth (Longitudinal Section)

A developing tooth is shown embedded in a socket, the **dental alveolus (23)** in the **bone (9)** of the jaw. The stratified squamous nonkeratinized **oral epithelium (1, 11)** covers the developing tooth. The underlying connective tissue in the digestive tube is called the **lamina propria (2, 12)**. A downgrowth from the oral epithelium (1, 11) invades the lamina propria (2, 12) and the primitive connective tissue as the **dental lamina (3)**. A layer of primitive **connective tissue (8, 17)** surrounds the developing tooth and forms a compact layer around the tooth, the **dental sac (8, 17)**.

The dental lamina (3) from the oral epithelium (1, 11) proliferates and gives rise to a cap-shaped enamel organ that consists of the **external enamel epithelium (4)**, the extracellular **stellate reticulum (5, 14)**, and the enamel-forming **ameloblasts** of the **inner enamel epithelium (6)**. The ameloblasts of the inner enamel epithelium (6) secrete the hard **enamel (7, 13)** around the **dentin (16)**. The enamel (7, 13) appears as a narrow band of dark red-staining material.

At the concave or the opposite end of the enamel organ, the **dental papilla (21)** originates from the primitive connective tissue **mesenchyme (21)** and forms the dental pulp or core of the developing tooth. **Blood vessels (20)** and nerves extend into and innervate the dental papilla (21) from below. The mesenchymal cells in the dental papilla (21) differentiate into **odontoblasts (15, 19)** and form the outer margin of the dental papilla (21). The odontoblasts (15) secrete an uncalcified dentin called **predentin (18)**. As predentin (18) calcifies, it forms a layer of pink-staining dentin (16) that lies adjacent to the dark-staining enamel (7, 13).

At the base of the tooth, the external enamel epithelium (4) and the ameloblasts of the inner enamel epithelium (6) continue to grow downward and form the bilayered **epithelial root sheath (of Hertwig) (10, 22)**. The cells of the epithelial root sheath (10, 22) induce the adjacent mesenchyme (21) cells to differentiate into odontoblasts (15, 19) and to form dentin (16).

FIGURE 11.12 ■ Developing Tooth: Dentinoenamel Junction in Detail

A section of the dentinoenamel junction from a developing tooth is illustrated at high magnification. On the left side of the figure is a small area of **stellate reticulum (1)** of enamel adjacent to the tall columnar **ameloblasts (2)** that secrete the **enamel (3)**. During enamel (3) formation, the apical extensions of ameloblasts become transformed into terminal processes (of Tomes). The mature enamel (3) consists of calcified, elongated **enamel rods (4)** or prisms that are barely visible in the dark-stained enamel (3). The enamel rods (4) extend through the thickness of the enamel (3).

The right side of the figure shows the nuclei of **mesenchymal cells** in the **dental papilla (5)**. The **odontoblasts (6)** are located adjacent to the dental papilla (5). The odontoblasts (6) secrete the uncalcified organic matrix of **predentin (8)**, which later calcifies into **dentin (9)**. The odontoblasts (6) exhibit slender apical extensions called **odontoblast processes (of Tomes) (7)**. These processes penetrate both the predentin (8) and dentin (9).

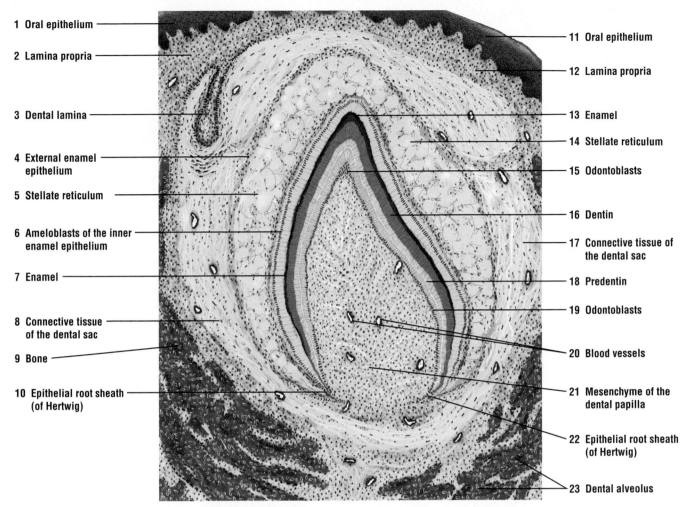

1 Oral epithelium

2 Lamina propria

3 Dental lamina

4 External enamel epithelium

5 Stellate reticulum

6 Ameloblasts of the inner enamel epithelium

7 Enamel

8 Connective tissue of the dental sac

9 Bone

10 Epithelial root sheath (of Hertwig)

11 Oral epithelium

12 Lamina propria

13 Enamel

14 Stellate reticulum

15 Odontoblasts

16 Dentin

17 Connective tissue of the dental sac

18 Predentin

19 Odontoblasts

20 Blood vessels

21 Mesenchyme of the dental papilla

22 Epithelial root sheath (of Hertwig)

23 Dental alveolus

FIGURE 11.11 ■ Developing tooth (longitudinal section). Stain: hematoxylin and eosin. Low magnification.

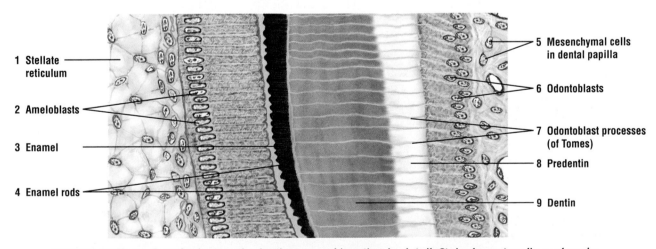

1 Stellate reticulum

2 Ameloblasts

3 Enamel

4 Enamel rods

5 Mesenchymal cells in dental papilla

6 Odontoblasts

7 Odontoblast processes (of Tomes)

8 Predentin

9 Dentin

FIGURE 11.12 ■ Developing tooth: dentinoenamel junction in detail. Stain: hematoxylin and eosin. High magnification.

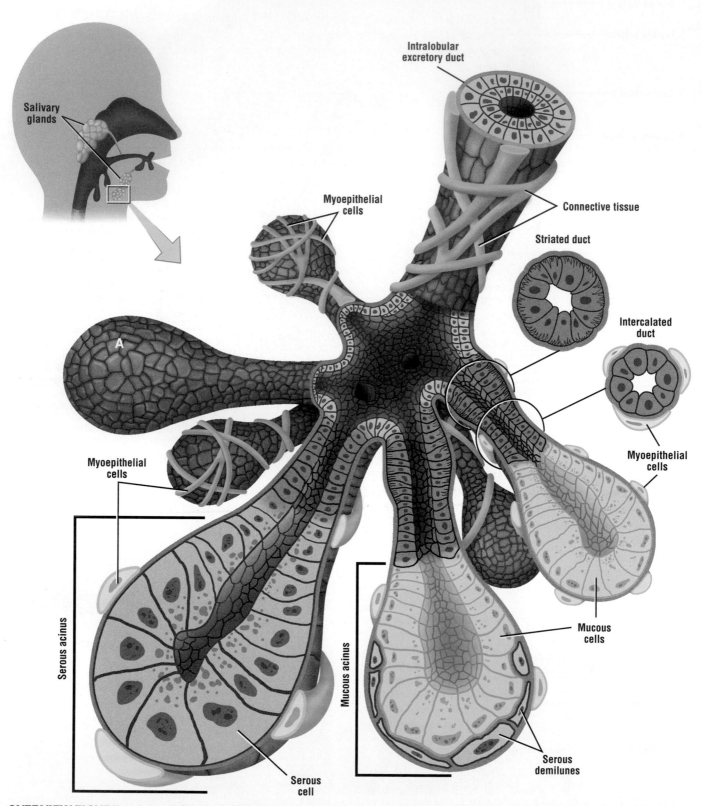

OVERVIEW FIGURE 11.2 ■ Salivary glands. The different types of acini (serous, mucous, and serous demilunes), different duct types (intercalated, striated, and interlobular), and myoepithelial cells of a salivary gland are illustrated.

The Major Salivary Glands

There are three major **salivary glands:** the parotid, submandibular, and sublingual. Salivary glands are located outside of the oral cavity and convey their secretions into the mouth via large **excretory ducts.** The paired **parotid glands** are the largest of the salivary glands, located anterior and inferior to the external ear. The smaller, paired **submandibular** (**submaxillary**) **glands** are located inferior to the mandible in the floor of the mouth. The smallest salivary glands are the **sublingual glands,** which are aggregates of smaller glands located inferior to the tongue.

Salivary glands are composed of cellular **secretory units** called **acini** (singular, acinus) and numerous **excretory ducts.** The secretory units are small, saclike dilations located at the end of the first segment of the excretory duct system, the **intercalated ducts.**

Cells of the Salivary Gland Acini

Cells that comprise the secretory acini of salivary glands are of two types: serous or mucous (Overview Figure 11.2, Salivary Glands).

Serous cells in the acini are pyramidal in shape. Their spherical or round nuclei are displaced basally by secretory granules accumulated in the upper or apical regions of the cytoplasm.

Mucous cells are similar in shape to serous cells, except their cytoplasm is completely filled with a light-staining, secretory product called **mucus.** As a result, the accumulated secretory granules flatten the nucleus and displace it to the base of the cytoplasm.

In some salivary glands, both mucous and serous cells are present in the same secretory acinus. In these mixed acini, where mucous cells predominate, serous cells form a crescent or moon-shaped cap over the mucous cells called a **serous demilune.** The secretions from serous cells in the demilunes enter the lumen of the acinus through tiny intercellular canaliculi between mucous cells.

Myoepithelial cells are flattened cells that surround both serous and mucous acini. Myoepithelial cells are also highly branched and **contractile.** They are sometimes called basket cells because they surround the acini with their branches like a basket. Myoepithelial cells are located between the cell membrane of the secretory cells in acini and the surrounding basement membrane.

Salivary Gland Ducts

Connective tissue fibers subdivide the salivary glands into numerous **lobules,** in which are found the secretory units and their excretory ducts.

Intercalated Ducts

Both serous and mucous, as well as mixed secretory, acini initially empty their secretions into the **intercalated ducts.** These are the smallest ducts in the salivary glands with small lumina lined by low cuboidal epithelium. Contractile myoepithelial cells surround some portions of intercalated ducts.

Striated Ducts

Several intercalated ducts merge to form the larger **striated ducts.** These ducts are lined by columnar epithelium and, with proper staining, exhibit tiny basal striations. The striations correspond to the basal infoldings of the cell membrane and the cellular interdigitations. Located in these basal infoldings of the cell membrane are numerous and elongated mitochondria.

Excretory Intralobular Ducts

Striated ducts, in turn, join to form larger **intralobular ducts** of gradually increasing size, surrounded by increased layers of connective tissue fibers.

Interlobular and Interlobar Ducts

Intralobular ducts join to form the larger **interlobular ducts** and **interlobar ducts.** The terminal portion of these large ducts conveys saliva from salivary glands to the oral cavity. Larger interlobular ducts may be lined with stratified epithelium, either low cuboidal or columnar (Overview Figure 11.2: Salivary Glands).

FIGURE 11.13 ■ Parotid Salivary Gland

The parotid salivary gland is a large serous gland that is classified as a compound tubuloacinar gland. This illustration depicts a section of the parotid gland at lower magnification, with details of specific structures represented at a higher magnification in separate boxes below.

The parotid gland is surrounded by a capsule from which arise numerous **interlobular connective tissue septa (6)** that subdivide the gland into lobes and lobules. Located in the connective tissue septa (6) between the lobules are **arteriole (9)**, **venule (1)**, and **interlobular excretory ducts (2, 13, IV)**.

Each salivary gland lobule contains secretory cells that form the **serous acini (5, 8, I)** and whose pyramid-shaped cells are arranged around a lumen. The spherical nuclei of the serous cells (I) are located at the base of the slightly basophilic cytoplasm. In certain sections, the lumen in serous acini (5, 8, I) is not always visible. At a higher magnification, small **secretory granules (I)** are visible in the cell apices of the serous acini (5, 8, I). The number of secretory granules in these cells varies with the functional activity of the gland. All serous acini (5, 8, I) are surrounded by thin, contractile **myoepithelial cells (7, I)** that are located between the basement membrane and the serous cells (5, 8, I). Because of their small size, in some sections only the nuclei are visible in the myoepithelial cells (7, I). Some parotid gland lobules may contain numerous **adipose cells (3)** that appear as clear oval structures surrounded by darker staining serous acini (5, 8, I).

The secretory serous acini (5, 8, I) empty their product into narrow channels, the **intercalated ducts (10, 12, II)**. These ducts have small lumina, are lined by a simple squamous or low cuboidal epithelium, and are often surrounded by myoepithelial cells (see Figure 11.14). The secretory product from the intercalated ducts (10, 12, II) drains into larger **striated ducts (11, III)**. These ducts have larger lumina and are lined by simple columnar cells that exhibit basal striations (11, III). The striations that are seen in the striated ducts (11, III) are formed by deep infolding of the basal cell membrane.

The striated ducts (11, III), in turn, empty their product into the **intralobular excretory ducts (4)** that are located within the lobules of the gland. These ducts join larger interlobular excretory ducts (2, 13, IV) in the connective tissue septa (6) that surround the salivary gland lobules. The lumina of interlobular excretory ducts (2, 13, IV) become progressively wider and the epithelium taller as the ducts increase in size. The epithelium of excretory ducts can increase from columnar to pseudostratified or even stratified columnar in large excretory (lobar) ducts that drain the lobes of the parotid gland.

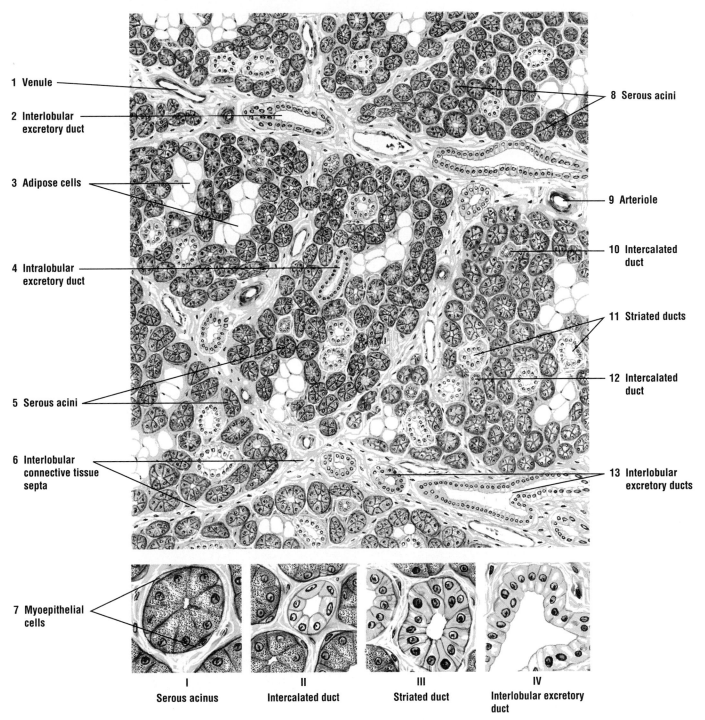

1 Venule

2 Interlobular excretory duct

3 Adipose cells

4 Intralobular excretory duct

5 Serous acini

6 Interlobular connective tissue septa

7 Myoepithelial cells

8 Serous acini

9 Arteriole

10 Intercalated duct

11 Striated ducts

12 Intercalated duct

13 Interlobular excretory ducts

I
Serous acinus

II
Intercalated duct

III
Striated duct

IV
Interlobular excretory duct

FIGURE 11.13 ■ Parotid salivary gland. Stain: hematoxylin and eosin. Upper: medium magnification. Lower: high magnification.

FIGURE 11.14 ■ Submandibular Salivary Gland

The submandibular salivary gland is also a compound tubuloacinar gland. However, the submandibular gland is a mixed gland, containing both serous and mucous acini, with serous acini predominating. The presence of both serous and mucous acini distinguishes the submandibular gland from the parotid gland, which is a purely serous gland.

This illustration depicts several lobules of the submandibular gland in which a few **mucous acini (5, 11, 13, II)** are intermixed with **serous acini (6, I).** The detailed features of different acini and ducts of the gland are illustrated at higher magnification in separate boxes below.

The serous acini (6, I) are similar to those in the parotid gland (Figure 11.13). These acini are characterized by smaller, darker-stained pyramidal cells, spherical basal nuclei, and apical secretory granules. The mucous acini (5, 11, 13, II) are larger than the serous acini (6, I), have larger lumina, and exhibit more variation in size and shape. The mucous cells (5, 11, 13, II) are columnar with pale or almost colorless cytoplasm after staining. The nuclei of mucous cells (5, 11, 13, II) are flattened and pressed against the base of the cell membrane.

In mixed acini (serous and mucous), the mucous acini are normally surrounded or capped by one or more serous cells, forming a crescent-shaped **serous demilunes (7, 10).** The thin, contractile **myoepithelial cells (8)** surround the serous (I) and mucous (II) acini and the **intercalated ducts (III).**

The duct system of the submandibular gland is similar to that of the parotid gland. The small intralobular **intercalated ducts (12, 14, 17, III)** have small lumina and are shorter, whereas the **striated ducts (4, 15, IV)** with distinct **basal striations (18)** in the cells are longer than in the parotid gland. This figure also illustrates a mucous acinus (13) that opens into an intercalated duct (14), which then joins a larger striated duct (15). Interlobular excretory ducts (16) are located in the **interlobular connective tissue septa (3)** that divide the gland into lobules and lobes. Also located in the connective tissue septa (3) are nerves, an **arteriole (1), venule (2),** and **adipose cells (9).**

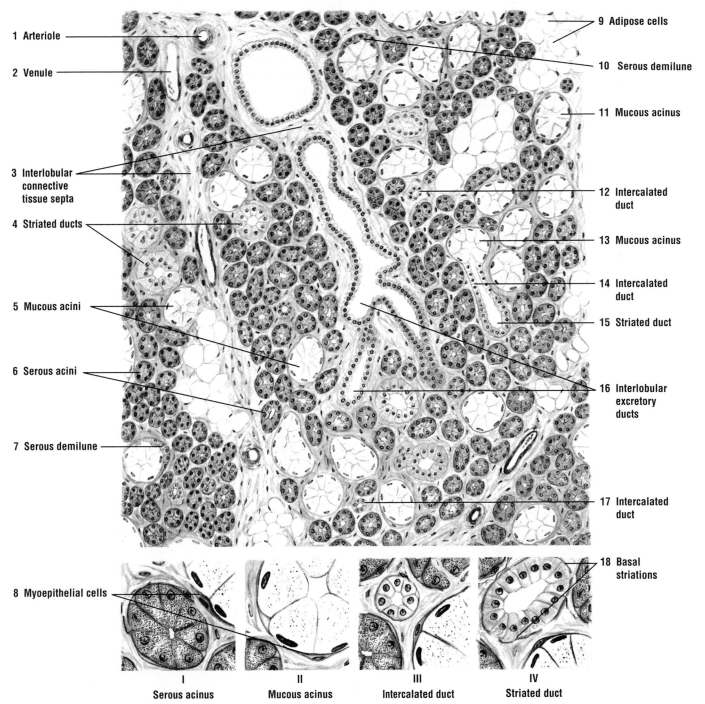

1 Arteriole

2 Venule

3 Interlobular connective tissue septa

4 Striated ducts

5 Mucous acini

6 Serous acini

7 Serous demilune

8 Myoepithelial cells

9 Adipose cells

10 Serous demilune

11 Mucous acinus

12 Intercalated duct

13 Mucous acinus

14 Intercalated duct

15 Striated duct

16 Interlobular excretory ducts

17 Intercalated duct

18 Basal striations

I Serous acinus

II Mucous acinus

III Intercalated duct

IV Striated duct

FIGURE 11.14 ■ Submandibular salivary gland. Stain: hematoxylin and eosin. Upper: medium magnification. Lower: high magnification.

FIGURE 11.15 ■ Sublingual Salivary Gland

The sublingual salivary gland is also a compound, mixed tubuloacinar gland that resembles the submandibular gland because it contains both **serous (11)** and **mucous acini (9, I, II)**. Most of the acini, however, are mucous (9, I, II) that are capped with peripheral **serous demilunes (1, 13, II)**. The light-stained mucous acini (9, I) are conspicuous in this section. Purely serous acini (11) are less numerous in the sublingual gland; however, the composition of each gland varies. In this medium-magnification illustration, serous acini (11) appear frequently, whereas in other sections of the sublingual gland, serous acini (11) may be absent. At higher magnification, the contractile **myoepithelial cells (7, I)** are seen around individual serous and mucous acini (I).

In comparison with other salivary glands, the duct system of the sublingual gland is somewhat different. The **intercalated ducts (2, III)** are short or absent, and not readily observed in a given section. In contrast, the nonstriated **intralobular excretory ducts (6, 8, IV)** are more prevalent in the sublingual glands. These excretory ducts (6, 8, IV) are equivalent to the striated ducts of the submandibular and parotid glands but lack the extensive membrane infolding and basal striations.

The **interlobular connective tissue septa (4)** are also more abundant in the sublingual than in the parotid and submandibular glands. An **arteriole (3)**, **venule (5)**, nerve fibers, and **interlobular excretory ducts (12)** are seen in the septa. The epithelial lining of the interlobular excretory ducts (12) varies from low columnar in the smaller ducts to pseudostratified or stratified columnar in the larger ducts. In addition, the oval-shaped **adipose cells (10)** are seen scattered in the connective tissue of the gland.

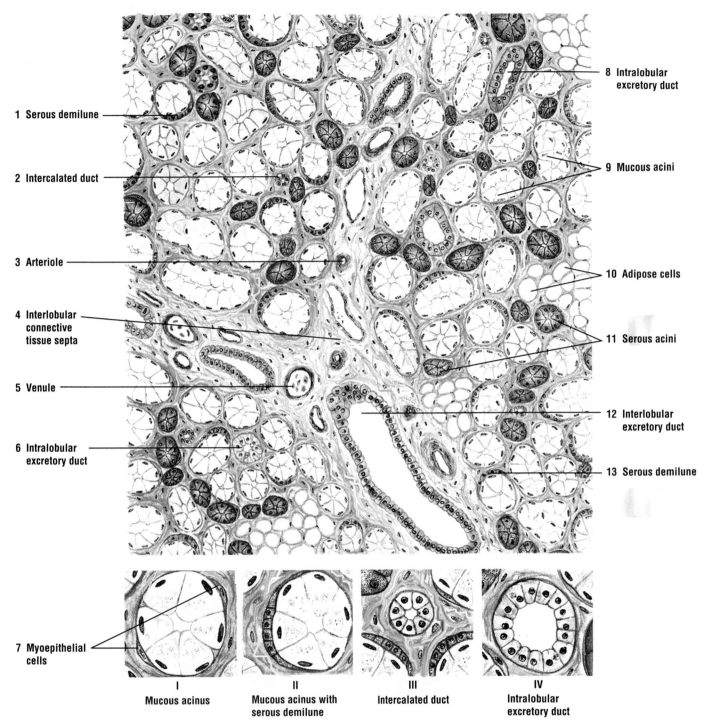

1 Serous demilune

2 Intercalated duct

3 Arteriole

4 Interlobular connective tissue septa

5 Venule

6 Intralobular excretory duct

7 Myoepithelial cells

8 Intralobular excretory duct

9 Mucous acini

10 Adipose cells

11 Serous acini

12 Interlobular excretory duct

13 Serous demilune

I	II	III	IV
Mucous acinus	Mucous acinus with serous demilune	Intercalated duct	Intralobular excretory duct

FIGURE 11.15 ■ Sublingual salivary gland. Stain: hematoxylin and eosin. Upper: medium magnification. Lower: high magnification.

FIGURE 11.16 ■ Serous Salivary Gland: Parotid Gland

This photomicrograph illustrates a section of the parotid salivary gland. In humans, the parotid gland is entirely composed of **serous acini (1)** and excretory ducts. In this illustration, the cytoplasm of serous cells in the serous acini (1) is filled with tiny secretory granules. A small **intercalated duct (2)** with its cuboidal epithelium is surrounded by the serous acini (1). Also visible on the right side of the illustration is a larger, lighter-stained excretory duct, the **striated duct (3)**.

FIGURE 11.17 ■ Mixed Salivary Gland: Sublingual Gland

The sublingual salivary gland exhibits both **mucous acini (2)** and **serous acini (3)**. The mucous acini (2) are larger and lighter staining than the serous acini (3), and their cytoplasm is filled with **mucus (1)**. The serous acini (3) are darker staining with tiny secretory granules located in the apical cytoplasm. The serous acini (3) that surround the mucous acini (2) form crescent-shaped structures called **serous demilunes (4)**. A tiny excretory **intercalated duct (5)**, lined by cuboidal epithelium, and a larger **striated duct (6)** with columnar epithelium, are also visible in the gland.

FUNCTIONAL CORRELATIONS: Salivary Glands, Saliva, and Salivary Ducts

Salivary glands produce about 1 L/day of watery secretion called **saliva,** which enters the oral cavity via different large excretory ducts. **Myoepithelial cells** surround the secretory acini and the intercalated ducts in the salivary glands. On contraction, these cells expel the secretory products from different acini.

Saliva is a mixture of secretions produced by cells in different salivary glands. Although the major composition of saliva is **water,** it also contains ions, mucus, enzymes, and antibodies (immunoglobulins). The sight, smell, thought, taste, or actual presence of food in the mouth causes an **autonomic stimulation** of the salivary glands that increases production of saliva and stimulates its release into the oral cavity.

Saliva performs numerous important functions. It moistens the chewed food and provides solvents that allow it to be tasted. Saliva lubricates the bolus of chewed food for easier swallowing and assistance in its passage through the esophagus to the stomach. Saliva also contains numerous **electrolytes** (calcium, potassium, sodium, chloride, bicarbonate ions, and others). A digestive enzyme, **salivary amylase,** is present in the saliva. It is mainly produced by the **serous acini** in the salivary glands. Salivary amylase initiates the breakdown of starch into smaller carbohydrates during the short time that food is present in the oral cavity. Once in the stomach, food is acidified by gastric juices, an action that decreases amylase activity and carbohydrate digestion.

Saliva also functions in controlling **bacterial flora** in the mouth and protecting the oral cavity against pathogens. Another salivary enzyme, **lysozyme,** also secreted by serous cells, hydrolyzes cell walls of bacteria and inhibits their growth in the oral cavity. In addition, saliva contains salivary **antibodies.** The antibodies, primarily immunoglobulin A (IgA), are produced by the **plasma cells** in the connective tissue of salivary glands. The antibodies form complexes with antigens and assist in immunologic defense against oral bacteria. Salivary acinar cells secrete a component that binds to and transports the immunoglobulins from plasma cells in the connective tissue into saliva.

As saliva flows through the duct system of salivary glands, the different salivary ducts modify its ionic content by selective transport, resorption, or secretions of ions. The **intercalated ducts** secrete bicarbonate ions into the ducts and absorb chloride from its contents. The **striated ducts** actively reabsorb sodium from saliva, while potassium and bicarbonate ions are added to the salivary secretions. The numerous infoldings of the basal cell membrane or striations seen in the striated ducts contain numerous elongated mitochondria. These structures are characteristic features of cells that transport fluids and electrolytes across cell membranes.

The striated ducts of each lobule drain into interlobular or excretory ducts that eventually form the main duct for each gland, which ultimately empties into the oral cavity.

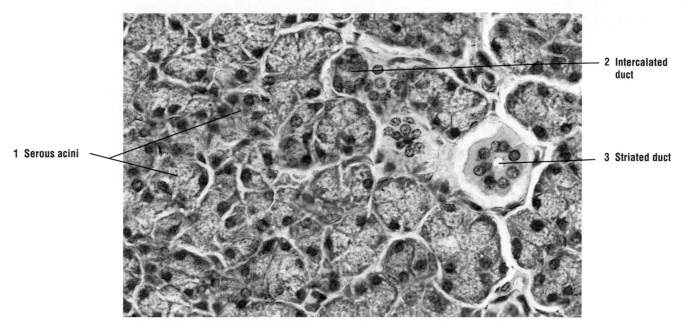

1 Serous acini

2 Intercalated duct

3 Striated duct

FIGURE 11.16 ■ Serous salivary gland: parotid gland. Stain: hematoxylin and eosin. ×165.

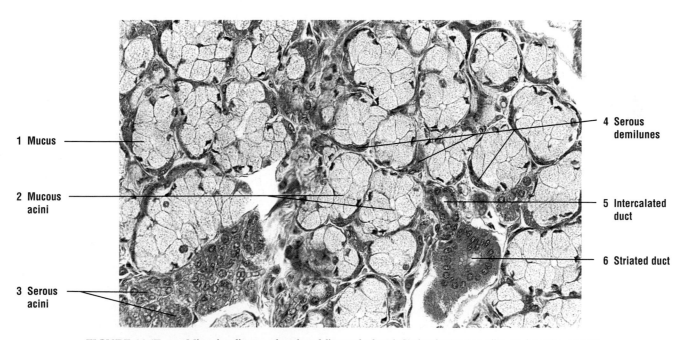

1 Mucus

2 Mucous acini

3 Serous acini

4 Serous demilunes

5 Intercalated duct

6 Striated duct

FIGURE 11.17 ■ Mixed salivary gland: sublingual gland. Stain: hematoxylin and eosin. ×165.

The Digestive System

- Hollow tube from oral cavity to anal canal
- Salivary glands, liver, and pancreas are accessory organs located outside of the tube
- Secretory products from accessory organs delivered to the tube via excretory ducts

The Oral Cavity

- Lined by stratified squamous epithelium for protection
- Food masticated here, and saliva lubricates food for swallowing

The Lips

- Lined by thin skin covered by stratified squamous keratinized epithelium
- Blood vessels close to the surface impart red color
- Contain hairs, sebaceous and sweat glands, and mucus-secreting labial glands
- Core contains skeletal muscle orbicularis oris

The Tongue

- Consists of interlacing skeleton muscle fibers
- Surface covered by surface elevations, called filiform, fungiform, and circumvallate papillae
- Filiform papillae are the most numerous and smallest that cover tongue; lack taste buds
- Fungiform papillae less numerous, larger with mushroom-like shape, and contain taste buds
- Circumvallate papillae are the largest, are in the back of tongue, and have furrows, underlying serous glands, and taste buds
- Foliate papillae are rudimentary in humans
- Posterior lingual glands in the connective tissue open onto dorsal surface of tongue

Taste Buds

- Located in foliate, fungiform, circumvallate papillae, pharynx, palate, and epiglottis
- Contain taste pores and occupy the thickness of the epithelium
- Neuroepithelial cells associated with afferent axons are the receptors for taste
- Also contain supportive sustentacular cells, whereas basal cells can serve as stem cells
- Substances that are tasted are first dissolved in saliva and then enter taste pore
- Serous glands wash peripheral taste buds in the furrows of circumvallate papillae
- Basic four taste sensations are sour, salt, bitter, and sweet
- Tip of tongue is sensitive to sweet and sour; posterior tongue to bitter, and lateral to sour taste

Lymphoid Aggregations: Tonsils

- Diffuse lymphoid tissue and nodules in the oral pharynx
- Palatine and lingual tonsils are covered by stratified squamous epithelium and show crypts
- Pharyngeal tonsil is single and covered by pseudostratified ciliated epithelium
- Some lymph nodules contain germinal centers

Teeth

- Developing teeth found in dental alveolus in the jawbone
- Downward growth from oral epithelium forms dental lamina, which gives rise to ameloblasts
- Mesenchyme gives rise to dental papilla and odontoblasts
- Odontoblasts secrete dentin, whereas ameloblasts produce enamel of tooth

The Major Salivary Glands

- Parotid, submandibular, and sublingual are major salivary glands that produce saliva
- Composed of secretory acini and excretory ducts that bring saliva from outside into oral cavity
- Cells are either serous or mucous; serous cells form serous demilunes around mucous acini
- Contractile myoepithelial cells surround serous and mucous acini and intercalated ducts
- Serous, mucous, and mixed secretory acini empty secretions into intercalated ducts
- Intercalated ducts merge into larger striated ducts with basal membrane infoldings
- Striated ducts form larger interlobular ducts that empty into interlobar excretory ducts
- Glands produce about 1 L of saliva per day, which is mostly water
- Saliva formed after autonomic stimulation
- Saliva contains electrolytes and carbohydrate-digesting enzyme salivary amylase
- Saliva contains antibodies produced by connective tissue plasma cells and lysozyme to control oral bacteria
- Saliva is modified by selective transport of ions in the intercalated ducts and striated ducts
- Sodium is reabsorbed from saliva, and potassium ions and bicarbonate ions are added to saliva

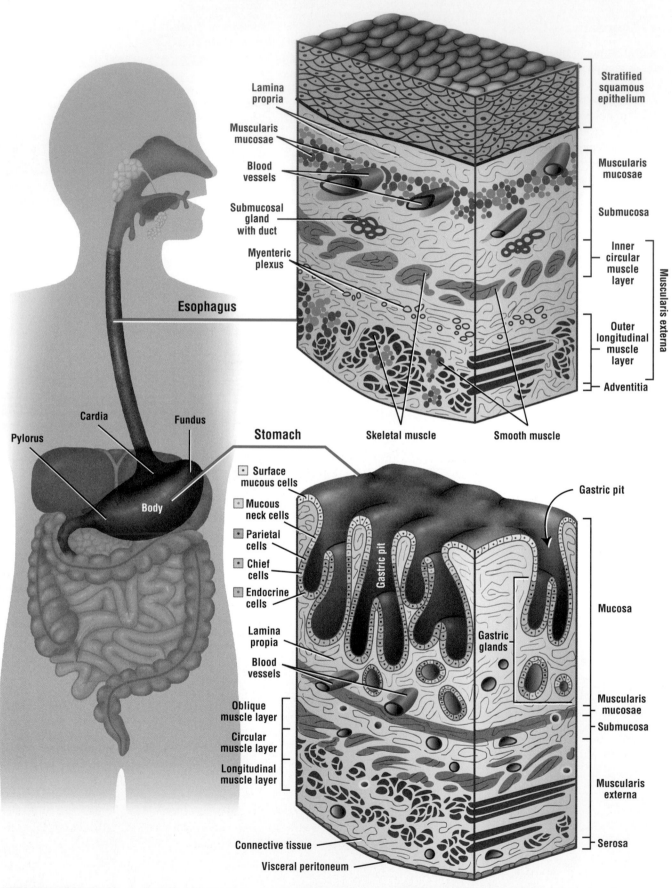

Lamina propria

Muscularis mucosae

Blood vessels

Submucosal gland with duct

Myenteric plexus

Esophagus

Stratified squamous epithelium

Muscularis mucosae

Submucosa

Inner circular muscle layer

Outer longitudinal muscle layer

Muscularis externa

Adventitia

Cardia

Pylorus

Fundus

Body

Stomach

Skeletal muscle

Smooth muscle

Surface mucous cells

Mucous neck cells

Parietal cells

Chief cells

Endocrine cells

Lamina propia

Blood vessels

Oblique muscle layer

Circular muscle layer

Longitudinal muscle layer

Connective tissue

Visceral peritoneum

Gastric pit

Gastric glands

Gastric pit

Mucosa

Muscularis mucosae

Submucosa

Muscularis externa

Serosa

OVERVIEW FIGURE 12 ■ Detailed illustration comparing the structural differences of the four layers (mucosa, submucosa, muscularis externa, and adventitia or serosa) in the wall of the esophagus and stomach.

Digestive System: Esophagus and Stomach

General Plan of the Digestive System

The digestive (gastrointestinal) tract is a long hollow tube that extends from the esophagus to the rectum. It includes the esophagus, stomach, small intestine (duodenum, jejunum, ileum), large intestine (colon), and rectum. The wall of the digestive tube exhibits four layers that show a basic histologic organization. The layers are the mucosa, submucosa, muscularis externa, and serosa or adventitia. Because of the different functions of the digestive organs in the digestive process, the morphology of these layers exhibits variations.

The **mucosa** is the innermost layer of the digestive tube. It consists of a covering **epithelium** and glands that extend into the underlying layer of loose connective tissue called the **lamina propria.** An inner circular and outer longitudinal layer of smooth muscle, called the **muscularis mucosae,** forms the outer boundary of the mucosa.

The **submucosa** is located below the mucosa. It consists of dense irregular connective tissue with numerous blood and lymph vessels and a **submucosal** (Meissner's) **nerve plexus.** This nerve plexus contains postganglionic parasympathetic neurons. The neurons and axons of the submucosal nerve plexus control the motility of the mucosa and secretory activities of associated mucosal glands. In the initial portion of the small intestine, the duodenum, the submucosa contains numerous branched mucous glands.

The **muscularis externa** is a thick, smooth muscle layer located inferior to the submucosa. Except for the large intestine, this layer is composed of an inner layer of circular smooth muscle and outer layer of longitudinal smooth muscle. Situated between the two smooth muscle layers of the muscularis externa is connective tissue and another nerve plexus called the **myenteric** (Auerbach's) **nerve plexus.** This plexus also contains some postganglionic parasympathetic neurons and controls the motility of smooth muscles in the muscularis externa.

The **serosa** is a thin layer of loose connective tissue that surrounds the visceral organs. The visceral organs may or may not be covered by a thin outer layer of squamous epithelium called **mesothelium.** If mesothelium covers the visceral organs, the organs are within the abdominal or pelvic cavities (**intraperitoneal**) and the outer layer is called serosa. The serosa covers the outer surface of the abdominal portion of the esophagus, stomach, and small intestine. It also covers parts of the colon (ascending and descending colon) only on the anterior and lateral surfaces because their posterior surfaces are bound to the posterior abdominal body wall and are not covered by the mesothelium (Overview Figure 12).

When the digestive tube is not covered by mesothelium, it then lies outside of the peritoneal cavity and is called **retroperitoneal.** In this case, the outermost layer adheres to the body wall and consists only of a connective tissue layer called **adventitia.**

The characteristic features of each layer of the digestive tube and their functions are discussed in detail with each illustration of the different organs.

Esophagus

The **esophagus** is a soft tube approximately 10 inches long that extends from the **pharynx** to the **stomach.** It is located posterior to the trachea and in the mediastinum of the **thoracic cavity.** After descending in the thoracic cavity, the esophagus penetrates the muscular **diaphragm.** A short section of the esophagus is present in the abdominal cavity before it terminates at the stomach.

In the thoracic cavity, the esophagus is surrounded only by the connective tissue, which is called the adventitia. In the abdominal cavity, a simple squamous mesothelium lines the outermost wall of the short segment of the esophagus to form the serosa.

Internally, the esophageal lumen is lined with moist, **nonkeratinized stratified squamous epithelium.** When the esophagus is empty, the lumen exhibits numerous but temporary **longitudinal folds** of mucosa. In the lamina propria of esophagus near stomach are the esophageal cardiac glands. In the submucosa are small esophageal glands. Both glands secrete mucus to protect the mucosa and to facilitate the passage of food material through the esophagus. The outer wall of the esophagus, the muscularis externa, contains a mixture of different types of muscle fibers. In the upper third of the esophagus, the muscularis externa contains striated **skeletal muscle fibers.** In the middle third of the esophagus, the muscularis externa contains both **skeletal** and **smooth muscle** fibers, while the lower third of the esophagus is composed entirely of **smooth muscle** fibers (see Overview Figure 12).

Stomach

The stomach is an expanded hollow organ situated between the esophagus and small intestine. At the esophageal-stomach junction, there is an abrupt transition from the stratified squamous epithelium of the esophagus to the **simple columnar epithelium** of the stomach. The luminal surface of the stomach is pitted with numerous tiny openings called **gastric pits.** These are formed by the luminal epithelium that invaginates the underlying connective tissue **lamina propria** of the **mucosa.** The tubular **gastric glands** are located below the luminal epithelium and open directly into the gastric pits to deliver their secretions into the stomach lumen. The gastric glands descend through the lamina propria to the **muscularis mucosae.**

Below the mucosa of the stomach is the dense connective tissue **submucosa** containing large blood vessels and nerves. The thick muscular wall of the stomach, the **muscularis externa,** exhibits three muscle layers instead of the two that are normally seen in the esophagus and small intestine. The outer layer of the stomach is covered by the **serosa** or visceral peritoneum.

Anatomically, the stomach is divided into the narrow **cardia,** where the esophagus terminates, an upper dome-shaped **fundus,** a lower **body** or **corpus,** and a funnel-shaped, terminal region called the **pylorus.**

The fundus and the body comprise about two thirds of the stomach and have identical histology. As a result, the stomach has only three distinct histologic regions. The fundus and body form the major portions of stomach. Their mucosae consist of different cell types and deep **gastric glands** that produce most of the **gastric secretions** or juices for digestion. Also, all stomach regions exhibit **rugae,** the longitudinal folds of the mucosa and submucosa. These folds are temporary and disappear when the stomach is distended with fluid or solid material (Overview Figure 12).

FIGURE 12.1 ■ Wall of Upper Esophagus (Transverse Section)

The esophagus is a long, hollow tube whose wall consists of the mucosa, submucosa, muscularis externa, and adventitia. In this illustration, the upper portion of the esophagus has been sectioned in a transverse plane.

The **mucosa (1)** of the esophagus consists of three parts: an inner lining of nonkeratinized **stratified squamous epithelium (1a);** an underlying thin layer of fine connective tissue, the **lamina propria (1b);** and a layer of longitudinal smooth muscle fibers, the **muscularis mucosae (1c),** shown in this illustration in transverse plane. The **connective tissue papillae (9)** of the lamina propria (1b) indent the epithelium (1a). Found in the lamina propria (1b) are small **blood vessels (8),** diffuse lymphatic tissue, and a small **lymphatic nodule (7).**

The **submucosa (3)** in the esophagus is a wide layer of moderately dense irregular connective tissue that often contains **adipose tissue (12).** The **mucous acini** of **esophageal glands proper (2)** are present in the submucosa (3) at intervals throughout the length of the esophagus. The **excretory ducts (10)** of the esophageal glands (2) pass through the muscularis mucosae (1c) and the lamina propria (1b) to open into the esophageal lumen. The dark-staining ductal epithelium of the glands merges with the stratified squamous surface epithelium (1a) of the esophagus (see Figure 12.2). Numerous blood vessels, such as the **vein** and **artery (11),** are found in the connective tissue of the submucosa (3).

Located inferior to the submucosa (3) is the **muscularis externa (4),** composed of two well-defined muscle layers, an **inner circular muscle layer (4a)** and the **outer longitudinal muscle layer (4b),** whose muscle fibers are shown here sectioned in a transverse plane. A thin layer of **connective tissue (13)** lies between the inner circular muscle layer (4a) and the outer longitudinal muscle layer (4b).

The muscularis externa (4) of the esophagus is highly variable in different species. In humans, the muscularis externa (4) in the upper third of the esophagus consists primarily of striated skeletal muscles. In the middle third of the esophagus, the inner circular layer (4a) and the outer longitudinal layer (4b) exhibit a mixture of both smooth muscle and skeletal muscle fibers. In the lower third of the esophagus, only smooth muscle is present.

The **adventitia (5)** of the esophagus consists of a loose connective tissue layer that blends with the adventitia of the trachea and the surrounding structures. **Adipose tissue (14),** large blood vessels, **artery** and **vein (15),** and **nerve fibers (6)** are numerous in the connective tissue of the adventitia (5).

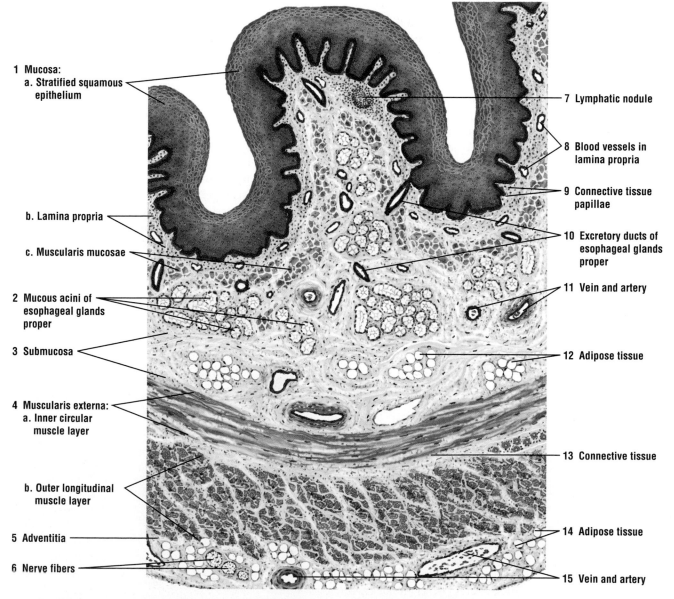

1 Mucosa:
  a. Stratified squamous epithelium

  b. Lamina propria

  c. Muscularis mucosae

2 Mucous acini of esophageal glands proper

3 Submucosa

4 Muscularis externa:
  a. Inner circular muscle layer

  b. Outer longitudinal muscle layer

5 Adventitia

6 Nerve fibers

7 Lymphatic nodule

8 Blood vessels in lamina propria

9 Connective tissue papillae

10 Excretory ducts of esophageal glands proper

11 Vein and artery

12 Adipose tissue

13 Connective tissue

14 Adipose tissue

15 Vein and artery

FIGURE 12.1 ■ Wall of upper esophagus (transverse section). Stain: hematoxylin and eosin. Low magnification.

FIGURE 12.2 ■ Upper Esophagus (Transverse Section)

The next two histologic sections illustrate the difference between the upper and lower esophageal wall.

The different layers of the esophagus are easily distinguishable. The mucosa of the upper esophagus (as in Figure 12.1) consists of a stratified squamous nonkeratinized **epithelium (1)**, a connective tissue **lamina propria (2)**, and a layer of smooth muscle **muscularis mucosae (3)** (transverse plane). A small **lymphatic nodule (4)** is visible in the lamina propria (2). In the **submucosa (7)** are cells of adipose tissue and **mucous acini of the esophageal glands proper (6)** with their **excretory ducts (5)**. The muscularis externa of the upper esophagus consists of an **inner circular layer (10)** and an **outer longitudinal layer (14)** of skeletal muscles, separated by a layer of **connective tissue (11)**. The outermost layer around the esophagus is the connective tissue **adventitia (8)** with adipose tissue, **nerves (13)**, a **vein (9)**, and **an artery (12)**.

FIGURE 12.3 ■ Lower Esophagus (Transverse Section)

This illustration shows the terminal portion of the esophagus after it has penetrated the diaphragm and entered the peritoneal cavity near the stomach.

The layers in the wall of the lower esophagus are similar to those in the upper region except for regional modifications (see Figure 12.2). As in the upper esophagus, the **mucosa (1)** of the lower esophagus consists of stratified squamous nonkeratinized **epithelium (1a)**, the connective tissue **lamina propria (1b)**, and a smooth muscle layer **muscularis mucosae (1c)** (transverse section). Also visible are the **connective tissue papillae (2)** of the lamina propria (1b) that indent the lining epithelium (1a) and a **lymphatic nodule (3)**.

The connective tissue **submucosa (6)** also contains mucous acini of the **esophageal glands proper (5)**, their **excretory ducts (4)**, and **adipose tissue (7)**. In some regions of the esophagus, these glands may be absent.

The major differences between the upper and lower esophagus are seen in the next two layers. The **muscularis externa (10)** in the lower esophagus consists entirely of smooth muscle layers, an **inner circular muscle layer (10a)** and an **outer longitudinal muscle layer (10b)**. The outermost layer of the lower esophagus is the **serosa (8)** or visceral peritoneum. Serosa (8) consists of a connective tissue layer lined by a simple squamous layer mesothelium. In contrast, the adventitia that surrounds the esophagus in the thoracic region consists only of a connective tissue layer.

In the upper esophagus, less connective tissue is present in the lamina propria (1b), around the smooth muscle fibers of muscularis externa (10), and in the serosa (8).

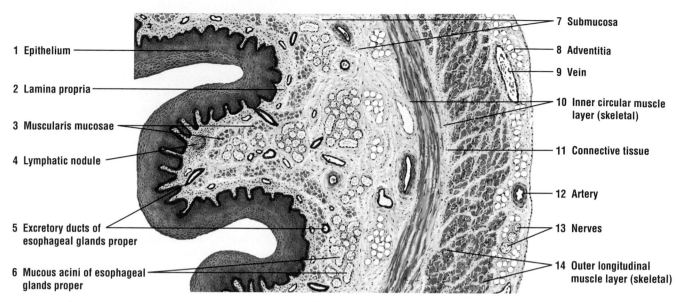

1 Epithelium

2 Lamina propria

3 Muscularis mucosae

4 Lymphatic nodule

5 Excretory ducts of esophageal glands proper

6 Mucous acini of esophageal glands proper

7 Submucosa

8 Adventitia

9 Vein

10 Inner circular muscle layer (skeletal)

11 Connective tissue

12 Artery

13 Nerves

14 Outer longitudinal muscle layer (skeletal)

FIGURE 12.2 ■ Upper esophagus (transverse section). Stain: hematoxylin and eosin. Low magnification.

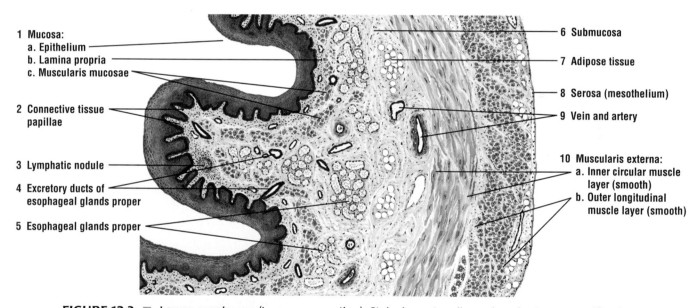

1 Mucosa:
   a. Epithelium
   b. Lamina propria
   c. Muscularis mucosae

2 Connective tissue papillae

3 Lymphatic nodule

4 Excretory ducts of esophageal glands proper

5 Esophageal glands proper

6 Submucosa

7 Adipose tissue

8 Serosa (mesothelium)

9 Vein and artery

10 Muscularis externa:
   a. Inner circular muscle layer (smooth)
   b. Outer longitudinal muscle layer (smooth)

FIGURE 12.3 ■ Lower esophagus (transverse section). Stain: hematoxylin and eosin. Low magnification.

FIGURE 12.4 ■ Upper Esophagus: Mucosa and Submucosa (Longitudinal Section)

This higher-magnification illustration of the upper esophagus has been sectioned longitudinally. The smooth muscle fibers of the muscularis mucosae (9) exhibit a longitudinal orientation, and the fibers of the inner circular muscle layer are cut in a transverse section.

The esophagus is lined with stratified squamous **epithelium (7).** Squamous cells form the outermost layers of the epithelium, the numerous polyhedral cells form the intermediate layers, and low columnar cells form the basal layer. Mitotic activity can be seen in the deeper layers of the epithelium. The connective tissue **lamina propria (8)** contains numerous blood vessels, aggregates of lymphocytes, and a small **lymphatic nodule (2). Connective tissue papillae (1)** from the lamina propria (8) indent the surface epithelium (7). The **muscularis mucosae (9)** is illustrated as bundles of smooth muscle fibers sectioned in a longitudinal plane.

The underlying **submucosa (3, 10)** contains **mucous acini of esophageal glands proper (4).** Small **excretory ducts (11)** from these glands (4), lined with simple epithelium, join the larger excretory ducts that are lined with stratified epithelium. One of the excretory ducts joins the stratified squamous epithelium (7) of the esophageal lumen. In the submucosa (3, 10) are also **blood vessels (12), nerves (5),** and **adipose cells (6).**

In the upper esophagus, the **inner circular muscle layer (13)** of the muscularis externa consists of skeletal muscle. A portion of this layer is illustrated in a transverse plane at the bottom of the figure.

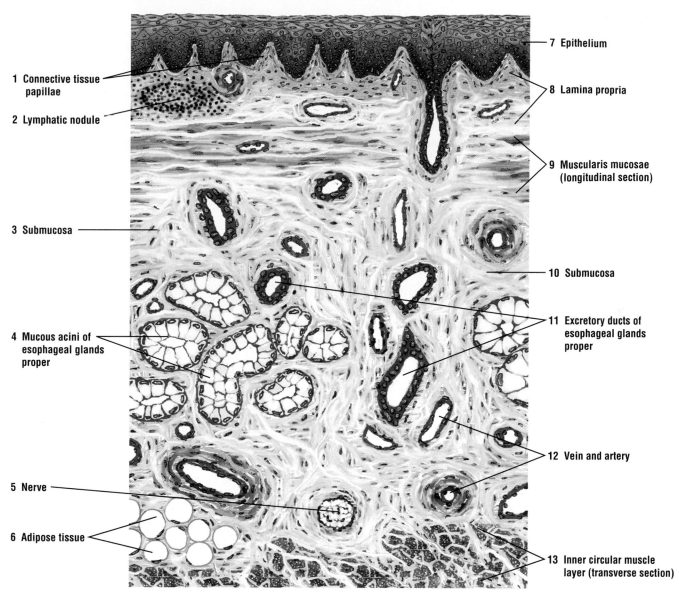

1 Connective tissue
  papillae

2 Lymphatic nodule

3 Submucosa

4 Mucous acini of
  esophageal glands
  proper

5 Nerve

6 Adipose tissue

7 Epithelium

8 Lamina propria

9 Muscularis mucosae
  (longitudinal section)

10 Submucosa

11 Excretory ducts of
   esophageal glands
   proper

12 Vein and artery

13 Inner circular muscle
   layer (transverse section)

FIGURE 12.4 ■ Upper esophagus: mucosa and submucosa (longitudinal view). Stain: hematoxylin and eosin. Medium magnification.

FIGURE 12.5 ◾ Lower Esophagus Wall (Transverse Section)

A low-magnification photomicrograph illustrates the lower portion of the esophagus and all layers of the mucosa. The mucosa consists of a thick but nonkeratinized **stratified squamous epithelium (1)**, a connective tissue **lamina propria (2)**, and a thin strip of smooth muscle **muscularis mucosae (3)**.

FUNCTIONAL CORRELATIONS: Esophagus

The major function of the esophagus is to convey liquids or a mass of chewed food (**bolus**) from the oral cavity to the stomach. For this function, the lumen of the esophagus is lined by a protective **nonkeratinized stratified squamous epithelium.** Aiding in this function are esophageal glands located in the connective tissue of the wall. There are two types of glands in the wall of the esophagus. The **esophageal cardiac glands** are present in the **lamina propria** of the upper and lower regions of the esophagus. These glands have a similar morphology to those found in the cardia of the stomach, where the esophagus terminates. **Esophageal glands proper** are located in the connective tissue of the submucosa. Both types of glands produce the secretory product **mucus,** which is conducted in **excretory ducts** through the epithelium to lubricate the esophageal lumen. The swallowed material is moved from one end of the esophagus to the other by strong muscular contractions called **peristalsis.** At the lower end of the esophagus, a muscular **gastroesophageal sphincter** constricts the lumen and prevents regurgitation of swallowed material into the esophagus.

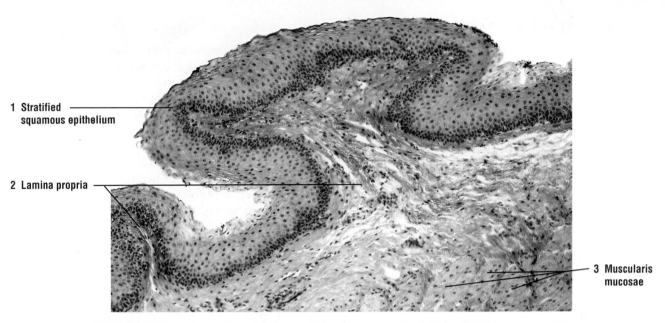

1 Stratified
squamous epithelium

2 Lamina propria

3 Muscularis
mucosae

FIGURE 12.5 ■ Lower esophageal wall (transverse section). Stain: Mallory-azan × 30.

FIGURE 12.6 ■ Esophageal-Stomach Junction

At its terminal end, the esophagus joins the stomach and forms the esophageal-stomach junction. The nonkeratinized **stratified squamous epithelium (1)** of the **esophagus** abruptly changes to simple columnar, mucus-secreting **gastric epithelium (10)** of the cardia region of the **stomach.**

At the esophageal-stomach junction, the **esophageal glands proper (7)** may be seen in the **submucosa (8).** **Excretory ducts (4, 6)** from these glands course through the **muscularis mucosae (5)** and the **lamina propria (2)** of the esophagus into its lumen. In the lamina propria (2) of the esophagus near the stomach region are the **esophageal cardiac glands (3).** Both the esophageal glands proper (7) and the cardiac glands (3) secrete mucus.

The lamina propria of the esophagus (2) continues into the **lamina propria** of the **stomach (12),** where it becomes filled with **glands (16, 17)** and diffuse lymphatic tissue. The lamina propria of the stomach (12) is penetrated by shallow **gastric pits (11)** into which empty the gastric glands (16, 17).

The upper region of the stomach contains two types of glands. The simple tubular **cardiac glands (17)** are limited to the transition region, the cardia of the stomach. These glands are lined with pale-staining, mucus-secreting columnar cells. Below the cardiac region of the stomach are the simple tubular **gastric glands (16),** some of which exhibit basal branching.

In contrast to the cardiac glands (17), the gastric glands (16) contain four different cell types: the pale-staining **mucous neck cells (13);** large, eosinophilic **parietal cells (14);** basophilic **chief** or **zymogenic cells (15);** and several different types of endocrine cells (not illustrated), collectively called the enteroendocrine cells.

The **muscularis mucosae** of the **stomach (18)** also continues with the muscularis mucosae of the esophagus (5). In the esophagus, the muscularis mucosae (5) is usually a single layer of longitudinal smooth muscle fibers, whereas in the stomach, a second layer of smooth muscle is added, called the inner circular layer.

The **submucosa (8, 19)** and the **muscularis externa (9, 21)** of the esophagus are continuous with those of the stomach. **Blood vessels (20)** are found in the submucosa (8, 19), from which smaller blood vessels are distributed to other regions of the stomach.

FIGURE 12.7 ■ Esophageal-Stomach Junction (Transverse Section)

A low-magnification photomicrograph illustrates the esophagus-stomach junction. The esophagus is characterized by a thick, protective, nonkeratinized **stratified squamous epithelium (1).** Inferior to the epithelium (1) is the **lamina propria (2),** below which is the smooth muscle **muscularis mucosae (3).** The lamina propria (2) indents the undersurface of the esophageal epithelium to form the connective tissue papillae. The esophageal-stomach junction is characterized by an abrupt transition from the stratified epithelium (1) of the esophagus to the **simple columnar epithelium (4)** of the stomach. The surface of the stomach also exhibits numerous **gastric pits (5)** into which open the **gastric glands (6).** The **lamina propria (7)** of the stomach, in contrast to that of the esophagus, is seen as thin strips of connective tissue between the tightly packed gastric glands (6).

Esophagus

Stomach

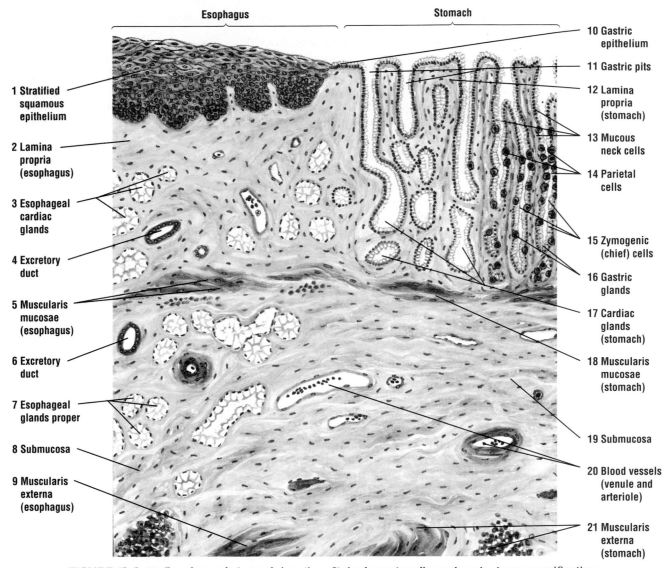

1 Stratified squamous epithelium

2 Lamina propria (esophagus)

3 Esophageal cardiac glands

4 Excretory duct

5 Muscularis mucosae (esophagus)

6 Excretory duct

7 Esophageal glands proper

8 Submucosa

9 Muscularis externa (esophagus)

10 Gastric epithelium

11 Gastric pits

12 Lamina propria (stomach)

13 Mucous neck cells

14 Parietal cells

15 Zymogenic (chief) cells

16 Gastric glands

17 Cardiac glands (stomach)

18 Muscularis mucosae (stomach)

19 Submucosa

20 Blood vessels (venule and arteriole)

21 Muscularis externa (stomach)

FIGURE 12.6 ■ Esophageal-stomach junction. Stain: hematoxylin and eosin. Low magnification.

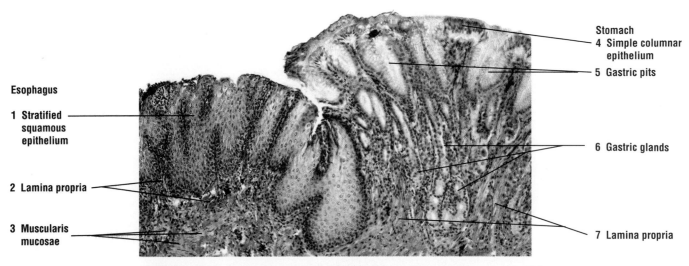

Esophagus

1 Stratified squamous epithelium

2 Lamina propria

3 Muscularis mucosae

Stomach

4 Simple columnar epithelium

5 Gastric pits

6 Gastric glands

7 Lamina propria

FIGURE 12.7 ■ Esophageal-stomach junction. Stain: Mallory-azan × 30.

FIGURE 12.8 ■ Stomach: Fundus and Body Regions (Transverse Section)

The three histologic regions of the stomach are the cardia, the fundus and body, and the pylorus. The fundus and body constitute the most extensive region in the stomach. The stomach wall exhibits four general regions: the **mucosa (1, 2, 3)**, **submucosa (4)**, **muscularis externa (5, 6, 7)**, and **serosa (8)**.

The **mucosa** consists of the **surface epithelium (1)**, **lamina propria (2)**, and **muscularis mucosae (3)**. The surface of the stomach is lined by **simple columnar epithelium (1, 11)** that extends into and lines the **gastric pits (10)**, which are tubular infoldings of the surface epithelium (11). In the fundus, the gastric pits (10) are not deep and extend into the mucosa about one fourth of its thickness. Beneath the epithelium is the loose connective tissue **lamina propria (2, 12)** that fills the spaces between the gastric glands. A thin smooth muscle **muscularis mucosae (3, 15)**, consisting of an inner circular and an outer longitudinal layer, forms the outer boundary of the mucosa. Thin strands of smooth muscle from the muscularis mucosae (3, 15) extend into lamina propria (2, 12) between the **gastric glands (13, 14)** toward the surface epithelium (1, 11), which are illustrated at higher magnification in Figure 12.9, label 8.

The gastric glands (13, 14) are packed in the lamina propria (2, 12) and occupy the entire mucosa (1, 2, 3). The gastric glands open into the bottom of the gastric pits (10). The surface epithelium of the gastric mucosa, from the cardiac to the pyloric region, consists of the same cell type. However, the cells that constitute the gastric glands distinguish the regional differences of the stomach. Two distinct cell types can be identified in the gastric glands. The acidophilic **parietal cells (13)** are located in the upper portions of the glands, whereas the basophilic **chief (zymogenic) (14)** cells occupy the lower regions. The subglandular regions of the lamina propria may (2, 12) contain either lymphatic tissue or small **lymphatic nodules (16)**.

The mucosa of the empty stomach exhibits temporary folds called **rugae (9)**. Rugae (9) are formed during the contractions of the smooth muscle layer, the muscularis mucosae (3, 15). As the stomach fills, the rugae disappear and form a smooth mucosa.

The **submucosa (4)** lies below the muscularis mucosae (3, 15). In the empty stomach, submucosa (4) can extend into the rugae (9). The submucosa (4) contains dense irregular connective tissue and more **collagen fibers (17)** than the lamina propria (2, 12). In addition, the submucosa (4) contains lymph vessels, **capillaries (21)**, large **arterioles (18)**, and **venules (19)**. Isolated clusters of parasympathetic ganglia of the **submucosal (Meissner's) nerve plexus (20)** can be seen deeper in the submucosa.

The **muscularis externa (5, 6, 7)** consists of three layers of smooth muscle, each oriented in a different plane: an inner **oblique (5)**, a middle **circular (6)**, and an outer **longitudinal (7)** layer. The oblique layer is not complete and is not always seen in sections of the stomach wall. In this illustration, the circular layer has been sectioned longitudinally and the longitudinal layer transversely. Located between the circular and longitudinal smooth muscle layers is a **myenteric (Auerbach's) nerve plexus (22)** of parasympathetic ganglia and nerve fibers.

The **serosa (8)** consists of a thin outer layer of connective tissue that overlies the muscularis externa (5, 6, 7) and is covered by a simple squamous mesothelium of the **visceral peritoneum (8)**. The serosa can contain **adipose cells (23)**.

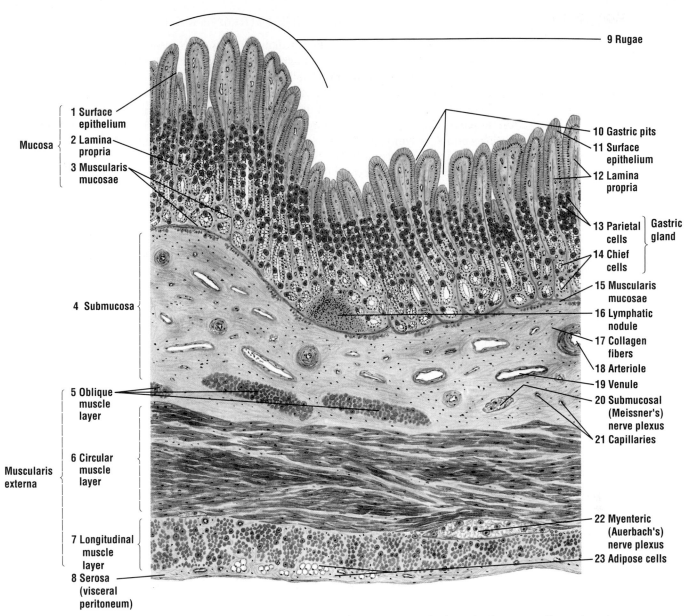

9 Rugae

1 Surface epithelium

2 Lamina propria

3 Muscularis mucosae

Mucosa

10 Gastric pits

11 Surface epithelium

12 Lamina propria

13 Parietal cells

14 Chief cells

Gastric gland

15 Muscularis mucosae

16 Lymphatic nodule

4 Submucosa

17 Collagen fibers

18 Arteriole

19 Venule

20 Submucosal (Meissner's) nerve plexus

21 Capillaries

5 Oblique muscle layer

6 Circular muscle layer

Muscularis externa

7 Longitudinal muscle layer

22 Myenteric (Auerbach's) nerve plexus

23 Adipose cells

8 Serosa (visceral peritoneum)

FIGURE 12.8 ■ Stomach: fundus and body regions (transverse section). Stain: hematoxylin and eosin. Low magnification.

FIGURE 12.9 ■ Stomach: Mucosa of the Fundus and Body (Transverse Section)

The mucosa and submucosa of the fundic region of the stomach are illustrated at a higher magnification. The simple columnar **surface epithelium (1, 13)** extends into the **gastric pits (11),** into which open the tubular **gastric glands (5).** The **lamina propria (6)** fills the spaces between the packed gastric glands (5) and extends from the surface epithelium (1) to the **muscularis mucosae (9).**

The lamina propria (6), which consists of fine reticular and collagen fibers, is better seen in the **mucosal ridges (2).** Scattered throughout the lamina propria (6) are the fibroblast nuclei, accumulations of lymphoid tissue in the form of a **lymphatic nodule (17),** lymphocytes, and other loose connective tissue cells.

The gastric glands (5) extend the length of the mucosa. In the deeper regions of the mucosa, the gastric glands may branch. As a result, the gastric glands appear as transverse and oblique sections. Each gastric gland consists of three regions. At the junction of the gastric pit with the gastric gland is the **isthmus (14),** lined by surface epithelial cells (1, 13) and **parietal cells (4).** Lower in the gland is the **neck (15),** containing mainly **mucous neck cells (3)** and some parietal cells (4). The base or **fundus (16)** is the deep portion of the gland, composed predominantly of **chief (zymogenic) cells (7)** and a few parietal cells (4). The fundic glands also contain undifferentiated cells and enteroendocrine cells (not illustrated) that secrete different hormones to regulate the digestive system.

Three types of cells can be identified in the fundic gastric glands. The mucous neck cells (3) are located just below the gastric pits (11) and are interspersed between the parietal cells (4) in the neck region of the glands. The parietal cells (4) stain uniformly acidophilic (pink), which distinguishes them from other cells in the fundic glands. In contrast, the chief cells (zymogenic) (7) are basophilic and are distinguishable from the acidophilic parietal cells (4).

The muscularis mucosae (9) in the stomach is composed of two thin strips of smooth muscle, the **inner circular layer (9a)** and **outer longitudinal layer (9b).** In this illustration, the inner circular layer (9a) is sectioned longitudinally and the outer layer (9b) is sectioned transversely. Extending upward from the muscularis mucosae (9) to the surface epithelium (1, 13) are strands of **smooth muscle (8, 12).**

Below the muscularis mucosa (9) is the **submucosa (10)** with denser connective tissue. **Collagen fibers (18)** and the nuclei of **fibroblasts (19)** are seen in the submucosa (10). The submucosa (10) also contains **arterioles (20), venules (21),** lymphatics, and capillaries, in addition to adipose cells.

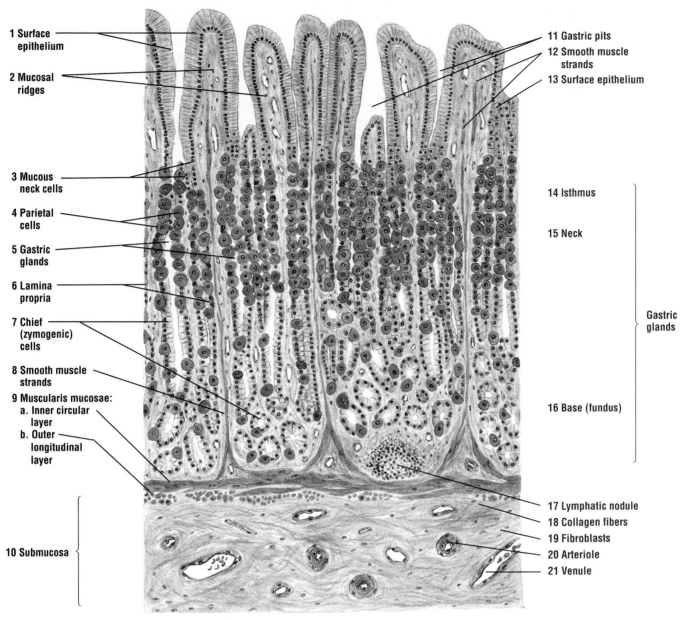

1 Surface epithelium

2 Mucosal ridges

3 Mucous neck cells

4 Parietal cells

5 Gastric glands

6 Lamina propria

7 Chief (zymogenic) cells

8 Smooth muscle strands

9 Muscularis mucosae:
  a. Inner circular layer
  b. Outer longitudinal layer

10 Submucosa

11 Gastric pits

12 Smooth muscle strands

13 Surface epithelium

14 Isthmus

15 Neck

16 Base (fundus)

Gastric glands

17 Lymphatic nodule

18 Collagen fibers

19 Fibroblasts

20 Arteriole

21 Venule

FIGURE 12.9 ■ Stomach: mucosa of the fundus and body (transverse section). Stain: hematoxylin and eosin. Medium magnification.

FIGURE 12.10 ■ Stomach: Fundus and Body Regions

This low-magnification photomicrograph illustrates the mucosa of the stomach wall. The fundus and body regions of the stomach have identical histology. The stomach surface is lined by mucus-secreting, **simple columnar epithelium (1)** that extends down into the **gastric pits (2).** In the fundus and body, the gastric pits (2) are shallow. Draining into the gastric pits (2) are the **gastric glands (5)** with different cell types. The cells of the gastric glands (5) are packed, and their lumina are not clearly visible. The large, pale-staining cells in the gastric glands (5) are the acid-secreting **parietal cells (3),** which are more numerous in the upper regions of the gastric glands (5). The darker-staining cells are the **chief (zymogenic) cells (6),** and they are mostly located in the basal regions of the gastric glands (5). Between the gastric glands (5) are strips of the connective tissue **lamina propria (7).** A thin strip of the smooth muscle, the **muscularis mucosae (8),** separates the mucosa from the **submucosa (4)** of the stomach.

FUNCTIONAL CORRELATIONS: Gastric Pits and Cells of Gastric Glands

The **cardia** and **pylorus** are located at opposite ends of the stomach. The cardia surrounds the entrance of the esophagus into the stomach. At the esophageal-stomach junction are the **cardiac glands.** The pylorus is the most inferior region of the stomach. It terminates at the border of the initial portion of the small intestine called the duodenum. In the cardia, the **gastric pits** are shallow, whereas in the pylorus, the gastric pits are deep. However, gastric glands in these two regions have similar histology and their cells are predominantly **mucus-secreting.**

In contrast, the gastric glands in the fundus and body of the stomach contain three major cell types. Located in the upper region of gastric glands near the gastric pits are **mucous neck cells.** The large polygonal cells with a distinctive eosinophilic cytoplasm are the **parietal cells.** These cells are primarily located in the upper half of the gastric glands and are squeezed between other gastric gland cells. Located predominantly in the lower region of the gastric glands are basophilic staining cuboidal **chief (zymogenic) cells.**

In addition to cells that are present in gastric glands, the mucosa of the digestive tract also contains a wide distribution of **enteroendocrine** or gastrointestinal endocrine cells. These cells are widely distributed in different digestive organs and are located among and between existing exocrine cells. Unless sections of digestive organs are prepared with special stains, these cells are poorly seen in normal histologic sections.

1 Simple columnar
    epithelium

2 Gastric pits

5 Gastric glands

3 Parietal cells

6 Chief (zymogenic)
    cells

7 Lamina propria

8 Muscularis mucosae

4 Submucosa

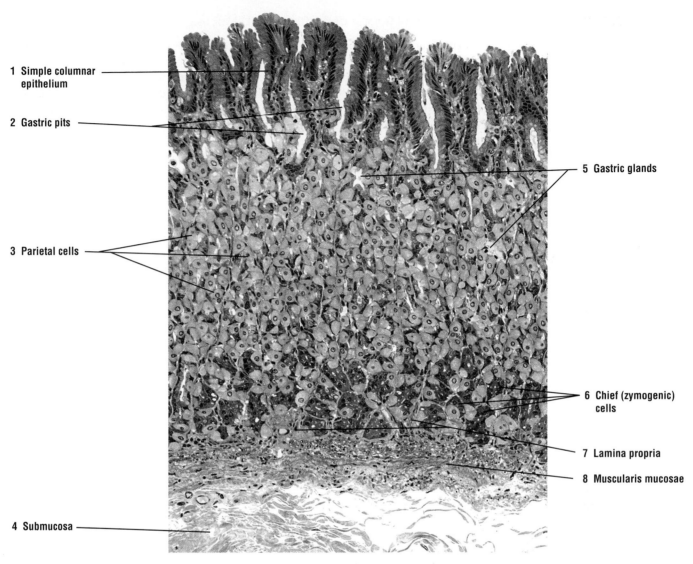

FIGURE 12.10 ■ Stomach: fundus and body regions (plastic section). Stain: hematoxylin and eosin. ×50.

FIGURE 12.11 ■ Stomach: Superficial Region of Gastric (Fundic) Mucosa

Higher magnification of the superficial region of the stomach shows the cells that constitute the mucosa of the fundus and body.

The columnar **surface epithelium** (1) exhibits basal oval nuclei and a lightly stained cytoplasm owing to the presence of mucigen droplets. The surface epithelium (1) is separated from the **lamina propria (3, 7, 8)** by a thin **basement membrane (2).** The lamina propria (3, 7, 8) is vascular and contains **blood vessels (9).** The surface epithelium (1) also extends downward into the **gastric pits (4).**

The **gastric glands (5)** lie in the lamina propria (3, 7, 8) below the gastric pits (4). The neck region of the gastric glands (5) is lined with **mucous neck cells (10)** that have round, basal nuclei. The constricted necks of the gastric glands (5) open by a short transition region into the bottom of the gastric pits (4).

The **parietal cells (6, 11)** are large cells with a pyramidal shape, round nuclei, and highly acidophilic cytoplasm that are interspersed among the mucous neck cells (10). Some pyramidal cells (6, 11) may be binucleate (two nuclei). The free surfaces of parietal cells (6, 11) open into the lumen of the gastric glands (5). The parietal cells (6, 11) are the most conspicuous cells in the gastric mucosa and are found predominantly in the upper third to upper half of the gastric glands (5).

Deeper in the lower half of the gastric glands (5) are found the basophilic **chief** or **zymogenic cells (12),** which also border on the lumen of the gland. Parietal cells (6, 11) are also seen here.

1 Surface epithelium

2 Basement membrane

3 Lamina propria

4 Gastric pits

5 Gastric glands
   (neck region)

6 Parietal cells

7 Lamina propria

8 Lamina propria

9 Blood vessels

10 Mucous neck cells

11 Parietal cells

12 Chief (zymogenic)
    cells

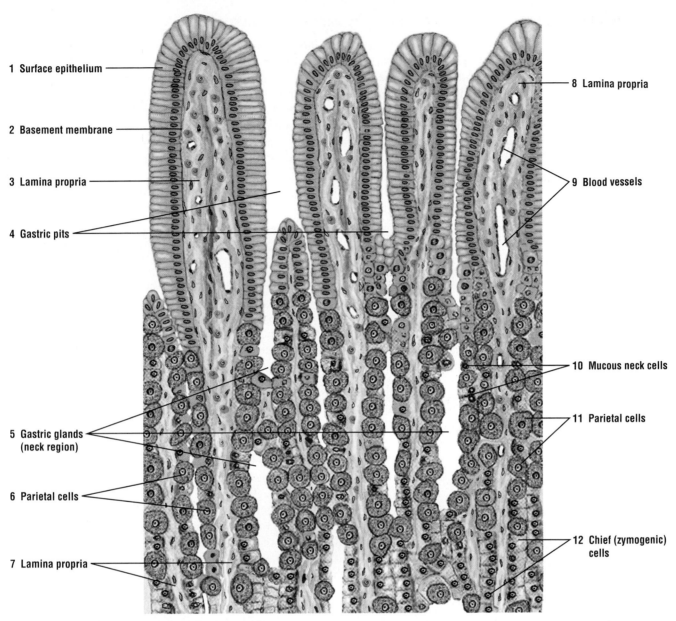

FIGURE 12.11 ■ Stomach: superficial region of gastric (fundic) mucosa. Stain: hematoxylin and eosin. High magnification.

FIGURE 12.12 ■ Stomach: Basal Region of Gastric (Fundic) Mucosa

The **gastric glands (1, 9)** in the body and fundus of the stomach show **basal branching (9).** In the upper regions of the gastric glands, the **chief** or **zymogenic cells (6, 10)** border the lumen of gastric glands (1, 9). In the basal region of the gastric mucosa, the **parietal cells (2)** are wedged against the basement membrane and are not always in direct contact with the lumen.

The connective tissue **lamina propria (3, 7)** surrounds the gastric glands (1). A small **lymphatic nodule (4)** is located in the lamina propria (3) adjacent to the gastric glands (1, 9). The two layers of the **muscularis mucosae (5),** the inner circular layer and the outer longitudinal layer, are seen below the gastric glands (1, 9). **Strands of smooth muscle (8)** extend upward from the muscularis mucosae (5) into the lamina propria (3, 7) between the gastric glands (1, 9).

Adjacent to the muscularis mucosae (5) is the connective tissue **submucosa (11).**

FUNCTIONAL CORRELATIONS

Stomach

The stomach has numerous functions. The stomach **receives, stores, mixes,** and **digests** ingested food products and secretes different hormones that regulate digestive functions. Some functions are **mechanically** and **chemically** specifically designed to reduce the mass of ingested food material, or **bolus,** to a semiliquid mass called **chyme.** The mechanical reduction of the bolus is performed by strong, muscular peristaltic contractions of the stomach wall when food enters the stomach. With the pylorus closed, the muscular contractions churn and mix the stomach contents with **gastric juices** produced by the **gastric glands. Neurons** and **axons** located in the **submucosal nerve plexus** and **myenteric nerve plexus** of the stomach wall regulate the peristaltic activity. The stomach also performs some absorptive functions; however, these are primarily limited to absorption of water, alcohol, salts, and certain drugs.

Gastric Gland Cells in the Body and Fundus of the Stomach

Chemical reduction or digestion of food in the stomach is the main function of gastric secretions produced by different cells in the gastric glands, especially cells located in the fundus and body regions of the stomach. The main components of the gastric secretions are **pepsin, hydrochloric acid, mucus, intrinsic factor, water, lysozyme,** and different **electrolytes.**

The **surface** or **luminal cells** that line the stomach secrete thick layers of **mucus,** whose main function is to cover, lubricate, and protect the stomach surface from the corrosive actions of acidic gastric juices secreted by different cells in the gastric glands.

The major component of gastric juice is the **hydrochloric acid,** produced by **parietal cells** that are located in the upper regions of the gastric glands. In humans, parietal cells also produce **gastric intrinsic factor,** a glycoprotein that is necessary for absorption of **vitamin B_{12}** from the small intestine. Vitamin B_{12} is necessary for **erythrocyte** (red blood cell) production (**erythropoiesis**) in the red bone marrow. Deficiency of this vitamin leads to the development of **pernicious anemia,** a disorder of erythrocyte formation.

Chief or **zymogenic cells** are filled with secretory granules that contain the proenzyme **pepsinogen,** an inactive precursor of **pepsin.** Release of pepsinogen during gastric secretion into the acidic environment of the stomach converts the inactive pepsinogen into a highly active, proteolytic enzyme pepsin. This enzyme digests large protein molecules into smaller peptides, converting almost all of the proteins into smaller molecules. Pepsin is primarily responsible for converting the solid food material into fluid chyme. The secretory activities of the chief and parietal cells are controlled by the autonomic nervous system and the hormone gastrin, secreted by the enteroendocrine cells of the pyloric region of the stomach.

Enteroendocrine cells secrete a variety of **polypeptides** and **proteins** with hormonal activity that influences different functions of the digestive tract. They are called enteroendocrine cells because they produce gastric hormones and are located in the digestive organs. The enteroendocrine cells are also called **APUD cells** because they can take up the precursors of amines and decarboxylate them. These are not confined to the gastrointestinal tract; they are also found in the respiratory organs and other organs of the body where they are also known by different names. Additional details, description, and illustration of known enteroendocrine (APUD) cells are found in Chapter 13.

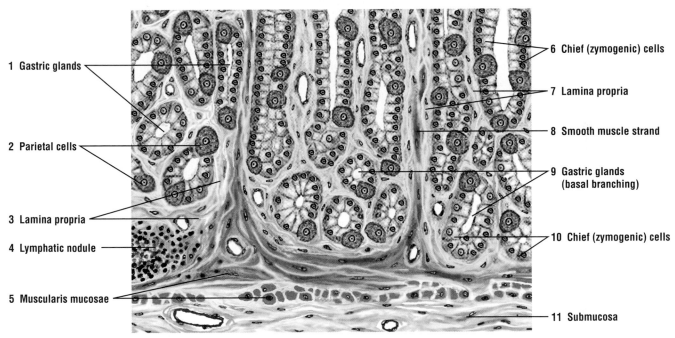

1 Gastric glands

2 Parietal cells

3 Lamina propria

4 Lymphatic nodule

5 Muscularis mucosae

6 Chief (zymogenic) cells

7 Lamina propria

8 Smooth muscle strand

9 Gastric glands (basal branching)

10 Chief (zymogenic) cells

11 Submucosa

FIGURE 12.12 ■ Stomach: basal region of gastric (fundic) mucosa. Stain: hematoxylin and eosin. High magnification.

FIGURE 12.13 ■ Pyloric Region of the Stomach

In the mucosa of the pyloric region of the stomach, the **gastric pits (3, 8)** are deeper than those in the body or fundus regions. The gastric pits (3, 8) extend into the mucosa to about one half or more of its thickness. The surface of the stomach is lined by simple **columnar mucous epithelium (1)** that also extends into and lines all the gastric pits (3, 8).

The **pyloric glands (5, 9)** open into the bottom of the gastric pits (3, 8). The pyloric glands (5, 9) are either branched or coiled tubular glands containing mucous secretions, illustrated in both transverse (5) and longitudinal (9) sections. Similar to the cardia region of the stomach, only one type of cell is found in the epithelium of these glands. The tall columnar cell stains lightly because of its mucigen content. As seen in other mucous cells, the flattened or oval nuclei are located at the base. Enteroendocrine cells are also present in this region and can be demonstrated with a special stain.

The remaining structures in the pyloric region of the stomach are similar to those of other regions. The **lamina propria (4)** contains diffuse lymphatic tissue and an occasional **lymphatic nodule (11)**. Located below the lymphatic nodule (11) is the smooth muscle **muscularis mucosae (6)**. Individual **smooth muscle fibers (2, 10)** from the circular layer of the **muscularis mucosae (6)** pass upward between the pyloric glands (5, 9) into the lamina propria (4) and the upper region of the mucosa. Located below the muscularis mucosae (6) is the dense irregular connective tissue **submucosa (7),** in which are found blood vessels **arteriole (13)** and **venule (12)** of different size.

FUNCTIONAL CORRELATIONS: Cells in Pyloric Gastric Glands

Pyloric glands contain the same cell types as those present in cardiac glands of the stomach. Mucus-secreting cells predominate in these glands. In addition to producing **mucus,** these cells also secrete an enzyme called **lysozyme** that destroys bacteria in the stomach.

1 Surface columnar
   mucous epithelium

2 Muscle fibers from
   muscularis mucosae

3 Gastric pits

4 Lamina propria

5 Pyloric glands
   (transverse section)

6 Muscularis mucosae

7 Submucosa

8 Gastric pits

9 Pyloric glands
   (longitudinal
   section)

10 Muscle fibers from
    muscularis
    mucosae

11 Lymphatic nodule

12 Venule

13 Arteriole

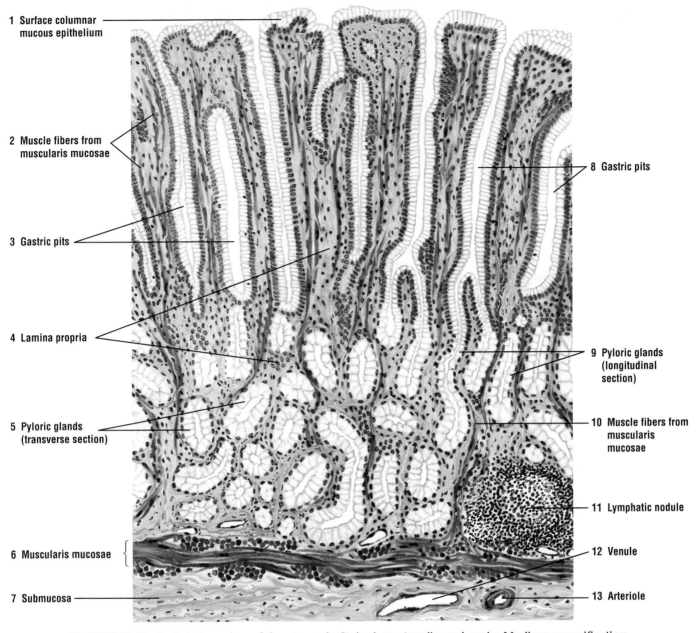

FIGURE 12.13 ■ Pyloric region of the stomach. Stain: hematoxylin and eosin. Medium magnification.

FIGURE 12.14 ■ Pyloric-Duodenal Junction

The **pylorus** (**1**) of the stomach is separated from the **duodenum** (**11**) of the small intestine by a thick smooth muscle layer called the **pyloric sphincter** (**8**) that is formed by the thickened circular layer of the muscularis externa of the **stomach** (**9**).

At the junction with the duodenum (11), the **mucosal ridges** (**4**) of the stomach around **gastric pits** (**3**) become broader and more irregular and their shape more variable. Coiled tubular **pyloric (mucous) glands** (**6**), located in the **lamina propria** (**5**), open at the bottom of the gastric pits (3). **Lymphatic nodules** (**16**) are seen between the stomach (1) and the duodenum (11).

The mucus-secreting **stomach epithelium** (**2**) changes to **intestinal epithelium** (**12**) in the duodenum. The intestinal epithelium (12) consists of goblet cells and columnar cells with striated borders (microvilli) that are present throughout the length of the small intestine. The duodenum (11) contains **villi** (**13**), a specialized surface modification. Each villus (singular) (13) is a leaf-shaped surface projection. Between individual villi are **intervillous spaces** (**14**) of the intestinal lumen.

Short, simple tubular **intestinal glands** (crypts of Lieberkühn) (**15**) are present in the lamina propria of the duodenum. These glands consist primarily of goblet cells and cells with striated borders (microvilli) of the surface epithelium.

Duodenal glands (Brunner's) (**18**) occupy most of the **submucosa** (**19**) in the upper duodenum (11) and are the characteristic features of the duodenum. The ducts of the duodenal glands (18) penetrate the **muscularis mucosae** of the **duodenum** (**17**) and enter the base of the intestinal glands (15), disrupting the muscularis mucosae (17) in this region. Except for the esophageal (submucosal) glands proper, the duodenal glands (18) are the only submucosal glands in the digestive tract. In the **muscularis externa of the stomach** (**9**) and in the **muscularis externa of the duodenum** (**20**) are neurons and axons of the **myenteric nerve plexuses** (**10, 21**).

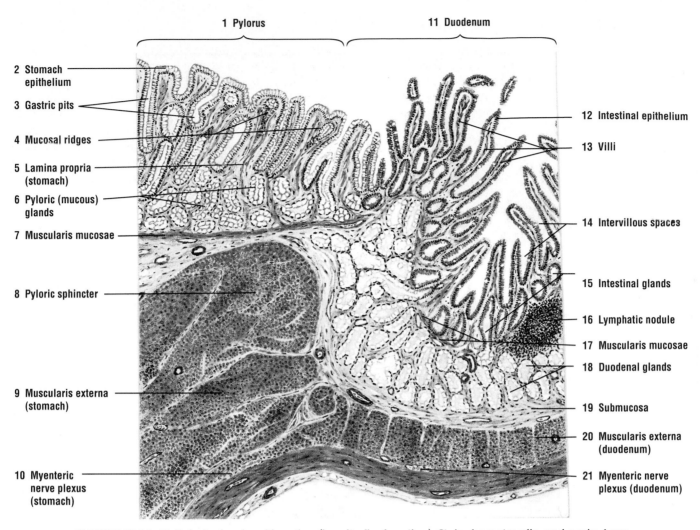

1 Pylorus

11 Duodenum

2 Stomach epithelium

3 Gastric pits

4 Mucosal ridges

5 Lamina propria (stomach)

6 Pyloric (mucous) glands

7 Muscularis mucosae

8 Pyloric sphincter

9 Muscularis externa (stomach)

10 Myenteric nerve plexus (stomach)

12 Intestinal epithelium

13 Villi

14 Intervillous spaces

15 Intestinal glands

16 Lymphatic nodule

17 Muscularis mucosae

18 Duodenal glands

19 Submucosa

20 Muscularis externa (duodenum)

21 Myenteric nerve plexus (duodenum)

FIGURE 12.14 ■ Pyloric-duodenal junction (longitudinal section). Stain: hematoxylin and eosin. Low magnification.

CHAPTER 12 ■ Summary

Digestive System: Esophagus and Stomach

General Plan of the Digestive System

- Hollow tube extending from oral cavity to rectum
- Wall exhibits basic organization of the entire tube

Mucosa: Composition

- Covering epithelium
- Loose connective tissue called lamina propria
- Smooth muscle layer muscularis mucosae, with inner circular and outer longitudinal layers

Submucosa

- Dense irregular connective tissue layer with blood vessels, nerves, and lymphatic vessels
- Contains submucosal nerve plexus that controls muscularis mucosae

Muscularis Externa

- Thick, smooth muscle layer inferior to submucosa
- Normally contains an inner circular and an outer longitudinal smooth muscle layers
- Myenteric nerve plexus located between inner and outer muscle layers
- Myenteric nerve plexus controls motility of smooth muscles in muscularis externa

Serosa

- Thin layer of tissue, mesothelium, that covers the visceral organs
- Covers abdominal esophagus, stomach, small intestine, and anterior wall of colon

Adventitia

- Covers thoracic part of esophagus and posterior wall of ascending and descending colon

Esophagus

- Soft tube that extends from pharynx to stomach, posterior to the trachea
- Penetrates diaphragm and enters stomach
- Lumen lined by nonkeratinized stratified squamous epithelium
- In the upper third, muscularis externa contains skeletal muscle
- In the middle, both smooth and skeletal muscle found in muscularis externa
- In lower third, muscularis externa contains smooth muscle
- Mucous esophageal glands are present in both the lamina propria and submucosa for lubrication
- Adventitia surrounds the esophagus in the thoracic cavity
- Muscularis mucosae and submucosa from esophagus continue with those of stomach layers

Stomach

- Transition from esophagus to stomach is abrupt and from stratified squamous to simple columnar
- Receives, stores, mixes, and digests ingested food products to form liquid chyme
- Converts bolus of ingested food into semiliquid mass chyme
- Consists of cardia, fundus, body, and pyloric regions
- Surface pitted by gastric pits, which are connected to gastric glands in the lamina propria
- Surface is lined by mucus-secreting simple columnar epithelium for protection
- Gastric glands produce gastric juices rich in hydrochloric acid and protein-digesting enzymes
- Muscularis externa shows internal oblique, middle circular, and outer longitudinal muscle layers
- Fundus and body form the major regions, and are histologically identical
- Submucosal and myenteric nerve plexuses regulate peristaltic activity

Gastric Glands and Cells

- In fundus and body produce the chemicals for digestion of stomach contents
- In body and fundus, parietal cells are large, acidophilic, and are in the upper gland region
- Deeper region of the glands contains chief or zymogen cells
- When contracted or empty, temporary rugae seen in the wall
- In cardia and pylorus, surface epithelium and simple tubular gastric glands produce mucus
- Glands in the pylorus produce mucus and bacteria-destroying enzyme lysozyme

- Parietal cells in fundus and body produce hydrochloric acid and gastric intrinsic factor
- Gastric intrinsic factor essential for absorption of vitamin B_{12} and erythropoiesis
- Chief or zymogen cells produce pepsinogen that is converted to pepsin in acid environment
- Enteroendocrine cells secrete variety of polypeptides and proteins for digestive functions
- In pylorus, gastric pits are deeper than in fundus or body
- Mucus-secreting stomach cells change to intestinal epithelium in the duodenum

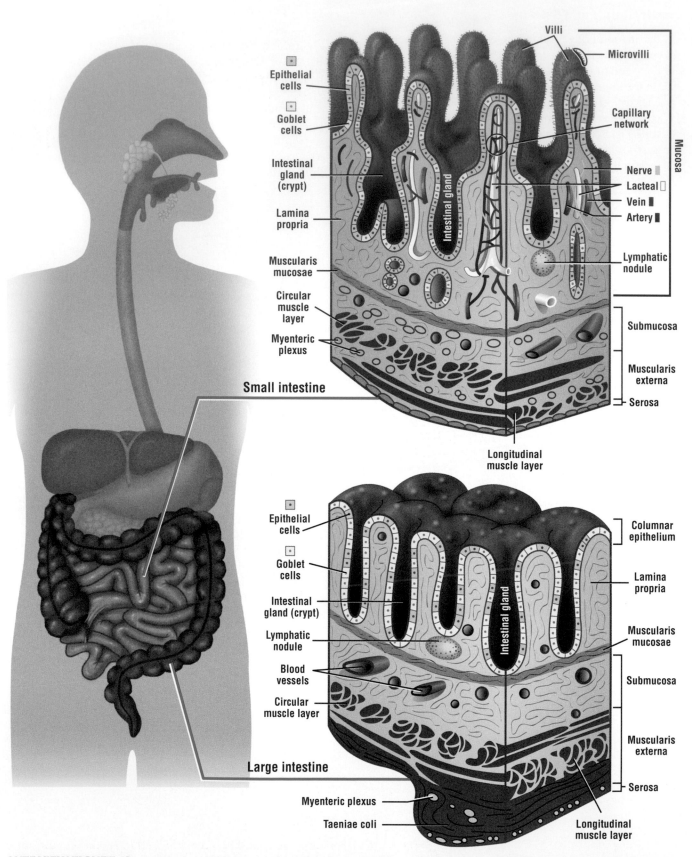

Small intestine

Villi

Microvilli

Epithelial cells

Goblet cells

Capillary network

Intestinal gland (crypt)

Intestinal gland

Mucosa

Nerve

Lacteal

Vein

Artery

Lamina propria

Muscularis mucosae

Lymphatic nodule

Circular muscle layer

Myenteric plexus

Submucosa

Muscularis externa

Serosa

Longitudinal muscle layer

Large intestine

Epithelial cells

Goblet cells

Columnar epithelium

Intestinal gland (crypt)

Lamina propria

Intestinal gland

Lymphatic nodule

Blood vessels

Muscularis mucosae

Submucosa

Circular muscle layer

Muscularis externa

Serosa

Myenteric plexus

Taeniae coli

Longitudinal muscle layer

OVERVIEW FIGURE 13 ■ Structural differences between the wall of the small intestine and large intestine, with emphasis on different layers of the wall.

Digestive System: Small and Large Intestines

Small Intestine

The **small intestine** is a long, convoluted tube about 5 to 7 m long; it is the longest section of the digestive tract. The small intestine extends from the junction with the stomach to join with the **large intestine** or **colon.** For descriptive purposes, the small intestine is divided into three parts: the **duodenum, jejunum,** and **ileum.** Although the microscopic differences among these three segments are minor, they allow for identification of the segments.

The main function of the small intestine is the digestion of gastric contents and absorption of nutrients into blood capillaries and lymphatic lacteals.

Surface Modifications of Small Intestine for Absorption

The mucosa of the small intestine exhibits specialized structural modifications that increase the cellular surface areas for absorption of nutrients and fluids. These modifications include the plicae circulares, villi, and microvilli.

In contrast to the rugae of stomach, the **plicae circulares** are permanent spiral folds or elevations of the mucosa (with a submucosal core) that extend into the intestinal lumen. The plicae circulares are most prominent in the proximal portion of the small intestine, where most absorption takes place; they decrease in prominence toward the ileum.

Villi are permanent fingerlike projections of lamina propria of the mucosa that extend into the intestinal lumen. They are covered by **simple columnar epithelium** and are also more prominent in the proximal portion of the small intestine. The height of the villi decreases toward the ileum of the small intestine. The connective tissue core of each villus contains a lymphatic capillary called a **lacteal,** blood capillaries, and individual strands of smooth muscles (see Overview Figure 13).

Each villus has a core of **lamina propria** that is normally filled with blood vessels, lymphatic capillaries, nerves, smooth muscle, and loose irregular connective tissue. In addition, the lamina propria is a storehouse for **immune cells** such as lymphocytes, plasma cells, tissue eosinophils, macrophages, and mast cells.

Smooth muscle fibers from the muscularis mucosae extend into the core of individual villi and are responsible for their movements. This action increases the contacts of the villi with the digested food products in the intestine.

Microvilli are cytoplasmic extensions that cover the apices of the intestinal absorptive cells. They are visible under a light microscope as a **striated (brush) border.** The microvilli are coated by a glycoprotein coat glycocalyx, which contains such **brush border enzymes** as lactase, peptidases, sucrase, lipase, and others that are important for digestion.

Cells, Glands, and Lymphatic Nodules in the Small Intestine

Intestinal glands (crypts of Lieberkühn) are located between the villi throughout the small intestine. These glands open into the intestinal lumen at the base of the villi. The simple columnar epithelium that lines the villi is continuous with that of the intestinal glands. In the glands are found stem cells, absorptive cells, goblet cells, Paneth cells, and some enteroendocrine cells.

Absorptive cells are the most common cell types in the intestinal epithelium. These cells are tall columnar with a prominent striated (brush) border of **microvilli.** A thick **glycocalyx** coat covers and protects the microvilli from the corrosive chemicals.

Goblet cells are interspersed among the columnar absorptive cells of the intestinal epithelium. They increase in number toward the distal region of the small intestine (ileum).

Enteroendocrine or **APUD** (amine precursor uptake and decarboxylation) cells are scattered throughout the epithelium of the villi and intestinal glands.

Duodenal (Brunner's) glands are primarily found in the submucosa of the initial portion of the duodenum and are highly characteristic of this region of the small intestine. These are branched, tubuloacinar glands with light-staining mucous cells. The ducts of duodenal glands penetrate the muscularis mucosae to discharge their secretory product at the base of intestinal glands.

Undifferentiated cells exhibit mitotic activity and are located in the base of intestinal glands. They function as stem cells and replace worn-out columnar absorptive cells, goblet cells, and intestinal gland cells.

Paneth cells are located at the base of intestinal glands. They are characterized by the presence of deep-staining eosinophilic granules in their cytoplasm.

Peyer's patches are numerous aggregations of closely packed, permanent **lymphatic nodules.** They are found primarily in the wall of the terminal portion of small intestine, the ileum. These nodules occupy a large portion of the lamina propria and submucosa of the ileum.

M cells are highly specialized epithelial cells that cover the Peyer's patches and large lymphatic nodules; they are not found anywhere else in the intestine. M cells phagocytose luminal antigens and present them to the lymphocytes and macrophages in the lamina propria, which are then stimulated to produce specific antibodies against the antigens.

Regional Differences in the Small Intestine

The **duodenum** is the shortest segment of the small intestine. The villi in this region are broad, tall, and numerous, with fewer goblet cells in the epithelium. Branched duodenal (Brunner's) glands with mucus-secreting cells in the submucosa characterize this region.

The **jejunum** exhibits shorter, narrower, and fewer villi than the duodenum. There are also more goblet cells in the epithelium.

The **ileum** contains few villi that are narrow and short. In addition, the epithelium contains more goblet cells than in the duodenum or jejunum. The lymphatic nodules are particularly large and numerous in the ileum, where they aggregate in the lamina propria and submucosa to form the prominent Peyer's patches.

Large Intestine (Colon)

The large intestine is situated between the anus and the terminal end of the ileum. It is shorter and less convoluted than the small intestine. It consists of an initial segment called the cecum, and the ascending, transverse, descending, and sigmoid colon, as well as the rectum and anus.

Chyme enters the large intestine from the ileum through the ileocecal valve. Unabsorbed and undigested food residues from the small intestine are forced into the large intestine by strong peristaltic actions of smooth muscles in the muscularis externa. The residues that enter the large intestine are in a semifluid state; however, by the time they reach the terminal portion of the large intestine, these residues become semisolid **feces.**

FIGURE 13.1 ■ Small Intestine: Duodenum (Longitudinal Section)

The wall of the duodenum consists of four layers: the mucosa with the **lining epithelium (7a), lamina propria (7b),** and the **muscularis mucosae (9, 12);** the underlying connective tissue **submucosa** with the mucous **duodenal (Brunner's) glands (3, 13);** the two smooth muscle layers of the **muscularis externa (14);** and the visceral peritoneum **serosa (15).** These layers are continuous with those of the stomach, small intestine, and large intestine (colon).

The small intestine is characterized by fingerlike extensions called **villi (7)** (singular, villus); a lining epithelium **(7a)** of columnar cells lined with microvilli that form the striated borders;

light-staining **goblet cells (2)**; and short, tubular **intestinal glands (crypts of Lieberkühn) (4, 8)** in the lamina propria (7b). Duodenal glands (3, 13) in the submucosa (13) characterize the duodenum. These glands are absent in the rest of the small intestine (jejunum and ileum) and large intestine.

The villi (7) are mucosal surface modifications. Between the villi (7) are the **intervillous spaces (1).** The lining epithelium (7a) covers each villus and the intestinal glands (4, 8). Each villus (7) contains a core of lamina propria (7b), strands of **smooth muscle fibers (10)** that extend upward into the villi from the muscularis mucosae (9, 12), and a central lymphatic vessel called the **lacteal (11)** (see Figure 13.7 for details).

The intestinal glands (4, 8) are located in the lamina propria (7b) and open into the intervillous spaces (1). In certain sections of the duodenum, the submucosal duodenal glands (13) extend into the lamina propria (3). The lamina propria (7b) also contains fine connective tissue fibers with reticular cells, diffuse lymphatic tissue, and **lymphatic nodules (5).**

The submucosa (13) in the duodenum is almost completely filled with branched, tubular duodenal glands (13). The duodenal glands (13) disrupt the muscularis mucosae (9, 12) when they penetrate into the lamina propria (3). The secretions from the duodenal glands (3) enter at the bottom of the intestinal glands (3, 4, 8).

In a cross section of the duodenum, the muscularis externa (14) consists of an **inner circular layer (14a)** and an **outer longitudinal layer (14b)** of smooth muscle. However, in this figure, the duodenum has been cut in a longitudinal plane, and the direction of fibers in these two smooth muscle layers is reversed. Parasympathetic ganglion cells of the **myenteric (Auerbach's) nerve plexus (6),** found in the small and large intestine, are visible in the connective tissue between the two muscle layers of the muscularis externa (14). Similar but smaller plexuses of ganglion cells are also found in the submucosa (not illustrated) in the small and large intestine.

The serosa (visceral peritoneum) (15) contains the connective tissue cells, blood vessels, and adipose cells. The serosa forms the outermost layer of the first part of the duodenum.

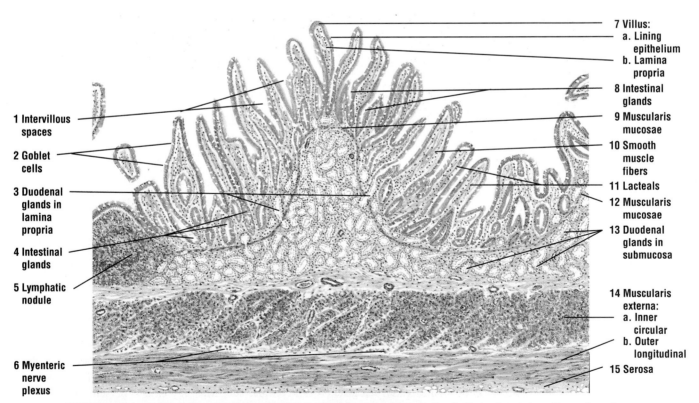

FIGURE 13.1 ■ Duodenum of the small intestine (longitudinal section). Stain: hematoxylin and eosin. Low magnification.

FIGURE 13.2 ■ Small Intestine: Duodenum (Transverse Section)

A low-magnification photomicrograph illustrates a transverse section of the duodenum. The luminal surface of the duodenum exhibits **villi (2)** that are covered by **simple columnar epithelium (1)** with a brush border. The core of each villus (2) contains **lamina propria (4, 6)** in which are found connective tissue cells, lymphatic cells, plasma cells, macrophages, smooth muscle cells, and others. In addition, the lamina propria (4, 6) contains blood vessels and the dilated, blind-ending lymphatic channels called **lacteals (3).** Between the villi (2) are the **intestinal glands (7)** that extend to the **muscularis mucosae (8).** Inferior to the muscularis mucosae (8) is the dense irregular connective tissue of **submucosa (9).** In the duodenum, the submucosa (9) is filled with light-staining, mucus-secreting **duodenal glands (5),** whose ducts pierce the muscularis mucosae (8) to deliver their secretory product at the base of the intestinal glands (7). Surrounding the submucosa (9) and the duodenal glands (5) is the **muscularis externa (10).**

FUNCTIONAL CORRELATIONS: Duodenum

A characteristic feature of the duodenum are the branched tubuloacinar **duodenal (Brunner's) glands** in the submucosa. Their excretory ducts penetrate the muscularis mucosae to deliver their secretions at the base of intestinal glands. Duodenal glands secrete or release their product into the lumen in response to the entrance of acidic chyme from the stomach and parasympathetic stimulation by the vagus nerve.

The main function of the duodenal glands is to protect the duodenal mucosa from the highly corrosive action of the gastric contents. Also, alkaline **mucus** and **bicarbonate secretions** from the duodenal gland secretions that enter the duodenum buffer or neutralize the acidic chyme to provide a more favorable environment for digestive enzymes that enter the duodenum from the pancreas.

Duodenal glands are also believed to produce a polypeptide hormone called **urogastrone.** This hormone inhibits hydrochloric acid secretion by the parietal cells in the stomach and increases epithelial proliferation in the small intestine.

FIGURE 13.3 ■ Small Intestine: Jejunum (Transverse Section)

The histology of the lower duodenum, jejunum, and ileum is similar to that of the upper duodenum (see Figure 13.1). The only exception is the duodenal (Brunner's) glands; these are usually limited to the submucosa in the upper part of the duodenum and are not found in the jejunum and ileum.

This figure illustrates the prominent and permanent fold of the **plica circularis (10)** that extends into the jejunal lumen. The core of the plica circularis (10) is formed by the dense irregular connective tissue **submucosa (3, 15)** that contains numerous **arteries** and **veins (13).** Numerous fingerlike extensions, the **villi (12),** cover the plica (10). Between the villi (12) are the **intervillous spaces (11),** and at the bottom of the villi (12) are the **intestinal glands (14)** located in the **lamina propria (5).** The intestinal glands (crypts of Lieberkühn) (4) open into the intervillous spaces (11).

In the lumen, each villus (12) exhibits a columnar **lining epithelium (1)** with striated border and goblet cells. Below the lining epithelium (1) in the lamina propria (5) is a **lymphatic nodule (6)** with a germinal center. Individual strands of smooth muscle fibers from the **muscularis mucosae (2)** extend in the lamina propria of the villi (12). Each villus also contains a central **lacteal (4)** and capillaries (see Figure 13.7).

The small intestine is surrounded by the **muscularis externa** that contains an **inner circular smooth muscle (7)** layer and an **outer longitudinal smooth muscle (8)** layer. Parasympathetic ganglion cells of the **myenteric plexus (16)** are present in the connective tissue between the muscle layers of the muscularis externa (7, 8). A similar submucosal plexus is present in the submucosa of the small intestine, but is not illustrated in this figure.

A visceral peritoneum or **serosa (17)** surrounds the small intestine. Under the serosal lining are connective tissue fibers, blood vessels, and **adipose cells (9).**

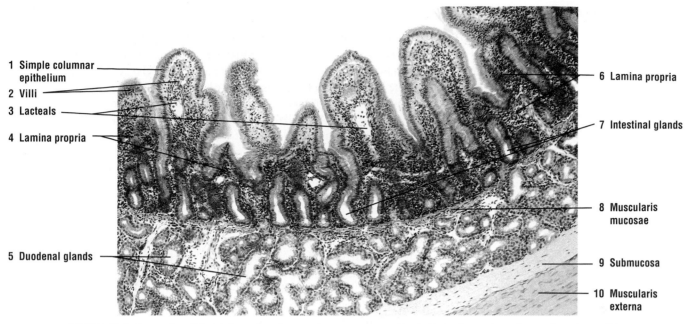

1 Simple columnar epithelium
2 Villi
3 Lacteals
4 Lamina propria
5 Duodenal glands

6 Lamina propria
7 Intestinal glands
8 Muscularis mucosae
9 Submucosa
10 Muscularis externa

FIGURE 13.2 ■ Small intestine: duodenum (transverse section). Stain: hematoxylin and eosin. ×25.

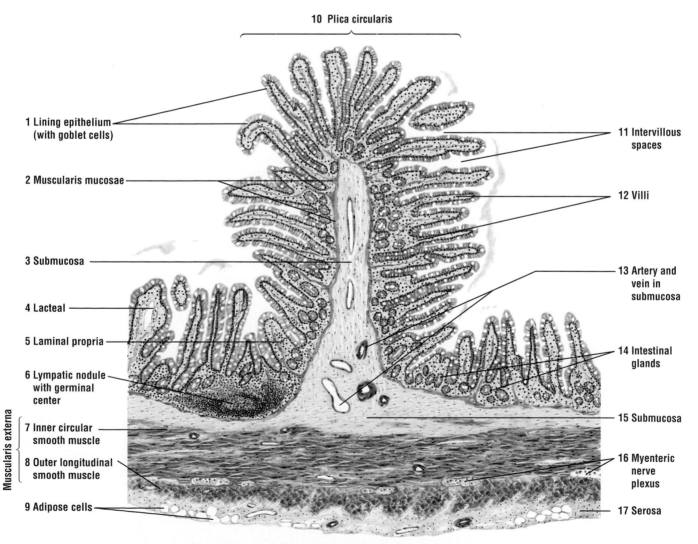

10 Plica circularis

1 Lining epithelium (with goblet cells)
2 Muscularis mucosae
3 Submucosa
4 Lacteal
5 Laminal propria
6 Lymphatic nodule with germinal center
Muscularis externa
7 Inner circular smooth muscle
8 Outer longitudinal smooth muscle
9 Adipose cells

11 Intervillous spaces
12 Villi
13 Artery and vein in submucosa
14 Intestinal glands
15 Submucosa
16 Myenteric nerve plexus
17 Serosa

FIGURE 13.3 ■ Small intestine: jejunum (transverse section). Stain: hematoxylin and eosin. Low magnification.

FIGURE 13.4 ■ Intestinal Glands With Paneth Cells and Enteroendocrine Cells

Adjacent to the **muscularis mucosae (5, 10)** are the **intestinal glands (7)** with **goblet cells (2)** and cells with striated borders. At the base of the intestinal glands (7) are pyramid-shaped cells with large, acidophilic granules that fill most of the cytoplasm and displace the nucleus toward the base of the cell. These are the **Paneth cells (4, 9);** they are found throughout the small intestine.

Enteroendocrine cells (3, 8) are interspersed among the intestinal gland cells, **mitotic gland cells (1, 6),** goblet cells (2), and Paneth cells (4, 9). Enteroendocrine cells contain fine granules that are located in the basal cytoplasm and close to the lamina propria and the blood vessels. Most enteroendocrine cells take up and decarboxylate precursors of biogenic monoamines and are, therefore, designated as amine precursor uptake and decarboxylation (APUD) cells. The APUD cells are found in the epithelia of the gastrointestinal tract (stomach, small and large intestines), respiratory tract, pancreas, and thyroid glands.

FIGURE 13.5 ■ Small Intestine: Jejunum With Paneth Cells

A low-magnification photomicrograph illustrates the mucosa of the jejunum. The **villi (1)** are lined by **simple columnar epithelium (2)** with a brush border. Between the columnar cells are the mucus-filled **goblet cells (3).** Located in the **lamina propria (6)** of each villus are lymphatic cells, macrophages, smooth muscle cells, **blood vessels (7),** and lymphatic lacteals (not visible). Between the villi are the **intestinal glands (8),** whose bases contain red-staining or eosinophilic secretory granules of **Paneth cells (9).** The intestinal glands (8) end near the **muscularis mucosae (4),** inferior to which is the **submucosa (5).**

FUNCTIONAL CORRELATIONS: Paneth Cells and Enteroendocrine Cells in the Small Intestine

Paneth cells, located in the bases of intestinal glands, are exocrine cells and produce **lysozyme,** an antibacterial enzyme that digests bacterial cell walls and destroys them. Paneth cells may also have some phagocytic functions. Thus, these cells have an important function in controlling the microbial flora in the small intestine.

Enteroendocrine cells in the small intestine secrete numerous **regulatory hormones,** including **gastric inhibitory peptide, secretin,** and **cholecystokinin (pancreozymin).** To release these hormones directly into the capillaries, the secretory granules in these cells are located in the base of the cells, which are adjacent to the lamina propria and the capillaries. Once these regulatory hormones enter the bloodstream, they control the release of gastric and pancreatic secretions, induce intestinal motility, and stimulate contraction of the gallbladder to release bile, among other functions.

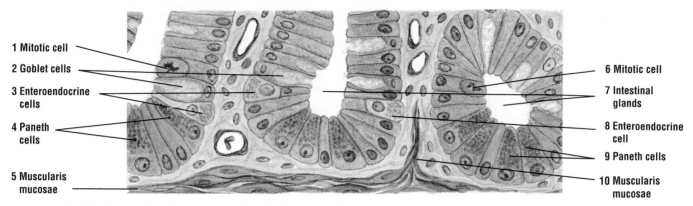

1 Mitotic cell

2 Goblet cells

3 Enteroendocrine cells

4 Paneth cells

5 Muscularis mucosae

6 Mitotic cell

7 Intestinal glands

8 Enteroendocrine cell

9 Paneth cells

10 Muscularis mucosae

FIGURE 13.4 ■ Intestinal glands with Paneth cells and enteroendocrine cells. Stain: hematoxylin and eosin. High magnification.

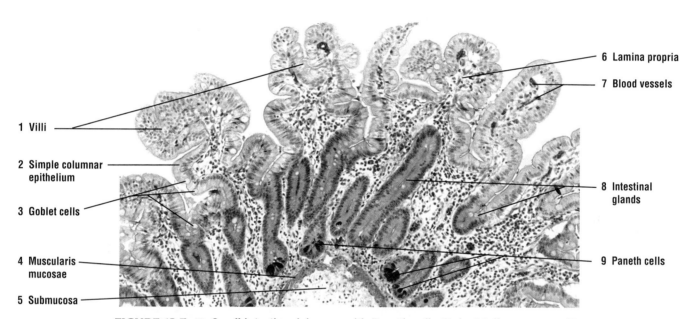

1 Villi

2 Simple columnar epithelium

3 Goblet cells

4 Muscularis mucosae

5 Submucosa

6 Lamina propria

7 Blood vessels

8 Intestinal glands

9 Paneth cells

FIGURE 13.5 ■ Small intestine: jejunum with Paneth cells. Stain: Mallory-azan. ×40.

FIGURE 13.6 ■ Small Intestine: Ileum With Lymphatic Nodules (Peyer's Patches) (Transverse Section)

A characteristic feature of the ileum is the aggregations of **lymphatic nodules (5, 12)** called **Peyer's patches (5, 12).** Each Peyer's patch is an aggregation of numerous lymphatic nodules that are located in the wall of the ileum opposite the mesenteric attachment. Most of the lymphatic nodules (5, 12) exhibit **germinal centers (5).** The lymphatic nodules (5, 12) usually coalesce, and the boundaries between them become indistinct.

The lymphatic nodules (5, 12) originate in the diffuse lymphatic tissue of the **lamina propria (10).** Villi are absent in the area of the intestinal lumen where the nodules reach the surface of the mucosa. Typically, the lymphatic nodules (5, 12) extend into the **submucosa (6),** disrupt the **muscularis mucosae (13),** and spread out in the loose connective tissue of the submucosa (6).

Also illustrated are the **surface epithelium (1)** that covers the **villi (2, 8), intestinal glands (4, 11), lacteals** in the **villi (3, 9),** the **inner circular layer (14a)** and **outer longitudinal layer (14b)** of the **muscularis externa (14),** and the **serosa (7).**

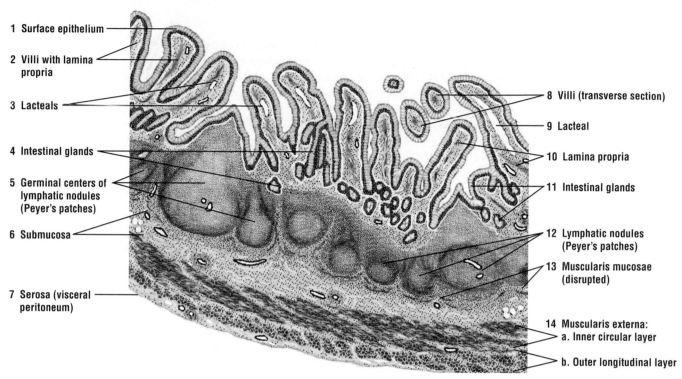

1 Surface epithelium

2 Villi with lamina propria

3 Lacteals

4 Intestinal glands

5 Germinal centers of lymphatic nodules (Peyer's patches)

6 Submucosa

7 Serosa (visceral peritoneum)

8 Villi (transverse section)

9 Lacteal

10 Lamina propria

11 Intestinal glands

12 Lymphatic nodules (Peyer's patches)

13 Muscularis mucosae (disrupted)

14 Muscularis externa:
a. Inner circular layer
b. Outer longitudinal layer

FIGURE 13.6 ■ Small intestine: ileum with lymphatic nodules (Peyer's patches) (transverse section). Stain: hematoxylin and eosin. Low magnification.

FIGURE 13.7 ■ Small Intestine: Villi

Several **villi (1)** are sectioned longitudinally and transversely, and illustrated at a higher magnification. The simple columnar **surface epithelium (2)** that covers the villi (1) contains mucus-secreting **goblet cells (7)** and absorptive cells with **striated borders (microvilli) (3).** To show mucus, the section was stained for carbohydrates. As a result, the goblet cells (7) are stained magenta red.

A thin **basement membrane (8)** is visible between the surface epithelium (2) and the **lamina propria (4).** In the core of the lamina propria (4) are found connective tissue cells and collagen fibers, blood cells, and **smooth muscle fibers (5).** Also present in each villus (but not always seen in sections) is a **central lacteal (6),** a lymphatic vessel lined with endothelium. Arterioles, one or more venules, and **capillaries (9)** are also visible in the villi.

FUNCTIONAL CORRELATIONS: Peyer's Patches in the Ileum

The lamina propria and submucosa contain numerous and large aggregates of large lymphatic nodules, called Peyer's patches. Overlying these lymphatic patches are specialized epithelial cells, called the **M cells.** The cell membranes of M cells show deep invaginations that contain both macrophages and lymphocytes. The lymphatic nodules of Peyer's patches contain numerous **B lymphocytes,** some **T lymphocytes, macrophages,** and **plasma cells.** M cells continually sample the **antigens** of the intestinal lumen, ingest the antigens, and present them to the underlying lymphocytes and macrophages in the lamina propria. The antigens that reach the underlying lymphocytes and macrophages then initiate the proper immunologic responses to these foreign molecules.

Small Intestine

The small intestine performs numerous digestive functions, including (1) continuation and completion of **digestion** (initiated in the oral cavity and stomach) of food products (chyme) by chemicals and enzymes produced in the liver and pancreas, and by cells in its own mucosa; (2) selective **absorption** of nutrients into the blood and lymph capillaries; (3) **transportation** of chyme and digestive waste material to the large intestine; and (4) release of different **hormones** into the bloodstream to regulate the secretory functions and motility of digestive organs.

On the surface epithelium, **goblet cells** secrete **mucus** that lubricates, coats, and protects the intestinal surface from the corrosive actions of digestive chemicals and enzymes. The outer **glycocalyx** coat on absorptive cells not only protects the intestinal surface from digestion, but also contains numerous enzymes required for the terminal digestion of food products. These enzymes are produced by absorptive epithelial cells.

Absorption of nutrients into the cell interior occurs via diffusion, facilitated diffusion, osmosis, and active transport. Intestinal cells absorb **amino acids, glucose,** and **fatty acids**—the end products of protein, carbohydrate, and fat digestion, respectively. Amino acids, water, various ions, and glucose are transported through intestinal cells into the **blood capillaries** present in the lamina propria of the villi, from which they pass to the liver via the portal vein. Most of the long-chain fatty acids and monoglycerides, however, do not enter the capillaries, but instead enter the tiny, blind-ending lymphatic vessels, called **lacteals,** that are also located in the lamina propria of each villus. The presence of smooth muscle fibers in the villi causes contractions of the villi and move the contents of the lacteals from the villi into larger lymph vessels in the submucosa and into the mesenteries.

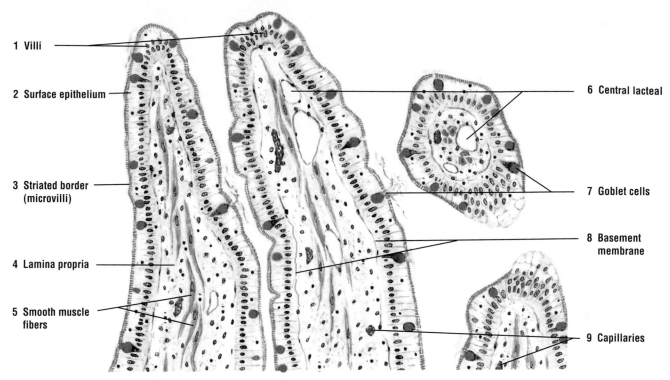

1 Villi

2 Surface epithelium

3 Striated border (microvilli)

4 Lamina propria

5 Smooth muscle fibers

6 Central lacteal

7 Goblet cells

8 Basement membrane

9 Capillaries

FIGURE 13.7 ■ Villi of small intestine (longitudinal and transverse sections). Stain: periodic acid-Schiff. Medium magnification.

FIGURE 13.8 ■ Large Intestine: Colon and Mesentery (Transverse Section)

The wall of the colon has the same basic layers as the small intestine. The **mucosa (4–7)** consists of simple columnar **epithelium (4)**, **intestinal glands (5)**, **lamina propria (6)**, and **muscularis mucosae (7)**. The underlying **submucosa (8)** contains connective tissue cells and fibers, various blood vessels, and nerves. Two smooth muscle layers make up the **muscularis externa (13)**. The **serosa (visceral peritoneum** and **mesentery) (3, 17)** covers the transverse colon and sigmoid colon. There are several modifications in the colon wall that distinguish it from other regions of the digestive tract (tube).

The colon does not have villi or plicae circulares, and the luminal surface of the mucosa is smooth. In the undistended colon, the mucosa (4–7) and submucosa (8) exhibit **temporary folds (12)**. In the lamina propria (6) and the submucosa (8) of the colon are **lymphatic nodules (9, 11)**.

The smooth muscle layers in the muscularis externa (13) of the colon are modified. The **inner circular muscle layer (16)** is continuous in the colon wall, whereas the outer muscle layer is condensed into three broad, longitudinal bands called **taeniae coli (1, 10)**. A very thin **outer longitudinal muscle layer (15)**, which is often discontinuous, is found between the taeniae coli (1, 10). The parasympathetic ganglion cells of the **myenteric (Auerbach's) nerve plexus (2, 14)** are found between the two smooth muscle layers of the muscularis externa (13).

The transverse and sigmoid colon are attached to the body wall by a **mesentery (18).** As a result, the serosa (3, 17) is the outermost layer.

FIGURE 13.9 ■ Large Intestine: Colon Wall (Transverse Section)

A low-magnification photomicrograph illustrates a portion of the colon wall. The simple columnar epithelium contains the **absorptive columnar cells (1)** and the mucus-filled **goblet cells (2, 6)**, which increase in number toward the terminal end of the colon. The **intestinal glands (4)** in the colon are deep and straight, and extend through the **lamina propria (3)** to the **muscularis mucosae (8)**. The lamina propria (3) and **submucosa (9)** are filled with aggregations of lymphatic cells and **lymphatic nodules (5, 7)**.

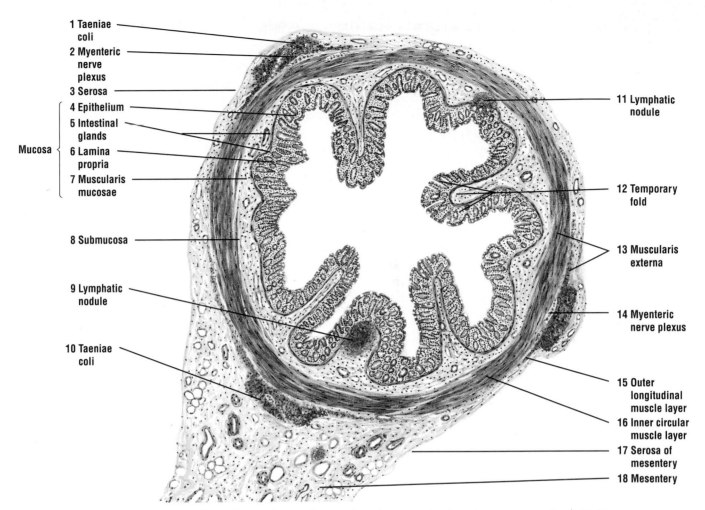

1 Taeniae coli
2 Myenteric nerve plexus
3 Serosa
4 Epithelium
5 Intestinal glands
6 Lamina propria
7 Muscularis mucosae

Mucosa

8 Submucosa
9 Lymphatic nodule
10 Taeniae coli

11 Lymphatic nodule
12 Temporary fold
13 Muscularis externa
14 Myenteric nerve plexus
15 Outer longitudinal muscle layer
16 Inner circular muscle layer
17 Serosa of mesentery
18 Mesentery

FIGURE 13.8 ■ Large intestine: colon and mesentery (panoramic view, transverse section). Stain: hematoxylin and eosin. Low magnification.

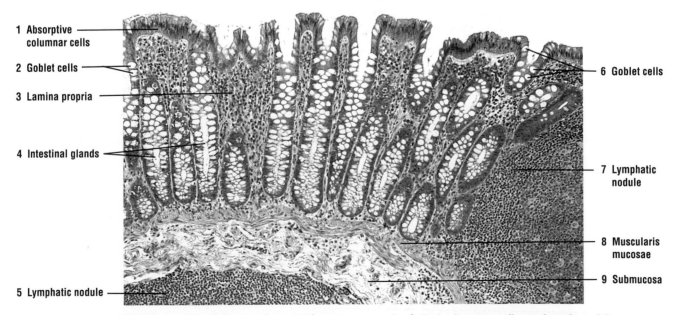

1 Absorptive columnar cells
2 Goblet cells
3 Lamina propria
4 Intestinal glands
5 Lymphatic nodule

6 Goblet cells
7 Lymphatic nodule
8 Muscularis mucosae
9 Submucosa

FIGURE 13.9 ■ Large intestine: colon wall (transverse section). Stain: hematoxylin and eosin. ×30.

FIGURE 13.10 ■ Large Intestine: Colon Wall (Transverse Section)

A section of undistended colon wall shows the **temporary fold (9)** of the mucosa **(2–4)** and **submucosa (5, 12)**. The four layers of the wall that are continuous with those of the small intestine are the mucosa **(2–4)**, submucosa **(5, 12)**, **muscularis externa (6)**, and **serosa (7)**.

Villi are absent in the colon, but the **lamina propria (3)** is indented by long **intestinal glands** (crypts of Lieberkühn) **(1, 10)** that extend through the lamina propria **(3)** to the **muscularis mucosae (4, 11)**.

The **lining epithelium (2)**, with numerous goblet cells, is simple columnar and continues into the intestinal glands **(1, 10)**. Some of the intestinal glands **(1, 10)** are sectioned in longitudinal, transverse, or oblique planes.

The lamina propria **(2)**, as in the small intestine, contains abundant diffuse lymphatic tissue. A distinct **lymphatic nodule (13)** can be seen deep in the lamina propria **(2)**. Some of the larger lymphatic nodules may extend through the muscularis mucosae **(4, 11)** into the submucosa **(5, 12)**.

The muscularis externa **(6)** is atypical. The longitudinal layer of the muscularis externa **(6)** is arranged into strips or bands of smooth muscle called the **taeniae coli (15)**. As in the circular layer, the taeniae coli **(15)** are supplied by **blood vessels (16)**. The parasympathetic ganglia of the **myenteric plexus (8, 14)** are located between the muscle layers of the muscularis externa **(6)**.

The serosa **(7)** covers the connective tissue and **adipose cells (17)** in the transverse and sigmoid colon. The ascending and descending colon are retroperitoneal, and their posterior surface is lined with adventitia.

FUNCTIONAL CORRELATIONS: Large Intestine

The principal functions of the large intestine are to absorb **water** and **minerals (electrolytes)** from the indigestible material that was transported from the ileum of the small intestine and to compact them into feces for elimination from the body. Consistent with these functions, the epithelium of the large intestine contains **columnar absorptive cells** (similar to those in the epithelium of the small intestine) and mucus-secreting **goblet cells,** which produce mucus for lubricating the lumen of the large intestine to facilitate passage of the feces. No digestive enzymes are produced by the cells of large intestine.

Histologic Differences Between the Small and Large Intestines (Colon)

The large intestine lacks plicae circulares and villi that characterize the small intestine. Intestinal glands are present in the large intestine and are similar to those of the small intestine. However, they are deeper (longer) and lack the Paneth cells in their bases. The epithelium of the large intestine also contains different enteroendocrine cells.

Although present in the small intestine, **goblet cells** are more numerous in the large intestine epithelium. Also, the number of goblet cells increases from the cecum toward the terminal portion of the sigmoid colon. The lamina propria of the large intestine contains many solitary lymphatic nodules, lymphocyte accumulations, plasma cells, and macrophages.

In contrast to the small intestine, the muscularis externa of the large intestine and cecum shows a unique arrangement. The inner circular smooth muscle layer is present. However, the outer longitudinal muscle layer is arranged into three longitudinal muscle strips called **taenia coli.** The contractions or tonus in the taenia coli forms sacculations in the large intestine, called **haustra** (see Overview Figure 13).

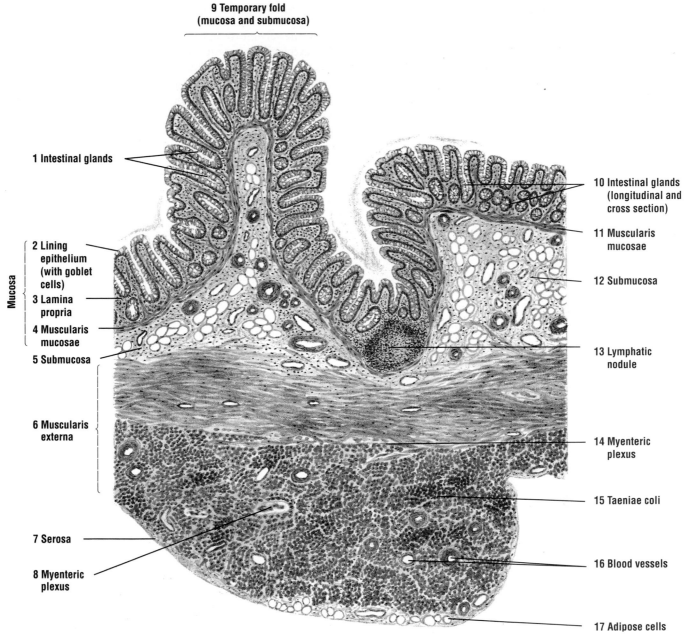

**9 Temporary fold
(mucosa and submucosa)**

1 Intestinal glands

Mucosa

2 Lining
epithelium
(with goblet
cells)
3 Lamina
propria
4 Muscularis
mucosae
5 Submucosa

6 Muscularis
externa

7 Serosa

8 Myenteric
plexus

10 Intestinal glands
(longitudinal and
cross section)

11 Muscularis
mucosae

12 Submucosa

13 Lymphatic
nodule

14 Myenteric
plexus

15 Taeniae coli

16 Blood vessels

17 Adipose cells

FIGURE 13.10 ■ Large intestine: colon wall (transverse section). Stain: hematoxylin and eosin. Medium
magnification.

FIGURE 13.11 ■ Appendix (Panoramic View, Transverse Section)

This figure illustrates a cross section of the vermiform appendix at low magnification. Its morphology is similar to that of the colon, except for certain modifications.

In comparing the mucosa of the appendix with that of the colon, the **lining epithelium (1)** contains numerous goblet cells, the underlying **lamina propria (3)** shows **intestinal glands (5)** (crypts of Lieberkühn), and there is a **muscularis mucosae (2).** The intestinal glands (5) in the appendix are less well developed, shorter, and often spaced farther apart than those in the colon. **Diffuse lymphatic tissue (6)** in the lamina propria (3) is abundant and is present often in the **submucosa (8).**

Lymphatic nodules (4, 9) with germinal centers are numerous and highly characteristic of the appendix. These nodules originate in the lamina propria (3) and may extend from the surface epithelium (1) to the submucosa (8).

The submucosa (8) has numerous **blood vessels (11).** The **muscularis externa (7)** consists of the **inner circular layer (7a)** and **outer longitudinal layer (7b).** The **parasympathetic ganglia (12)** of the **myenteric plexus (12)** are located between the inner (7a) and outer (7b) smooth muscle layers of the muscularis externa.

The outermost layer of the appendix is the **serosa (10)** under which are seen **adipose cells (13).**

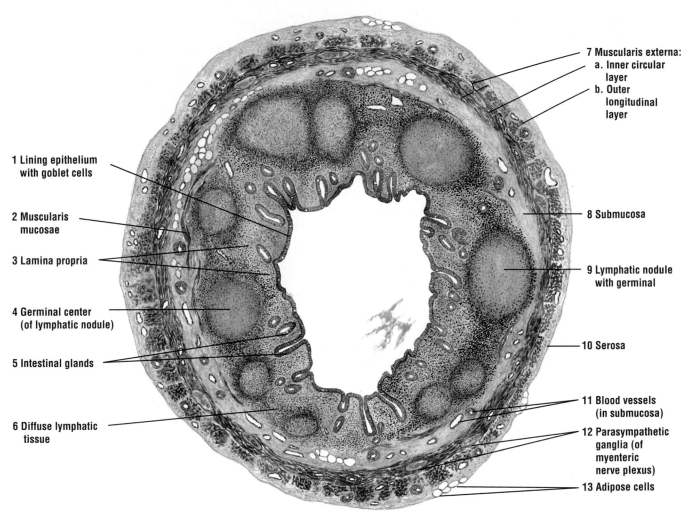

1 Lining epithelium with goblet cells

2 Muscularis mucosae

3 Lamina propria

4 Germinal center (of lymphatic nodule)

5 Intestinal glands

6 Diffuse lymphatic tissue

7 Muscularis externa:
a. Inner circular layer
b. Outer longitudinal layer

8 Submucosa

9 Lymphatic nodule with germinal

10 Serosa

11 Blood vessels (in submucosa)

12 Parasympathetic ganglia (of myenteric nerve plexus)

13 Adipose cells

FIGURE 13.11 ■ Appendix (panoramic view, transverse section). Stain: hematoxylin and eosin. Low magnification.

FIGURE 13.12 ■ Rectum (Panoramic View, Transverse Section)

The histology of the upper rectum is similar to that of the colon.

The **surface epithelium (1)** of the **lumen (5)** is lined by simple columnar cells with striated borders and goblet cells. The **intestinal glands (4), adipose cells (12),** and **lymphatic nodules (10)** in the **lamina propria (2)** are similar to those in the colon. The intestinal glands are longer, closer together, and filled with goblet cells. Beneath the lamina propria (2) is the **muscularis mucosae (11).**

The **longitudinal folds (3)** in the upper rectum and colon are temporary. These folds (3) contain a core of **submucosa (8)** covered by the mucosa. Permanent longitudinal folds (rectal columns) are found in the lower rectum and the anal canal.

Taeniae coli of the colon continue into the rectum, where the **muscularis externa (13)** acquires the typical **inner circular (13a)** and **outer longitudinal (13b)** smooth muscle layers. Between these two smooth muscle layers are the **parasympathetic ganglia** of the **myenteric (Auerbach's) plexus (14).**

Adventitia (9) covers a portion of the rectum, and serosa covers the remainder. Numerous **blood vessels (6, 7, 15)** are found in both the submucosa (8) and adventitia (9).

FIGURE 13.13 ■ Anorectal Junction (Longitudinal Section)

The portion of the anal canal above the **anorectal junction (7)** represents the lowermost part of the rectum. The part of the anal canal below the anorectal junction (7) shows the transition from the **simple columnar epithelium (1)** to the **stratified squamous epithelium (8)** of the skin. The change from the rectal mucosa to the anal mucosa occurs at the anorectal junction (7).

The rectal mucosa is similar to the mucosa of the colon. The **intestinal glands (3)** are somewhat shorter and spaced farther apart. As a result, the **lamina propria (2)** is more prominent, diffuse lymphatic tissue is more abundant, and solitary **lymphatic nodules (11)** are more numerous.

The **muscularis mucosae (4)** and the intestinal glands (3) of the digestive tract terminate in the vicinity of the anorectal junction (7). The lamina propria (2) of the rectum is replaced by the dense irregular connective tissue of the **lamina propria of the anal canal (9).** The **submucosa (5)** of the rectum merges with the connective tissue in the lamina propria of the anal canal, a region that is highly vascular. The **internal hemorrhoidal plexus (10)** of veins lies in the mucosa of the anal canal. Blood vessels from this region continue into the submucosa (5) of the rectum.

The circular smooth muscle layer of the **muscularis externa (6)** increases in thickness in the upper region of the anal canal and forms the **internal anal sphincter (6).** Lower in the anal canal, the internal anal sphincter (6) is replaced by skeletal muscles of the **external anal sphincter (12).** External to the external anal sphincter (12) is the skeletal **levator ani muscle (13).**

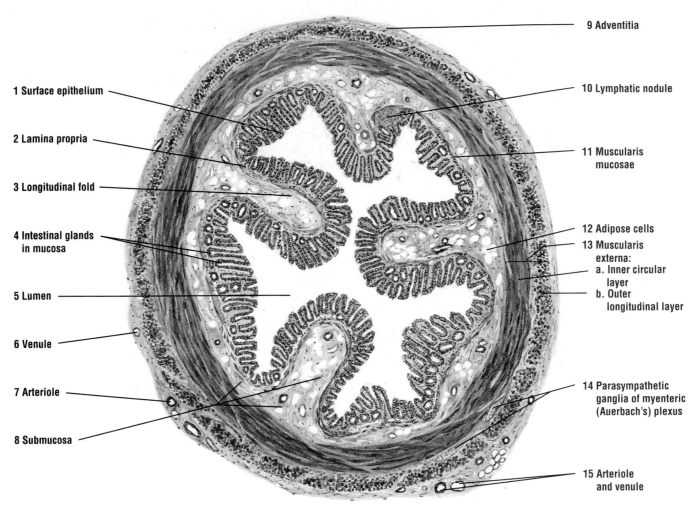

1 Surface epithelium

2 Lamina propria

3 Longitudinal fold

4 Intestinal glands
  in mucosa

5 Lumen

6 Venule

7 Arteriole

8 Submucosa

9 Adventitia

10 Lymphatic nodule

11 Muscularis
   mucosae

12 Adipose cells
13 Muscularis
   externa:
   a. Inner circular
     layer
   b. Outer
     longitudinal layer

14 Parasympathetic
   ganglia of myenteric
   (Auerbach's) plexus

15 Arteriole
   and venule

FIGURE 13.12 ■ Rectum (panoramic view, transverse section). Stain: hematoxylin and eosin. Low magnification.

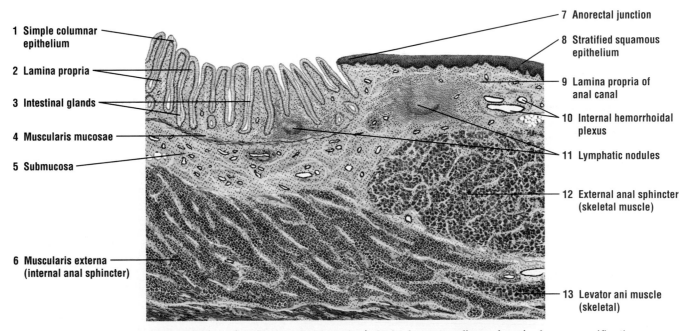

1 Simple columnar
  epithelium

2 Lamina propria

3 Intestinal glands

4 Muscularis mucosae

5 Submucosa

6 Muscularis externa
  (internal anal sphincter)

7 Anorectal junction

8 Stratified squamous
  epithelium

9 Lamina propria of
  anal canal

10 Internal hemorrhoidal
   plexus

11 Lymphatic nodules

12 External anal sphincter
   (skeletal muscle)

13 Levator ani muscle
   (skeletal)

FIGURE 13.13 ■ Anorectal junction (longitudinal section). Stain: hematoxylin and eosin. Low magnification.

CHAPTER 13 ■ Summary

Digestive System: Small and Large Intestines

Small Intestine

- Long, convoluted tube divided into duodenum, jejunum, and ileum
- Duodenum is the shortest segment with broad, tall, and numerous villi
- Digests gastric contents and absorbs nutrients into blood capillaries and lymphatic lacteals
- Transports chyme and waste products to large intestine
- Releases numerous hormones to regulate secretory functions and motility of digestive organs
- Amino acids, water, ions, glucose and other substances are absorbed and transported in blood capillaries
- Long-chain fatty acids and monoglycerides are transported by lymphatic lacteals
- Contains numerous permanent surface modifications that increase cellular contact for absorption
- Plicae circulares are spiral folds with submucosa core that extend into intestinal lumen
- Villi are fingerlike projections of lamina propria that extend into the intestinal lumen
- Microvilli are cytoplasmic extensions of absorptive cells that extend into intestinal lumen
- Microvilli are coated with brush border enzymes that digest food products before absorption
- Villi contain a core of connective tissue with capillaries, lacteal, and smooth muscle strands
- Lamina propria is filled with lymphocytes, plasma cells, macrophages, eosinophils, and mast cells
- Smooth muscle strands in lamina propria of villi induce their movement and contractions

Cells of Small Intestine

- Absorptive cells with microvilli covered by glycocalyx are most common in intestinal epithelium
- Goblet cells, interspersed between absorptive cells, increase in number toward distal region
- Enteroendocrine cells are scattered throughout the epithelium and intestinal glands
- Secretory granules of enteroendocrine cells located at base of cells and close to capillaries
- Enteroendocrine cells secrete numerous regulatory hormones for the digestive system
- Undifferentiated cells in the base of intestinal glands replace worn-out luminal cells
- Paneth cells with pink eosinophilic granules in cytoplasm are located in the intestinal glands
- Paneth cells produce the antibacterial enzyme lysozyme to control microbial flora in intestine
- M cells are specialized cells that cover the lymphatic Peyer's patches

Glands of Small Intestine

- Intestinal glands located between villi throughout the small intestine
- Intestinal glands open into the intestinal lumen at the base of the villi
- Duodenal glands in the submucosa of duodenum are characteristic of this region
- Duodenal glands penetrate muscularis mucosae to discharge mucus and bicarbonate secretions
- Bicarbonate secretions enter base of intestinal glands and protect duodenum from acidic chyme
- Polypeptide urogastrone from duodenal glands inhibits hydrochloric acid secretions

Lymphatic Accumulations in Small Intestine

- Peyer's patches are numerous aggregations of permanent lymphatic nodules
- Peyer's patches found primarily in the lamina propria and submucosa of terminal part of intestine
- Overlying Peyer's patches are specialized M cells, which are not anywhere else in the intestine
- M cells show deep invaginations that contain macrophages and lymphocytes
- M cells sample intestinal antigens and present them to underlying lymphocytes for response

Large Intestine

- Situated between anus and the terminal end of ileum
- Shorter and less convoluted than small intestine
- Consists of cecum, ascending, transverse, descending, and sigmoid sections
- Semifluid chyme enters through ileocecal valve
- At terminal end, semifluid residues become hardened or semisolid feces
- Main function is the absorption of water and electrolytes
- Epithelium consists of simple columnar epithelium with increased number of goblet cells

- Goblet cells produce mucus for lubricating the canal to facilitate passage of feces
- No enzymes or chemicals produced, but enteroendocrine cells are present in the epithelium
- No plicae circulares, villi, or Paneth cells are present; intestinal glands are deeper
- Increased numbers of solitary lymphatic nodules with cells are present in lamina propria
- Muscularis externa contains inner circular layer with outer layer arranged in three strips, taenia coli
- Contractions of taenia coli form sacculations or haustra

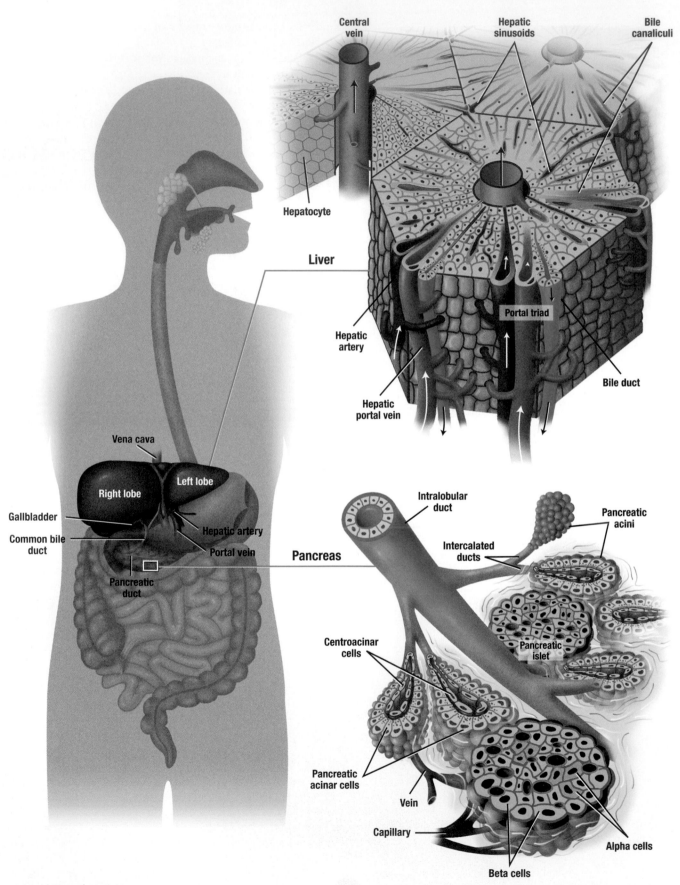

OVERVIEW FIGURE 14 ■ A section from the liver and the pancreas is illustrated, with emphasis on the details of the liver lobule and the duct system of the exocrine pancreas.

CHAPTER **14**

Digestive System: Liver, Gallbladder, and Pancreas

The accessory organs of the digestive system are located outside of the digestive tube. Excretory glands from the salivary glands open into the oral cavity. The **liver, gallbladder,** and **pancreas** are also **accessory organs** of the digestive tract that deliver their secretory products to the small intestine by excretory ducts. The **common bile duct** from the liver and the main pancreatic duct from the pancreas join in the duodenal loop to form a single duct common to both organs. This duct then penetrates the duodenal wall and enters the lumen of the small intestine. The gallbladder joins the common bile duct via the cystic duct. Thus, **bile** from the gallbladder and **digestive enzymes** from the pancreas enter the duodenum via a common duct.

Liver

The liver is located in a very strategic position. All nutrients and liquids that are absorbed in the intestines enter the liver through the **hepatic portal vein,** except the complex lipid products, which are transported by the lymph vessels. The absorbed products first percolate through the liver capillaries called **sinusoids.** Nutrient-rich blood in the hepatic portal vein is first brought to the liver before it enters the general circulation. Because venous blood from the digestive organs in the hepatic portal vein is poor in oxygen, the **hepatic artery** from the aorta supplies liver cells with oxygenated blood, forming a dual blood supply to the liver.

The liver exhibits repeating hexagonal units called **liver (hepatic) lobules.** In the center of each lobule is the **central vein,** from which radiate plates of liver cells, called **hepatocytes,** and sinusoids toward the periphery. Here, the connective tissue forms **portal canals** or **portal areas,** where branches of the hepatic artery, hepatic portal vein, **bile duct,** and lymph vessels can be seen. In human liver, three to six portal areas can be seen per lobule. Venous and arterial blood from the peripheral portal areas first mix in the liver sinusoids as it flows toward the central vein. From here, blood enters the general circulation through the hepatic veins that leave the liver and enter the inferior vena cava.

The hepatic sinusoids are tortuous, dilated blood channels lined by a discontinuous layer of **fenestrated endothelial cells** that also exhibit fenestrations and discontinuous basal lamina. The hepatic sinusoids are separated from the underlying hepatocytes by a subendothelial **perisinusoidal space** (of Disse). As a result, ingested material carried in the sinusoidal blood has a direct access through the discontinuous endothelial wall with the hepatocytes. The structure and the tortuous path of sinusoids through the liver allows for an efficient exchange of materials between hepatocytes and blood. In addition to the endothelial cells, the hepatic sinusoids also contain macrophages, called Kupffer cells, located on the luminal side of the endothelial cells.

Hepatocytes secrete bile into tiny channels called **bile canaliculi** located between individual hepatocytes. The canaliculi converge at the periphery of liver lobules in the portal areas as **bile ducts.** The bile ducts then drain into larger hepatic ducts that carry bile out of the liver. Within the liver lobules, bile flows in bile canaliculi toward the bile duct in the portal area, whereas blood in the sinusoids flows toward the central vein. As a result, bile and blood do not mix.

313

Gallbladder

The gallbladder is a small, hollow organ attached to the inferior surface of the liver. Bile is produced by liver hepatocytes and then flows to and is stored in the gallbladder. Bile leaves the gallbladder via the cystic duct and enters the duodenum via the **common bile duct** through the **major duodenal papilla,** a fingerlike protrusion of the duodenal wall into the lumen.

The gallbladder is not a gland because its main function is to store and concentrate bile by absorbing its water. Bile is released into the digestive tract as a result of hormonal stimulation after a meal. When the gallbladder is empty, the mucosa exhibits deep **folds.**

Exocrine Pancreas

The pancreas is a soft, elongated organ located posterior to the stomach. The **head** of the pancreas lies in the duodenal loop and the **tail** extends across the abdominal cavity to the spleen. Most of the pancreas is an **exocrine gland.** The exocrine secretory units or acini contain pyramid-shaped **acinar cells,** whose apices are filled with secretory granules. These granules contain the precursors of several pancreatic **digestive enzymes** that are secreted into the excretory ducts in an inactive form.

The secretory acini are subdivided into **lobules** and bound together by loose connective tissue. The **excretory ducts** in the exocrine pancreas start from within the center of individual acini as pale-staining centroacinar cells, which continue into the short **intercalated ducts.** The intercalated ducts merge to form **intralobular ducts** in the connective tissue, which, in turn, join to form larger **interlobular ducts** that empty into the **main pancreatic duct.** Excretory ducts of the pancreas do not have striated ducts.

Endocrine Pancreas

The endocrine units of the pancreas are scattered among the exocrine acini as isolated, pale-staining vascularized units called **pancreatic islets** (of Langerhans). Each islet is surrounded by fine fibers of reticular connective tissue. With special immunocytochemical processes, four cell types can be identified in each pancreatic islet: **alpha, beta, delta,** and **pancreatic polypeptide (PP) cells.**

Alpha cells constitute about 20% of the islets and are located primarily around the islet periphery. The beta cells are most numerous, constituting about 70% of the islet cells, and are primarily concentrated in the center of the islet. The remaining cell types are few in number and are located in various places throughout the islets.

FIGURE 14.1 ■ Pig Liver (Panoramic View, Transverse Section)

In the pig's liver, connective tissue from the hilus extends between the liver lobes as **interlobular septa (5, 9)** and defines the **hepatic (liver) lobules (7).** To illustrate the connective tissue boundaries that form each hepatic lobule (7), a section of pig's liver was stained with Mallory-azan stain, which stains the connective tissue septa (5, 9) dark blue.

A complete hepatic lobule (on the left) and parts of adjacent hepatic lobules (7) are illustrated. The blue-staining interlobular septa (5, 9) contain interlobular branches of the **portal vein (4, 11), bile duct (2, 12),** and **hepatic artery (3, 13),** which are collectively considered **portal areas** or portal canals. At the periphery of each lobule can be seen several portal areas within the interlobular septa (5, 9). Within the interlobular septa (5, 9) are also found small lymphatic vessels and nerves, which are small and only occasionally seen.

In the center of each hepatic lobule (7) is the **central vein (1, 8).** Radiating from each central vein (1, 8) toward the lobule periphery are **plates of hepatic cells (6).** Located between the hepatic plates (6) are blood channels called **hepatic sinusoids (10).** Arterial and venous blood mixes in the hepatic sinusoids (10) and then flows toward the central vein (1, 8) of each lobule (7).

Bile is produced by the liver cells. Bile flows through the very small bile canaliculi between the hepatocytes into the interlobular **bile ducts (2, 12)** (see Figure 14.5).

The interlobular vessels and bile ducts (2–4, 11–13) are highly branched in the liver. In a cross section of the liver lobule, more than one section of these structures can be seen within a portal area.

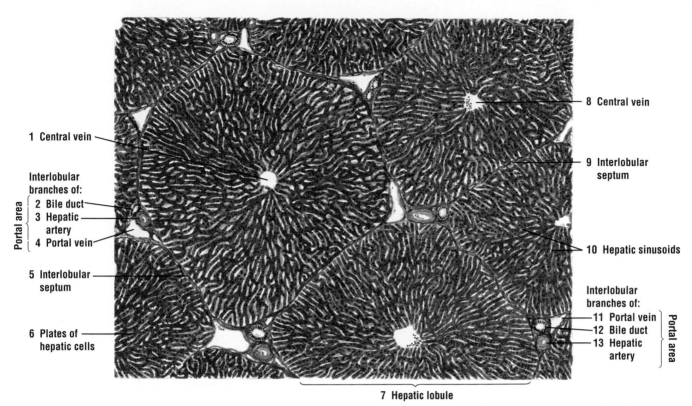

1 Central vein

Interlobular
branches of:
Portal area
  2 Bile duct
  3 Hepatic artery
  4 Portal vein

5 Interlobular septum

6 Plates of hepatic cells

8 Central vein

9 Interlobular septum

10 Hepatic sinusoids

Interlobular
branches of:
Portal area
  11 Portal vein
  12 Bile duct
  13 Hepatic artery

7 Hepatic lobule

FIGURE 14.1 ■ Pig liver lobules (panoramic view, transverse section). Stain: Mallory-azan. Low magnification.

FIGURE 14.2 ■ Primate Liver (Panoramic View, Transverse Section)

In the primate or human liver, the connective tissue septa between individual **hepatic lobules (8)** are not as conspicuous as in the pig, and the liver sinusoids are continuous between lobules. Despite these differences, **portal areas** containing interlobular branches of the **portal veins (2, 11)**, **hepatic arteries (3, 13)**, and **bile ducts (1, 12)** are visible around the lobule (8) peripheries in the **interlobular septa (4, 10)**.

This figure illustrates numerous hepatic lobules (8). In the center of each hepatic lobule (8) is the **central vein (6, 9)**. The **hepatic sinusoids (5)** appear between the **plates of hepatic cells (7)** that radiate from the central veins (6, 9) toward the periphery of the hepatic lobule (8). As illustrated in Figure 14.1, branches of the interlobular vessels and bile ducts are seen within the portal areas of a hepatic lobule (8).

FUNCTIONAL CORRELATIONS

Liver

The liver performs hundreds of functions. Hepatocytes perform more functions than any other cell in the body, and perform both endocrine and exocrine roles.

Exocrine Functions

One major **exocrine function** of hepatocytes is to synthesize and release 500 to 1,200 mL of **bile** into the **bile canaliculi** per day. From these canaliculi, bile flows through a system of ductules and ducts to enter the gallbladder, where it is stored and concentrated by removal of water. Release of bile from the liver and gall bladder is primarily regulated by hormones. Bile flow is increased when a hormone such as **cholecystokinin** is released by the mucosal enteroendocrine cells, stimulated when dietary fats in the chyme enter the duodenum. This hormone causes contraction of smooth muscles in the gallbladder wall and relaxation of the sphincter, allowing the bile to enter the duodenum.

Bile salts in the bile **emulsify fats** in the small intestine (duodenum). This process allows for more efficient digestion of fats by the fat-digesting **pancreatic lipases** produced by the pancreas. The digested fats are subsequently absorbed by cells in the small intestine and enter the blind-ending lymphatic **lacteal** channels located in individual villi. From the lacteals, fats are carried into larger lymphatic ducts that eventually drain into the major veins.

Hepatocytes also excrete **bilirubin**, a toxic chemical formed in the body after degradation of worn-out erythrocytes by liver macrophages, called **Kupffer cells.** Bilirubin is taken up by hepatocytes from the blood and excreted into bile.

Hepatocytes also have an important role in the immune system. **Antibodies** produced by plasma cells in the intestinal lamina propria are taken from blood by hepatocytes and transported into bile canaliculi and bile. From here, antibodies enter the intestinal lumen, where they control the intestinal bacterial flora.

Endocrine Functions

Hepatocytes are also **endocrine cells.** The arrangement of hepatocytes in a liver lobule allows them to take up, metabolize, accumulate, and store numerous products from the blood. Hepatocytes then release many of the metabolized or secreted products back into the bloodstream, as the blood flows through the sinusoids and comes in direct contact with individual hepatocytes.

The endocrine functions of the liver hepatocytes involve synthesis of numerous **plasma proteins,** including albumin and the blood-clotting factors prothrombin and fibrinogen. The liver also stores fats, various vitamins, and carbohydrates as **glycogen.** When the cells of the body need **glucose,** glycogen that is stored in the liver is converted back into glucose and released into the bloodstream.

Hepatocytes also **detoxify** the blood of drugs and harmful substances as it percolates through the sinusoids. **Kupffer cells** in the sinusoids are specialized liver phagocytes derived from blood monocytes. These large, branching cells filter and phagocytose particulate material, cellular debris, and worn-out or damaged erythrocytes that flow through the sinusoids.

The liver also performs vital functions early in life. In the fetus, the liver is the site of **hemopoiesis,** or blood cell production.

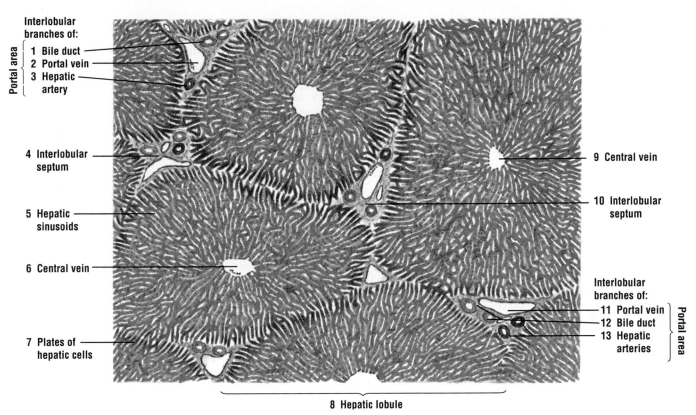

Interlobular
branches of:

Portal area

1 Bile duct
2 Portal vein
3 Hepatic
   artery

4 Interlobular
   septum

5 Hepatic
   sinusoids

6 Central vein

7 Plates of
   hepatic cells

9 Central vein

10 Interlobular
    septum

Interlobular
branches of:

11 Portal vein
12 Bile duct
13 Hepatic
    arteries

Portal area

8 Hepatic lobule

FIGURE 14.2 ■ Primate liver lobules (panoramic view, transverse section). Stain: hematoxylin and eosin. Low magnification.

FIGURE 14.3 ■ Bovine Liver: Liver Lobule (Transverse Section)

A lower-magnification photomicrograph of a bovine liver illustrates several hepatic (liver) lobules. The portal area of the hepatic lobule contains the branches of the **portal vein (5), hepatic artery (6),** and normally a bile duct, which is not seen in this micrograph. From the **central vein (1)** radiate the **plates of hepatic cells (2)** toward the lobule periphery. Located between the plates of hepatic cells (2) are the blood channels called **sinusoids (3).** The sinusoids (3) convey blood from the portal vein (5) and hepatic artery (6) to the central vein (1). Both the central vein (1) and the sinusoids (3) are lined by a discontinuous and fenestrated type of **endothelium (4).**

FIGURE 14.4 ■ Hepatic (Liver) Lobule (Sectional View, Transverse Section)

A section of hepatic lobule between the **central vein (9)** and the peripheral connective tissue **interlobular septum (1, 6)** of the portal area is illustrated in greater detail. In the interlobular septum (1, 6) are transverse sections of a **portal vein (4), hepatic arteries (3), bile ducts (5),** and a **lymphatic vessel (2).** Multiple cross sections of hepatic arteries (3) and bile ducts (5) are attributable either to their branching in the septum or their passage into and out of the septum.

Branches of the portal vein (4) and hepatic artery (3) penetrate the interlobular septum (1, 6) and form the **sinusoids (8, 10).** The sinusoids (8, 10) are situated between **plates of hepatic cells (7)** and follow their branchings and anastomoses. Discontinuous **endothelial cells (10)** line the sinusoids (8, 10) and the central vein (9). **Blood cells** (erythrocytes and leukocytes) in the **sinusoids (8)** drain toward the central vein (9) of each lobule. Present in the sinusoids (10) are also fixed macrophages called the Kupffer cells (see Figure 14.6).

FIGURE 14.5 ■ Bile Canaliculi in Liver Lobule (Osmic Acid Preparation)

Preparation of a liver section with osmic acid and staining with hematoxylin and eosin reveals the **bile canaliculi (3, 5).** Bile canaliculi (3, 5) are tiny channels between individual liver (hepatic) cells in the **hepatic plates (4).** The canaliculi (3, 5) follow an irregular course between the hepatic plates (4) and branch freely within the hepatic plates (4).

The **sinusoids (6)** are lined by discontinuous **endothelial cells (1).** All sinusoids (6) drain toward and open into the **central vein (2).**

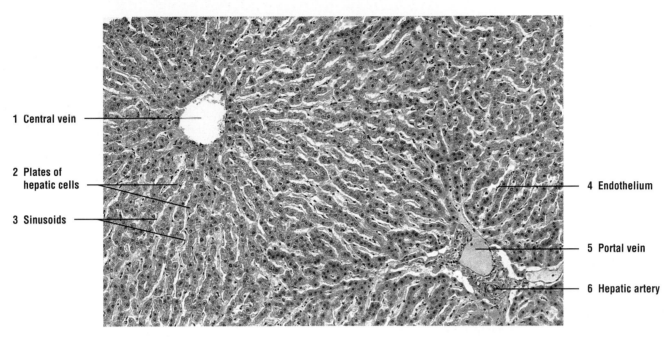

1 Central vein

2 Plates of hepatic cells

3 Sinusoids

4 Endothelium

5 Portal vein

6 Hepatic artery

FIGURE 14.3 ■ Bovine liver: liver lobule (transverse section). Stain: hematoxylin and eosin. ×30.

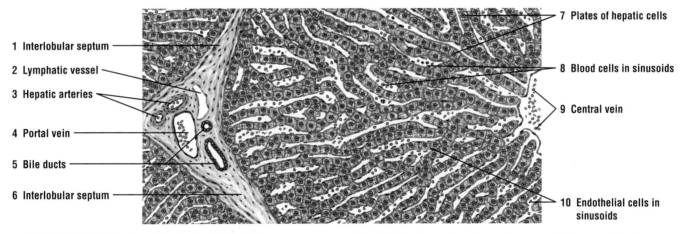

1 Interlobular septum

2 Lymphatic vessel

3 Hepatic arteries

4 Portal vein

5 Bile ducts

6 Interlobular septum

7 Plates of hepatic cells

8 Blood cells in sinusoids

9 Central vein

10 Endothelial cells in sinusoids

FIGURE 14.4 ■ Liver lobule (sectional view, transverse section). Stain: hematoxylin and eosin. High magnification.

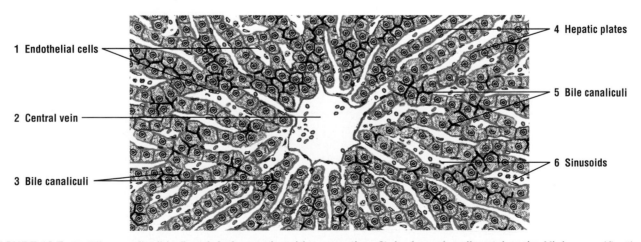

1 Endothelial cells

2 Central vein

3 Bile canaliculi

4 Hepatic plates

5 Bile canaliculi

6 Sinusoids

FIGURE 14.5 ■ Bile canaliculi in liver lobule: osmic acid preparation. Stain: hematoxylin and eosin. High magnification.

FIGURE 14.6 ■ Kupffer Cells in Liver Lobule (India Ink Preparation)

The majority of cells that line the liver **sinusoids (5)** are **endothelial cells (2).** These small cells have an attenuated cytoplasm and a small nucleus. To demonstrate the phagocytic cells in the liver sinusoids (5), an animal was intravenously injected with India ink. The phagocytic **Kupffer cells (3, 7)** ingest the carbon particles from the ink, which fill their cytoplasm with dark deposits. As a result, Kupffer cells (3, 7) become prominent in the sinusoids (5) between the **hepatic plates (6).** Kupffer cells (3, 7) are large cells with several processes and an irregular or stellate outline that protrudes into the sinusoids (5). The nuclei of Kupffer cells (3, 7) are obscured by the ingested carbon particles.

On the periphery of the lobule is visible a section of the connective tissue **interlobular septum (1)** and a part of the **bile duct (4)** that is lined with cuboidal cells.

FIGURE 14.7 ■ Glycogen Granules in Liver Cells (Hepatocytes)

The cytoplasm of liver cells varies in appearance depending on nutritional status. After a meal, liver **hepatocytes (1)** store increased amounts of glycogen in their cytoplasm. With the periodic acid-Schiff stain, the **glycogen granules (2, 4)** in the hepatocyte (1) cytoplasm stain bright red and exhibit an irregular distribution within the cytoplasm.

Also visible in this illustration are hepatic **sinusoids (3)** and flattened **endothelial cells (5)** that line their lumina.

FIGURE 14.8 ■ Reticular Fibers in Liver Lobule

Fine **reticular fibers (6, 8)** provide most of the supporting connective tissue of the liver. In this illustration, the reticular fibers stain black and the liver cells stain pale pink or violet. The reticular fibers (6, 8) line the **sinusoids (8),** support the endothelial cells, and form a denser network of reticula fibers in the wall of the **central vein (7).** The reticular fibers (6, 8) also merge with the **collagen fibers** in the **interlobular septum (1),** where they surround the **portal vein (2)** and the **bile duct (3).**

Also visible in the reticular network are the pink-staining **nuclei of hepatocytes (4)** and the **hepatic plates (5)** that radiate from the central vein (7) toward the interlobular septum (1).

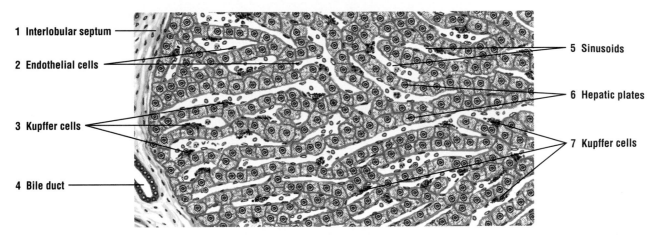

1 Interlobular septum
2 Endothelial cells
3 Kupffer cells
4 Bile duct
5 Sinusoids
6 Hepatic plates
7 Kupffer cells

FIGURE 14.6 ■ Kupffer cells in a liver lobule (India ink preparation). Stain: hematoxylin and eosin. High magnification.

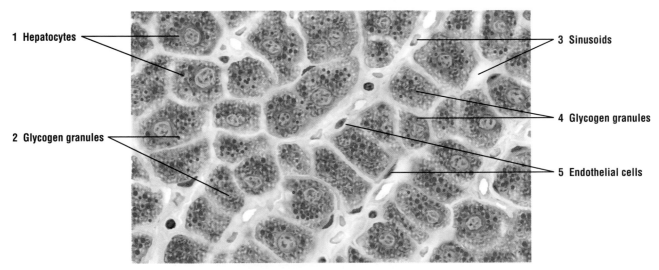

1 Hepatocytes
2 Glycogen granules
3 Sinusoids
4 Glycogen granules
5 Endothelial cells

FIGURE 14.7 ■ Glycogen granules in liver cells. Stain: periodic acid-Schiff with blue counterstain for nuclei. Oil immersion.

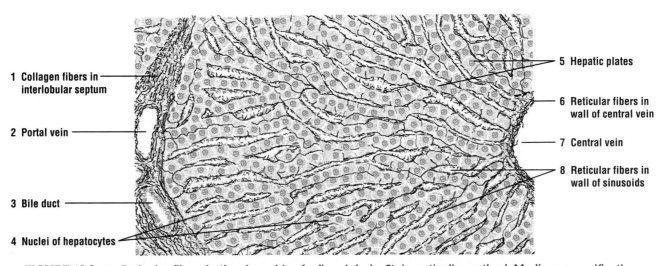

1 Collagen fibers in interlobular septum
2 Portal vein
3 Bile duct
4 Nuclei of hepatocytes
5 Hepatic plates
6 Reticular fibers in wall of central vein
7 Central vein
8 Reticular fibers in wall of sinusoids

FIGURE 14.8 ■ Reticular fibers in the sinusoids of a liver lobule. Stain: reticulin method. Medium magnification.

FIGURE 14.9 ■ Wall of the Gallbladder

The gallbladder is a muscular sac. Its wall consists of mucosa, muscularis, and adventitia or serosa. The wall of the gallbladder does not contain a muscularis mucosae or submucosa.

The mucosa consists of a **simple columnar epithelium** (1) and the underlying connective tissue **lamina propria** (2) that contains loose connective tissue, some diffuse lymphatic tissue, and blood vessels, **venule and arteriole** (9). In the nondistended state, the gallbladder wall shows temporary **mucosal folds** (7) that disappear when the gallbladder becomes distended with bile. The mucosal folds (7) resemble the villi in the small intestine; however, they vary in size and shape and display an irregular arrangement. Between the mucosal folds (7) are found **diverticula** or **crypts** (3, 8) that often form deep indentations in the mucosa. In cross section, the diverticula or crypts (3, 8) in the lamina propria (2) resemble tubular glands. However, there are no glands in the gallbladder proper, except in the neck region of the organ.

External to the lamina propria (2) is the muscularis of the gallbladder with bundles of randomly oriented **smooth muscle fibers** (10) that do not show distinct layers and interlacing **elastic fibers** (4).

Surrounding the bundles of smooth muscle fibers (10) is a thick layer of dense **connective tissue** (6) that contains large blood vessels, **artery and vein** (11), lymphatics, and **nerves** (5).

Serosa (12) covers the entire unattached gallbladder surface. Where the gallbladder is attached to the liver surface, this connective tissue layer is the adventitia.

FUNCTIONAL CORRELATIONS: The Gallbladder

The primary functions of the gallbladder are to collect, store, concentrate, and expel **bile** when it is needed for emulsification of fat. Bile is continually produced by liver hepatocytes and transported via the excretory ducts to the gallbladder for storage. Here, sodium is actively transported through the simple columnar epithelium of the gallbladder into the extracellular connective tissue, creating a strong osmotic pressure. Water and chloride ions passively follow, producing concentrated bile.

Release of bile into the duodenum is under hormonal control. In response to the entrance of dietary fats into the proximal duodenum, the hormone **cholecystokinin (CCK)** is released into the bloodstream by **enteroendocrine cells** located in the intestinal mucosa. CCK is carried in the bloodstream to the gallbladder, where it causes strong rhythmic contractions of the smooth muscle in its wall. At the same time, the smooth **sphincter muscles** around the neck of gallbladder relax. The combination of these two actions forces the bile into the duodenum via the **common bile duct.**

1 Simple columnar epithelium

2 Lamina propria

3 Diverticula or crypts

4 Elastic fibers

5 Nerves

6 Connective tissue

7 Mucosal folds

8 Diverticula or crypts

9 Venule and arteriole

10 Smooth muscle fibers

11 Artery and vein

12 Serosa

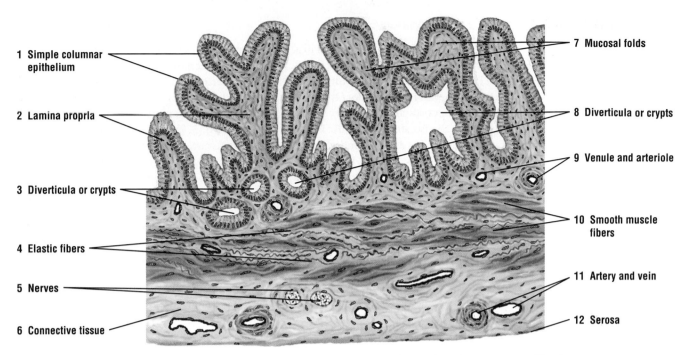

FIGURE 14.9 ■ Wall of gallbladder. Stain: hematoxylin and eosin. Low magnification.

FIGURE 14.10 ■   Pancreas (Sectional View)

The pancreas has both endocrine and exocrine components. The exocrine component forms the majority of the pancreas and consists of closely packed secretory **serous acini** and **zymogenic cells (1)** arranged into small lobules. The lobules are surrounded by thin intralobular and **interlobular connective tissue septa (4, 13)** that contain **blood vessels (5, 9), interlobular ducts (12)**, nerves, and occasionally, a sensory receptor called a **Pacinian corpuscle (11).** Within the serous acini (1) are the isolated **pancreatic islets (of Langerhans) (3, 7).** The pancreatic islets (3, 7) represent the endocrine portion and are the characteristic features of the pancreas.

Each pancreatic acinus (1) consists of pyramid-shaped, protein-secreting **zymogenic** cells (1) that surround a small central lumen. The excretory ducts of the individual acini are visible as pale-staining **centroacinar cells (6, 10)** within their lumina. The secretory products leave the acini via **intercalated (intralobular) ducts (2)** that have small lumina lined with low cuboidal epithelium. The centroacinar cells (6, 10) are continuous with the epithelium of the intercalated ducts (2).

The intercalated ducts (2) drain into interlobular ducts (12) located in the interlobular connective tissue septa (4, 13). The interlobular ducts (12) are lined by a simple cuboidal epithelium that becomes taller and stratified in larger ducts.

Pancreatic islets (3, 7) are demarcated from the surrounding exocrine acini (1) tissue by a thin layer of reticular fibers. The islets (3, 7) are larger than the acini and are compact clusters of epithelial cells permeated by **capillaries (8).** The cells of a pancreatic islet (3, 7) are illustrated at higher magnification in Figures 14.11 and 14.12.

FUNCTIONAL CORRELATIONS: Exocrine Pancreas

The exocrine and endocrine functions of the pancreas are performed by separate exocrine and endocrine cells. The pancreas produces numerous digestive enzymes that exit the gland through a major excretory duct, whereas the different hormones are transported via blood vessels.

Both hormones and vagal stimulation regulate pancreatic exocrine secretions. Two intestinal hormones, **secretin** and **cholecystokinin (CCK),** secreted by the **enteroendocrine (APUD) cells** in the duodenal mucosa into the bloodstream, regulate pancreatic secretions.

In response to the presence of acidic chyme in the small intestine (duodenum), the release of the hormone secretin stimulates exocrine pancreatic cells to produce large amounts of a watery fluid rich in **sodium bicarbonate ions.** This fluid, which has little or no enzymatic activity, is primarily produced by **centroacinar cells** in the acini and by cells that line the smaller **intercalated ducts.** The main function of this bicarbonate fluid is to neutralize the acidic chyme, stop the action of pepsin from the stomach, and create a neutral pH in the duodenum for the action of the digestive pancreatic enzymes.

In response to the presence of fats and proteins in the small intestine, CCK is released into the bloodstream. CCK stimulates the acinar cells in the pancreas to secrete large amounts of digestive enzymes: **pancreatic amylase** for carbohydrate digestion, **pancreatic lipase** for lipid digestion, **deoxyribonuclease** and **ribonuclease** for digestion of nucleic acids, and the **proteolytic enzymes trypsinogen, chymotrypsinogen,** and **procarboxypeptidase.**

Pancreatic enzymes are first produced in the acinar cells in an inactive form and are only activated in the duodenum by the hormone **enterokinase** secreted by the intestinal mucosa. This hormone converts trypsinogen to trypsin, which then converts all other pancreatic enzymes into active digestive enzymes.

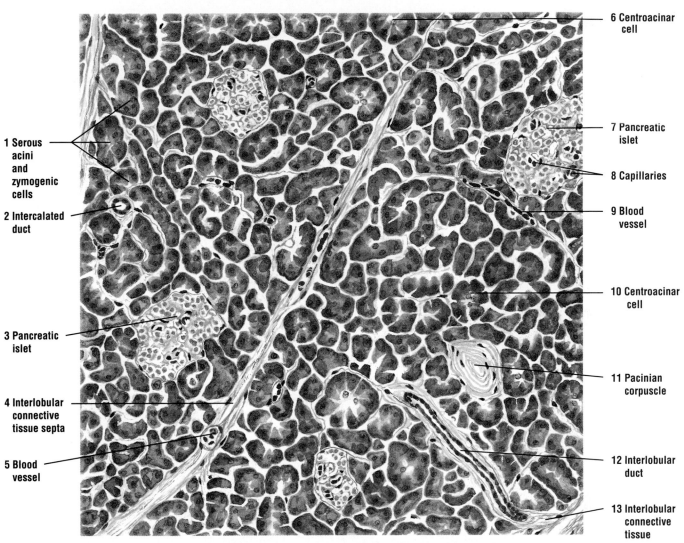

1 Serous acini and zymogenic cells

2 Intercalated duct

3 Pancreatic islet

4 Interlobular connective tissue septa

5 Blood vessel

6 Centroacinar cell

7 Pancreatic islet

8 Capillaries

9 Blood vessel

10 Centroacinar cell

11 Pacinian corpuscle

12 Interlobular duct

13 Interlobular connective tissue

FIGURE 14.10 ■ Exocrine and endocrine pancreas (sectional view). Stain: hematoxylin and eosin. Low magnification.

FIGURE 14.11 ■ Pancreatic Islet

A pale-staining, **pancreatic islet (of Langerhans) (2)** is illustrated at a higher magnification. The endocrine cells of the islet (2) are arranged in cords and clumps, between which are found connective tissue fibers and a **capillary (3)** network. A thin **connective tissue capsule (4)** separates the endocrine pancreas from the exocrine **serous acini (5)**. Some serous acini (5) contain pale-staining **centroacinar cells (5),** which are part of the duct system that connect to the **intercalated duct (1)**. Myoepithelial cells do not surround the secretory acini in the pancreas.

In routine histologic preparations, the individual hormone-secreting cells of the pancreatic islet (1) cannot be identified.

FIGURE 14.12 ■ Pancreatic Islet (Special Preparation)

This pancreas has been prepared with a special stain to distinguish the glucagon-secreting **alpha (A) cells (1)** from the insulin-secreting **beta (B) cells (3)**. The cytoplasm of alpha cells (1) stains pink, whereas the cytoplasm of beta cells (3) stains blue. The alpha cells (1) are situated more peripherally in the islet and the beta cells (3) more in the center. Also, beta cells (3) predominate, constituting about 70% of the islet. Delta (D) cells (not illustrated) are also present in the islets. These cells are least abundant, have a variable cell shape, and may occur anywhere in the pancreatic islet.

Capillaries (2) around the endocrine cells demonstrate the rich vascularity of the pancreatic islets. The thin **connective tissue capsule (4)** separates the islet cells from the **serous acini (6)**. **Centroacinar cells (5)** are visible in some of the acini.

FUNCTIONAL CORRELATIONS: Endocrine Pancreas

The endocrine components of the pancreas are scattered throughout the organ as islands of endocrine cells called **pancreatic islets** (of Langerhans). Pancreatic islets secrete two major hormones that regulate blood glucose levels and glucose metabolism.

Alpha cells in the pancreatic islets produce the hormone **glucagon,** which is released in response to low levels of glucose in the blood. Glucagon elevates blood glucose levels by accelerating the conversion of glycogen, amino acids, and fatty acids in the liver cells into glucose.

Beta cells in pancreatic islets produce the hormone **insulin,** whose release is stimulated by elevated blood glucose levels after a meal. Insulin lowers blood glucose levels by accelerating membrane transport of glucose into liver cells, muscle cells, and adipose cells. Insulin also accelerates the conversion of glucose into glycogen in liver cells. The effects of insulin on blood glucose levels are opposite to that of glucagon.

Delta cells secrete the hormone **somatostatin.** This hormone decreases and inhibits secretory activities of both alpha (glucagon-secreting) and beta (insulin-secreting) cells through local action within the pancreatic islets.

Pancreatic polypeptide cells (PP) produce the hormone **pancreatic polypeptide,** which inhibits production of pancreatic enzymes and alkaline secretions.

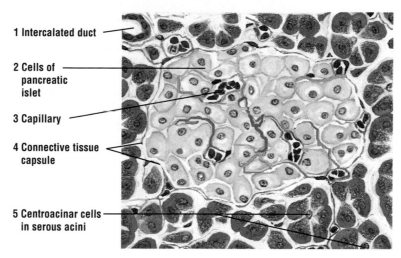

1 Intercalated duct

2 Cells of
   pancreatic
   islet

3 Capillary

4 Connective tissue
   capsule

5 Centroacinar cells
   in serous acini

FIGURE 14.11 ■ Pancreatic islet. Stain: hematoxylin and eosin. High magnification.

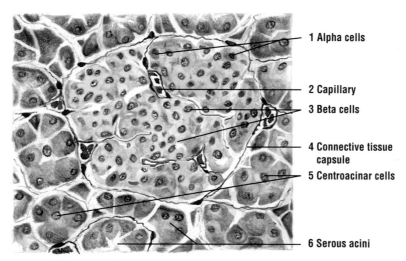

1 Alpha cells

2 Capillary

3 Beta cells

4 Connective tissue
   capsule

5 Centroacinar cells

6 Serous acini

FIGURE 14.12 ■ Pancreatic islet (special preparation). Stain: Gomori's chrome alum hematoxylin and phloxine. High magnification.

FIGURE 14.13 ■ Pancreas: Endocrine (Pancreatic Islet) and Exocrine Regions

A higher-magnification photomicrograph of the pancreas illustrates both exocrine and endocrine components. In the center is the light-staining endocrine **pancreatic islet (3)**. A thin **connective tissue capsule (2)** separates the pancreatic islet (3) from the exocrine **secretory acini (5).** The pancreatic islet (3) is vascularized by blood vessels and **capillaries (6).** The exocrine secretory acini (5) consist of pyramid-shaped cells arranged around small lumina in whose centers are seen one or more light-staining **centroacinar cells (4).**

The smallest excretory duct in the pancreas is the **intercalated duct (1)** lined by a simple cuboidal epithelium.

1 Intercalated duct

2 Connective tissue
  capsule

3 Pancreatic islet

4 Centroacinar
  cells

5 Secretory
  acini

6 Capillaries

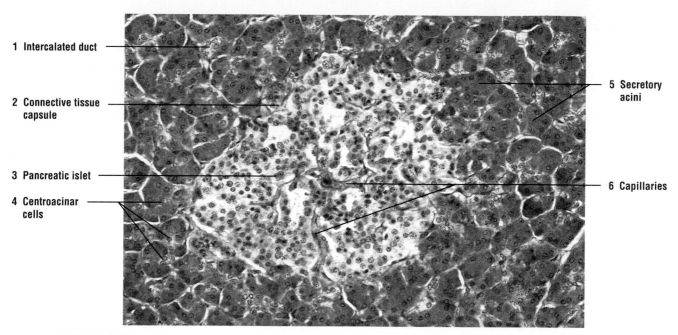

FIGURE 14.13 ■ Pancreas: endocrine (pancreatic islet) and exocrine regions. Stain: periodic acid-Schiff and hematoxylin. ×80.

Digestive System

Liver

- Located outside of the digestive tube in strategic position
- All absorbed nutrients pass through liver via portal vein and hepatic sinusoids
- Has dual blood supply: portal vein and hepatic artery
- Is organized into repeating liver lobules, with central vein in the center of lobule
- Plates of liver cells (hepatocytes) radiate to lobule periphery from central vein
- Portal vein, hepatic artery, and bile duct in lobule periphery are portal areas
- Venous and arterial blood mix in sinusoids and flow toward central vein
- Hepatic sinusoids lined by discontinuous and fenestrated endothelium
- Substances in blood contact hepatocytes via subendothelial perisinusoidal spaces

Gallbladder, Hepatocytes, and Exocrine Functions

- As exocrine function, hepatocytes secrete bile into bile canaliculi
- Bile flows opposite to blood to bile ducts in portal areas
- Bile is stored in gallbladder, where water is removed and bile is concentrated
- Hormone cholecystokinin regulates release of bile from liver and gallbladder
- Enteroendocrine cells in intestinal mucosa release cholecystokinin as fats in chyme enter duodenum
- Cholecystokinin causes gallbladder contraction and expulsion of bile
- Bile emulsifies fats for more efficient digestion by pancreatic lipases
- Fats are absorbed into lymphatic lacteals in the villi of small intestine
- Hepatocytes excrete bilirubin into bile and move antibodies from blood into bile

Hepatocytes: Endocrine Functions, Detoxification, and Hemopoiesis

- Take up, metabolize, accumulate, and store products from blood
- Synthesize and release plasma proteins, including blood-clotting factors
- Store glycogen and release as glucose when needed
- Detoxify drugs and harmful substances in sinusoids
- Specialized liver macrophages, Kupffer cells, line the sinusoids
- Kupffer cells filter and phagocytose debris and worn-out red blood cells
- In fetus, hepatocytes are sites for hemopoiesis

Pancreas: Exocrine

- Head of organ lies in the duodenal loop
- Exocrine component forms majority of organ and is composed of serous acini
- Zymogen cells of acini filled with granules that contain digestive enzymes
- Acini contain pale-staining centroacinar cells in their lumina
- Centroacinar cells continuous with cells of intercalated ducts
- Hormones secretin and cholecystokinin regulate secretions
- Intestinal enteroendocrine cells release hormones when acidic chyme is present
- Secretin stimulates sodium bicarbonate production by centroacinar cells and intercalated duct cells
- Alkaline sodium bicarbonate fluid neutralizes acidic chyme
- Cholecystokinin released when fats and proteins are present in chyme
- Cholecystokinin stimulates production of pancreatic digestive enzymes
- Enzymes first produced in inactive form and activated in duodenum

Pancreas: Endocrine

- Endocrine portion in form of isolated pancreatic islets among exocrine acini
- Each pancreatic islet is surrounded and separated by fine reticular fibers
- Four cell types present in pancreatic islets: alpha, beta, delta, and PP cells
- Alpha cells produce glucagon in response to low sugar levels
- Glucagon elevates blood glucose by accelerating conversion of glycogen in liver
- Beta cells produce insulin during elevated glucose levels
- Insulin lowers blood glucose by inducing glucose transport into liver, muscle, and adipose cells
- Delta cells produce somatostatin, which inhibits activity of both alpha and beta cells
- PP (pancreatic polypeptide) cells inhibit enzymatic and alkaline pancreatic secretions

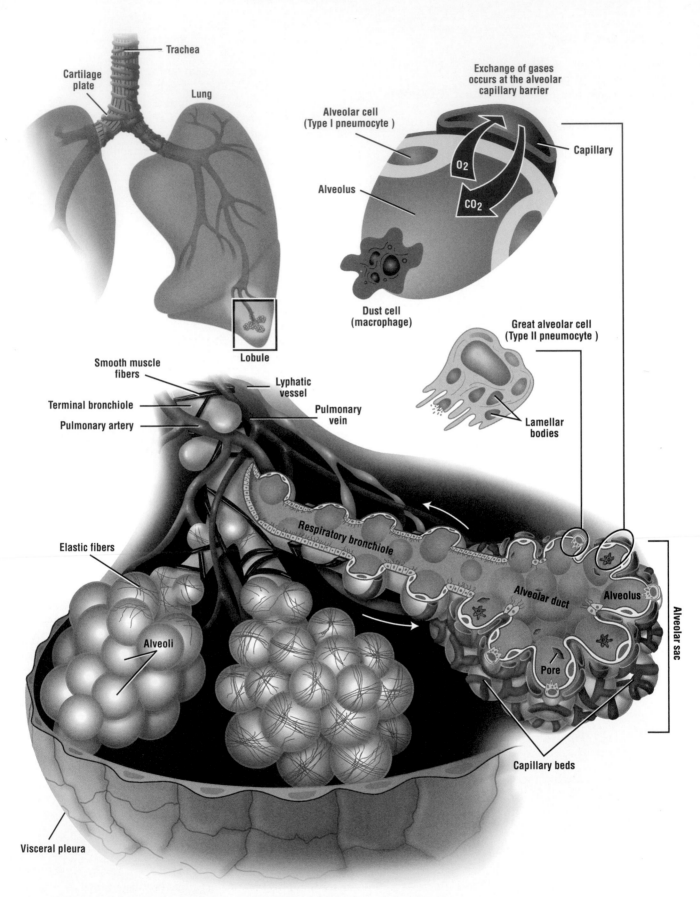

OVERVIEW FIGURE 15 ■ A section of the lung is illustrated in three dimensions and in transverse section, with emphasis on the internal structure of the respiratory bronchiole and alveolar cells.

Respiratory System

Components of the Respiratory System

The respiratory system consists of **lungs** and numerous **air passages,** or tubes, of various sizes that lead to and from each lung. In addition, the system consists of a conducting portion and a respiratory portion.

The **conducting portion** of the respiratory system consists of passageways outside (extrapulmonary) and inside (intrapulmonary) the lungs that conduct air for gaseous exchange to and from the lungs. In contrast, the **respiratory portion** consists of passageways within the lungs that not only conduct the air, but also allow for **respiration,** or gaseous exchange.

The extrapulmonary passages, which include the trachea, bronchi, and larger bronchioles, are lined by a distinct **pseudostratified ciliated epithelium** containing numerous **goblet cells.** As the passageways enter the lungs, the bronchi undergo extensive branching and their diameters become progressively smaller. There is also a gradual decrease in the height of the lining epithelium, amount of cilia, and number of goblet cells in these tubules. The **bronchioles** represent the terminal portion of the conducting passageways. These give rise to the **respiratory bronchioles,** which represent the transition zone between conducting and respiratory portions.

The **respiratory portion** consists of respiratory bronchioles, alveolar ducts, alveolar sacs, and alveoli. Gaseous exchange in the lungs takes place in the **alveoli,** the terminal air spaces of the respiratory system. In the alveoli, goblet cells are absent and the lining epithelium is thin **simple squamous.**

Olfactory Epithelium

Air that enters the lungs first passes by the roof or superior region of the nasal cavity. Located in the roof of the nose is a highly specialized epithelium, called the **olfactory epithelium,** which detects and transmits odors. This epithelium consists of three cell types: supportive (sustentacular), basal, and olfactory (sensory). Located below the epithelium in the connective tissue are the serous olfactory glands.

Olfactory cells are the **sensory bipolar neurons** that are distributed between the more apical supportive cells and the basal cells of the olfactory epithelium. The olfactory cells span the thickness of the epithelium and end at the surface of the olfactory epithelium as small, round bulbs, called the **olfactory vesicles.** Radiating from each olfactory vesicle are long, **nonmotile olfactory cilia** that lie parallel to the epithelial surface; these nonmotile cilia function as odor receptors. In contrast to respiratory epithelium, the olfactory epithelium has no goblet cells or motile cilia.

In the connective tissue directly below the olfactory epithelium are **olfactory nerves** and **olfactory glands.** Olfactory (Bowman's) glands produce a serous fluid that bathes the olfactory cilia and serves as a solvent to dissolve the odor molecules for detection by the olfactory cells.

Conducting Portion of Respiratory System

The conducting portion of the respiratory system consists of the nasal cavities, pharynx, larynx, trachea, extrapulmonary bronchi, and a series of intrapulmonary bronchi and bronchioles with decreasing diameters that end as **terminal bronchioles. Hyaline cartilage** provides structural support and ensures that the larger air passageways are always patent (open). Incomplete C-shaped **hyaline cartilage rings** encircle the **trachea.** Elastic and smooth muscle fibers, called the trachealis muscle, bridge the space between the ends of the hyaline cartilage. The cartilage rings of the trachea face posteriorly and are located adjacent to the esophagus.

As the trachea divides into smaller **bronchi** and the bronchi enter the lungs, the hyaline cartilage rings are replaced by irregular **hyaline cartilage plates** that encircle the bronchi. As the bronchi continue to divide and decrease in size, the cartilage plates also decrease in size and number. When the diameters of bronchioles decrease to about 1 mm, cartilage plates completely disappear from conducting passageways. Terminal bronchioles represent the final conducting passageways and have diameters ranging from 0.5 mm to 1.0 mm. There are between 20 and 25 generations of branching before the passageways reach the size of terminal bronchioles.

The larger bronchioles are lined by tall, **ciliated pseudostratified epithelium** that is similar to that of the trachea and bronchi. As the tubular size decreases, the epithelial height is gradually reduced, and the epithelium becomes **simple ciliated epithelium.** The epithelium of larger bronchioles also contains numerous **goblet cells.** The number of these cells gradually decreases with the decreasing tubular size, and the goblet cells are not present in the epithelium of terminal bronchioles.

Smaller bronchioles are lined only by **simple cuboidal epithelium.** In place of the goblet cells, another type of cells, called **Clara cells,** is found with the ciliated cels in the terminal and respiratory bronchioles. Clara cells are nonciliated, secretory cuboidal cells that increase in number as the number of ciliated cells decreases.

Respiratory Portion of the Respiratory System

The respiratory portion of the respiratory system is the distal continuation of the conducting portion and starts with the air passageways where respiration or gaseous exchange occurs. Terminal bronchioles give rise to **respiratory bronchioles,** which exhibit thin-walled outpocketings called **alveoli** and where respiration can take place. The respiratory bronchioles represent the **transitional zone** between air conduction and gaseous exchange or respiration.

Respiration can only occur in **alveoli** because the barrier between inspired air in the alveoli and venous blood in capillaries is extremely thin. Other intrapulmonary structures in which respiration occurs are the **alveolar ducts** and **alveolar sacs.**

In addition to the cells in the passageways, there are other cell types in the lung. The alveoli contain two cell types. The most abundant cells are the **squamous alveolar cells** or **type I pneumocytes.** These are extremely squamous cells that line all alveolar surfaces. Interspersed among the squamous alveolar cells either singly or in small groups are the **type II pneumocytes.** Lung **macrophages,** derived from circulating blood monocytes, are also found both in the connective tissue of alveolar walls or interalveolar septa (**alveolar macrophages**) and in the alveoli (**dust cells**). Also present in the interalveolar septa are extensive capillary networks, pulmonary arteries, pulmonary veins, lymphatic ducts, and nerves (Overview Figure 15).

FIGURE 15.1 ■ Olfactory Mucosa and Superior Concha (Panoramic View)

The olfactory mucosa is located in the roof of the nasal cavity, on each side of the dividing septum, and on the surface of the **superior concha (1),** one of the bony shelves in the nasal cavity.

The **olfactory epithelium (2, 6)** (see Figures 15.2 and 15.3) is specialized for reception of smell. As a result, it appears different from the respiratory epithelium. Olfactory epithelium (2, 6) is pseudostratified tall columnar epithelium without goblet cells and without motile cilia, in contrast to the respiratory epithelium.

The underlying lamina propria contains the branched tubuloacinar **olfactory (Bowman's) glands (4, 5).** These glands produce a serous secretion, in contrast to the mixed mucous and serous secretions produced by glands in the rest of the nasal cavity. Small nerves that are located in the lamina propria are the **olfactory nerves (3, 7).** The olfactory nerves (3, 7) represent the aggregated afferent axons that leave the olfactory cells and continue into the cranial cavity, where they synapse in the olfactory (cranial) nerves.

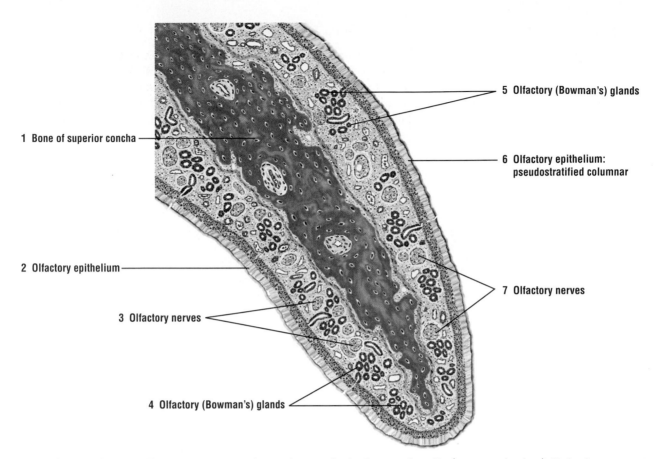

1 Bone of superior concha

2 Olfactory epithelium

3 Olfactory nerves

4 Olfactory (Bowman's) glands

5 Olfactory (Bowman's) glands

6 Olfactory epithelium: pseudostratified columnar

7 Olfactory nerves

FIGURE 15.1 ■ Olfactory mucosa and superior concha in the nasal cavity (panoramic view). Stain: hematoxylin and eosin. Low magnification.

FIGURE 15.2 ■ Olfactory Mucosa: Detail of a Transitional Area

This illustration depicts a transition between the **olfactory epithelium (1)** and **respiratory epithelium (9).** In the transition region, the histologic differences between these epithelia are obvious. The olfactory epithelium (1) is tall, pseudostratified columnar epithelium, composed of three different cell types: supportive, basal, and neuroepithelial olfactory cells. The individual cell outlines are difficult to distinguish in a routine histologic preparation; however, the location and shape of nuclei allow identification of the cell types.

The supportive or **sustentacular cells (3)** are elongated, with oval nuclei situated more apically or superficially in the epithelium. The **olfactory cells (4)** have oval or round nuclei that are located between the nuclei of the supportive cells (3) and **basal cells (5).** The apices and bases of the olfactory cells (4) are slender. The apical surfaces of the olfactory cells (4) contain slender, nonmotile microvilli that extend into the **mucus (2)** that covers the epithelial surface. The basal cells (5) are short cells located at the base of the epithelium between the supportive (3) and olfactory cells (4).

Extending from the bases of the olfactory cells (4) are axons that pass into the **lamina propria (6)** as bundles of unmyelinated **olfactory nerves** or **fila olfactoria (14).** The olfactory nerves (14) leave the nasal cavity and pass into the olfactory bulbs at the base of the brain.

The transition from the olfactory epithelium (1) to the respiratory epithelium (9) is abrupt. The respiratory epithelium (9) is pseudostratified columnar epithelium with distinct **cilia (10)** and many **goblet cells (11).** Also, in the illustrated transition area, the height of the respiratory epithelium (9) is similar to the olfactory epithelium (1). In other regions of the tract, the respiratory epithelium (9) is reduced in comparison to the olfactory epithelium (1).

The underlying lamina propria (6) contains capillaries, lymphatic vessels, **arterioles (8), venules (13),** and branched, tubuloacinar serous **olfactory (Bowman's) glands (7).** The olfactory glands (7) deliver their secretions through narrow excretory **ducts (12)** that penetrate the olfactory epithelium (1). The secretions from the olfactory glands (7) moisten the epithelial surface, dissolve the molecules of odoriferous substances, and stimulate the olfactory cells (4).

FIGURE 15.3 ■ Olfactory Mucosa in the Nose: Transition Area

In the superior region of the nasal cavity, the **respiratory epithelium** changes abruptly into **olfactory epithelium,** as shown in this higher-power photomicrograph.

The respiratory epithelium is lined by motile **cilia (1)** and contains **goblet cells (2).** The olfactory epithelium lacks cilia (1) and goblet cells (2). Instead, it exhibits nuclei of **supportive cells (5),** located near the epithelial surface, nuclei of odor receptive **olfactory cells (6),** located more in the center of the epithelium, and **basal cells (7),** located close to the **basement membrane (3).**

Below the olfactory epithelium in the connective tissue **lamina propria (4)** are **blood vessels (9), olfactory nerves (10),** and **olfactory (Bowman's) glands (8).**

FUNCTIONAL CORRELATIONS: Olfactory Epithelium

To detect odors, odoriferous substances must first be dissolved. The dissolved odor molecules then bind to odor receptor molecules on **olfactory cilia** and stimulate the odor-binding **receptors** on the cilia of the olfactory epithelium to conduct impulses. The unmyelinated afferent axons of olfactory cells leave the olfactory epithelium and form numerous small **olfactory nerve bundles** in the lamina propria. Impulses from olfactory cells are conducted in the nerves that pass through the ethmoid bone in the skull and synapse in the **olfactory bulbs** of the brain. Olfactory bulbs are located in the cranial cavity of the skull above the nasal cavity. From here, neurons relay the information to higher centers in the cortex for odor interpretation.

Olfactory epithelium is kept moist by a watery secretion produced by serous tubuloacinar **olfactory (Bowman's) glands** located directly below the epithelium in the lamina propria. This secretion, delivered via ducts, continually washes the surface of olfactory epithelium. In this manner, odor molecules dissolve in the secreted fluid and are continually washed away by new fluid, allowing the receptor cells to again detect and respond to new odors.

The supportive cells provide mechanical support for the olfactory cells, whereas the basal cells function as stem cells. Basal cells give rise to new olfactory cells and supportive cells of the olfactory epithelium.

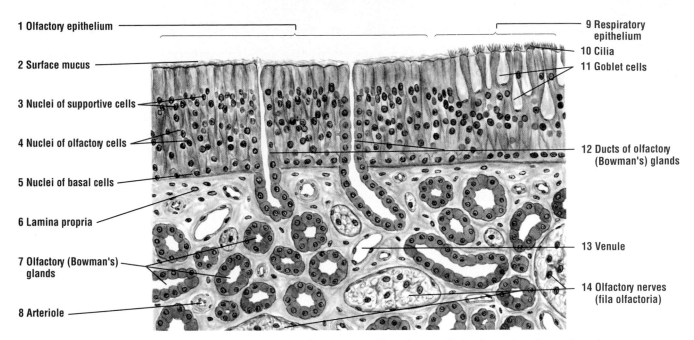

1 Olfactory epithelium

2 Surface mucus

3 Nuclei of supportive cells

4 Nuclei of olfactory cells

5 Nuclei of basal cells

6 Lamina propria

7 Olfactory (Bowman's) glands

8 Arteriole

9 Respiratory epithelium

10 Cilia

11 Goblet cells

12 Ducts of olfactory (Bowman's) glands

13 Venule

14 Olfactory nerves (fila olfactoria)

FIGURE 15.2 ■ Olfactory mucosa: details of a transitional area. Stain: hematoxylin and eosin. High magnification.

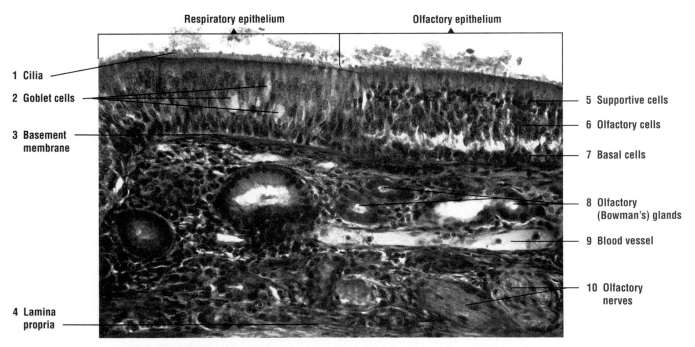

Respiratory epithelium

Olfactory epithelium

1 Cilia

2 Goblet cells

3 Basement membrane

4 Lamina propria

5 Supportive cells

6 Olfactory cells

7 Basal cells

8 Olfactory (Bowman's) glands

9 Blood vessel

10 Olfactory nerves

FIGURE 15.3 ■ Olfactory mucosa in the nose: transition area. Stain: Mallory-azan. ×80.

FIGURE 15.4 ■   Epiglottis (Longitudinal Section)

The epiglottis is the superior portion of the larynx that projects upward from the larynx's anterior wall. It has both a lingual and a laryngeal surface.

A central **elastic cartilage** of **epiglottis (3)** forms the framework of the epiglottis. Its **lingual mucosa (2)** (anterior side) is lined with a **stratified squamous nonkeratinized epithelium (1).** The underlying lamina propria merges with the connective tissue **perichondrium (4)** of the elastic cartilage of epiglottis (3).

The lingual mucosa (2) with its stratified squamous epithelium (1) covers the apex of the epiglottis and about half of the **laryngeal mucosa (7)** (posterior side). Toward the base of the epiglottis on the laryngeal surface (7), the lining stratified squamous epithelium (1) changes to **pseudostratified ciliated columnar epithelium (8).** Located below the epithelium in the **lamina propria (6)** on the laryngeal side (7) of the epiglottis are tubuloacinar **seromucous glands (6).**

In addition to the tongue, **taste buds (5)** and solitary lymphatic nodules may be observed in the lingual epithelium (2) or laryngeal epithelium (7).

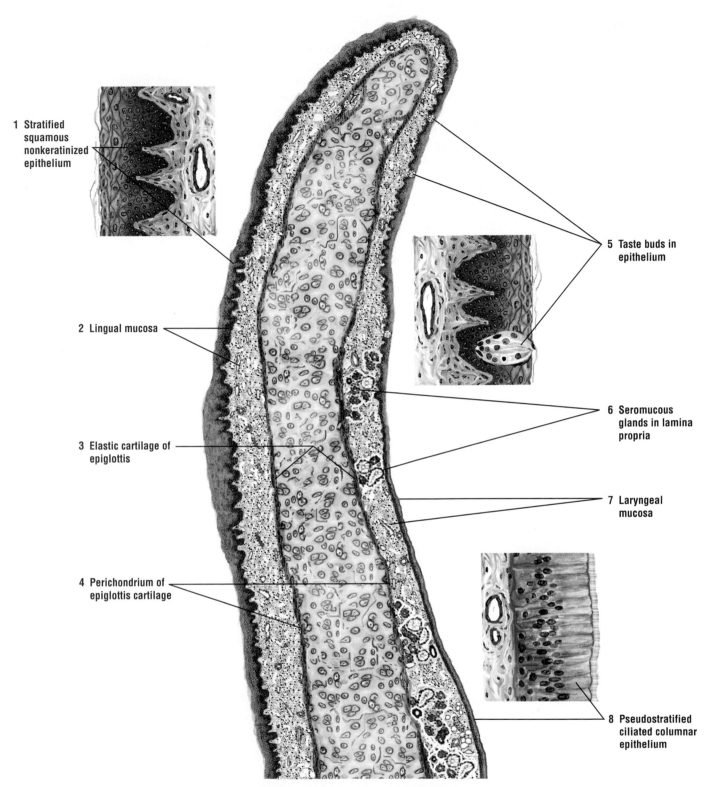

1 Stratified squamous nonkeratinized epithelium

2 Lingual mucosa

3 Elastic cartilage of epiglottis

4 Perichondrium of epiglottis cartilage

5 Taste buds in epithelium

6 Seromucous glands in lamina propria

7 Laryngeal mucosa

8 Pseudostratified ciliated columnar epithelium

FIGURE 15.4 ■ Epiglottis (longitudinal section). Stain: hematoxylin and eosin. Low magnification. Insets: high magnification.

FIGURE 15.5 ■ Larynx (Frontal Section)

This image illustrates a vertical section through one half of the larynx.

The **false (superior) vocal fold (9)**, also called vocal cord, is covered by the mucosa that is continuous with the posterior surface of the epiglottis. As in the epiglottis, the false vocal fold (9) is lined by **pseudostratified ciliated columnar epithelium (7)** with goblet cells. In the **lamina propria (3)** are numerous and mixed **seromucous glands (8)**. Excretory ducts from these mixed glands (8) open onto the epithelial surface (7). Numerous **lymphatic nodules (2), blood vessels (1),** and **adipose cells (1)** are also located in the lamina propria (3) of the false vocal fold (9).

The **ventricle (10)** is a deep indentation and recess that separates the false (superior) vocal fold (9) from the **true (inferior) vocal fold (11–13).** The mucosa in the wall of the ventricle (10) is similar to that of the false vocal fold (9). Lymphatic nodules (2) are more numerous in this area and are sometimes called the "laryngeal tonsils." The lamina propria (3) blends with the **perichondrium (5)** of the hyaline **thyroid cartilage (4).** There is no distinct submucosa. The lower wall of the ventricle (10) makes the transition to the true vocal fold (11–13).

The mucosa of the true vocal fold (11–13) is lined by nonkeratinized **stratified squamous epithelium (11)** and a thin, dense lamina propria devoid of glands, lymphatic tissue, or blood vessels. At the apex of the true vocal fold is the **vocalis ligament (12)** with dense elastic fibers that extend into the adjacent lamina propria and the skeletal **vocalis muscle (13).** The skeletal thyroarytenoid muscle and the thyroid cartilage (4) constitute the remaining wall.

The epithelium in the lower larynx changes to **pseudostratified ciliated columnar epithelium (15)**, and the lamina propria contains mixed **seromucous glands (14).** The hyaline **cricoid cartilage (6)** is the lowermost cartilage of the larynx.

1 Arteriole, venule, and adpiose cells

2 Lymphatic nodules

3 Lamina propria

4 Thyroid cartilage

5 Perichondrium

6 Cricoid cartilage

7 Pseudostratified ciliated epithelium

8 Seromucous glands

9 False vocal cord

10 Ventricle

11 Stratified squamous epithelium

12 Vocalis ligament

13 Vocalis muscle

True vocal fold

14 Seromucous glands

15 Pseudostratified ciliated epithelium

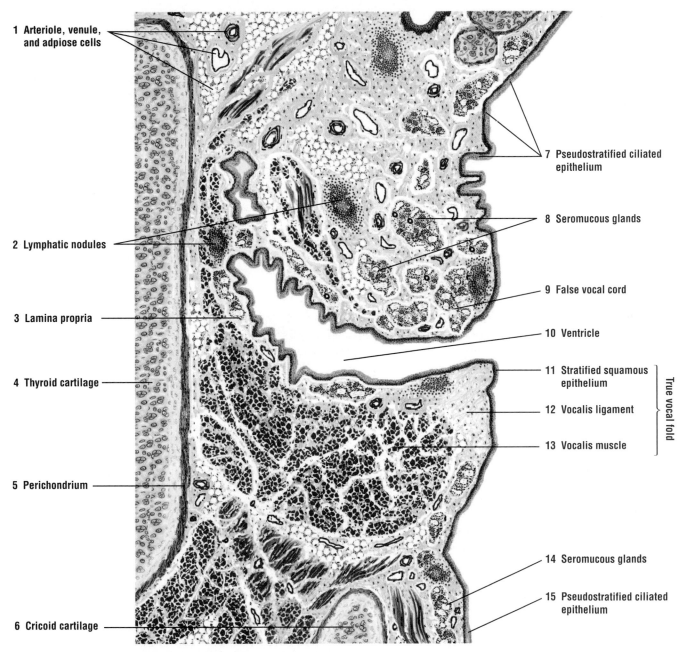

FIGURE 15.5 ■ Frontal section of larynx. Stain: hematoxylin and eosin. Low magnification.

FIGURE 15.6 ■ Trachea (Panoramic View, Transverse Section)

The wall of the trachea consists of mucosa, submucosa, hyaline cartilage, and adventitia. The trachea is kept patent (open) by C-shaped **hyaline cartilage (3)** rings. Hyaline cartilage (3) is surrounded by the dense connective tissue **perichondrium (9),** which merges with the **submucosa (4)** on one side and the **adventitia (1)** on the other. Numerous **nerves (6), blood vessels (8),** and **adipose tissue (2)** are located in the adventitia.

The gap between the posterior ends of the hyaline cartilage (3) is filled by the smooth **trachealis muscle (7).** The trachealis muscle (7) lies in the connective tissue deep to the **elastic membrane (14)** of the mucosa. Most of the trachealis muscle (7) fibers insert into the perichondrium (9) that covers the hyaline cartilage (3).

The lumen of the trachea is lined by **pseudostratified ciliated columnar epithelium (12)** with goblet cells. The underlying **lamina propria (13)** contains fine connective tissue fibers, diffuse lymphatic tissue, and occasional solitary lymphatic nodules. Located deeper in the lamina propria (13) is the longitudinal elastic membrane (14) formed by elastic fibers. The elastic membrane (14) divides the lamina propria (13) from the submucosa (4), which contains loose connective tissue that is similar to that of lamina propria (13). In the submucosa (4) are found the tubuloacinar **seromucous tracheal glands (10)** whose **excretory ducts (11)** pass through the lamina propria (13) to the tracheal lumen.

The mucosa exhibits **mucosal folds (5)** along the posterior wall of the trachea where the hyaline cartilage (3) is absent. The seromucous tracheal glands (10) that are present in the submucosa can extend and be seen in the adventitia (1).

FIGURE 15.7 ■ Tracheal Wall (Sectional View)

A section of tracheal wall between the **hyaline cartilage (1)** and the lining **pseudostratified ciliated columnar epithelium (8)** with **goblet cells (10)** is illustrated at a higher magnification. A thin **basement membrane (9)** separates the lining epithelium (8) from the **lamina propria (11).**

Below the lamina propria (11) is the connective tissue **submucosa (6),** in which are found the **seromucous tracheal glands (3).** A **serous demilune (7)** surrounds a mucous acinus of the seromucous tracheal glands (3). The **excretory duct (5)** of the tracheal glands (3) is lined by simple cuboidal epithelium and extends through the lamina propria (11) to the epithelial surface (8).

The adjacent hyaline cartilage (1) is surrounded by the connective tissue **perichondrium (2).** The larger **chondrocytes in lacunae (4)** that are located in the interior of the hyaline cartilage (1) become progressively flatter toward the perichondrium (2), which gradually blends with the surrounding connective tissue of the submucosa (6). An **arteriole** and **venule (12)** supply the connective tissue of the submucosa (6) and the lamina propria (11).

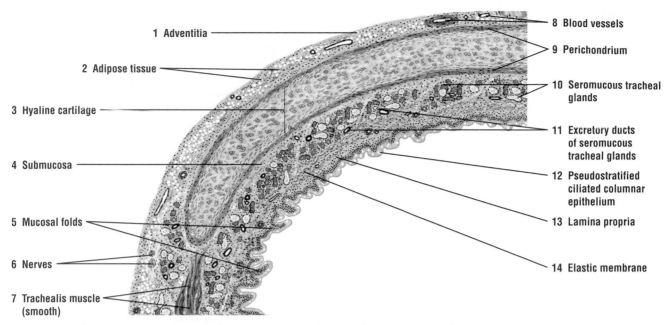

1 Adventitia

2 Adipose tissue

3 Hyaline cartilage

4 Submucosa

5 Mucosal folds

6 Nerves

7 Trachealis muscle (smooth)

8 Blood vessels

9 Perichondrium

10 Seromucous tracheal glands

11 Excretory ducts of seromucous tracheal glands

12 Pseudostratified ciliated columnar epithelium

13 Lamina propria

14 Elastic membrane

FIGURE 15.6 ■ Trachea (transverse section). Stain: hematoxylin and eosin. Low magnification.

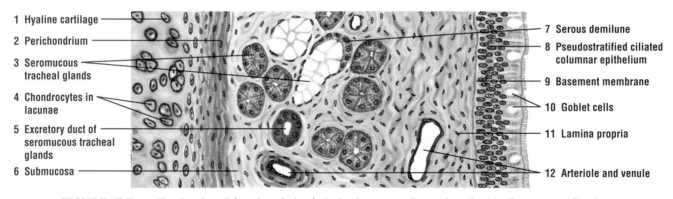

1 Hyaline cartilage

2 Perichondrium

3 Seromucous tracheal glands

4 Chondrocytes in lacunae

5 Excretory duct of seromucous tracheal glands

6 Submucosa

7 Serous demilune

8 Pseudostratified ciliated columnar epithelium

9 Basement membrane

10 Goblet cells

11 Lamina propria

12 Arteriole and venule

FIGURE 15.7 ■ Tracheal wall (sectional view). Stain: hematoxylin and eosin. Medium magnification.

FIGURE 15.8 ■ Lung (Panoramic View)

This illustration shows the major structures in the lung for air conduction and gaseous exchange (respiration).

The histology of the intrapulmonary bronchi is similar to that of the trachea and extrapulmonary bronchi, except that in the intrapulmonary bronchi, the C-shaped cartilage rings of the trachea are replaced by cartilage plates. All cartilage in the trachea and lung is hyaline cartilage.

The wall of an **intrapulmonary bronchus (5)** is identified by the surrounding **hyaline cartilage plates (7).** The bronchus (5) is also lined by pseudostratified columnar ciliated epithelium with goblet cells. The wall in the intrapulmonary bronchus (5) consists of a thin **lamina propria (4),** a narrow layer of **smooth muscle (3),** a **submucosa (2)** with **bronchial glands (6),** hyaline cartilage plates (7), and **adventitia (1).**

As the intrapulmonary bronchus (5) branches into smaller bronchi and bronchioles, the epithelial height and the cartilage around the bronchi decrease, until only an occasional piece of cartilage is seen. Cartilage disappears from the bronchi walls when their diameters decrease to about 1 mm.

In the **bronchiole (17),** pseudostratified columnar ciliated epithelium with occasional goblet cells lines the lumen. The lumen shows **mucosal folds (18)** caused by the contractions of the surrounding **smooth muscle (19)** layer. Bronchial glands and cartilage plates are no longer present, and the bronchiole (17) is surrounded by the **adventitia (16).** In this illustration, a **lymphatic nodule (15)** and a **vein (15)** adjacent to the adventitia (16) accompany the bronchiole (17).

The **terminal bronchioles (8, 10)** exhibit **mucosal folds (10)** and are lined by a columnar ciliated epithelium that lacks goblet cells. A thin layer of lamina propria and **smooth muscle (11)** and an adventitia surround the terminal bronchioles (8, 10).

The **respiratory bronchioles (12, 22)** with alveoli outpocketings are directly connected to the **alveolar ducts (13, 20)** and the **alveoli (23).** In the respiratory bronchioles (12, 22), the epithelium is low columnar or cuboidal and may be ciliated in the proximal portion of the tubules. A thin connective tissue layer supports the smooth muscle, the elastic fibers of the lamina propria, and the accompanying **blood vessels (21).** The **alveoli (12)** in the walls of the respiratory bronchioles (12, 22) appear as small evaginations or outpockets.

Each respiratory bronchiole (12, 22) divides into several alveolar ducts (13, 20). The walls of the alveolar ducts (13, 20) are lined by alveoli (23) that directly open into the alveolar duct. Clusters of alveoli (23) that surround and open into alveolar ducts (13, 20) are called **alveolar sacs (24).** In this illustration, a plane of section passes from a terminal bronchiole (8) to the respiratory bronchiole and into alveolar ducts (20).

The **pulmonary vein (9)** and **pulmonary artery (9)** also branch as they accompany the bronchi and bronchioles into the lung. Small blood vessels are also seen in the connective tissue **trabecula (25)** that separates the lungs into different segments.

The **serosa (14)** or visceral pleura surrounds the lungs. Serosa (14) consists of a thin layer of pleural **connective tissue (14a)** and a simple squamous layer of pleural **mesothelium (14b).**

1 Adventitia
2 Submucosa
3 Smooth muscle
4 Lamina propria
5 Intrapulmonary bronchus
6 Bronchial glands with excretory duct
7 Hyaline cartilage plates
8 Terminal bronchiole
9 Pulmonary vein and artery
10 Terminal bronchiole with mucosal folds
11 Smooth muscle
12 Respiratory bronchiole with alveoli
13 Alveolar ducts
14 Serosa:
   a. Connective tissue
   b. Mesothelium

15 Lymphatic nodule and vein
16 Adventitia
17 Bronchiole
18 Mucosal folds
19 Smooth muscle
20 Alveolar ducts
21 Blood vessels
22 Respiratory bronchiole
23 Alveoli opening into alveolar duct
24 Alveolar sacs
25 Trabecula with blood vessels

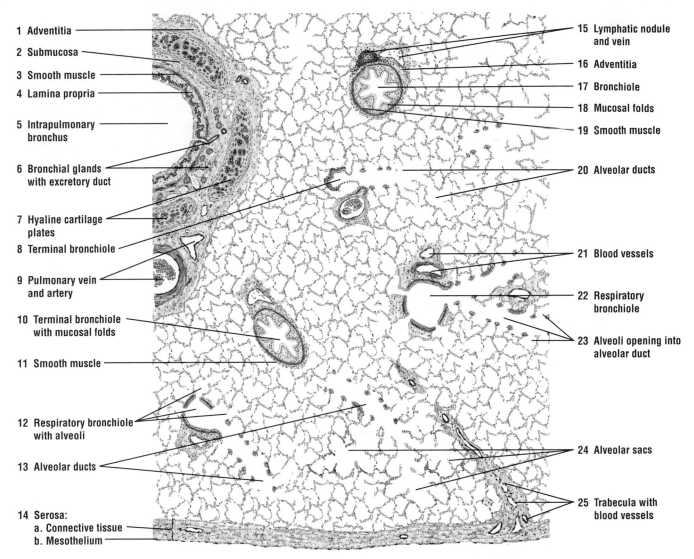

FIGURE 15.8 ■ Lung (panoramic view). Stain: hematoxylin and eosin. Low magnification.

FIGURE 15.9 ■ Intrapulmonary Bronchus

The trachea divides outside of the lungs and gives rise to primary or extrapulmonary bronchi. On entering the lungs, the primary bronchi divide and give rise to a series of smaller or intrapulmonary bronchi.

The intrapulmonary bronchi are lined by pseudostratified columnar ciliated **bronchial epithelium (6)** supported by a thin layer of **lamina propria (7)** of fine connective tissue with elastic fibers (not illustrated) and a few lymphocytes. A thin layer of **smooth muscle (10, 16)** surrounds the lamina propria (7) and separates it from the **submucosa (8).** The submucosa (8) contains numerous **seromucous bronchial glands (5, 18).** An **excretory duct (18)** from the bronchial gland (5, 18) passes through the lamina propria (7) to open into the bronchial lumen. In mixed seromucous bronchial glands (5, 18), serous demilunes may be seen.

In the lung, the hyaline cartilage rings of the trachea are replaced by the **hyaline cartilage plates (11, 14)** that surround the bronchus. A connective tissue **perichondrium (12, 15)** covers each cartilage plate (11, 14). The hyaline cartilage plates (11, 14) become smaller and farther apart as the bronchi continue to divide and decrease in size. Between the cartilage plates (11, 14), the submucosa (8) blends with the **adventitia (3).** Bronchial glands (5, 18) and **adipose cells (2)** are present in the submucosa (8) of larger bronchi.

Bronchial blood vessels (19) and a **bronchial arteriole (4)** are visible in the connective tissue around the bronchus. Accompanying the bronchus are also a larger **vein (9)** and an **artery (17).**

Surrounding the intrapulmonary bronchus, its connective tissue, and the hyaline cartilage plates (11, 14) are the lung **alveoli (1, 13).**

FIGURE 15.10 ■ Terminal Bronchiole (Transverse Section)

The bronchioles subdivide into smaller terminal bronchioles, whose diameters are approximately 1 mm or less. The terminal bronchioles are lined by **simple columnar epithelium (3).** In the smallest bronchioles, the epithelium may be simple cuboidal. The cartilage plates, bronchial glands, and goblet cells are absent from the terminal bronchioles. The terminal bronchioles represent the smallest passageways for conducting air.

Owing to smooth muscle contractions, **mucosal folds (7)** are prominent in the bronchioles. A well-developed **smooth muscle (5)** layer surrounds the thin **lamina propria (6),** which, in turn, is surrounded by the **adventitia (8).**

Adjacent to the bronchiole is a small branch of the **pulmonary artery (2).** The terminal bronchiole is surrounded by the lung **alveoli (1).** Surrounding the alveoli are the **thin interalveolar septa with capillaries (4).**

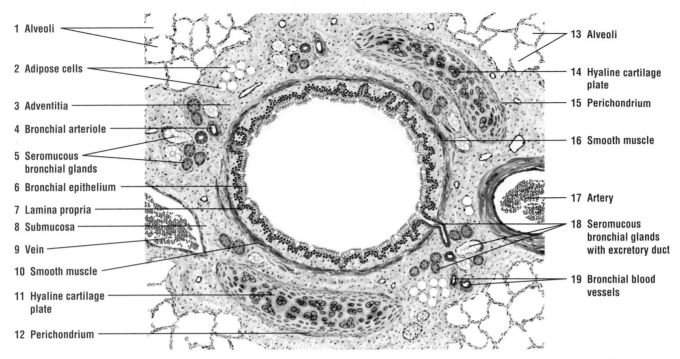

1 Alveoli

2 Adipose cells

3 Adventitia

4 Bronchial arteriole

5 Seromucous bronchial glands

6 Bronchial epithelium

7 Lamina propria

8 Submucosa

9 Vein

10 Smooth muscle

11 Hyaline cartilage plate

12 Perichondrium

13 Alveoli

14 Hyaline cartilage plate

15 Perichondrium

16 Smooth muscle

17 Artery

18 Seromucous bronchial glands with excretory duct

19 Bronchial blood vessels

FIGURE 15.9 ■ Intrapulmonary bronchus (transverse section). Stain: hematoxylin and eosin. Low magnification.

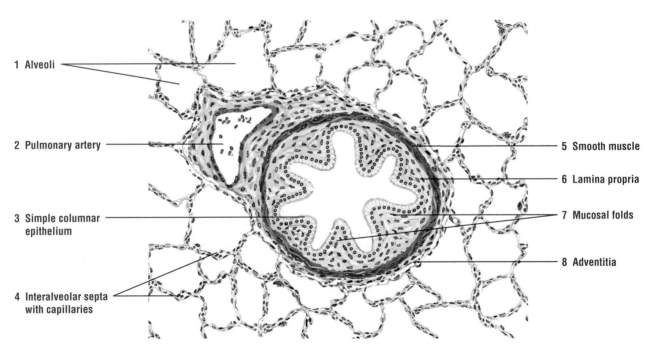

1 Alveoli

2 Pulmonary artery

3 Simple columnar epithelium

4 Interalveolar septa with capillaries

5 Smooth muscle

6 Lamina propria

7 Mucosal folds

8 Adventitia

FIGURE 15.10 ■ Terminal bronchiole (transverse section). Stain: hematoxylin and eosin. Low magnification.

FIGURE 15.11 ■ Respiratory Bronchiole, Alveolar Duct, and Lung Alveoli

The terminal bronchioles give rise to the respiratory bronchioles. The **respiratory bronchiole (2)** represents a transition zone between the conducting and respiratory portions of the respiratory system.

The wall of the respiratory bronchiole (2) is lined by **simple cuboidal epithelium (3).** Single **alveolar outpocketings (1, 6)** are found in the wall of each respiratory bronchiole (2). Cilia may be present in the epithelium of the proximal portion of the respiratory bronchiole (2) but disappear in the distal portion. A thin layer of **smooth muscle (7)** surrounds the epithelium. A small branch of the **pulmonary artery (4)** accompanies the respiratory bronchiole (2) into the lung.

Each respiratory bronchiole (2) gives rise to an **alveolar duct (9)** into which open numerous **alveoli (8)**. In the lamina propria that surrounds the rim of alveoli (8) in the alveolar duct (10) are **smooth muscle bundles (5).** These smooth muscle bundles (5) appear as knobs between adjacent alveoli.

FIGURE 15.12 ■ Alveolar Walls and Alveolar Cells

The **alveoli (3)** are evaginations or outpocketings of the respiratory bronchioles, alveolar ducts, and alveolar sacs, the terminal ends of the alveolar ducts. The alveoli (3) are lined by a layer of thin, simple squamous **alveolar cells (7)** or pneumocyte type I cells. The adjacent alveoli (3) share a common **interalveolar septum (4)** or alveolar wall.

The interalveolar septa (4) consist of simple squamous alveolar cells (7), fine connective tissue fibers and fibroblasts, and numerous **capillaries (1)** located in the thin interalveolar septa (4). The thin interalveolar septa (4) bring the capillaries (1) close to the squamous alveolar cells (7) of the adjacent alveoli (3).

In addition, the alveoli (3) also contain **alveolar macrophages (6)** or dust cells. Normally, the alveolar macrophages (6) contain several carbon or dust particles in their cytoplasm. Also found in the alveoli (3) are the **great alveolar cells (2, 5)** or type II pneumocytes. The greater alveolar cells (2, 5) are interspersed among the simple squamous alveolar cells (6) in the alveoli (3).

At the free ends of the interalveolar septa (4) and around the open ends of the alveoli (3) are narrow bands of **smooth muscle fibers (8).** These muscle fibers are continuous with the muscle layer that lines the respiratory bronchioles.

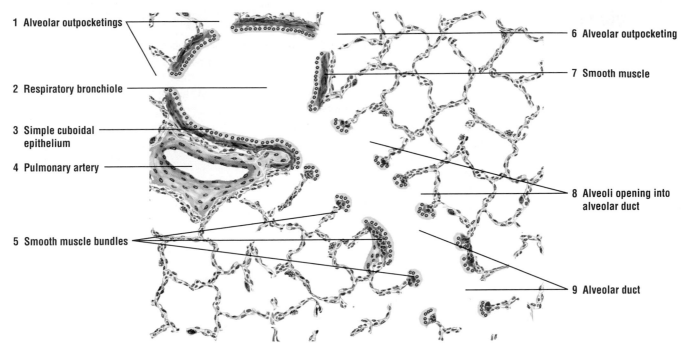

1 Alveolar outpocketings

2 Respiratory bronchiole

3 Simple cuboidal epithelium

4 Pulmonary artery

5 Smooth muscle bundles

6 Alveolar outpocketing

7 Smooth muscle

8 Alveoli opening into alveolar duct

9 Alveolar duct

FIGURE 15.11 ■ Respiratory bronchiole, alveolar duct, and lung alveoli. Stain: hematoxylin and eosin. Low magnification.

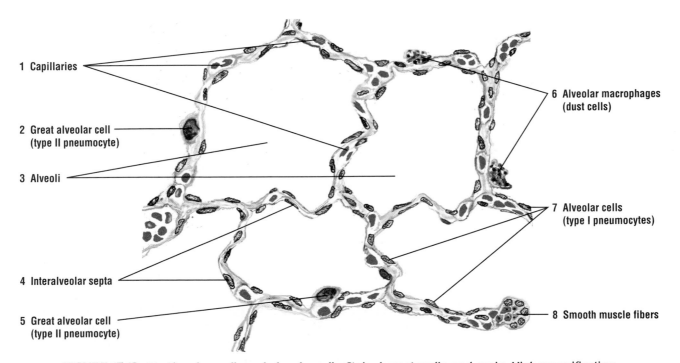

1 Capillaries

2 Great alveolar cell (type II pneumocyte)

3 Alveoli

4 Interalveolar septa

5 Great alveolar cell (type II pneumocyte)

6 Alveolar macrophages (dust cells)

7 Alveolar cells (type I pneumocytes)

8 Smooth muscle fibers

FIGURE 15.12 ■ Alveolar walls and alveolar cells. Stain: hematoxylin and eosin. High magnification.

FIGURE 15.13 ■ Lung: Terminal Bronchiole, Respiratory Bronchiole, and Alveoli

This photomicrograph of the lung shows the smallest air-conducting passage, the **terminal bronchiole (7)**. The terminal bronchiole (7) gives rise to thinner **respiratory bronchioles (3)**, whose walls are characterized by numerous **alveoli (2)**. Each respiratory bronchiole (3) gives rise to an **alveolar duct (1, 4, 8)** that continues into the **alveolar sacs (5)**. The terminal bronchiole (7) and the adjacent **blood vessel (6)** are surrounded by the alveoli (2).

FUNCTIONAL CORRELATIONS

Conducting Portion of the Respiratory System

The conducting portions of the respiratory system condition the inhaled air. **Mucus** is continuously produced by **goblet cells** in pseudostratified ciliated respiratory epithelium and **mucous glands** in the lamina propria. These secretions form a mucous layer that covers the luminal surfaces in most conducting tubes. As a result, the **moist mucosa** in the conducting portion of the respiratory system **humidifies** the air. The mucus and ciliated epithelium also filter and clean the air of particulate matter, infectious microorganisms, and other airborne matter. In addition, a rich and extensive **capillary network** beneath the epithelium in the connective tissue **warms** the inspired air as it passes the conducting portion and before it reaches the respiratory portion in the lungs.

Clara Cells

Clara cells are most numerous in the terminal bronchioles. These cells become the predominant cell type in the most distal part of the respiratory bronchioles. Clara cells have several important functions. They secrete one of the lipoprotein components of **surfactant,** which is a tension-reducing agent that is also found in the alveoli. Clara cells may also function as **stem cells** to replace lost or injured bronchial epithelial cells. These cells may also secrete proteins into the bronchial tree to protect the lung from inhaled toxic substances, oxidative pollutants, or inflammation.

Cells of Lung Alveoli

The lung alveoli contain numerous cell types. **Type I alveolar cells,** also called **type I pneumocytes**, are extremely thin simple squamous cells that line the alveoli in the lung and are the main sites for gaseous exchange. A thin **interalveolar septum** is located between adjacent alveoli. Located within the interalveolar septum between the delicate reticular and elastic fibers is a network of capillaries. Type I alveolar cells are in very close contact with the endothelial lining of capillaries, forming a very thin **blood-air barrier,** across which gaseous exchange takes place. The blood-air barrier consists of the surface lining and the cytoplasm of type I pneumocyte, the fused basement membrane of the pneumocyte and the endothelial cell, and the thin cytoplasm of the capillary endothelium.

Type II alveolar cells, also called **type II pneumocytes** or **septal cells,** are fewer in number and cuboidal in shape. They are found singly or in groups adjacent to the squamous type I alveolar cells within the alveoli. Their rounded apices project into the alveoli above the type I alveolar cells. These alveolar cells are secretory and contain dense-staining **lamellar bodies** in their apical cytoplasm. These cells synthesize and secrete a phospholipid-rich product called pulmonary **surfactant.** When it is released into the alveolus, surfactant spreads as a thin layer over the surfaces of type I alveolar cells, lowering the alveolar **surface tension.** The reduced surface tension in the alveoli decreases the force that is needed to inflate alveoli during inspiration. Therefore, surfactant stabilizes the alveolar diameters, facilitates their expansion, and prevents their collapse during respiration by minimizing the collapsing forces. During fetal development, the great alveolar cells secrete a sufficient amount of surfactant for respiration during the last 28 to 32 weeks of gestation. In addition to producing surfactant, the great alveolar cells can divide and function as **stem cells** for type I squamous alveolar cells in the alveoli. It is also believed that surfactant has some **bactericidal** effects in the alveoli that counteract potentially dangerous inhaled pathogens.

Alveolar macrophages or **dust cells** are monocytes that have entered the pulmonary connective tissue and alveoli. The primary function of these macrophages is to clean the alveoli of invading microorganisms and inhaled particulate matter by **phagocytosis.** These cells are seen either in the individual alveoli or in the thin alveolar septa. Their cytoplasm normally contains phagocytosed particulate particles.

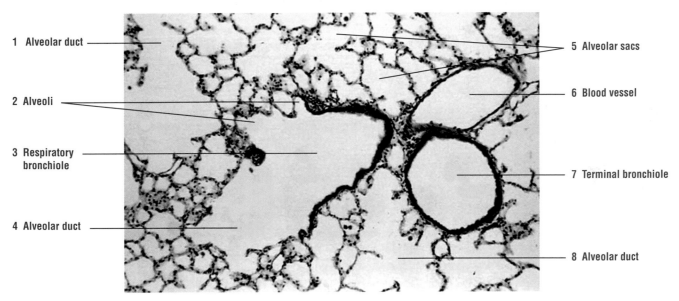

1 Alveolar duct

2 Alveoli

3 Respiratory bronchiole

4 Alveolar duct

5 Alveolar sacs

6 Blood vessel

7 Terminal bronchiole

8 Alveolar duct

FIGURE 15.13 ■ Lung: terminal bronchiole, respiratory bronchiole, alveolar ducts, alveoli, and blood vessel. Stain: hematoxylin and eosin. ×40.

Components of Respiratory System

- Conducting portion consists of solid passageways that move air in and out of lungs
- Pseudostratified ciliated epithelium with numerous goblet cells line the larger passageways
- As passageways branch, there is a decrease in epithelium height and tubule size
- Terminal bronchioles represent the terminal portion of conducting portion
- Respiratory bronchioles represent the transition zone between conducting and respiratory zones

Conducting Portion of Respiratory System: Extrapulmonary and Intrapulmonary

- Extrapulmonary structures are the nose, pharynx, larynx, trachea, and bronchi
- Conditions air by humidifying, warming, and filtering it owing to cilia and mucus in passageways
- Intrapulmonary structures include bronchi, bronchioles, and terminal bronchioles
- Incomplete hyaline cartilage C-rings encircle and keep trachea patent (open)
- In the lungs, hyaline cartilage plates replace C rings and encircle the larger bronchi
- Bronchioles of about 1 mm diameter no longer have cartilage
- As tubular size decreases, epithelium becomes simple ciliated and goblet cells disappear

Clara Cells

- Replace goblet cells and become predominant cells in terminal and respiratory bronchioles
- Are secretory, nonciliated cells that increase in number as ciliated cells decrease
- Secrete lipoprotein components of surfactant, a tension-reducing agent
- May also function as stem cells to replace lost or injured bronchial epithelial cells
- May secrete proteins into bronchial tree to protect lung from inflammation or toxic pollutants

Respiratory Portion of Respiratory System

- Starts with a passageway where initial respiration can take place
- Terminal bronchioles give rise to respiratory bronchioles
- Respiratory bronchioles exhibit thin-walled alveoli, where respiration can take place
- Gaseous exchange can take place only when alveoli are present
- Consists of respiratory bronchioles, alveolar ducts, alveolar sacs, and alveoli

- Goblet cells are absent from alveoli and the lining is very thin where respiration occurs

Cells of Lung Alveoli

- Type I alveolar cells (type I pneumocytes)
- Are very thin and line the lung alveoli
- With capillary endothelium, form the thin blood-air barrier
- Type II alveolar cells (type II pneumocytes)
- Are adjacent to type I cells
- Are secretory cells, whose apices project above type I cells
- Contain numerous secretory lamellar bodies
- Synthesize phospholipid surfactant for release into individual alveoli
- Surfactant reduces alveolar surface tension, allowing expansion and preventing collapse

Alveolar Macrophages

- Are monocytes that enter pulmonary connective tissue and alveoli
- Clean alveoli of invading organisms and phagocytose particular matter

Olfactory Epithelium

- Located in the roof of the nasal cavity and on each side of the superior concha
- Contains supportive, basal, and olfactory cells, the sensory bipolar neurons, without goblet cells
- Olfactory cells span the thickness of epithelium and are distributed in the middle of epithelium
- Surface of cells shows small, round olfactory vesicles with nonmotile olfactory cilia
- Olfactory cilia contain odor-binding receptors that are stimulated by odor molecules
- Below epithelium are serous olfactory glands that bathe olfactory cilia and provide odor solvents
- Olfactory nerves in lamina propria leave olfactory cells and continue into cranial cavity
- Supportive cells provide mechanical support; basal cells serve as stem cells for epithelium
- Transition from olfactory to respiratory epithelium is abrupt

Epiglottis

- Superior part of larynx that projects upward from larynx wall
- A central elastic cartilage forms core of the epiglottis
- Stratified squamous epithelium lines lingual (anterior) and part of laryngeal (posterior) surface
- Base of epiglottis lined with pseudostratified ciliated columnar epithelium
- Taste buds may be present in lingual or laryngeal epithelium

Larynx

- Pseudostratified ciliated columnar epithelium lines false vocal fold, as in posterior epiglottis
- Mixed seromucous glands, blood vessels, lymphatic nodules, and adipose cells in lamina propria
- Ventricle, a deep indentation, separates false vocal fold from true vocal fold
- True vocal fold lined by stratified squamous nonkeratinized epithelium
- Vocalis ligament is at the apex of true vocal fold and skeletal vocalis muscle is adjacent
- Hyaline thyroid cartilage and cricoid cartilage provide support for the larynx

- Epithelium in lower larynx changes back to pseudostratified ciliated columnar

Trachea

- Wall consists of mucosa, submucosa, hyaline cartilage, and adventitia
- Cartilage C rings keep trachea open with gaps between rings filled with trachealis muscle
- The lining is pseudostratified ciliated columnar epithelium with goblet cells
- Submucosa contains seromucous tracheal glands with ducts opening into trachea lumen

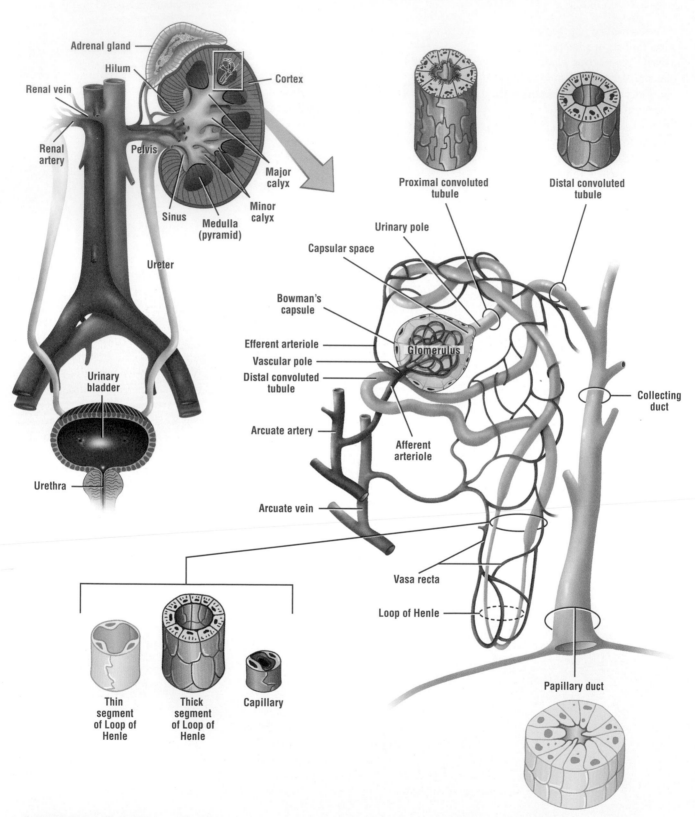

OVERVIEW FIGURE 16 ■ A sagittal section of the kidney shows the cortex and medulla, with blood vessels and the excretory ducts, including the pelvis and the ureter and a histologic comparison of blood vessels, the different tubules of the nephron, and the collecting ducts.

CHAPTER 16

Urinary System

The Kidney

The urinary system consists of two **kidneys,** two **ureters** that lead to a single urinary **bladder,** and a single **urethra.** The kidneys are large, bean-shaped organs located retroperitoneally adjacent to the posterior body wall. Superior to each kidney is the **adrenal gland** embedded in renal fat and connective tissue. The concave, medial border of the kidney is the **hilum,** which contains three large structures, the **renal artery, renal vein,** and the funnel-shaped **renal pelvis.** Surrounding these structures is loose connective tissue and a fat-filled space called the **renal sinus.**

Each kidney is covered by a dense irregular connective tissue capsule. A sagittal section through the kidney shows a darker, outer **cortex** and a lighter, inner **medulla,** which consists of numerous cone-shaped **renal pyramids.** The base of each pyramid faces the cortex and forms the corticomedullary boundary. The round apex of each pyramid extends downward to the renal pelvis to form the **renal papilla.** A portion of the cortex also extends on each side of the renal pyramids to form the **renal columns.**

Each renal papilla is surrounded by a funnel-shaped **minor calyx,** which collects urine from the papilla. The minor calyces join in the renal sinus to form a **major calyx.** Major calyces, in turn, join to form the larger funnel-shaped renal pelvis. The renal pelvis leaves each kidney through the hilum, narrows to become a muscular **ureter,** and descends toward the bladder on each side of the posterior body wall.

Uriniferous Tubules and Nephrons of the Kidney

The functional unit of each kidney is the microscopic **uriniferous tubule.** It consists of a **nephron** and a **collecting duct** into which empty the filtered contents of the nephron. Millions of nephrons are present in each kidney cortex. The nephron, in turn, is subdivided into two components, a renal corpuscle and renal tubules.

There are two types of nephrons. **Cortical nephrons** are located in the cortex of kidney, whereas the **juxtamedullary nephrons** are situated near the junction of the cortex and medulla of the kidney. Although all nephrons participate in urine formation, juxtamedullary nephrons produce a hypertonic environment in the interstitium of the kidney medulla that results in the production of concentrated (hypertonic) urine.

Renal Corpuscle

The renal corpuscle consists of a tuft of capillaries, called the **glomerulus,** surrounded by a double layer of epithelial cells, called the **glomerular (Bowman's) capsule.** The inner or **visceral layer** of the capsule consists of unique and highly modified branching epithelial cells, called **podocytes.** The podocytes are adjacent to and completely invest the glomerular capillaries. The outer or **parietal layer** of the glomerular capsule consists of simple squamous epithelium.

The renal corpuscle is the initial segment of each nephron. Blood is filtered in renal corpuscles through the capillaries of the glomerulus, and the filtrate enters the **capsular (urinary) space** located between the parietal and visceral cell layers of the glomerular capsule. Each renal corpuscle has a **vascular pole,** where the afferent arteriole enters and the efferent arteriole leaves the corpuscle. On the opposite end of the renal corpuscle is the **urinary pole.** Filtrate produced by the glomerulus that enters the capsular space leaves each renal corpuscle at the urinary pole, where the proximal convoluted tubule starts.

Filtration of blood in renal corpuscles is facilitated by glomerular endothelium. The endothelium in glomerular capillaries is **porous** (fenestrated) and highly permeable to many substances in the blood, except to the formed blood elements or plasma proteins. Thus, glomerular filtrate that enters the capsular space is not urine. Instead, it is an ultrafiltrate that is similar to plasma, except for the absence of proteins.

Renal Tubules

As the glomerular filtrate leaves the renal corpuscle at the urinary pole, it flows through different parts of the nephron before reaching the renal tubules called the collecting tubules and collecting ducts. The glomerular filtrate first enters the **renal tubule,** which extends from the glomerular capsule to the collecting tubule. This renal tubule has several distinct histologic and functional regions.

The portion of the renal tubule that begins at the renal corpuscle is highly twisted or tortuous and is therefore called the **proximal convoluted tubule.** Initially, this tubule is located in the cortex but then descends into the medulla to become continuous with the loop of Henle. The **loop of Henle** consists of several parts: a thick, descending portion of the proximal convoluted tubule; a thin descending and ascending segment; and a thick, ascending portion called the **distal convoluted tubule.** The distal convoluted tubule is shorter and less convoluted than the proximal convoluted tubule, and it ascends into the kidney cortex. Because the proximal convoluted tubule is longer than the distal convoluted tubule, it is more frequently observed near the renal corpuscles and in the renal cortex.

Glomerular filtrate then flows from the distal convoluted tubule to the **collecting tubule.** In juxtamedullary nephrons, the loop of Henle is very long; it descends from the kidney cortex deep into the medulla and then loops back to ascend into the cortex (Overview Figure 16).

The collecting tubule is not part of the nephron. A number of short collecting tubules join to form several larger **collecting ducts.** As the collecting ducts become larger and descend toward the papillae of the medulla, they are called **papillary ducts.** Smaller collecting ducts are lined by light-staining cuboidal epithelium. Deeper in the medulla, the epithelium in these ducts changes to columnar. At the tip of each papilla, the papillary ducts empty their contents into the minor calyx. The area on the papilla that exhibits openings of the papillary ducts is called the **area cribrosa** (Overview Figure 16).

The kidney cortex also exhibits numerous, lighter-staining **medullary rays** that extend vertically from the bases of the pyramids into the cortex. Medullary rays consist primarily of collecting ducts, blood vessels, and straight portions of a number of nephrons that penetrate the cortex from the base of the pyramids.

Renal Blood Supply

To understand the functional correlation of the kidney, it becomes important to understand the blood supply of the organ. Each kidney is supplied by a **renal artery** that divides in the hilus into several segmental branches, which branch into several **interlobar arteries.** The interlobar arteries continue in the kidney between the pyramids toward the cortex. At the corticomedullary junction, the interlobar arteries branch into **arcuate arteries,** which arch over the base of the pyramids and give rise to **interlobular arteries.** These branch further into the **afferent arteriole**s, which give rise to the **capillaries** in the **glomeruli** of renal corpuscles. **Efferent arterioles** leave the renal corpuscles and form a complex **peritubular capillary network** around the tubules in the cortex and long, straight capillary vessels or **vasa recta** in the medulla that loops back to the corticomedullary region. The vasa recta forms loops that are parallel to the loops of Henle. The interstitium is drained by interlobular veins that continue toward the arcuate veins.

FIGURE 16.1 ■ Kidney: Cortex, Medulla, Pyramid, and Minor Calyx (Panoramic View)

In the sagittal section, the kidney is subdivided into an outer darker-staining **cortex** and an inner lighter-staining **medulla.** Externally, the cortex is covered with a dense, irregular connective tissue **renal capsule (1).**

The cortex contains both distal and **proximal convoluted tubules (4, 11), glomeruli (2),** and **medullary rays (3).** Present also in the cortex are the **interlobular arteries (12)** and **interlobular veins (13).** The medullary rays (3) are formed by the straight portions of nephrons, blood vessels, and collecting tubules that join in the medulla to form the larger **collecting ducts (6).** The medullary rays do not extend to the kidney capsule (1) because of the **subcapsular convoluted tubules (10).**

The medulla comprises the renal pyramids. The **base** of each **pyramid (5)** is adjacent to the cortex and its apex forms the pointed **renal papilla (7)** that projects into the surrounding, funnel-like structure, the **minor calyx (16),** which represents the dilated portion of the ureter. The **area cribrosa (9)** is pierced by small holes, which are the openings of the collecting ducts (6) into the minor calyx (16).

The tip of the renal papilla (7) is usually covered with a simple **columnar epithelium (8).** As the columnar epithelium of the renal papilla (7) reflects onto the outer wall of the minor calyx (16), it becomes a **transitional epithelium (16).** A thin layer of connective tissue and smooth muscle (not illustrated) under this epithelium then merges with the connective tissue of the **renal sinus (15).**

Present in the renal sinus (15) are branches of the renal artery and vein called the **interlobar artery (17)** and the **interlobar vein (18).** The interlobar vessels (17, 18) enter the kidney and arch over the base of the pyramid (5) at the corticomedullary junction as the **arcuate artery and vein (14).** The arcuate vessels (14) give rise to smaller, interlobular arteries (12) and interlobular veins (13) that pass radially into the kidney cortex and give rise to the afferent glomerular arteries that give rise to the capillaries of the glomeruli (3).

FUNCTIONAL CORRELATIONS: Kidney

The kidneys are vital organs for maintaining the body's stable internal environment, or **homeostasis.** This function is performed by regulating the body's blood pressure, blood composition and pH, fluid volume, and acid-base balance. The kidneys also produce urine, which is formed in the kidneys as a result of three main functions: **filtration** of blood in the glomeruli, **reabsorption** of nutrients and other valuable substances from the filtrate that enters the proximal and distal convoluted tubules, and **secretion or excretion** of metabolic waste products or unwanted chemicals or substances into the filtrate. Approximately 99% of the glomerular filtrate produced by the kidneys that enters the tubules is reabsorbed into the system in the nephrons; the remaining 1% of the filtrate enters the bladder and is voided as urine.

In addition, kidney cells produce two important substances, an enzyme renin and a glycoprotein erythropoietin. **Renin** regulates blood pressure to maintain proper filtration pressure in the kidney glomeruli. **Erythropoietin,** believed to be produced and released by the endothelial cells of the peritubular capillary network, stimulates erythrocyte production in red bone marrow.

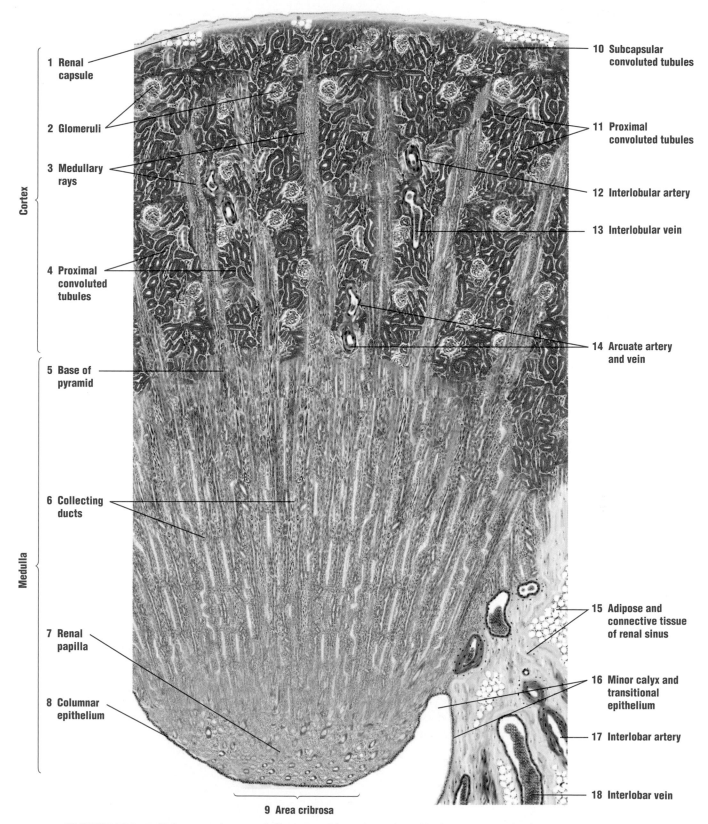

Cortex

1 Renal capsule

2 Glomeruli

3 Medullary rays

4 Proximal convoluted tubules

5 Base of pyramid

Medulla

6 Collecting ducts

7 Renal papilla

8 Columnar epithelium

9 Area cribrosa

10 Subcapsular convoluted tubules

11 Proximal convoluted tubules

12 Interlobular artery

13 Interlobular vein

14 Arcuate artery and vein

15 Adipose and connective tissue of renal sinus

16 Minor calyx and transitional epithelium

17 Interlobar artery

18 Interlobar vein

FIGURE 16.1 ■ Kidney: cortex, medulla, pyramid, and renal papilla (panoramic view). Stain: hematoxylin and eosin. Low magnification.

FIGURE 16.2 ■ Kidney Cortex and Upper Medulla

A higher magnification of the kidney shows greater detail of the cortex. The **renal corpuscles (5, 9)** consist of a **glomerulus (5a)** and the **glomerular (Bowman's) capsule (5b)**. The glomerulus (5a) is a tuft of capillaries that is formed from the afferent **glomerular arteriole (11),** and is supported by fine connective tissue and surrounded by the glomerular capsule (5b).

The internal or **visceral layer (9a)** of the glomerular capsule (5b) surrounds the glomerular capillaries with modified epithelial cells called **podocytes (9a)**. At the **vascular pole (8)** of the renal corpuscle (9), the epithelium of the visceral layer (9a) reflects to form the simple squamous **parietal layer (9b)** of the glomerular capsule (5b). The space between the visceral layer (9a) and the parietal layer (9b) of the renal corpuscle (9) is the **capsular space (10)**.

Two types of convoluted tubules, sectioned in various planes, surround the renal corpuscles (5, 9). These are the **proximal convoluted tubules (1)** and **distal convoluted tubules (2, 4)**. The convoluted tubules are the initial and terminal segments of the nephron. The proximal convoluted tubules (1) are longer than the distal convoluted tubules (2, 4) and are, therefore, more numerous in the cortex. The proximal convoluted tubules (1) exhibit a small, uneven lumen, and a single layer of cuboidal cells with eosinophilic, granular cytoplasm. A brush border (microvilli) lines the cells but is not always well preserved in the sections. Also, the cell boundaries in the proximal convoluted tubules (1) are not distinct because of extensive basal and lateral cell membrane interdigitations with the neighboring cells.

The urinary capsular space (10) in the renal corpuscle (5, 9) is continuous with the lumen of the proximal convoluted tubule at the urinary pole (see Figure 16.3). At the urinary pole, the squamous epithelium of the parietal layer (9b) of the glomerular capsule (5b) changes to cuboidal epithelium of the proximal convoluted tubule (1).

The distal convoluted tubules (2, 4) are shorter and are fewer in number in the cortex. The distal convoluted tubules (2, 4) also exhibit larger lumina with smaller, cuboidal cells. The cytoplasm stains less intensely than in the proximal convoluted tubules (1), and the brush border is not present on the cells. Similar to the proximal convoluted tubules (1), the distal convoluted tubules (2, 4) show deep basal and lateral cell membrane infoldings and interdigitations.

Also found in the cortex are the medullary rays. The medullary rays include the following three types of tubules: **straight (descending) segments of the proximal tubules (14), straight (ascending) segments of the distal tubules (6),** and the **collecting tubules (12)**. The straight (descending) segments of the proximal tubules (14) are very similar to the proximal convoluted tubules (1), and the straight (ascending) segments of the distal tubules (6) are very similar to distal convoluted tubules (2, 4). The collecting tubules (12) in the cortex are distinct because of their lightly stained cuboidal cells and cell membranes.

The medulla contains only straight portions of the tubules and the segments of the loop of Henle (thick and thin descending segments, and thin and thick ascending segments). The **thin segments of the loops of Henle (15)** are lined by simple squamous epithelium and resemble the **capillaries (13)**. The distinguishing features of the thin loops of Henle (15) are the thicker epithelial lining and absence of blood cells in their lumina. In contrast, most capillaries (13) have blood cells in the lumina.

Also visible in the cortex are the **interlobular blood vessels (3)** and the larger **interlobar vein and artery (7)**. The interlobular blood vessels (3) give rise to the afferent glomerular arteriole (11) that enters the glomerular capsule (5b) at the vascular pole (8) and forms the capillary tuft of the glomerulus (5a).

FUNCTIONAL CORRELATIONS: Kidney Cells and Tubules

Mesangial Cells

In addition to podocytes that surround the capillaries, there are other specialized cells in the glomerulus, called **mesangial cells,** that are also attached to the capillaries. Mesangial cells synthesize the extracellular matrix and provide structural support for the glomerular capillaries. As blood is filtered, numerous proteinaceous macromolecules are trapped in the basal lamina of the glomerulus. Mesangial cells function as **macrophages** in the intraglomerular regions and phagocytose material that accumulates on the glomerular filter, thus preventing its clogging with debris. These cells also appear to be contractile and can regulate glomerular blood flow as a result of the presence of receptors for vasoactive substances. Some of the mesangial cells are also located outside of the renal corpuscle in the vascular pole region. Here, they are called the extraglomerular mesangial cells that form part of the juxtaglomerular apparatus.

Proximal Convoluted Tubules

All nephrons participate in urine formation. The cells of the **proximal convoluted tubules** show numerous deep infoldings of the basal cell membrane, between which are located numerous elongated mitochondria, and lateral interdigitations with the neighboring cells. These features characterize cells that are involved in active transport of molecules and electrolytes from the filtrate across the cell membrane into the interstitium. The mitochondria supply the necessary ATP (energy) for active transport of Na^+ by the Na^+/K^+ ATPase (sodium pump) located in the basolateral regions of the cell membrane.

Reabsorption of most of the substances from the glomerular filtrate takes place in the proximal convoluted tubules. As the glomerular filtrate enters the proximal convoluted tubules, all **glucose, proteins,** and **amino acids,** almost all carbohydrates, and about 75 to 85% of water and sodium and chloride ions are absorbed from the glomerular filtrate into the surrounding **peritubular capillaries.** The presence of **microvilli** (brush border) on proximal convoluted tubule cells greatly increases the surface area and facilitates absorption of filtered material. In addition, the proximal convoluted tubules secrete certain metabolites, hydrogen, ammonia, dyes, and drugs such as penicillin from the body into the glomerular filtrate. The metabolic waste products urea and uric acid remain in the proximal convoluted tubules and are eliminated from the body in the urine.

The proximal convoluted tubule is longer than the distal convoluted tubule. As a result, the sections of this tubule are more frequently seen in the cortex near the renal corpuscles that those of distal convoluted tubules.

Loops of Henle

The **loops of Henle** of the juxtaglomerular nephrons produce the **hypertonic urine** by creating an osmotic gradient in the interstitium from the cortex of the kidney to the tips of the renal papillae. Sodium chloride and urea are transported and concentrated in the interstitial tissue of the kidney medulla by means of a complex **countercurrent multiplier system,** which creates a high interstitial osmolarity deep in the medulla. In the juxtamedullary nephrons, the loops of Henle are very long, extend deep into the medulla, and assist in maintaining the high osmotic gradient necessary for removing water from the filtrate into the interstitium. The hypertonicity (high osmotic pressure) of extracellular fluid in the medulla removes water from the glomerular filtrate as it flows through these tubules, with the **vasa recta** helping to maintain the osmotic concentration gradient in the medulla. These capillary loops are permeable to water and take up the water from the medullary interstitium to return it to systemic circulation.

Distal Convoluted Tubules

The **distal convoluted tubules** are shorter and less convoluted than the proximal tubules. Therefore, these tubules are less frequently observed in the cortex and near the renal corpuscles. In comparison with the proximal convoluted tubules, the distal convoluted tubules do not exhibit brush borders, the cells are smaller, and more nuclei are seen per tubule. The basolateral membranes of distal convoluted tubule cells show increased interdigitations and the presence of elongated mitochondria within these infoldings. The main function of the distal convoluted tubules is to actively reabsorb sodium ions from the tubular filtrate. This activity is directly linked with excretion of hydrogen and potassium ions into the tubular fluid.

Sodium reabsorption in the distal convoluted tubules is controlled by the hormone **aldosterone,** which is secreted by the adrenal cortex. In the presence of aldosterone, cells of the distal convoluted tubules actively absorb sodium and chloride ions from the filtrate and transport them across the cell membrane into the interstitium. Here, these ions are absorbed by the **peritubular capillaries** and returned back to the systemic circulation, thus decreasing sodium loss in urine. These functions of distal convoluted tubules are vital for maintaining the acid-base balance of body fluids and blood.

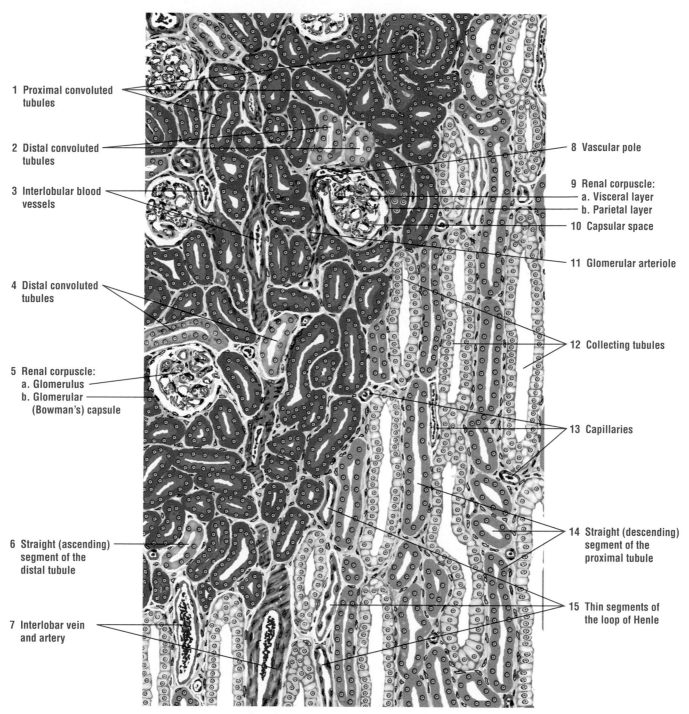

1 Proximal convoluted tubules

2 Distal convoluted tubules

3 Interlobular blood vessels

4 Distal convoluted tubules

5 Renal corpuscle:
  a. Glomerulus
  b. Glomerular (Bowman's) capsule

6 Straight (ascending) segment of the distal tubule

7 Interlobar vein and artery

8 Vascular pole

9 Renal corpuscle:
  a. Visceral layer
  b. Parietal layer

10 Capsular space

11 Glomerular arteriole

12 Collecting tubules

13 Capillaries

14 Straight (descending) segment of the proximal tubule

15 Thin segments of the loop of Henle

FIGURE 16.2 ■ Kidney cortex and upper medulla. Stain: hematoxylin and eosin. Low magnification.

FIGURE 16.3 ■ Kidney Cortex: Juxtaglomerular Apparatus

A higher magnification of the kidney cortex illustrates the renal corpuscle, convoluted tubules, and juxtaglomerular apparatus.

The renal corpuscle exhibits the **glomerular capillaries (2), parietal (10a)** and **visceral (10b)** epithelium of the **glomerular (Bowman's) capsule (10),** and the **capsular space (13).** The brush borders and acidophilic cells distinguish the **proximal convoluted tubules (6, 14)** from the **distal convoluted tubules (1, 15),** whose smaller, less intensely stained cells lack the brush borders. The cuboidal cells of the **collecting tubules (8)** exhibit cell outlines and pale cytoplasm. Distinct **basement membranes (9)** surround these tubules.

Each renal corpuscle exhibits a vascular pole where the **afferent glomerular arterioles (12)** enter and efferent glomerular arterioles exit. On the opposite side of the renal corpuscle is the **urinary pole (11).** Here, the capsular space (13) becomes continuous with the lumen of the proximal convoluted tubule (6, 14). The plane of section through both the vascular and urinary poles is only occasionally seen in the kidney cortex. However, this section shows the renal corpuscle where blood is filtered, glomerular filtrate accumulated, and initial stages where the filtrate is modified to form urine.

At the vascular pole, modified epithelioid cells with cytoplasmic granules replace the smooth muscle cells in the tunica media of the afferent glomerular arteriole (12). These cells are the **juxtaglomerular cells (4).** In the adjacent distal convoluted tubule, the cells that border the juxtaglomerular cells (4) are narrow and more columnar. This area of darker, more compact cell arrangement is called the **macula densa (5).** The juxtaglomerular cells (4) in the afferent glomerular arteriole (12) and the macula densa (5) cells in the distal convoluted tubule form the juxtaglomerular apparatus.

1 Distal convoluted tubule

2 Glomerular capillaries

3 Glomerular arteriole

4 Juxtaglomerular cells

5 Macula densa

6 Proximal convoluted tubule

7 Interlobular vessels:
   a. Venule
   b. Arteriole

8 Collecting tubule

9 Basement membrane

10 Glomerular (Bowman's) capsule:
   a. Parietal layer
   b. Visceral layer

11 Urinary pole

12 Afferent glomerular arteriole

13 Capsular space

14 Proximal convoluted tubule

15 Distal convoluted tubule

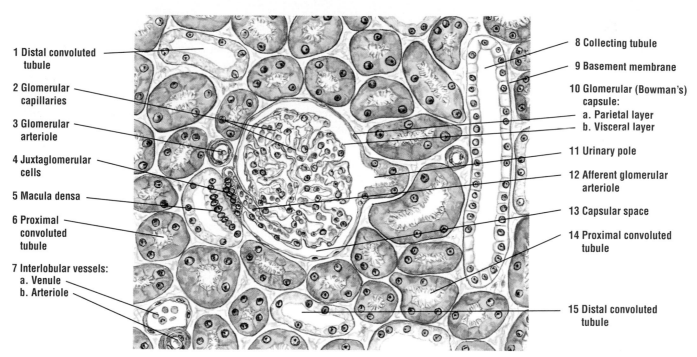

FIGURE 16.3 ■ Kidney cortex: juxtaglomerular apparatus. Stain: hematoxylin and eosin. Medium magnification.

FIGURE 16.4 ■ Kidney: Renal Corpuscle, Juxtaglomerular Apparatus, and Convoluted Tubules

This high-magnification photomicrograph shows a renal corpuscle with surrounding tubules. The renal corpuscle consists of **glomerulus (1)** and the **glomerular capsule (2)** with a **parietal layer (2a)** and a **visceral layer (2b)**. Between these layers is the **capsular space (5)**, with **podocytes (4, 7)** located on the surface of the visceral layer (2b). At the vascular pole of the renal corpuscle, blood vessels enter and leave the renal corpuscle. Adjacent to the vascular pole is the **juxtaglomerular apparatus (3)**. The juxtaglomerular apparatus (3) consists of modified smooth muscle cells of the afferent arteriole in the vascular pole, the **juxtaglomerular cells (3a),** and the **macula densa (3b)** of the **distal convoluted tubule (6, 9)**. Surrounding the renal corpuscle are the darker-staining **proximal convoluted tubules (8)** and the distal convoluted tubules (6, 9).

FUNCTIONAL CORRELATIONS: Juxtaglomerular Apparatus

Adjacent to the renal corpuscles and distal convoluted tubules lies a special group of cells called **juxtaglomerular apparatus.** This apparatus consists of two components, the juxtaglomerular cells and the macula densa.

Juxtaglomerular cells are a group of modified **smooth muscle cells** located in the wall of the **afferent arteriole** just before it enters the glomerular capsule to form the glomerulus. The cytoplasm of these cells contains membrane-bound secretory granules of the enzyme **renin.** The **macula densa** is a group of modified distal convoluted tubule cells. The macula densa cells and juxtaglomerular cells are separated by a thin basement membrane. The proximity of juxtaglomerular cells to the macula densa allows for integration of their functions.

The main function of the juxtaglomerular apparatus is to maintain the necessary blood pressure in the kidney for glomerular filtration. The cells of this apparatus act as both the baroreceptors and chemoreceptors. The juxtaglomerular cells monitor changes in the **systemic blood pressure** by responding to stretching in the walls of the afferent arterioles. The cells in the macula densa are sensitive to changes in sodium chloride concentration. A decrease in the blood pressure produces a decreased amount of glomerular filtrate and, consequently, a decreased sodium ion concentration in the filtrate as it flows past the macula densa in the distal convoluted tubule.

A decrease in systemic blood pressure or a decreased sodium concentration in the filtrate induces the juxtaglomerular cells to release the enzyme renin into the bloodstream. Renin converts the plasma protein **angiotensinogen** to **angiotensin I,** which in turn, is converted to **angiotensin II** by another enzyme present in the **endothelial cells** of lung capillaries. Angiotensin II is an active hormone and a powerful **vasoconstrictor** that initially produces arterial constriction, thereby increasing the systemic blood pressure. In addition, angiotensin II stimulates the release of the hormone **aldosterone** from the adrenal gland cortex.

Aldosterone acts primarily on the cells of distal convoluted tubules to increase their reabsorption of sodium and chloride ions from the glomerular filtrate. Water follows sodium chloride by osmosis and increases fluid volume in the circulatory system. The combination of these effects raises the systemic blood pressure, increases the glomerular filtration rate in the kidney, and eliminates the need for further release of renin. Aldosterone also facilitates the elimination of potassium and hydrogen ions and is an essential hormone for maintaining electrolyte balance in the body.

1 Glomerulus

2 Glomerular capsule
  a. Parietal layer
  b. Visceral layer

3 Juxtaglomerular apparatus
  a. Juxtaglomerular cells
  b. Macula densa

4 Podocyte

5 Capsular space

6 Distal convoluted tubules

7 Podocyte

8 Proximal convoluted tubules

9 Distal convoluted tubule

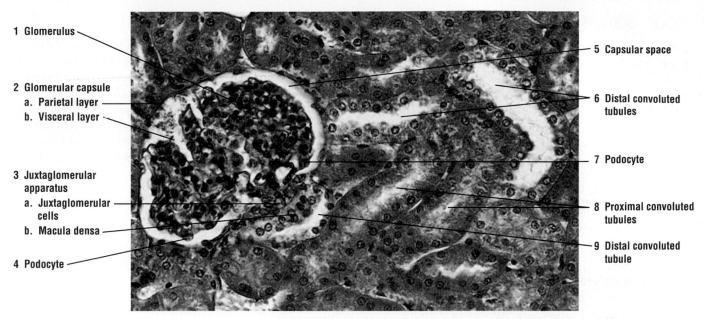

FIGURE 16.4 ■ Kidney cortex: renal corpuscle, juxtaglomerular apparatus, and convoluted tubules. Stain: hematoxylin and eosin. ×130.

FIGURE 16.5 ■ Kidney: Scanning Electron Micrograph of Podocytes

This scanning electron micrograph illustrates the very unique and unusual appearance of the visceral epithelium of the glomerular capsule and the podocytes, which surround all of the capillaries in the kidney glomeruli. The flattened **cell body** of the **podocyte (6)** extends thicker **primary processes (1, 3)** that surround the capillary walls. The primary processes (1, 3) give rise to the smaller **pedicles (2, 7),** which interdigitate with similar pedicles from other podocytes around the capillaries. Between the pedicles (2, 6) are the tiny **filtration slits (5).** Also visible are remnants of **proteinaceous debris (4)** that became lodged in the filtration slits (5) during blood filtration. Surrounding the podocytes in the renal corpuscle is the dark-appearing capsular space that would contain the glomerular filtrate in a functioning kidney.

FIGURE 16.6 ■ Kidney: Transmission Electron Micrograph of Podocyte and Glomerular Capillary

This transmission electron micrograph shows the association of a podocyte with glomerular capillaries in the renal corpuscle of kidney. The **nucleus (3)** and **cytoplasm** of the **podocyte (11)** are separated from the adjacent **basement membrane** of the **capillary (13).** The larger **primary process** of the **podocyte (12)** extends from the podocyte cytoplasm (11) to surround the wall of the capillary. The smaller **pedicles (2, 5)** from the primary process of the podocyte (12) are attached to the basement membrane of the capillary (13). Between the individual pedicles (2, 5) are the **filtration slits (1).** Separating the podocyte (3, 11) from the capillaries and adjacent podocytes is the clear **capsular space (4).** In the **lumen** of the **capillary (6, 8)** are the **nucleus** of the **endothelial cell (10)** and sections of an **erythrocyte (7)** and **leukocyte (9).** In the lumen of the capillary (6, 8) are also visible tiny **fenestrations** in the endothelium (**arrowheads**).

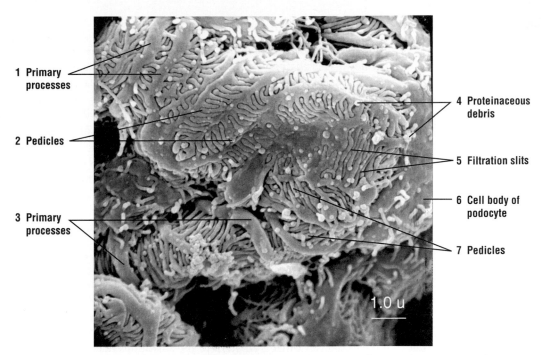

1 Primary processes

2 Pedicles

3 Primary processes

4 Proteinaceous debris

5 Filtration slits

6 Cell body of podocyte

7 Pedicles

1.0 u

FIGURE 16.5 ■ Kidney: scanning electron micrograph of podocytes (visceral epithelium of glomerular (Bowman's) capsule) surrounding the glomerular capillaries.

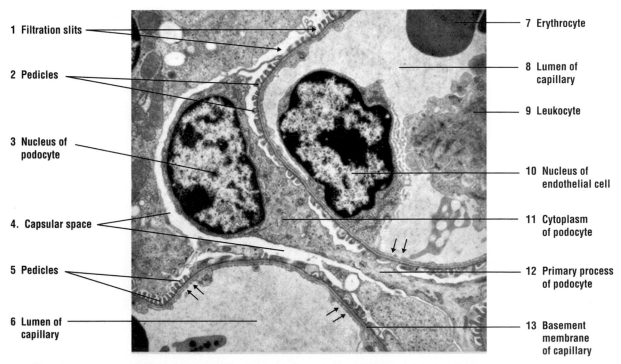

1 Filtration slits

2 Pedicles

3 Nucleus of podocyte

4. Capsular space

5 Pedicles

6 Lumen of capillary

7 Erythrocyte

8 Lumen of capillary

9 Leukocyte

10 Nucleus of endothelial cell

11 Cytoplasm of podocyte

12 Primary process of podocyte

13 Basement membrane of capillary

FIGURE 16.6 ■ Kidney: transmission electron micrograph of podocyte and adjacent capillaries in the renal corpuscle. ×6,500.

FIGURE 16.7 ■ Kidney Medulla: Papillary Region (Transverse Section)

The papilla in the kidney faces the minor calyx and contains the terminal portions of the collecting tubules, now called the **papillary ducts (3)**. The papillary ducts (3) exhibit large diameters and wide lumina, and are lined by tall, pale-staining columnar cells. Also present in the papilla are the **straight (ascending) segments of the distal tubules (7, 10)** and the **straight (descending) segments of the proximal tubules (1, 6, 11)**. Note that these straight segments in the medulla are very similar to the corresponding convoluted tubules in the cortex. Interspersed among the ascending (7, 10) and descending straight tubules (1, 6, 11) are the transverse sections of the **thin segments of the loop of Henle (5, 8)** that resemble the **capillaries (4, 9)** or small **venules (2)**. The capillaries (4, 9) and the small venules (2) differ from the thin segments of the loop of Henle (5, 8) by thinner walls and by the presence of blood cells in their lumina.

The **connective tissue (12)** surrounding the tubules is more abundant in the papillary region of the kidney, and the papillary ducts (3) are spaced further apart.

FIGURE 16.8 ■ Kidney Medulla: Terminal End of Papilla (Longitudinal Section)

Several collecting ducts merge in the papilla of the kidney medulla to form large, straight tubules called the **papillary ducts (6),** which are lined by simple cuboidal or columnar epithelium. Openings of the numerous papillary ducts (6) at the tip of the papilla produce a sievelike appearance in the papilla that is called the area cribrosa. The contents from the papillary ducts (6) continue into the minor calyx that is adjacent to and surrounds the tip of each papilla.

In this illustration, the papilla is lined by a stratified **covering epithelium (7)**. At the area cribrosa, the covering epithelium (7) is usually a tall simple columnar type that is continuous with the papillary ducts (6).

Thin segments of the loops of Henle (3, 5) descend deep into the papilla and are identifiable as thin ducts with empty lumina. **Venules (1)** and the **capillaries (4)** of the vasa recta are usually identified by the presence of blood cells in their lumina. Surrounding the blood vessels (1, 4) and the papillary ducts (6) is the **renal interstitium (connective tissue) (2)**.

FUNCTIONAL CORRELATIONS: Collecting Tubules, Collecting Ducts, and Antidiuretic Hormone

Glomerular filtrate flows from the distal convoluted tubules to **collecting tubules** and **collecting ducts.** Under normal conditions, these tubules are not permeable to water. However, during excessive water loss from the body or dehydration, **antidiuretic hormone (ADH)** is released from the posterior lobe (neurohypophysis) of the **pituitary gland** in response to increased blood osmolarity (decreased water). ADH causes the epithelium of collecting tubules and collecting ducts to become highly permeable to water. As a result, water leaves the ducts and enters the hypertonic interstitium. Water in the interstitium is collected and returned to the general circulation via the peritubular capillaries and vasa recta, and the glomerular filtrate in the collecting ducts becomes hypertonic (highly concentrated) urine.

In the absence of ADH, the cells of the collecting tubules remain impermeable to water, and increased volume of water remains in the collecting ducts. As a result, dilute urine is produced.

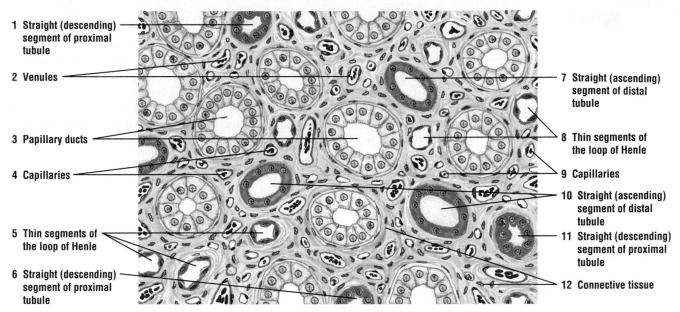

1 Straight (descending) segment of proximal tubule
2 Venules
3 Papillary ducts
4 Capillaries
5 Thin segments of the loop of Henle
6 Straight (descending) segment of proximal tubule
7 Straight (ascending) segment of distal tubule
8 Thin segments of the loop of Henle
9 Capillaries
10 Straight (ascending) segment of distal tubule
11 Straight (descending) segment of proximal tubule
12 Connective tissue

FIGURE 16.7 ■ Kidney medulla: papillary region (transverse section). Stain: hematoxylin and eosin. Medium magnification.

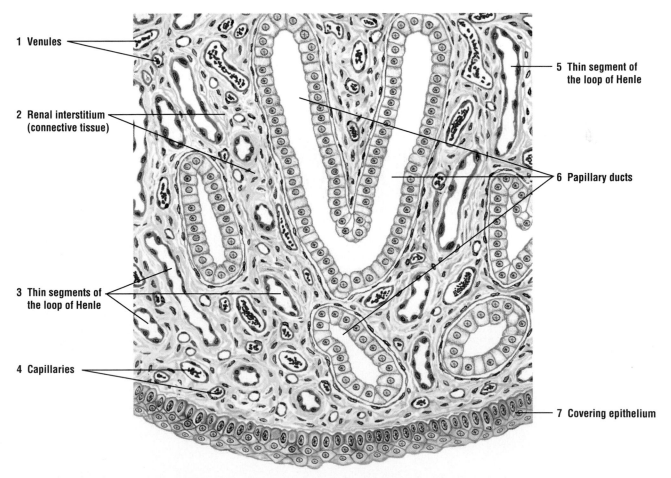

1 Venules
2 Renal interstitium (connective tissue)
3 Thin segments of the loop of Henle
4 Capillaries
5 Thin segment of the loop of Henle
6 Papillary ducts
7 Covering epithelium

FIGURE 16.8 ■ Kidney medulla: terminal end of papilla (longitudinal section). Stain: hematoxylin and eosin. Medium magnification.

FIGURE 16.9 ■ Kidney: Ducts of Medullary Region (Longitudinal Section)

The medullary region of the kidney consists primarily of various sized tubules, larger ducts, and blood vessels of the vasa recta. In this photomicrograph, different kidney tubules and blood vessels have been sectioned in a longitudinal plane. The tubules with large, light-staining cuboidal cells are the **collecting tubules (1).** Adjacent to the collecting tubules (1) are tubules with darker-staining cuboidal cells. These are the **thick segments of the loop of Henle (2).** Between the tubules are blood vessels of the **vasa recta (4)** and the **thin segments of the loop of Henle (3).** Blood vessels of the vasa recta (4) can be distinguished from the thin segments of the loop of Henle (3) by the presence of blood cells in their lumina.

FIGURE 16.10 ■ Ureter (Transverse Section)

An undistended **lumen** of the **ureter (4)** exhibits numerous longitudinal mucosal folds formed by the muscular contractions. The wall of the ureter consists of mucosa, muscularis, and adventitia.

The ureter mucosa consists of **transitional epithelium (7)** and a wide **lamina propria (5).** The transitional epithelium has several cell layers, the outermost layer characterized by large cuboidal cells. The intermediate cells are polyhedral in shape, whereas the basal cells are low columnar or cuboidal.

The lamina propria (5) contains fibroelastic connective tissue, which is denser with more fibroblasts under the epithelium and looser near the muscularis. Diffuse lymphatic tissue and occasional small lymphatic nodules may be observed in the lamina propria.

In the upper ureter, the muscularis consists of two muscle layers, an inner **longitudinal smooth muscle layer (3)** and a middle **circular smooth muscle layer (2);** these layers are not always distinct. An additional third outer longitudinal layer of smooth muscle is found in the lower third of the ureter near the bladder.

The **adventitia (9)** blends with the surrounding fibroelastic connective tissue and **adipose tissue (1, 10),** which contain numerous **arterioles (6), venules (8),** and small nerves.

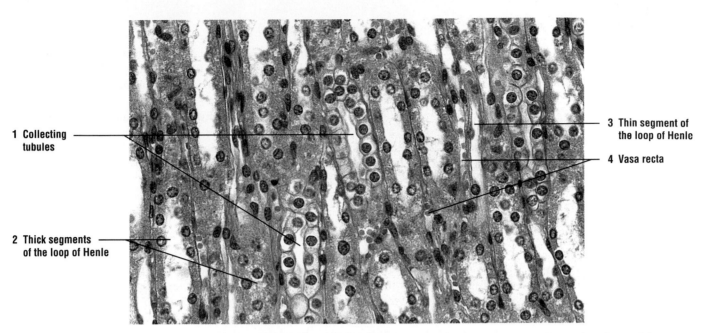

1 Collecting tubules

2 Thick segments of the loop of Henle

3 Thin segment of the loop of Henle

4 Vasa recta

FIGURE 16.9 ■ Kidney: ducts of medullary region (longitudinal section). Stain: hematoxylin and eosin. ×130.

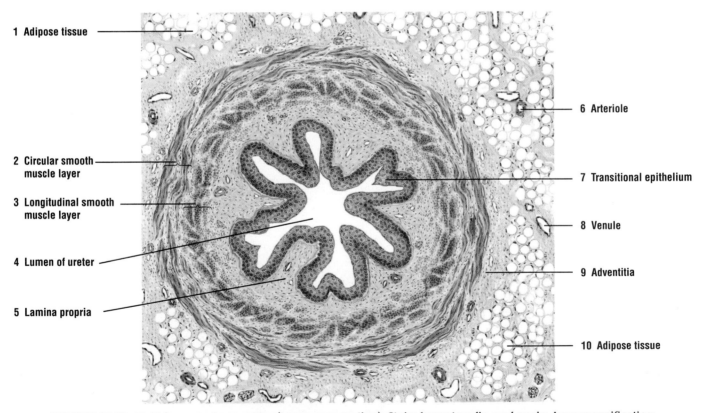

1 Adipose tissue

2 Circular smooth muscle layer

3 Longitudinal smooth muscle layer

4 Lumen of ureter

5 Lamina propria

6 Arteriole

7 Transitional epithelium

8 Venule

9 Adventitia

10 Adipose tissue

FIGURE 16.10 ■ Urinary system: ureter (transverse section). Stain: hematoxylin and eosin. Low magnification.

FIGURE 16.11 ■ Section of a Ureter Wall (Transverse Section)

This illustration shows a higher magnification of a ureter wall. The **transitional epithelium** (7) in an undistended ureter shows **mucosal folds** (6) and numerous layers with round cells. The superficial cells of the transitional epithelium (7) have a special **surface membrane** (5) that serves as an osmotic barrier between the urine and the underlying tissue.

A thin basement membrane separates the epithelium from the loose **lamina propria** (9).

The **muscularis** (2, 8) often appears as loosely arranged smooth muscle bundles surrounded by abundant connective tissue. The upper ureter has an inner **longitudinal smooth muscle layer** (8) and a middle circular **smooth muscle layer** (2). A third longitudinal smooth muscle layer is found in the lower third of the ureter.

The **adventitia** (4) with **adipose cells** (3) merges with the connective tissue of the posterior abdominal wall to which the ureter is attached.

FIGURE 16.12 ■ Ureter (Transverse Section)

The ureter is a muscular tube that conveys urine from the kidneys to the bladder by the contractions of the thick, smooth muscle layers found in its wall. This low-magnification photomicrograph shows a ureter in transverse section. The mucosa of the ureter is highly folded and lined by a thick **transitional epithelium** (1). Below the transitional epithelium (1) is the connective tissue **lamina propria** (2). The muscularis of the ureter contains two smooth muscle layers, an **inner longitudinal layer** (3) and a **middle circular muscle layer** (4). A third outer longitudinal layer (not shown) is added to the wall in the lower third of the ureter, near the bladder. A connective tissue **adventitia** (6), with **blood vessels** (5) and **adipose tissue** (7), surrounds the ureter.

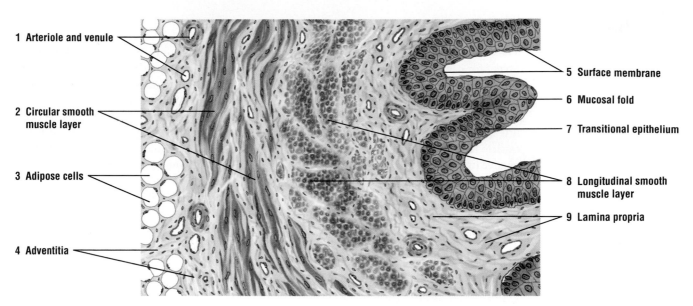

1 Arteriole and venule

2 Circular smooth muscle layer

3 Adipose cells

4 Adventitia

5 Surface membrane

6 Mucosal fold

7 Transitional epithelium

8 Longitudinal smooth muscle layer

9 Lamina propria

FIGURE 16.11 ■ Section of a ureter wall (transverse section). Stain: hematoxylin and eosin. Medium magnification.

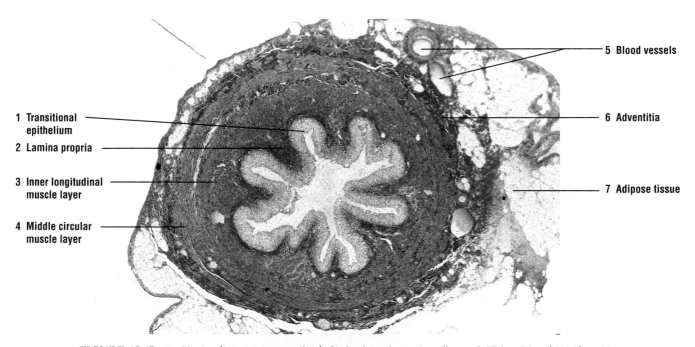

1 Transitional epithelium

2 Lamina propria

3 Inner longitudinal muscle layer

4 Middle circular muscle layer

5 Blood vessels

6 Adventitia

7 Adipose tissue

FIGURE 16.12 ■ Ureter (transverse section). Stain: iron hematoxylin and Alcian blue (IHAB). ×10.

FIGURE 16.13 ■ Urinary Bladder: Wall (Transverse Section)

The bladder has a thick muscular wall. The wall is similar to that of the lower third of the ureter, except for its thickness. In the wall are found three loosely arranged layers of smooth muscle, the inner longitudinal, middle circular, and outer longitudinal layers. However, similar to the ureter, the distinct muscle layers are difficult to distinguish. The three layers are arranged in anastomosing **smooth muscle bundles (1)** between which is found the **interstitial connective tissue (2).** In this illustration, the muscle bundles are sectioned in various planes (1) and the three distinct muscle layers are not distinguishable. The interstitial connective tissue (2) merges with the connective tissue of the **serosa (3). Mesothelium (3b)** covers the **connective tissue of serosa (3a)** and is the outermost layer. Serosa (3) lines the superior surface of the bladder, whereas its inferior surface is covered by the connective tissue adventitia, which merges with the connective tissue of adjacent structures.

The mucosa of an empty bladder exhibits numerous **mucosal folds (5)** that disappear during bladder distension. The **transitional epithelium (6)** is thicker than in the ureter and consists of about six layers of cells. The **lamina propria (7),** inferior to the epithelium, is wider than in the ureters. The loose connective tissue in the deeper zone contains more elastic fibers. Numerous **blood vessels (4, 8)** of various sizes are found in the serosa (3), between the smooth muscle bundles (1), and in the lamina propria (8).

FIGURE 16.14 ■ Urinary Bladder: Contracted Mucosa (Transverse Section)

The mucosa from an empty and contracted urinary bladder wall is illustrated at a higher magnification. Here, the superficial cells of the **transitional epithelium (4)** are low cuboidal or columnar and appear dome-shaped. Also, some superficial cells may be **binucleate (6)** (contain two nuclei). The outer **plasma membrane (5)** of the superficial cells in the epithelium is prominent. The deeper cells in the epithelium are round (4) and the basal cells more columnar (see also Figure 2-7).

The subepithelial **lamina propria (3)** contains fine connective tissue fibers, numerous fibroblasts, and blood vessels, **venule** and **arteriole (2).** The muscularis consists of three indistinct muscle layers that are visible as **smooth muscle bundles (1)** sectioned in longitudinal and transverse planes.

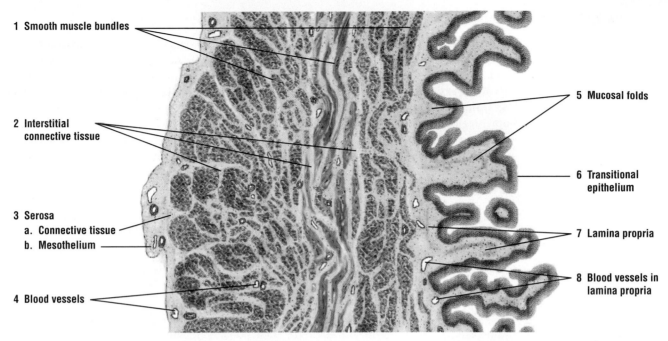

1 **Smooth muscle bundles**

2 **Interstitial connective tissue**

3 **Serosa**
   a. **Connective tissue**
   b. **Mesothelium**

4 **Blood vessels**

5 **Mucosal folds**

6 **Transitional epithelium**

7 **Lamina propria**

8 **Blood vessels in lamina propria**

FIGURE 16.13 ■ Urinary bladder: wall (transverse section). Stain: hematoxylin and eosin. Low magnification.

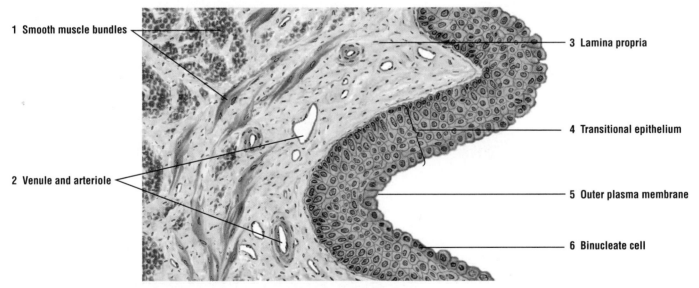

1 **Smooth muscle bundles**

2 **Venule and arteriole**

3 **Lamina propria**

4 **Transitional epithelium**

5 **Outer plasma membrane**

6 **Binucleate cell**

FIGURE 16.14 ■ Urinary bladder: contracted mucosa (transverse section). Stain: hematoxylin and eosin. Medium magnification.

FIGURE 16.15 ■ Urinary Bladder: Stretched Mucosa (Transverse Section)

When fluid fills the bladder, the **transitional epithelium (1)** changes its shape. Increased volume in the bladder appears to reduce the number of cell layers, the **surface cells (5)** appear squamous, and the thickness of the transitional epithelium (1) is reduced to about three layers. This is because the surface cells (5) flatten to accommodate the increasing surface area. In the stretched condition, the transitional epithelium (1) may resemble stratified squamous epithelium found in other regions of the body. Note also that the folds in the bladder wall disappear and the **basement membrane (2)** is not folded. As in an empty bladder (Figure 16.14) the underlying **connective tissue (6)** contains **venules (3)** and **arterioles (7).** Below the connective tissue (6) are **smooth muscle fibers (4, 8),** sectioned in cross (4) and longitudinal (8) planes.

FUNCTIONAL CORRELATIONS: Urinary Bladder

The **urinary bladder** is a hollow organ with a thick muscular wall. Its main function is to store urine. Because the lumen of the bladder is lined with a **transitional epithelium,** the wall of the organ can stretch or enlarge (change shape) as the bladder fills with urine. When the bladder is empty, the thick transitional epithelium may exhibit five or six layers of cells. The superficial cells in the epithelium are cuboidal, large, and dome-shaped, and bulge into the lumen. When the bladder fills with urine, however, the transitional epithelium is stretched, and the cells in the epithelium appear thinner and squamous to accommodate the increased volume of urine.

The changes in the appearance and cell shapes in the transitional epithelium are because of the unique thickened regions in the plasma membrane of superficial cells called **plaques.** The plaques are connected to thinner, shorter, and more flexible **interplaque regions.** These structures act like "hinges," and in an empty bladder, the interplaque regions allow the cell membrane to fold. When the bladder is filled with urine, these folds disappear, and the interplaque regions allow the cells to expand during full stretch. The plaques unfold and become part of the surface during stretching and flattening of the cells.

The exposed cell membrane of superficial cells in the transitional epithelium is also thicker. In addition, **desmosomes** and **occluding junctions** attach the cells to each other. The plaques are impermeable to water, salts, and urine, even when the epithelium is fully stretched. These unique properties of transitional epithelium in the urinary passages provide for an effective **osmotic barrier** between urine and the underlying connective tissue.

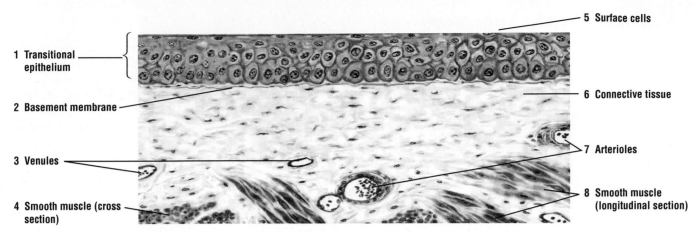

1 Transitional epithelium

5 Surface cells

2 Basement membrane

6 Connective tissue

3 Venules

7 Arterioles

4 Smooth muscle (cross section)

8 Smooth muscle (longitudinal section)

FIGURE 16.15 ■ Urinary bladder: mucosa stretched (transverse section). Stain: hematoxylin and eosin. Medium magnification.

Urinary System

The Kidney

- System consists of two kidneys, two ureters, a bladder, and a urethra
- Hilus contains renal artery, renal vein, and renal pelvis surrounded by renal sinus
- Darker outer region of kidney is cortex; lighter inner region is medulla
- Medulla contains numerous pyramids, which face the cortex at corticomedullary junction
- Round apex of each pyramid extends toward renal pelvis as renal papilla
- Cortex that extends on each side of renal pyramid constitutes the renal columns
- Each papilla is surrounded by a minor calyx that joins to form a major calyx
- Major calyces join to form the funnel-shaped renal pelvis that narrows into the muscular ureter
- Urine is formed as a result of blood filtration, and absorption from and excretion into the filtrate
- Almost all filtrate is reabsorbed into the systemic circulation and about 1% of filtrate is voided as urine
- Produces renin that regulates filtration pressure and erythropoietin for erythrocyte production

Uriniferous Tubules and Nephrons

- Functional unit of kidney is uriniferous tubule
- Consists of nephron and collecting duct
- Two types of nephrons: cortical nephrons in cortex and juxtamedullary nephrons in medulla
- Nephron is subdivided into renal corpuscle and renal tubules

Renal Corpuscle

- Blood is filtered in the glomerular capillaries of the corpuscle to form ultrafiltrate
- Consists of capillaries called glomerulus and double-layered glomerular (Bowman's) capsule
- Visceral layer of capsule contains podocytes that surround fenestrated glomerular capillaries
- Podocytes exhibit primary processes and pedicles that form filtration slits around capillaries
- Parietal layer is lined by simple squamous epithelium of the glomerular capsule
- Between parietal and visceral layers is the capsular (urinary) space that holds glomerular filtrate
- At vascular pole, afferent and efferent arterioles enter and exit the renal corpuscle
- At opposite urinary pole, ultrafiltrate enters the proximal convoluted tubule

Renal Tubules

- Glomerular filtrate leaves renal corpuscle and enters renal tubules that extend to collecting ducts
- Initial tubule is the proximal convoluted tubule that starts at the urinary pole of renal corpuscle
- Loop of Henle consists of thick descending, a thin loop, and thick ascending tubules
- Distal convoluted tubule ascends into kidney cortex and joins the collecting tubule
- Juxtamedullary nephrons have very long loops of Henle
- Collecting tubules not part of nephron, but join larger collecting ducts to form papillary ducts
- Deep in medulla, papillary ducts are lined by columnar epithelium and exit in area cribrosa
- Medullary rays in cortex are collecting ducts, blood vessels, and straight portions of nephrons

Renal Blood Supply

- Renal artery divides in the hilus into segmental arteries that become interlobar arteries
- At corticomedullary junction, interlobar arteries branch into arcuate arteries
- Arcuate arteries form interlobular arteries, from which arise afferent glomerular arterioles
- Glomerular arterioles form capillaries of glomeruli that exit renal corpuscles as efferent arterioles
- Efferent arterioles form peritubular capillaries and vasa recta in the medulla

Kidney Cells and Tubules

Mesangial Cells

- Found in the glomerulus attached to the glomerular capillaries
- Function as macrophages, and regulate blood pressure as a result of vasoactive receptors and contractility
- Extraglomerular cells form part of the juxtaglomerular apparatus

Proximal Convoluted Tubules

- Proximal convoluted tubules lined with brush border and absorb most of filtrate
- Basal infoldings of cell membrane contain numerous mitochondria and sodium pumps
- Mitochondria supply energy for ionic transport across cell membrane into the interstitium
- All glucose, proteins, and amino acids, almost all carbohydrates, and 75 to 85% of water absorbed here
- Secretion of metabolic waste, hydrogen, ammonia, dyes, and drugs into the filtrate for voiding
- Longer than distal convoluted tubules and more frequently seen in cortex near renal corpuscles

Loop of Henle

- In juxtamedullary nephrons produces hypertonic urine owing to the countercurrent multiplier system
- High interstitial osmolarity draws water from the filtrate
- Vasa recta capillaries take up water from interstitium and return it to systemic circulation

Distal Convoluted Tubules

- Shorter than proximal convoluted tubules, less frequent in cortex, and lack brush border
- Basolateral membrane shows infoldings and contains numerous mitochondria
- Under influence of aldosterone, sodium ions actively absorbed from the filtrate
- Peritubular capillaries return ions to systemic circulation to maintain vital acid-base balance

Juxtaglomerular Apparatus

- Located adjacent to renal corpuscle and distal convoluted tubule
- Consists of juxtaglomerular cells of afferent arteriole and macula densa of distal convoluted tubule
- Main function is to maintain proper blood pressure for blood filtration in renal corpuscles
- Juxtaglomerular cells respond to stretching in the wall of afferent arterioles, a baroreceptor
- Macula densa responds to changes in sodium chloride concentration in glomerular filtrate
- Decreased blood pressure and ionic content causes release of enzyme renin by juxtaglomerular cells
- Renin release eventually converts plasma proteins to angiotensin II, a powerful vasoconstrictor
- Angiotensin II stimulates release of aldosterone, which acts on the distal convoluted tubules
- Distal convoluted tubules absorb NaCl with water, increasing blood volume and pressure

Collecting Tubules, Collecting Ducts, and Antidiuretic Hormone (ADH)

- Glomerular filtrate flows from distal convoluted tubules to collecting tubules and ducts
- During excessive water loss or dehydration, ADH released from pituitary gland

- ADH causes epithelium of collecting duct to become highly permeable to water
- Water that is retained in interstitium is collected by peritubular capillaries and vasa recta
- In absence of ADH, increased water is retained in collecting ducts and urine is dilute

Ureter

- Lined by transitional epithelium and consists of mucosa, muscularis, and adventitia
- Upper part lined by inner longitudinal and middle circular smooth muscle layers
- Third longitudinal smooth muscle layer added in the lower third of ureter
- Connective tissue adventitia surrounds the ureter

Bladder

- Thick muscular wall with three indistinct layers of smooth muscle
- Serosa lines superior surface and adventitia covers the inferior surface
- Transitional epithelium in empty bladder exhibits about six layers of cells
- When stretched, transitional epithelium appears stratified squamous
- Changes in epithelium caused by thicker plasma membrane of superficial cells and plaques
- Plaques act like hinges, allow cell to expand during stretching; cells become squamous
- Thicker plasma membrane and transitional epithelium provide osmotic barrier to urine

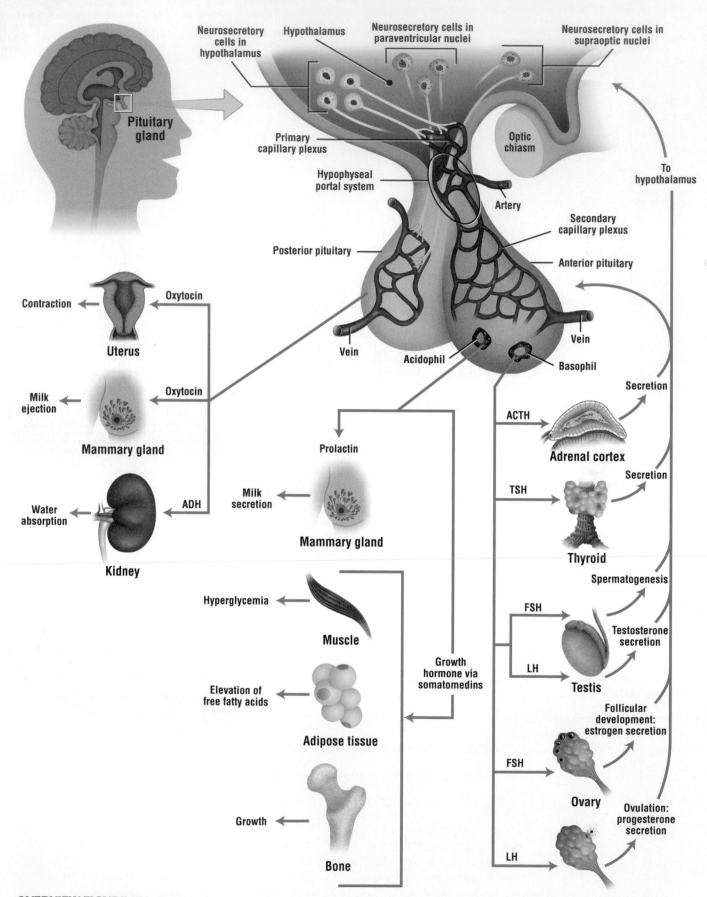

OVERVIEW FIGURE 17.1 ■ Hypothalamus and hypophysis (pituitary gland). A section of hypothalamus and hypophysis illustrates the neuronal, axonal, and vascular connections between the hypothalamus and the hypophysis. Also illustrated are the major target cells, tissues, and organs of the hormones that are produced by both the anterior (adenohypophysis) and posterior (neurohypophysis) pituitary gland.

CHAPTER 17

Endocrine System

SECTION 1 ■ Endocrine System and Hormones

The endocrine system consists of cells, tissues, and organs that synthesize and secrete **hormones** directly into blood and lymph capillaries. As a result, endocrine glands and organs are **ductless** because they do not have excretory ducts. Furthermore, the cells in most endocrine tissues and organs are arranged into **cords** and **clumps,** and are surrounded by an extensive **capillary network.**

Hormones produced by endocrine cells include peptides, proteins, steroids, amino acid derivatives, and catecholamines. Because hormones act at a distance from the site of their release, the hormones first enter the bloodstream to be transported to the **target organs.** Here, they influence the structure and the programmed function of the target organ cells by binding to specific hormone receptors. **Hormone receptors** can be located either on the plasma membrane, cytoplasm, or nucleus of target cells. Nonsteroidal receptors for protein and peptide hormones are usually located on cell surfaces. Their interaction and activation by the hormone results in production of an intracellular **second messenger,** which is **cyclic adenosine monophosphate** or cyclic AMP for numerous hormones. Cyclic AMP then activates a specific sequence of enzymes and various cellular events in specific response to the particular hormone.

Other receptors are intracellular and are activated by hormones that diffuse through cellular and nuclear membranes. Steroidal hormones and thyroid hormones are soluble in lipids and can easily cross these membranes. Once inside the target cells, these steroid hormones combine with specific protein receptors. The resulting hormone-receptor complex binds in the nucleus to a particular DNA sequence that either activates or inhibits specific genes. The activated genes initiate the synthesis of messenger RNA, which enters the cytoplasm to produce hormone-specific proteins. The new proteins induce cellular changes that are specifically associated with the influence of the particular hormone. The hormones that combine with the intracellular receptors do not use the second messenger. Instead, they directly influence gene expression of the affected cell.

Numerous organs contain individual endocrine cells or endocrine tissues. Such mixed (endocrine-exocrine) organs are the pancreas, kidneys, reproductive organs of both sexes, placenta, and gastrointestinal tract. Endocrine cells and tissues are discussed with the specific exocrine organs in their respective chapters.

There are also complete endocrine organs or glands (Overview Figure 17.1). These include the **hypophysis** or **pituitary gland** (described below), **thyroid gland, adrenal (suprarenal) glands,** and **parathyroid glands** (described in Section 2).

Embryologic Development of Hypophysis (Pituitary Gland)

The structure and function of the hypophysis reflect its dual embryologic origin. During development, the epithelium of the **pharyngeal roof** (oral cavity) forms an outpocketing called the **hypophyseal (Rathke's) pouch.** As development proceeds, the hypophyseal pouch detaches from the oral cavity and becomes the cellular or glandular portion of the hypophysis, now called the **adenohypophysis (anterior pituitary).** At the same time, the downgrowth from the developing brain (diencephalon) forms the neural portion of the hypophysis, called the **neurohypophysis (posterior pituitary).** The two separately developed structures then unite to form a single gland, the hypophysis. The hypophysis remains attached to a ventral extension of the brain, called the **hypothalamus.** A short stalk, called the **infundibulum,** is a neural pathway that attaches the hypophysis to the hypothalamus. The neurons in the hypothalamus control the release of hormones from the adenohypophysis, as well as secrete hormones that are stored in and released from the neurohypophysis.

After development, the hypophysis rests in a bony depression of the sphenoid bone of the skull, called the **sella turcica,** located inferior to the hypothalamus.

Subdivisions of the Hypophysis

The epithelial-derived adenohypophysis has three subdivisions: the pars distalis, pars tuberalis, and pars intermedia. The **pars distalis** is the largest part of the hypophysis. The **pars tuberalis** surrounds the neural stalk. The **pars intermedia** is a thin cell layer between the pars distalis and the neurohypophysis. It represents the remnant of the hypophyseal pouch and is rudimentary in humans, but prominent in other mammals.

The neurohypophysis, situated posterior to the adenohypophysis, also consists of three parts: the median eminence, infundibulum, and pars nervosa. The **median eminence** is located at the base of the hypothalamus from which extends the pituitary stalk or **infundibulum,** in which are located the unmyelinated axons that extend from the neurons in the hypothalamus. The large portion of the neurohypophysis is the **pars nervosa.** This region contains the unmyelinated axons of secretory hypothalamic neurons, their endings with hormones, and the supportive cells, called **pituicytes.**

Vascular and Neural Connections of Hypophysis

Adenohypophysis

Because the adenohypophysis does not develop from neural tissue, its connection to the **hypothalamus** of the brain is via a rich vascular network. **Superior hypophyseal arteries** from the internal carotid artery supply the pars tuberalis, median eminence, and infundibulum. These arteries form a fenestrated **primary capillary plexus** in the median eminence at the base of the hypothalamus. Secretory neurons that are located in the hypothalamus synthesize hormones that have a direct influence on cell functions in the adenohypophysis. The axons from these neurons terminate on the capillaries of the primary capillary plexus, into which they release their hormones.

Small venules then drain the primary capillary plexus and deliver the blood with the hormones to a **secondary capillary plexus** that surrounds the cells in the pars distalis of the adenohypophysis. The venules that connect the primary capillary plexus of the hypothalamus with the secondary capillary plexus in the adenohypophysis form the **hypophyseal portal system.** To ensure efficient transport of hormones from the blood to the cells, the capillaries in the primary and secondary capillary plexuses are **fenestrated** (contain small pores).

Neurohypophysis

In contrast, the neurohypophysis has a direct neural connection with the brain. As a result, there are no neurons or hormone-producing cells in the neurohypophysis, and it remains connected to the brain by a multitude of unmyelinated axons and supportive cells, the pituicytes. The **neurons** (cell bodies) of these axons are located in the **supraoptic** and **paraventricular nuclei** of the hypothalamus. The unmyelinated axons that extend from the hypothalamus into the neurohypophysis form the **hypothalamohypophysial tract** and the bulk of the neurohypophysis.

Neurons in the hypothalamus first synthesize the hormones that are released from the neurohypophysis. These hormones bind to the carrier glycoprotein **neurophysin** and are then transported from the hypothalamus down the axons to the neurohypophysis. Here, the hormones accumulate and are stored in the distended terminal ends of unmyelinated axons as **Herring bodies.** When needed, hormones from the neurohypophysis are directly released into the fenestrated capillaries of the pars nervosa by nerve impulses from the hypothalamus.

FIGURE 17.1 ■ Hypophysis (Panoramic View, Sagittal Section)

The hypophysis (pituitary gland) consists of two major subdivisions, the adenohypophysis and neurohypophysis. The adenohypophysis is further subdivided into **pars distalis (anterior lobe)**

(5), **pars tuberalis (7),** and **pars intermedia (9).** The neurohypophysis is divided into **pars nervosa (11), infundibulum (6),** and the median eminence (not illustrated). The pars tuberalis (7) surrounds the infundibulum (6) and is visible above and below the infundibulum (6) in a sagittal section. The infundibulum (6) connects the hypophysis with the hypothalamus at the base of the brain.

The pars distalis (5) contains two main cell types, chromophobe cells and chromophil cells. The chromophils are subdivided into **acidophils (alpha cells) (4)** and **basophils (beta cells) (2),** illustrated at a higher magnification in Figure 17.2.

Pars intermedia (9) and pars nervosa (11) form the posterior lobe of the hypophysis. Pars nervosa (11) consists primarily of unmyelinated axons and supporting pituicytes. A **connective tissue capsule (1, 10)** surrounds the pars distalis (5) and pars nervosa (11) portions of the gland.

The pars intermedia (9) is situated between the pars distalis (5) and the pars nervosa (11), and represents the residual lumen of Rathke's pouch. The pars intermedia (9) normally contains **colloid-filled vesicles (9a)** that are surrounded by cells of pars intermedia (9).

Both the pars distalis (5) and pars nervosa (11) are supplied by numerous **blood vessels (8)** and **capillaries (3)** of different sizes.

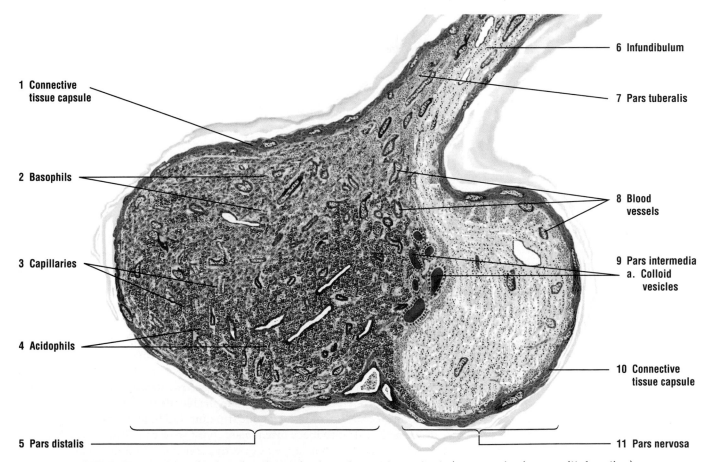

FIGURE 17.1 ■ Hypophysis: adenohypophysis and neurohypophysis (panoramic view, sagittal section). Stain: hematoxylin and eosin. Low magnification.

FIGURE 17.2 ■ Hypophysis: Sections of Pars Distalis, Pars Intermedia, and Pars Nervosa

With higher magnification, numerous **sinusoidal capillaries** (1) and different cell types are visible in the **pars distalis. Chromophobe cells** (2) have a light-staining, homogeneous cytoplasm and are normally smaller than the chromophils. The cytoplasm of chromophils stains reddish in the **acidophils** (3) and blueish in the **basophils** (4).

The **pars intermedia** contains **follicles** (6) and colloid-filled **cystic follicles** (7). Follicles lined with basophils (8) are often present in the pars intermedia.

The **pars nervosa** is characterized by unmyelinated axons and the supportive **pituicytes** (5) with oval nuclei.

FUNCTIONAL CORRELATIONS: Hypophysis

Hormones produced by neurons in the **hypothalamus** directly influence and control the synthesis and release of six specific hormones from the adenohypophysis. **Releasing hormones** are produced by neurons in the hypothalamus for **each hormone** that is released from the adenohypophysis. For two hormones, growth hormone and prolactin, **inhibitory hormones,** as well as releasing hormones, are produced.

The releasing and inhibitory hormones secreted from the hypothalamic neurons are carried from the primary capillary plexus to the second capillary plexus in the adenohypophysis via the **hypophyseal portal system.** On reaching the adenohypophysis, the hormones bind to specific receptors on cells and either stimulate the cells to secrete and release a specific hormone into the circulation or inhibit this function.

In contrast, the neurohypophysis does not secrete hormones. Instead, the neurohypophysis stores and releases only two hormones, **oxytocin** and **vasopressin** (antidiuretic hormone or ADH) that were synthesized in the hypothalamus by the neurons in the **paraventricular nuclei** and **supraoptic nuclei.** These hormones are then transported along unmyelinated axons and stored in the axon terminals of the neurohypophysis as **Herring bodies,** from which they are released into the capillaries of the par nervosa as needed. Herring bodies are visible with a light microscope.

Cells of the Adenohypophysis

The cells of the adenohypophysis were initially classified as **chromophobes** and **chromophils,** based on the affinity of their cytoplasmic granules for specific stains. The pale-staining chromophobes are believed to be either degranulated chromophils with few granules or undifferentiated stem cells. The chromophils were further subdivided into **acidophils** and **basophils** because of their staining properties. Immunocytochemical techniques now identify these cells on the basis of their specific hormones. In the adenohypophysis, there are two types of acidophils, **somatotrophs** and **mammotrophs,** and three types of basophils, **gonadotrophs, thyrotrophs,** and **corticotrophs.**

The hormones released from these cells are carried in the bloodstream to the target organs, where they bind to specific receptors that influence the structure and function of the target cells. Once the target cells are activated, a **feedback mechanism** (positive or negative) can further control the synthesis and release of these hormones by directly acting on cells in the adenohypophysis or neurons in the hypothalamus.

FIGURE 17.3 ■ Hypophysis: Pars Distalis (Sectional View)

This illustration shows the two main populations of cells in the pars distalis of the adenohypophysis. The cells here are arranged in clumps. Between the clumps are seen the numerous **capillaries (5), blood vessels (3),** and thin **connective tissue fibers (6)** that separate the clumps. Cell types in the pars distalis can be identified with special fixation and staining affinity of the cytoplasmic granules.

The **chromophobes (4)** usually exhibit pale nuclei and pale cytoplasm with poorly defined cell outlines. The aggregation of chromophobes in groups or clumps is seen in this illustration.

The **acidophils (2)** are more numerous and can be distinguished by their red-staining granules in the cytoplasm and blue nuclei.

The **basophils (1)** are less numerous and appear as cells that contain blue-staining granules in their cytoplasm. The degree of granularity and the stain density vary in different cells.

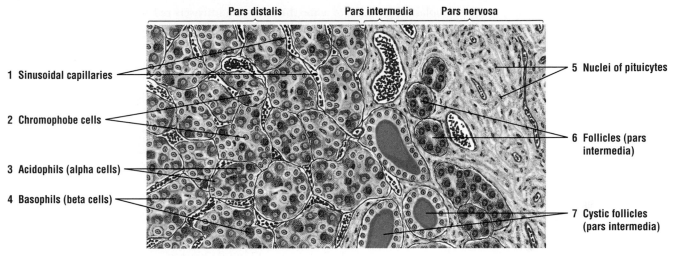

Pars distalis   **Pars intermedia**   **Pars nervosa**

1 Sinusoidal capillaries

2 Chromophobe cells

3 Acidophils (alpha cells)

4 Basophils (beta cells)

5 Nuclei of pituicytes

6 Follicles (pars intermedia)

7 Cystic follicles (pars intermedia)

FIGURE 17.2 ■ Hypophysis: sections of pars distalis, pars intermedia, and pars nervosa. Stain: hematoxylin and eosin. Medium magnification.

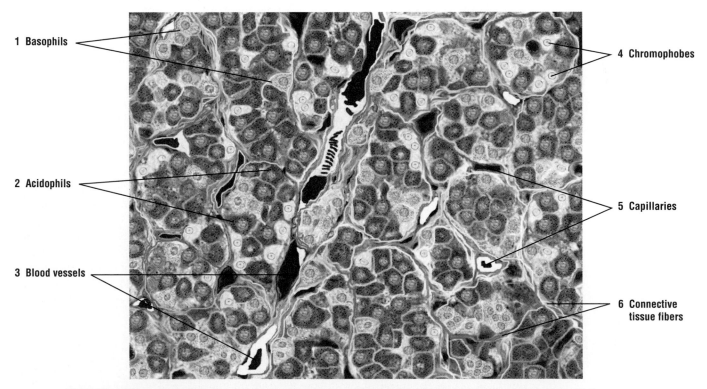

1 Basophils

2 Acidophils

3 Blood vessels

4 Chromophobes

5 Capillaries

6 Connective tissue fibers

FIGURE 17.3 ■ Pars distalis of adenohypophysis: acidophils, basophils, and chromophobes. Stain: azan. High magnification.

FIGURE 17.4 ■ Cell Types in the Hypophysis

Groups of different cell types of the hypophysis are illustrated at higher magnification after modified azan staining. The nuclei of all cells are stained orange-red.

The **chromophobes** (**a**) exhibit a clear and very light orange cytoplasm. The appearance of clear cytoplasm indicates that the cells do not have granules, and as a result, their cell boundaries are indistinct.

The cytoplasmic granules of **acidophils** (**b**) stain intensely red, and the cell outlines are distinct. A sinusoid capillary surrounds the acidophils.

The **basophils** (**c**) exhibit variable cell shapes and granules that vary in size.

The **pituicytes** (**d**) of pars nervosa have variable cell shape and cell size. The small, orange-stained cytoplasm is diffuse and barely visible.

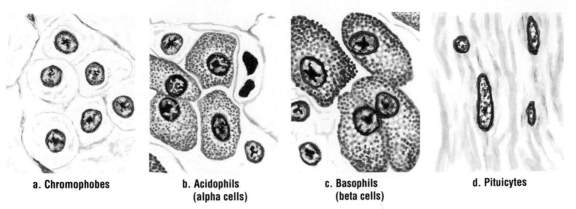

a. Chromophobes

b. Acidophils
(alpha cells)

c. Basophils
(beta cells)

d. Pituicytes

FIGURE 17.4 ■ Cell types in the hypophysis. Stain: modified azan. Oil immersion.

FIGURE 17.5 ■ Hypophysis: Pars Distalis, Pars Intermedia, and Pars Nervosa

A higher-power photomicrograph illustrates the cellular pars distalis and pars intermedia of the adenohypophysis, and the light staining pars nervosa of the neurohypophysis. With this stain, different cell types can be identified in the pars distalis. The red-staining or eosinophilic cells are the **acidophils (5).** The cells with bluish cytoplasm are the **basophils (4).** The light, unstained cells scattered among the acidophils (5) and basophils (4) are the **chromophobes (7).** The pars intermedia exhibits small **cysts** or **vesicles (6)** filled with colloid.

The pars nervosa is filled with unmyelinated, light-staining axons of secretory cells, whose cell bodies are located in the hypothalamus. Most of the red-staining nuclei in the pars nervosa are the supportive cell **pituicytes (2).** Accumulations of neurosecretory material at the end of the axon terminals in the pars nervosa are the irregular-shaped, red-staining structures called the **Herring bodies (3).** Herring bodies (3) are closely associated with capillaries and **blood vessels (1).** Surrounding the secretory cells and axon terminals in the neurohypophysis are blood vessels (1) and fenestrated capillaries.

FUNCTIONAL CORRELATIONS: Cells and Hormones of the Adenohypophysis

Acidophils

Somatotrophs secrete **somatotropin,** also called growth hormone or GH. This hormone stimulates cellular metabolism, general body growth, uptake of amino acids, and protein synthesis. Somatotropin also stimulates the liver to produce **somatomedins,** also called insulin-like growth factor (IGF-I). These hormones increase proliferation of cartilage cells (chondrocytes) in the **epiphyseal plates** of developing or growing long bones to increase bone length. There is also an increase in the growth of the skeletal muscle and increased release of fatty acids from the adipose cells for energy production by body cells. Growth hormone inhibiting hormone, also called **somatostatin,** inhibits the release of growth hormone from somatotrophs in the pituitary gland.

Mammotrophs produce the lactogenic hormone **prolactin** that stimulates development of mammary glands during pregnancy. After parturition (birth), prolactin maintains milk production in the developed mammary glands during lactation. Release of prolactin from mammotrophs is inhibited by prolactin release inhibitory hormone, also called dopamine.

Basophils

Thyrotrophs secrete **thyroid-stimulating hormone** (**thyrotropin,** or **TSH**). TSH stimulates synthesis and secretion of the hormones **thyroxin** and **triiodothyronine** from the thyroid gland.

Gonadotrophs secrete **follicle-stimulating hormone (FSH)** and **luteinizing hormone (LH).** In females, FSH promotes growth and maturation of ovarian follicles and subsequent **estrogen** secretion by developing follicles. In males, FSH promotes **spermatogenesis** in the testes and secretion of **androgen-binding protein** into seminiferous tubules by **Sertoli cells.**

In females, LH in association with FSH induces **ovulation,** promotes the final maturation of ovarian follicles, and stimulates the formation of the **corpus luteum** after ovulation. LH also promotes secretion of estrogen and progesterone from the corpus luteum. In males, LH maintains and stimulates the **interstitial cells** (of Leydig) in the testes to produce the hormone **testosterone.** As a result, LH is sometimes called interstitial cell-stimulating hormone (ICSH).

Corticotrophs secrete **adrenocorticotropic hormone (ACTH).** ACTH influences the function of the cells in **adrenal cortex.** ACTH also stimulates the synthesis and release of glucocorticoids from the zona fasciculata and zona reticularis of adrenal cortex.

Pars Intermedia

In lower vertebrates (amphibians and fishes), the pars intermedia is well developed and produces **melanocyte-stimulating hormone (MSH).** MSH increases skin pigmentation by causing dispersion of melanin granules. In humans and most mammals, the pars intermedia is rudimentary.

FUNCTIONAL CORRELATIONS: Cells and Hormones of the Neurohypophysis

Oxytocin

The two hormones, oxytocin and antidiuretic hormone (ADH), that are released from the neurohypophysis are synthesized in the supraoptic and paraventricular nuclei of the hypothalamus. Release of oxytocin is stimulated by vaginal and cervical distension before birth, and nursing of the infant after birth. The main targets of **oxytocin** are the smooth muscles of the pregnant uterus. During labor, oxytocin is released to induce strong contractions of smooth muscles in the uterus, resulting in childbirth (parturition). After parturition, the suckling action of the infant on the nipple activates the **milk-ejection reflex** in the lactating mammary glands. Afferent impulses from the nipple stimulate neurons in the hypothalamus, causing oxytocin release. Oxytocin then stimulates the contraction of **myoepithelial cells** around the alveoli and ducts in the lactating mammary glands, ejecting milk into the excretory ducts and the nipple.

Antidiuretic Hormone (ADH) or Vasopressin

The main action of antidiuretic hormone (ADH) is to increase **water permeability** in the **distal convoluted tubules** and **collecting tubules** of the kidney. As a result, more water is reabsorbed from the filtrate into the interstitium and retained in the body, creating a more concentrated urine. A sudden decrease of blood pressure is also a stimulus for release of ADH. It is believed that in large doses, ADH may cause smooth muscle contraction in arteries and arterioles. However, physiologic doses of ADH appear to have minimal effects on blood pressure.

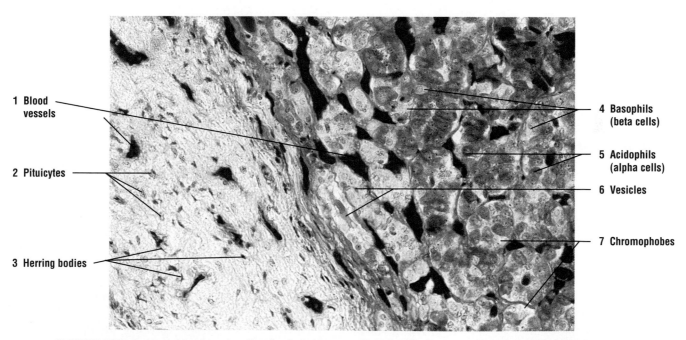

1 Blood vessels
2 Pituicytes
3 Herring bodies
4 Basophils (beta cells)
5 Acidophils (alpha cells)
6 Vesicles
7 Chromophobes

FIGURE 17.5 ■ Hypophysis: pars distalis, pars intermedia, and pars nervosa (human). Stain: Mallory-azan and orange G. ×80.

- Consists of cells, tissues, and organs that produce blood-borne chemicals
- Consists of ductless glands, arranged in cords and clumps, and surrounded by capillaries
- Hormones enter bloodstream and interact with target organs with specific receptors
- Hormone receptors located on cell membrane, in cytoplasm, or in nucleus
- Nonsteroidal hormones use second messenger (cyclic AMP) to activate specific responses
- Steroidal hormones enter target cells and in nucleus influence specific gene expression

Embryologic Development of Hypophysis (Pituitary Gland)

- Has dual embryologic origin, epithelial and neural
- Epithelial portion develops from pharyngeal roof and Rathke's pouch
- Pouch detaches and becomes the cellular portion, the adenohypophysis
- Downgrowth of brain forms the neural portion, the neurohypophysis
- Neurohypophysis remains attached to hypothalamus by a neural stalk, called infundibulum
- Neurons in hypothalamus control release of hormones from adenohypophysis

Subdivision of Hypophysis

- Adenohypophysis (anterior pituitary) has three subdivisions
- Pars distalis is the largest part
- Pars intermedia is remnant of the pouch and rudimentary in humans
- Pars tuberalis surrounds the neural stalk
- Neurohypophysis (posterior pituitary) consists of three parts
- Median eminence is located at base of hypothalamus
- Infundibulum is the neural stalk that connects neurohypophysis to hypothalamus
- Pars nervosa is the largest portion that consists of unmyelinated axons and pituicytes

Vascular and Neural Connections of Hypophysis

Adenohypophysis

- Connection between hypothalamus of brain and adenohypophysis is vascular
- Superior hypophyseal arteries form fenestrated primary capillary plexus in median eminence
- Secretory neurons in hypothalamus terminate on capillary plexus and release hormones
- Small venules connect to secondary capillary plexus in adenohypophysis, forming a portal system
- Hypothalamus produces releasing hormones and inhibitory hormones for adenohypophysis
- Releasing or inhibitory hormones are carried via the portal system to cells in pars distalis
- Releasing hormones bind to specific receptors in cells of pars distalis

Cells and Hormones of Adenohypophysis

- Based on stains, there are three cell types: acidophils, basophils, and chromophobes
- Acidophils subdivided into somatotrophs and mammotrophs
- Basophils subdivided into thyrotrophs, gonadotrophs, and corticotrophs

Somatotrophs

- Secrete somatotropin for growth hormone for cell metabolism and general body growth
- Somatotropin also stimulates liver to produce somatomedins
- Somatomedins influence cartilage cells in epiphyseal plates to increase growth in length
- Somatostatin inhibits release of growth hormone from somatotrophs

Mammotrophs

- Produce prolactin that stimulates mammary gland development during pregnancy
- Prolactin maintains milk production after parturition

Thyrotrophs

- Release thyroid-stimulating hormone (TSH) that stimulates thyroid gland hormones
- Thyroid gland produces thyroxin and triiodothyronine

Gonadotrophs

- Secrete both follicle-stimulating hormone (FSH) and leuteinizing hormone (LH)
- In females, FSH stimulates follicular development, maturation, and estrogen production
- In males, FSH promotes spermatogenesis and androgen-binding protein secretion by Sertoli cells
- In females, LH induces follicular maturation, ovulation, and corpus luteum formation
- Corpus luteum secretes estrogen and progesterone
- In males, LH stimulates interstitial cells in testes to produce testosterone (androgens)

Corticotrophs

- Secrete adrenocorticotropic hormone (ACTH) to regulate adrenal cortex functions
- Feedback mechanism controls further synthesis and release of specific hormones
- Pars intermedia in humans is rudimentary; in lower vertebrates produces melanocyte-stimulating hormone (MSH)

Neurohypophysis

- Does not have any secretory cells; secretory neurons are located in hypothalamus of brain
- Has a direct neural connection to hypothalamus via axons
- Contains unmyelinated axons of hypothalamohypophysial tract and supportive cells called pituicytes
- Neurons of axons located in supraoptic and paraventricular nuclei of hypothalamus
- Neurons synthesize hormones that are transported in and stored at axon terminals as Herring bodies

- Releases two hormones from axon terminals, oxytocin and antidiuretic hormone (ADH)

Oxytocin

- Release stimulated by vaginal and cervical distension during labor
- Stimulates contraction of smooth uterine muscles during childbirth
- Activates milk ejection in lactating glands by stimulating contraction of myoepithelial cells

Antidiuretic Hormone (ADH)

- Increases permeability to water in distal convoluted tubules and collecting tubules of kidney
- Creates more concentrated urine after water is reabsorbed from glomerular filtrate
- Is also released during decreased blood pressure and, in large doses, contracts arterial walls

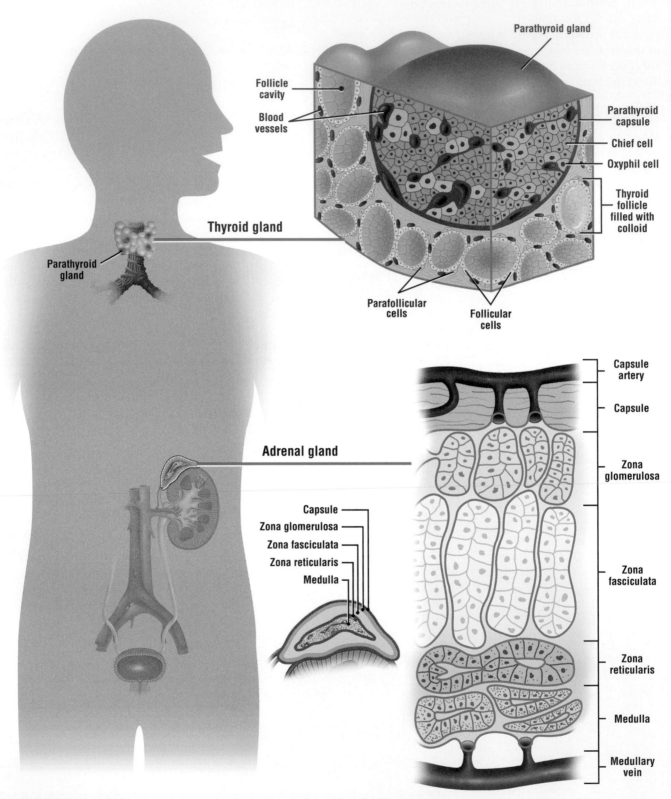

OVERVIEW FIGURE 17.2 ■ Thyroid gland, parathyroid gland, and adrenal gland. The microscopic organization and general location in the body of the thyroid, parathyroid, and adrenal glands are illustrated.

SECTION 2 ■ Thyroid Gland, Parathyroid Glands, and Adrenal Gland

The location in the body and histologic appearance of the thyroid gland, parathyroid glands, and adrenal glands are illustrated in the Overview Figure 17.2.

Thyroid Gland

The **thyroid gland** is located in the anterior neck inferior to the larynx. It is a single gland that consists of large right and left lobes, connected in the middle by an isthmus. Most endocrine cells, tissues, or organs are arranged in cords or clumps, and store their secretory products within their cytoplasm. The thyroid gland is a unique endocrine organ in that its cells are arranged into spherical structures, called **follicles.** Each follicle is surrounded by reticular fibers and a vascular network of capillaries that allows for easy entrance of thyroid hormones into the bloodstream. The follicular epithelium can be simple squamous, cuboidal, or low columnar, depending on the state of activity of the thyroid gland.

Follicles are the structural and functional units of the thyroid gland. The cells that surround the follicles, the **follicular cells,** also called principal cells, synthesize, release, and store their product outside of their cytoplasm, or extracellularly, in the lumen of the follicles as a gelatinous substance, called **colloid.** Colloid is composed of **thyroglobulin,** an iodinated glycoprotein that is the inactive storage form of the thyroid hormones.

In addition to follicular cells, the thyroid gland also contains larger, pale-staining **parafollicular** cells. These cells are found either peripherally in the follicular epithelium or within the follicle. When parafollicular cells are located in the confines of a follicle, they are always separated from the follicular lumen by neighboring follicular cells.

Parathyroid Glands

Mammals generally have four **parathyroid glands.** These small oval glands are situated on the posterior surface of the thyroid gland, but separated from the thyroid gland by a thin connective tissue **capsule.** Normally, one parathyroid gland is located on superior pole and one on the inferior pole of each lobe of the thyroid gland. In contrast to the thyroid gland, cells of the parathyroid glands are arranged into cords or clumps, surrounded by a rich network of capillaries.

There are two types of cells in the parathyroid glands: functional **principal** or **chief cells** and **oxyphil cells.** Oxyphil cells are larger, are found singly or in small groups, and are less numerous than the chief cells. In routine histologic sections, these cells stain deeply acidophilic. On rare occasions, small colloid-filled follicles may be seen in the parathyroid glands.

Adrenal (Suprarenal) Glands

The **adrenal glands** are endocrine organs situated near the superior pole of each kidney. Each adrenal gland is surrounded by a dense irregular connective tissue capsule and embedded in the adipose tissue around the kidneys. Each adrenal gland consists of an outer **cortex** and an inner **medulla.** Although these two regions of the adrenal gland are located in one organ and are linked by a common blood supply, they have separate and distinct embryologic origins, structures, and functions.

Cortex

The adrenal cortex exhibits three concentric zones: zona glomerulosa, zona fasciculata, and zona reticularis.

The **zona glomerulosa** is a thin zone inferior to the adrenal gland capsule. It consists of cells arranged in small clumps.

The **zona fasciculata** is intermediate and the thickest zone of the adrenal cortex. This zone exhibits vertical columns of one cell thickness adjacent to straight capillaries. This layer is characterized by pale-staining cells owing to the increased presence of numerous lipid droplets.

The **zona reticularis** is the innermost zone that is adjacent to the adrenal medulla. The cells in this zone are arranged in cords or clumps.

In all three zones, the secretory cells are adjacent to fenestrated capillaries. The cells of these zones in the adrenal cortex produce three classes of steroid hormones: **mineralocorticoids, glu-cocorticoids,** and **sex hormones.**

Medulla

The medulla lies in the center of the adrenal gland. The cells of the adrenal medulla, also arranged in small cords, are modified postganglionic sympathetic neurons that have lost their axons and dendrites during development. Instead, they have become secretory cells that synthesize and secrete **catecholamines** (primarily epinephrine and norepinephrine). Preganglionic axons of the sympathetic neurons innervate the adrenal medulla cells, which are surrounded by an extensive capillary network. As result, the release of epinephrine and norepinephrine from the adrenal medulla is under direct control of the sympathetic division of the **autonomic nervous system.**

FIGURE 17.6 ■ Thyroid Gland: Canine (General View)

The thyroid gland is characterized by variable-sized **follicles (2, 4, 12)** that are filled with an aci-dophilic **colloid** (2, 12). The follicles are usually lined by a simple cuboidal epithelium consisting of **follicular** (principal) cells **(3, 7).** The follicles that are sectioned tangentially (4) do not exhibit a lumen. The follicular cells (3, 7) synthesize and secrete the thyroid hormones. In routine histo-logic preparations, colloid often retracts from the follicular wall (12).

The thyroid gland also contains another cell type called the **parafollicular cells (1, 8).** These cells occur as single cells or in clumps on the periphery of the follicles. The parafollicular cells (1, 8) stain light and are visible in the canine thyroid. Parafollicular cells (1, 8) synthesize and secrete the hormone calcitonin.

Connective tissue septa (5, 9) from the thyroid gland capsule extend into the gland's interior and divide the gland into lobules. Numerous blood vessels, **arterioles (6), venules (10),** and **cap-illaries (13)** are seen in the connective tissue septa (5, 9) and around follicles (2, 12). Little **inter-follicular connective tissue (11)** is found between individual follicles.

1 Parafollicular cells

2 Follicle with colloid

3 Follicular cells

4 Follicle (tangential section)

5 Connective tissue septa

6 Arteriole

7 Follicular cells

8 Parafollicular cells

9 Connective tissue septa

10 Venule

11 Interfollicular connective tissue

12 Follicle with retracted colloid

13 Capillaries

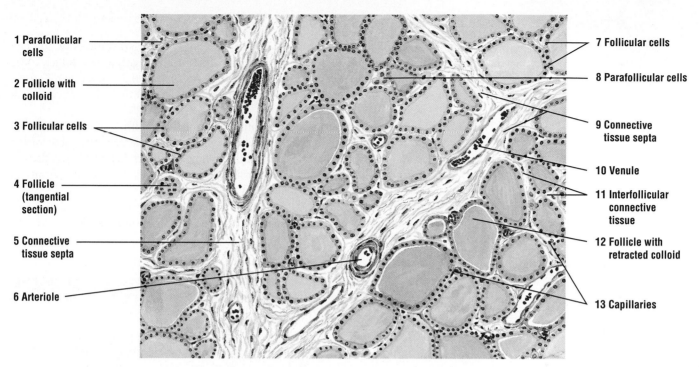

FIGURE 17.6 ■ Thyroid gland: canine (general view). Stain: hematoxylin and eosin. Low magnification.

FIGURE 17.7 ■ Thyroid Gland Follicles: Canine (Sectional View)

A higher magnification of the thyroid gland shows the details of thyroid **follicles (2, 9).** The height of the **follicular cells (5, 11)** depends on their function. In highly active follicles, the epithelium is cuboidal (9). In less active follicles, the epithelium appears flat (5). All thyroid follicles (2, 9) are filled with **colloid (2),** some of which show retraction **(12)** from the follicular wall or distortion **(12)** as a result of slide preparation.

The **parafollicular cells (1, 10)** are located within the follicular epithelium (1) or in small clumps (10) adjacent to the thyroid follicles (2, 9). These cells (1, 10) are larger and oval or varied in shape with lighter staining cytoplasm than that of the follicular cells (5, 11). The parafollicular cells (1, 10) are not directly located on the follicular lumen. Instead, they are separated from the lumen by the processes of neighboring follicular cells (5, 11).

Surrounding the thyroid follicles (2, 9), the follicular cells (5, 11), and the parafollicular cells (1, 10) is a thin **interfollicular connective tissue (3, 8)** with numerous **blood vessels (6)** and **capillaries (4).**

FUNCTIONAL CORRELATIONS: Thyroid Gland

Formation of Thyroid Hormones

The secretory functions of **follicular cells,** which are responsible for the production of thyroid hormones in the thyroid gland, are controlled by **thyroid-stimulating hormone (TSH)** released from the adenohypophysis. **Iodide** is an essential element for production of the active thyroid hormones triiodothyronine (T_3) and tetraiodothyronine or thyroxine (T_4) that are released into the bloodstream by the thyroid gland.

Low levels of thyroid hormones in the blood stimulate the release of TSH from the adenohypophysis. In response to TSH stimulus, the follicular cells in the thyroid gland take up **iodide** from the circulation via the iodide pump located in the follicular basal cell membrane. Iodide is then oxidized to iodine in the follicular cells and transported into the follicular lumen. In the lumen, iodine combines with amino acid tyrosine groups to form **iodinated thyroglobulin,** of which the **hormones triiodothyronine (T_3)** and **tetraiodothyronine or thyroxine (T_4)** are the principal products. T_3 and T_4 remain bound to the iodinated thyroglobulin in thyroid follicles in an inactive form until needed. TSH released from the adenohypophysis stimulates the thyroid gland cells to release the thyroid hormones into the bloodstream.

Release of Thyroid Hormones

Release of thyroid hormones involves endocytosis (uptake) of thyroglobulin by follicular cells, hydrolysis of the iodinated thyroglobulin by lysosomes, and release of the principal **thyroid hormones (T_3 and T_4)** at the base of follicular cells into the surrounding capillaries. The presence of thyroid hormones in the general circulation accelerates the metabolic rate of the body and increases cell metabolism, growth, differentiation, and development throughout the body. In addition, thyroid hormones increase the rate of protein, carbohydrate, and fat metabolism.

Parafollicular Cells

The thyroid gland also contains **parafollicular** cells. These cells appear on the periphery of the follicular epithelium as single cells or as cell clusters between the follicles. Parafollicular cells are not part of thyroid follicles and are not in contact with colloid.

The parafollicular cells synthesize and secrete the hormone **calcitonin (thyrocalcitonin)** into capillaries. The main function of calcitonin is to lower blood calcium levels in the body. This is primarily accomplished by reducing the number of **osteoclasts** in the bones, inhibiting bone resorption, and thereby reducing calcium release. Calcitonin also promotes increased excretion of calcium and phosphate ions from the kidneys into the urine. The production and release of calcitonin by the parafollicular cells depends only on blood calcium levels and is completely independent of the pituitary gland hormones.

1 Parafollicular
cells

2 Follicles with
colloid

3 Interfollicular
connective tissue

4 Capillary

5 Follicular cells

6 Blood vessel

7 Follicle (tangential
section)

8 Interfollicular
connective tissue

9 Follicle with
colloid

10 Parafollicular
cells

11 Follicular cells

12 Retracted or
distorted colloid

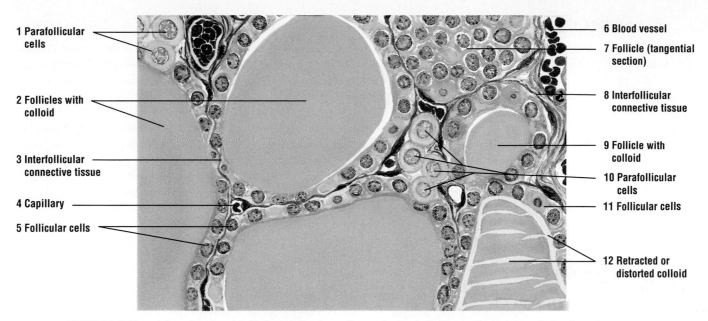

FIGURE 17.7 ■ Thyroid gland follicles, follicular cells, and parafollicular cells (sectional view). Stain: hematoxylin and eosin. High magnification.

FIGURE 17.8 ■ Thyroid and Parathyroid Glands: Canine (Sectional View)

The **thyroid gland (1)** is closely associated with the **parathyroid gland (3)**. A thin **connective tissue capsule (2)** with **capillaries (9)** and **blood vessels (8)** separates the two glands. Connective tissue **trabeculae (6)** from the surrounding capsule (2) extend into the parathyroid gland (3) and bring larger blood vessels (8) into its interior, where they branch into capillaries (9) around the parathyroid cells (3).

The parathyroid gland (3) cells are arranged into anastomosing cords and clumps, instead of the **follicles with colloid (4),** lined by **follicular cells (5),** of the thyroid gland (1). However, occasionally an isolated small follicle with colloid material may be observed in the parathyroid gland (3). The parathyroid gland (3) contains two cell types, the **chief (principal) cells (7)** and the **oxyphil cells (10)**. The chief cells (7) are the most numerous cells. They are round and have a pale, slightly acidophilic cytoplasm. The oxyphil cells (10) are larger and less numerous than the chief cells (7), and exhibit an acidophilic cytoplasm with smaller, darker-staining nuclei (10). The oxyphil cells (10) are found singly or in small clumps. The oxyphil cells (10) increase in number with age.

FIGURE 17.9 ■ Thyroid Gland and Parathyroid Gland

This photomicrograph shows a section of parathyroid gland adjacent to the thyroid gland. A thin **connective tissue septum (3)** separates the two glands. Different size **follicles** with **colloid (1)** and lined by **follicular cells (2)** characterize the thyroid gland.

Instead of follicles, the parathyroid gland contains two cell types. **Chief cells (4)** are smaller and more numerous, whereas the **oxyphil cells (5)** are larger and less numerous, and exhibit a highly eosinophilic cytoplasm. Numerous **blood vessels (6)** surround the secretory cells in both organs.

FUNCTIONAL CORRELATIONS: Parathyroid Glands

The **chief cells** of the parathyroid glands produce **parathyroid hormone (parathormone)**. The main function of this hormone is to maintain proper calcium levels in the extracellular body fluids. This is accomplished by elevating calcium levels in the blood. This action is opposite or antagonistic to that of calcitonin, which is produced by parafollicular cells in the thyroid glands.

Release of parathyroid hormone stimulates proliferation and increases the activity of the **osteoclasts** in bones. This activity releases more calcium from the bone into the bloodstream, thereby maintaining proper calcium levels. As the calcium concentration in the bloodstream increases, further production of parathyroid hormone is suppressed.

Parathyroid hormone also targets the kidneys and intestines. The distal convoluted tubules in the kidneys increase reabsorption of calcium from the glomerular filtrate and elimination of phosphate, sodium, and potassium ions into urine. Parathyroid hormone also influences the kidneys to form the hormone **calcitriol,** the active form of vitamin D, resulting in increased calcium absorption from the gastrointestinal tract into the bloodstream.

The secretion and release of parathyroid hormone depends primarily on the concentration of calcium levels in the blood and not on pituitary hormones. Because parathyroid hormone maintains optimal levels of calcium in the blood, parathyroid glands are essential to life.

The function of **oxyphil cells** in the parathyroid glands is presently not known.

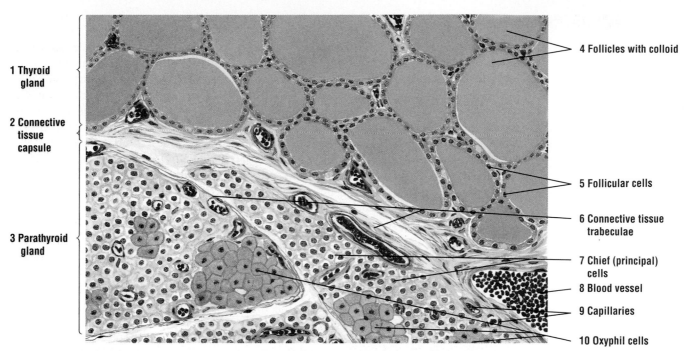

1 Thyroid gland

2 Connective tissue capsule

3 Parathyroid gland

4 Follicles with colloid

5 Follicular cells

6 Connective tissue trabeculae

7 Chief (principal) cells

8 Blood vessel

9 Capillaries

10 Oxyphil cells

FIGURE 17.8 ■ Thyroid and parathyroid glands: canine (sectional view). Stain: hematoxylin and eosin. Low magnification.

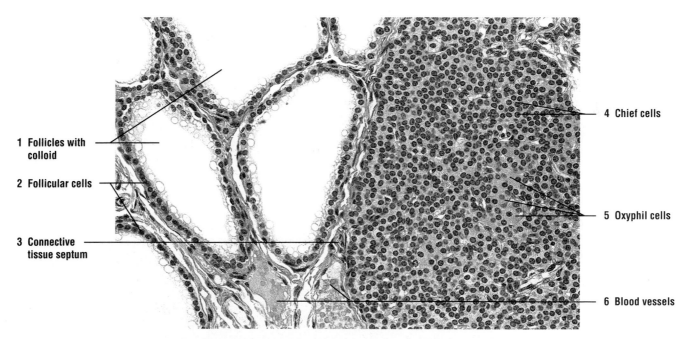

1 Follicles with colloid

2 Follicular cells

3 Connective tissue septum

4 Chief cells

5 Oxyphil cells

6 Blood vessels

FIGURE 17.9 ■ Thyroid gland and parathyroid gland. Stain: hematoxylin and eosin. ×80.

FIGURE 17.10 ■ Adrenal (Suprarenal) Gland

The adrenal (suprarenal) gland consists of an outer **cortex (1)** and an inner **medulla (5),** surrounded by a thick connective tissue **capsule (6)** that contains branches of adrenal blood vessels, veins, nerves (largely unmyelinated), and lymphatics. A **connective tissue septum** with a **blood vessel (2)** passes from the capsule (6) into the cortex. Other connective tissue septa carry the blood vessels to the medulla (5). Fenestrated sinusoidal **capillaries (8, 10)** and large **blood vessels (14)** are found throughout the cortex (1) and medulla (5).

The adrenal cortex (1) is subdivided into three concentric zones. Directly under the connective tissue capsule (6) is the outer **zona glomerulosa (7).** The **cells (7)** in zona glomerulosa (7) are arranged into ovoid groups or clumps and surrounded by numerous sinusoidal capillaries (8). The cytoplasm of these cells (7) stains pink and contains few lipid droplets.

The middle and the widest cell layer is the **zona fasciculata (3, 9).** The **cells of the zona fasciculata (9)** are arranged in vertical columns or radial plates. Because of the increased amount of lipid droplets in their cytoplasm, the cells of the zona fasciculata (9) appear light or vacuolated after a normal slide preparation. Sinusoidal capillaries (10) between the cell columns follow a similar vertical or radial course.

The third and the innermost cell layer is the **zona reticularis (4, 11).** This cell layer borders on the adrenal medulla (5). The **cells (11)** of the zona reticularis (4) form anastomosing cords surrounded by sinusoidal capillaries.

The medulla (5) is not sharply demarcated from the cortex. The cytoplasm of the **secretory cells of the medulla (13)** appears clear. After tissue fixation in potassium bichromate, called the chromaffin reaction, fine brown granules become visible in the cells of the medulla. These granules indicate the presence of the catecholamines epinephrine and norepinephrine in the cytoplasm.

The medulla also contains **sympathetic neurons (12)** that are seen singly or in small groups. The neurons (12) exhibit a vesicular nucleus, prominent nucleolus, and a small amount of peripheral chromatin.

Sinusoidal capillaries drain the contents of the medulla (5) into the prominent medullary blood vessels (14).

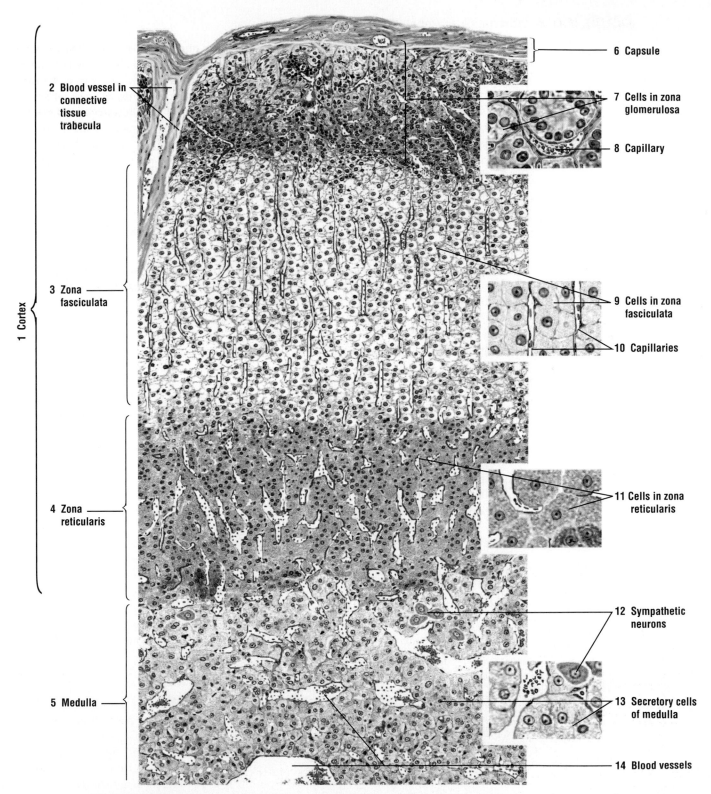

1 Cortex

2 Blood vessel in connective tissue trabecula

3 Zona fasciculata

4 Zona reticularis

5 Medulla

6 Capsule

7 Cells in zona glomerulosa

8 Capillary

9 Cells in zona fasciculata

10 Capillaries

11 Cells in zona reticularis

12 Sympathetic neurons

13 Secretory cells of medulla

14 Blood vessels

FIGURE 17.10 ■ Cortex and medulla of adrenal (suprarenal) gland. Stain: hematoxylin and eosin. Low magnification.

FIGURE 17.11 ■ Adrenal (Suprarenal) Gland: Cortex and Medulla

A lower-magnification photomicrograph illustrates a section of the adrenal gland. The cortex is surrounded by a dense connective tissue **capsule (1).** Beneath the capsule (1) is the **zona glomerulosa (2),** containing irregular ovoid clumps of cells. The intermediate and widest zone is the **zona fasciculata (3).** Here, the cells are arranged into light-staining, narrow cords, between which are found capillaries and fine connective tissue fibers. The innermost zone of the adrenal cortex is the **zona reticularis (4),** in which the cells are arranged into groups of branching cords and clumps.

The adrenal **medulla (5)** is located adjacent to the zona reticularis (4). In the medulla (5), the cells are larger and also arranged into clumps. Large **blood vessels (6)** (veins) drain the medulla (5).

FUNCTIONAL CORRELATIONS: Adrenal Gland Cortex and Medulla

Adrenal Gland Cortex

The adrenal gland cortex is under the influence of the pituitary gland hormone ACTH (adrenocorticotropic hormone). Cells of the adrenal gland cortex synthesize and release three types of steroids: mineralocorticoids, glucocorticoids, and androgens.

The cells of the **zona glomerulosa** in the adrenal cortex produce **mineralocorticoid hormones,** primarily **aldosterone.** Aldosterone release is initiated via the **renin-angiotensin** pathway in response to decreased arterial blood pressure and low levels of sodium in the plasma. These changes are detected by the **juxtaglomerular apparatus** (juxtaglomerular cells and macula densa) located in the kidney cortex near the renal corpuscles.

Aldosterone has a major influence on fluid and electrolyte balance in the body, with the main target being the distal convoluted tubules in the kidneys. The primary function of aldosterone is to increase **sodium reabsorption** from the glomerular filtrate by cells in the distal convoluted tubules of the kidney and increase potassium excretion into urine. As water follows sodium, there is an increase in fluid volume in the circulation. The increased volume increases blood pressure and restores normal electrolyte balance.

The cells of the zona fasciculata—and probably those of the zona reticularis—secrete **glucocorticoids,** of which **cortisol** and **cortisone** are the most important. Glucocorticoids are released into the circulation in response to stress. These steroids stimulate protein, fat, and carbohydrate metabolism, especially by increasing circulating blood **glucose** levels. Glucocorticoids also suppress inflammatory responses by reducing the number of circulating lymphocytes from lymphoid tissues and decreasing their production of antibodies. In addition, cortisol suppresses the tissue response to injury by decreasing cellular and humoral immunity.

Although the cells of the zona reticularis are believed to produce sex steroids, they are mainly weak androgens and have little physiologic significance. Glucocorticoid secretion, and the secretory functions of zona fasciculata and zona reticularis, are regulated by feedback control from the pituitary gland and adrenocorticotropic hormone (ACTH).

Adrenal Gland Medulla

The functions of the adrenal medulla are controlled by the hypothalamus through the sympathetic division of the autonomic nervous system. Cells in the adrenal medulla are activated in response to fear or acute emotional stress, causing them to release the catecholamines **epinephrine** and **norepinephrine.** Release of these chemicals prepares the individual for a "fight" or "flight" response, resulting in increased heart rate, increased cardiac output and blood flow, and a surge of glucose into the bloodstream from the liver for added energy. Catecholamines produce the maximal use of energy and physical effort to overcome the stress.

1 Capsule

2 Zona glomerulosa

3 Zona fasciculata

4 Zona reticularis

5 Medulla

6 Blood vessels

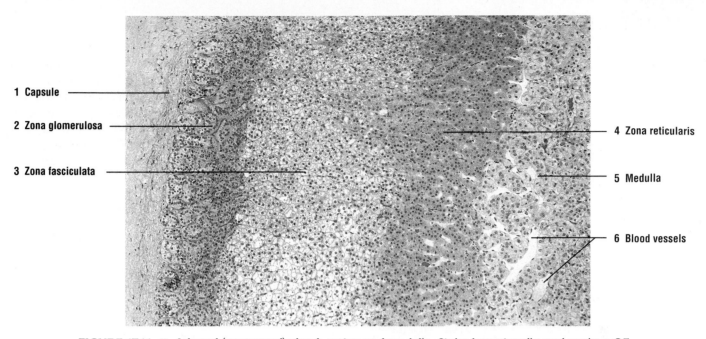

FIGURE 17.11 ■ Adrenal (suprarenal) gland: cortex and medulla. Stain: hematoxylin and eosin. ×25

Thyroid Gland

- Located in anterior neck region and consists of two large, connected lobes
- Consists of follicles surrounded by follicular cells that fill the lumen with gelatinous colloid material
- Colloid contains thyroglobulin, an iodinated inactive storage form of thyroid hormones
- Follicular cells controlled by thyroid-stimulating hormone (TSH)
- Iodide essential element in production of thyroid hormones
- Low levels of thyroid hormones stimulates release of TSH from adenohypophysis
- Iodide is taken up from blood, oxidized to iodine, and transported into follicular lumen
- Iodine combines with tyrosine groups to form iodinated thyroglobulin
- Triiodothyronine (T_3) and tetraiodothyronine (T_4) are the principal thyroid gland hormones
- Release of thyroid hormones involves endocytosis of thyroglobulin and hydrolysis of thyroglobulin
- Thyroid hormones increase metabolic rate, growth, differentiation, and development of body
- Parafollicular cells are located in follicular peripheries of thyroid gland
- Parafollicular cells secrete calcitonin to lower blood calcium by reducing number of osteoclasts
- Parafollicular cells act independent of pituitary gland hormones, instead depend on calcium level

Parathyroid Glands

- Mammals have four glands, situated on posterior surface of thyroid
- Instead of follicles, cells arranged in cords or clumps
- Two cell types, principal or chief cells and oxyphil cells
- Chief cells produce parathyroid hormone (parathormone)
- Main function is to maintain proper calcium levels by counterbalancing calcitonin action
- Parathyroid hormone stimulates osteoclasts and increases their activity to release more calcium into blood
- Parathyroid hormone induces kidney and intestines to absorb and retain more calcium
- Release of hormone depends on calcium levels and not pituitary hormones
- Are essential to life owing to maintenance of proper calcium levels
- Function of oxyphil cells not presently known

Adrenal Glands

- Located near superior pole of each kidney
- Have separate and distinct embryologic origin, structure, and function
- Covered with a connective tissue capsule and consist of outer cortex and inner medulla
- Fenestrated capillaries and large vessels throughout both regions
- Cortex subdivided into three zones: zona glomerulosa, zona fasciculata, and zona reticularis

Cortex

- Under direct influence of ACTH from pituitary gland
- Release three types of steroid hormones: mineralocorticoids, glucocorticoids, and androgens
- Cells in zona glomerulosa secrete mineralocorticoids, primarily aldosterone
- Aldosterone release is caused by decreased arterial blood pressure and low sodium levels
- Juxtaglomerular apparatus in kidney initiates the renin-angiotensin pathway to increase blood pressure
- Aldosterone increases sodium reabsorption and increased water retention by distal convoluted tubules
- Increased fluid volume increases blood pressure and inhibits further release of aldosterone
- Cells of zona fasciculata secrete glucocorticoids, of which cortisol and cortisone are important
- Glucocorticoids are released in response to stress, increase metabolism and glucose levels, and suppress inflammatory responses
- Cells of zona reticularis produce weak androgens

Medulla

- Cells are modified postganglionic sympathetic neurons that became secretory
- Action controlled by sympathetic division of autonomic nervous system, not pituitary gland
- Cells contain catecholamines (epinephrine and norepinephrine) and respond to acute stress
- Prepares the individual for flight or fight response by activating maximal use of energy and physical effort

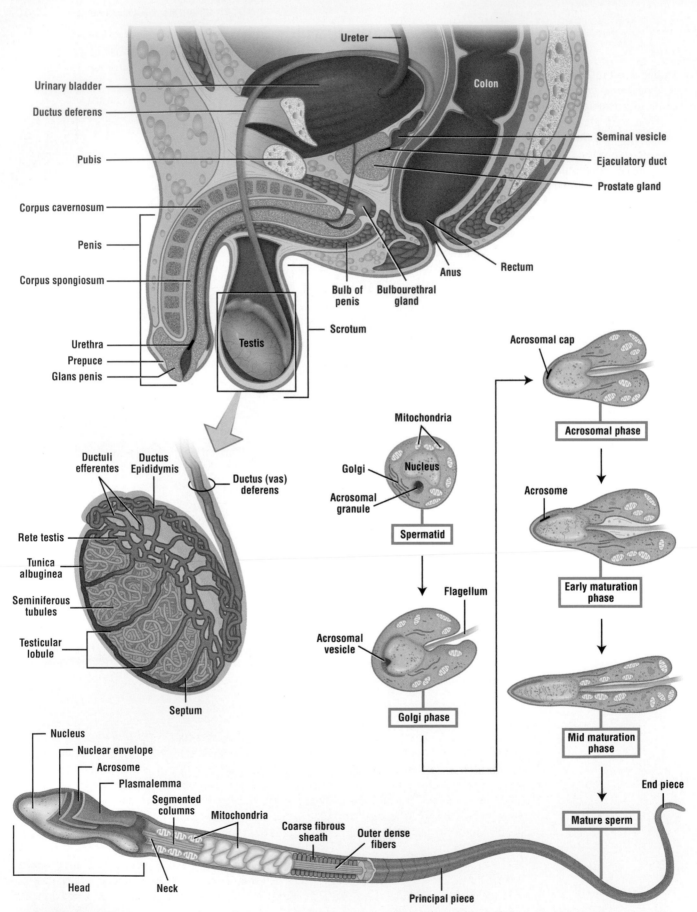

OVERVIEW FIGURE 18 ■ Location of the testes and the accessory male reproductive organs, with emphasis on the internal organization of the testis, the different phases of spermiogenesis, and the structure of a mature sperm.

Male Reproductive System

SECTION 1 ■ The Reproductive System

The male reproductive system consists of a pair of testes, numerous excurrent ducts, and different accessory glands that produce a variety of secretions that are added to sperm to form semen. The **testes** contain spermatogenic **stem cells** that continuously divide to produce new generations of cells that are eventually transformed into **spermatozoa,** or **sperm.** From the testes, the sperm move through excurrent ducts to the **epididymis** for storage and maturation. During sexual excitation and ejaculation, sperm leave the epididymis via the **ductus (vas) deferens** and exit the reproductive system through the penile **urethra.**

The **accessory glands**—prostate gland, seminal vesicles, and bulbourethral glands—of the male reproductive system are discussed and illustrated in detail in Section 2.

Scrotum

The paired testes are located outside the body cavity in the **scrotum.** In the scrotum, the temperature of the testes is about 2° to 3°C lower than normal body temperature. This lower temperature is vital for normal functioning of the testes and **spermatogenesis,** or sperm production. Perspiration and evaporation of sweat from the scrotal surface maintains the testes in a cooler environment.

Equally important in lowering testicular temperature is the special arrangement of blood vessels that supply the testes. Testicular arteries that descend into the scrotum are surrounded by a complex plexus of veins that ascend from the testes and form the **pampiniform plexus.** Blood returning from the testes in the pampiniform plexus is cooler than the blood in the testicular arteries. By a **countercurrent heat-exchange mechanism,** arterial blood is cooled by venous blood before it enters the testes, helping to maintain a lower temperature in testes.

Testes

A thick connective tissue capsule, the **tunica albuginea,** surrounds each testis. Posteriorly, the tunica albuginea thickens and extends inward into each testis to form the **mediastinum testis.** A thin connective tissue **septum** extends from the mediastinum testis and subdivides each testis into about 250 incomplete compartments or **testicular lobules,** each containing one to four coiled **seminiferous tubules.** Each seminiferous tubule is lined by stratified **germinal epithelium,** containing proliferating **spermatogenic (germ) cells** and nonproliferating **supporting (sustentacular)** or **Sertoli cells.** In the seminiferous tubules, spermatogenic cells divide, mature, and are transformed into sperm (Overview Figure 18).

Surrounding each seminiferous tubule are fibroblasts, musclelike cells, nerves, blood vessels, and lymphatic vessels. In addition, between the seminiferous tubules are clusters of epithelioid cells, the **interstitial cells (of Leydig).** These cells are steroid-secreting cells that produce the male sex hormone **testosterone.**

Formation of Sperm: Spermatogenesis

The process of sperm formation is called **spermatogenesis.** This includes mitotic divisions of spermatogenic cells, which produce replacement stem cells and other spermatogenic cells that eventually give rise to **primary spermatocytes** and **secondary spermatocytes.** Both primary and secondary spermatocytes undergo **meiotic divisions** that reduce the number of chromosomes and the amount of DNA. Division of secondary spermatocytes produces cells called **spermatids** that contain 23 single chromosomes (22+X or 22+Y). Spermatids do not undergo any further divisions, but instead are transformed into sperm by a process called **spermiogenesis.**

Once the spermatogenic cells in the germinal epithelium differentiate, they are held together by **intercellular bridges** during further differentiation and development. The intercellular bridges are broken when the developed spermatids are released into the seminiferous tubules as mature sperm.

Transformation of Spermatids: Spermiogenesis

Spermiogenesis is a complex morphologic process by which the spherical spermatids are transformed into elongated sperm cells. During spermiogenesis, the size and shape of the spermatids are altered, and the nuclear chromatin condenses. In the **Golgi phase,** small granules accumulate in the Golgi apparatus of the spermatid and form an **acrosomal granule** within a membrane-bound **acrosomal vesicle.** During the **acrosomal phase**, both the acrosomal vesicle and acrosomal granule spread over the condensing spermatid nucleus at the anterior tip of the spermatid as an **acrosome.** The acrosome functions as a specialized type of lysosome and contains several hydrolytic enzymes, such as hyaluronidase and protease with trypsinlike activity, that assist the sperm in penetrating the cells (corona radiata) and the membrane (zona pellucida) that surround the ovulated oocyte. During the **maturation phases,** the plasma membrane moves posteriorly from the nucleus to cover the developing **flagellum** (sperm tail). The mitochondria migrate to and form a tight sheath around the middle piece of the flagellum. The final maturation phase is characterized by the shedding of the excess or residual cytoplasm of the spermatid and release of the sperm cell into the lumen of the seminiferous tubule. Sertoli cells then phagocytose the residual cytoplasm.

The mature sperm cell is composed of a **head** and an acrosome that surrounds the anterior portion of the nucleus, a **neck,** a **middle piece** characterized by the presence of a compact mitochondrial sheath, and a main or **principal piece** (Overview Figure 18).

Excurrent Ducts

Newly released sperm pass from the seminiferous tubules into the intertesticular excurrent ducts that connect each testis with the overlying epididymis. These excurrent ducts consist of the **straight tubules** (tubuli recti) and the **rete testis,** the epithelial-lined spaces in the mediastinum testis. From the rete testis, the sperm enter approximately 12 short tubules, the **ductuli efferentes** (efferent ducts), which conduct sperm from the rete testis to the initial segment or the head of the **epididymis.**

The extratesticular duct that conducts the sperm to the penile urethra is the **ductus epididymis,** which is continuous with the **ductus (vas) deferens** and **ejaculatory ducts** in the prostate gland. During sexual excitation and ejaculation, strong contractions of the **smooth muscle** that surrounds the **ductus epididymis** expel the sperm (Overview Figure 18).

FUNCTIONAL CORRELATIONS: Testes

Spermatogonia

The function of the testes is to produce both sperm and testosterone. Testosterone is an essential hormone for development and maintenance of male sexual characteristics and normal functioning of the accessory reproductive glands.

The spermatogenic cells in the seminiferous tubules divide, differentiate, and produce sperm by a process called **spermatogenesis.** This process involves the following:

- Mitotic divisions of spermatogonia to form stem cells
- Formation of **primary** and **secondary spermatocytes** from spermatogenic cells
- **Meiotic divisions** of primary and secondary spermatocytes to reduce the somatic chromosome numbers by one half and formation of **spermatids,** which are germ cells with only 23 single chromosomes (22+X or 22+Y)
- Morphologic transformation of spermatids into mature sperm by a process called **spermiogenesis**

Sertoli Cells

Sertoli cells are the supportive cells of the testes that are located among the spermatogenic cells in the seminiferous tubules. They perform numerous important functions in the testes, among which are the following:

- Physical support, protection, and nutrition of the developing sperm (spermatids)
- Phagocytosis of excess cytoplasm (residual bodies) from the developing spermatids
- Release of mature sperm, called spermiation, into the lumen of seminiferous tubules
- Secretion of fructose-rich testicular fluid for nourishment and transport of sperm to the excurrent ducts
- Production and release of androgen-binding protein (ABP) that binds to and increases the concentration of testosterone in the lumen of the seminiferous tubules that is necessary for spermatogenesis. ABP secretion is under the control of follicle-stimulating hormone (FSH) from the pituitary gland
- Secretion of the hormone inhibin, which suppresses the release of FSH from the pituitary gland
- Production and release of the anti-müllerian hormone, also called müllerian-inhibiting hormone, that suppresses the development of müllerian ducts in the male and inhibits the development of female reproductive organs

Blood-Testis Barrier

The adjacent cytoplasm of Sertoli cells are joined by occluding **tight junctions,** producing a **blood-testis barrier** that subdivides each seminiferous tubule into a **basal compartment** and an **adluminal compartment.** This important barrier segregates the spermatogonia from all successive stages of spermatogenesis in the adluminal compartment and excludes the plasma proteins and bloodborne antibodies from the lumen of seminiferous tubules. The more-advanced spermatogenic cells can be recognized by the body as foreign and cause an immune response. The barrier protects these cells from the immune system by restricting the passage of membrane **antigens** from developing sperm into the bloodstream. Thus, the blood-testis barrier prevents an autoimmune response to the individual's own sperm, antibody formation, and eventual induction of sterility. The blood-testis barrier also keeps harmful substances in the blood from entering the developing germinal epithelium.

FIGURE 18.1 ■ Testis (Sectional View)

Each testis is enclosed in a thick, connective tissue capsule called the **tunica albuginea (1)**, internal to which is a vascular layer of loose connective tissue called the **tunica vasculosa (2, 8)**. The connective tissue extends inward from the tunica vasculosa (2, 8) into the testis to form the **interstitial connective tissue (3, 12)**. The interstitial connective tissue (3, 12) surrounds, binds, and supports the **seminiferous tubules (4, 6, 9)**. Extending from the mediastinum testis (see Figure 18.2 below) toward the tunica albuginea (1) are thin fibrous **septa (7, 10)** that divide the testis into compartments called lobules. Within each lobule are found one to four seminiferous tubules (4, 6, 9). The septa (7, 10) are not solid, and there is intercommunication between lobules.

Located in the interstitial connective tissue (3, 12) around the seminiferous tubules (4, 6, 9) are **blood vessels (13)**, loose connective tissue cells, and clusters of epithelial **interstitial cells (of Leydig) (5, 11)**. The interstitial cells (5, 11) are the endocrine cells of the testis and secrete the male sex hormone testosterone into the bloodstream.

The seminiferous tubules (4, 6, 9) are long, convoluted tubules in the testis that are normally observed cut in transverse (4), longitudinal (6), or tangential (9) planes of section. The seminiferous tubules (4, 6, 9) are lined with a stratified epithelium called the **germinal epithelium (14).** The germinal epithelium (14) contains two cell types, the spermatogenic cells that produce sperm and the supportive Sertoli cells that nourish the developing sperm. The germinal epithelium (14) rests on the basement membrane of the seminiferous tubules (4, 6, 9) and its cells are illustrated in greater detail in Figures 18.3, 18.4, and 18.5.

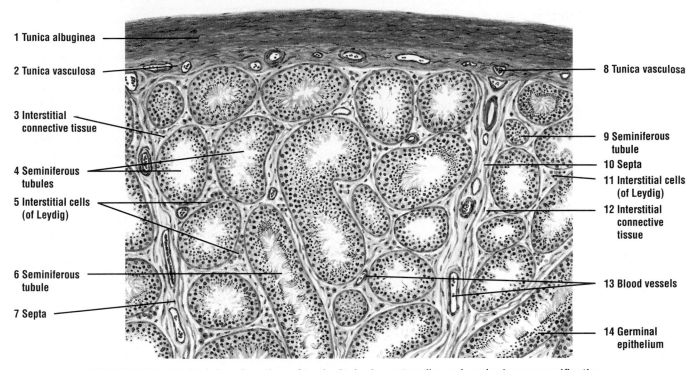

1 Tunica albuginea

2 Tunica vasculosa

3 Interstitial connective tissue

4 Seminiferous tubules

5 Interstitial cells (of Leydig)

6 Seminiferous tubule

7 Septa

8 Tunica vasculosa

9 Seminiferous tubule

10 Septa

11 Interstitial cells (of Leydig)

12 Interstitial connective tissue

13 Blood vessels

14 Germinal epithelium

FIGURE 18.1 ■ Peripheral section of testis. Stain: hematoxylin and eosin. Low magnification.

FIGURE 18.2 ■ Seminiferous Tubules, Straight Tubules, Rete Testis, and Ductuli Efferentes (Efferent Ductules)

In the posterior region of the testis, the tunica albuginea extends into the testis interior as the **mediastinum testis (10, 16).** In this illustration, the plane of section passes through the **seminiferous tubules (3, 5),** the connective tissue and blood vessels of the mediastinum testis (10, 16), and the excretory ducts, the **ductuli efferentes (efferent ductules) (9, 13).**

A few seminiferous tubules (3, 5) are visible on the left side. The tubules (3, 5) are lined with spermatogenic epithelium and sustentacular (Sertoli) cells. The **interstitial connective tissue (4)** is continuous with the mediastinum testis (10, 16) and contains the steroid (testosterone)-producing **interstitial cells (of Leydig) (1).** In the mediastinum testis (10, 16), the seminiferous tubules (3, 5) terminate in the **straight tubules (2, 6).** The straight tubules (2, 6) are short, narrow ducts lined with cuboidal or low columnar epithelium that are devoid of spermatogenic cells.

The straight tubules (2, 6) continue into the **rete testis (7, 8, 12)** of the mediastinum testis (10, 16). The rete testis (7, 8, 12) is an irregular, anastomosing network of tubules with wide lumina lined by a simple squamous to low cuboidal or low columnar epithelium. The rete testis (7, 8, 12) becomes wider near the ductuli efferentes (efferent ductules) (9, 13), into which the rete testis empties. The ductuli efferentes (9, 13) are straight but become highly convoluted in the head of the ductus epididymis. The ductuli efferentes (9, 13) connect the rete testis (7, 8, 12) with the epididymis (see Figure 18.6). Some tubules in the rete testis (12) and ductuli efferentes (9, 13) contain accumulations of **sperm (11, 14).**

The epithelium of the ductuli efferentes (9, 13) consists of groups of tall columnar cells that alternate with groups of shorter cuboidal cells. Because of the alternating cell heights, the lumina of the ductuli efferentes are uneven. The tall cells in the ductuli efferentes (9, 13) exhibit **cilia (15)** and the cuboidal cells exhibit microvilli.

FUNCTIONAL CORRELATIONS: Hormones of Male Reproductive Organs

Normal spermatogenesis is dependent on the action of **luteinizing hormone (LH)** and **follicle-stimulating hormone (FSH)** produced by **gonadotrophs** in the **adenohypophysis** of the pituitary gland. LH binds to receptors on **interstitial cells** (of Leydig) and stimulates them to synthesize the hormone **testosterone.** FSH stimulates **Sertoli cells** to synthesize and release **androgen-binging protein (ABP)** into the seminiferous tubules. ABP combines with testosterone and increases its concentration in the seminiferous tubules, which then stimulates spermatogenesis. Increased concentration of testosterone in the seminiferous tubules is essential for proper **spermatogenesis.** In addition, the structure and function of the accessory reproductive glands, as well as development and maintenance of male secondary sexual characteristics, are dependent on proper testosterone levels.

The hormone **inhibin,** also secreted by the Sertoli cells, has an inhibitory effect on the pituitary gland and suppresses or inhibits additional production of FSH.

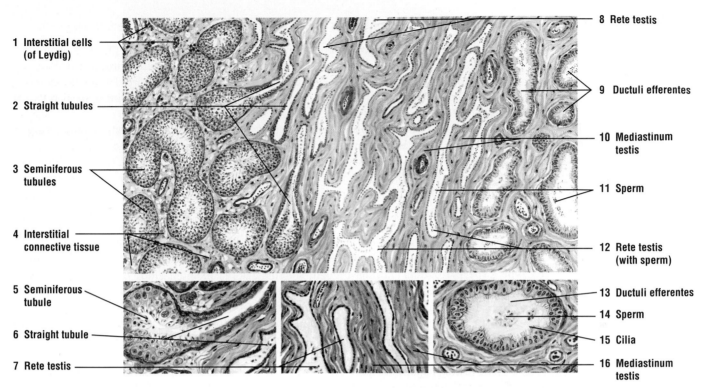

1 Interstitial cells (of Leydig)
2 Straight tubules
3 Seminiferous tubules
4 Interstitial connective tissue
5 Seminiferous tubule
6 Straight tubule
7 Rete testis
8 Rete testis
9 Ductuli efferentes
10 Mediastinum testis
11 Sperm
12 Rete testis (with sperm)
13 Ductuli efferentes
14 Sperm
15 Cilia
16 Mediastinum testis

FIGURE 18.2 ■ Seminiferous tubules, straight tubules, rete testis, and efferent ductules (ductuli efferentes). Stain: hematoxylin and eosin. Low magnification (inset: high magnification).

FIGURE 18.3 ■ Primate Testis: Spermatogenesis in Seminiferous Tubule (Transverse Section)

Different stages of spermatogenesis are illustrated in a **seminiferous tubule (3)**. Each seminiferous tubule (3) is surrounded by an outer layer of connective tissue with **fibroblasts (1)** and an inner **basement membrane (2)**. Between the seminiferous tubules (3) are the interstitial tissue with **fibroblasts (1, 18)**, **blood vessels (10)**, nerves, lymphatics, and the **interstitial cells (of Leydig) (11, 15)**.

The stratified germinal epithelium of the seminiferous tubule (3) consists of **supporting** or **Sertoli cells (6, 7, 14)** and **spermatogenic cells (5, 9, 12)**. Sertoli cells (6, 7, 14) are slender, elongated cells with irregular outlines that extend from the basement membrane (2) to the lumen of the seminiferous tubule (3). The nuclei of Sertoli cells (6, 7, 14) are ovoid or elongated and contain fine, sparse chromatin. A distinct nucleolus distinguishes Sertoli cells (6, 7, 14) from the spermatogenic cells (5, 9, 12) that surround Sertoli cells (6, 7, 14).

The immature spermatogenic cells, called the **spermatogonia (12)**, are adjacent to the basement membrane (2) of the seminiferous tubules (3). The spermatogonia (12) divide mitotically to produce several generations of cells. Three types of spermatogonia are recognized. The **pale type A spermatogonia (12a)** have a light-staining cytoplasm and a round or ovoid nucleus with pale, finely granular chromatin. The **dark type A spermatogonia (12b)** appear similar but with darker chromatin. The third type is type B spermatogonia.

Type A spermatogonia (12a) serve as stem cells for the germinal epithelium and give rise to other type A and type B spermatogonia. The final mitotic division of type B spermatogonia produces **primary spermatocytes (5, 16)**.

The primary spermatocytes (5, 16) are the largest germ cells in the seminiferous tubules (3) and occupy the middle region of the germinal epithelium. Their cytoplasm contains large nuclei with coarse clumps or thin threads of chromatin. The first meiotic division of the primary spermatocytes (Figure 18.4: I, 5) produces smaller secondary spermatocytes with less-dense nuclear chromatin (Figure 18.4: I, 3). The secondary spermatocytes (Figure 18.4: I, 3) undergo a second meiotic division shortly after their formation and are not frequently seen in the seminiferous tubules (3).

The second meiotic division produces **spermatids (4, 8, 9, 13, 17)** that are smaller cells than the primary or secondary spermatocytes (Figure 18.4: I, 2, 3, 5). The spermatids (4, 8, 9, 13, 17) are grouped in the adluminal compartment of the seminiferous tubule (3) and are closely associated with Sertoli cells (6, 13, 14). Here, the spermatids (4, 8, 9, 13, 17) differentiate into sperm by a process called spermiogenesis. The small, dark-staining heads of the maturing spermatids (4, 8) are embedded in the cytoplasm of Sertoli cells (6, 7, 14) with their tails extending into the lumen of the seminiferous tubule (3).

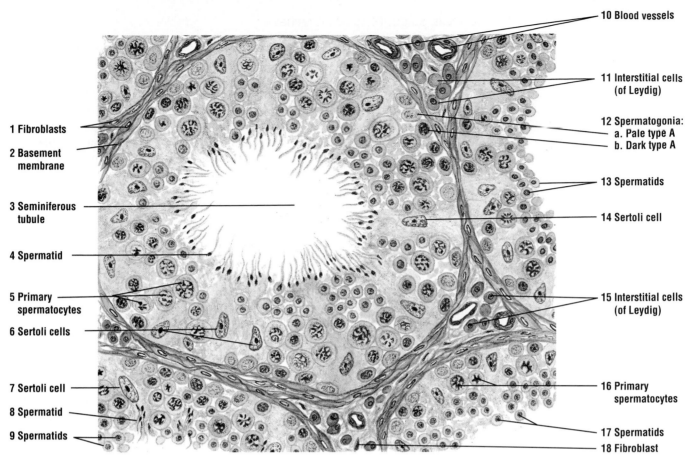

1 Fibroblasts
2 Basement membrane
3 Seminiferous tubule
4 Spermatid
5 Primary spermatocytes
6 Sertoli cells
7 Sertoli cell
8 Spermatid
9 Spermatids

10 Blood vessels
11 Interstitial cells (of Leydig)
12 Spermatogonia:
   a. Pale type A
   b. Dark type A
13 Spermatids
14 Sertoli cell
15 Interstitial cells (of Leydig)
16 Primary spermatocytes
17 Spermatids
18 Fibroblast

FIGURE 18.3 ■ Primate testis: spermatogenesis in seminiferous tubules (transverse section). Stain: hematoxylin and eosin. Medium magnification.

FIGURE 18.4 ■ Primate Testis: Stages of Spermatogenesis

Three stages of spermatogenesis are illustrated. In the left illustration (I), the **primary spermatocytes** (5) form the **secondary spermatocytes** (3), which undergo rapid meiotic division to form the **spermatids** (1, 2) that become embedded deep in the **Sertoli cell** (4) cytoplasm. Adjacent to the basement membrane are the **type A spermatogonia** (6).

In the middle illustration (II), the **spermatids** (7) are near the lumen of the seminiferous tubule before their release. Also visible are round **spermatids** (8) and **primary spermatocytes** (9) close to **Sertoli cells** (10). Near the base of the seminiferous tubule are the **spermatogonia** (11).

In the right illustration (III), the mature sperm have been released (spermiation) into the seminiferous tubule and the germinal epithelium contains only **spermatids** (8), **primary spermatocytes** (9), **spermatogonia** (11), and the supporting **Sertoli cells** (10).

FIGURE 18.5 ■ Testis: Seminiferous Tubules (Transverse Section)

This photomicrograph illustrates a **seminiferous tubule** (5) and parts of adjacent seminiferous tubules. A thick germinal epithelium lines each seminiferous tubule (5).

The **dark type A** (1a) and the **pale type B** (1b) **spermatogonia** (1) are located in the base of the tubule. The **primary spermatocytes** (2) and **spermatids** (7) in different stages of maturation are embedded in the germinal epithelium closer to the lumen. The tails of the spermatids (7) protrude into the lumen of the seminiferous tubules (5). The supportive **Sertoli cells** (6) are located throughout the germinal epithelium.

Each seminiferous tubule (5) is surrounded by a fibromuscular interstitial **connective tissue** (3). Here are found the testosterone-secreting **interstitial cells** (4).

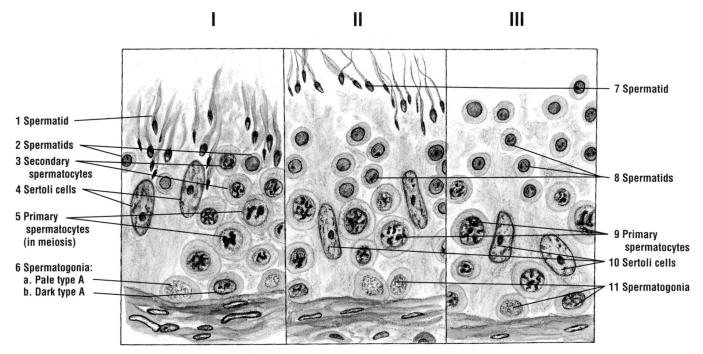

I   **II**   **III**

1 Spermatid

2 Spermatids

3 Secondary
  spermatocytes

4 Sertoli cells

5 Primary
  spermatocytes
  (in meiosis)

6 Spermatogonia:
  a. Pale type A
  b. Dark type A

7 Spermatid

8 Spermatids

9 Primary
  spermatocytes

10 Sertoli cells

11 Spermatogonia

FIGURE 18.4 ■ Primate testis: different stages of spermatogenesis. Stain: hematoxylin and eosin. High magnification.

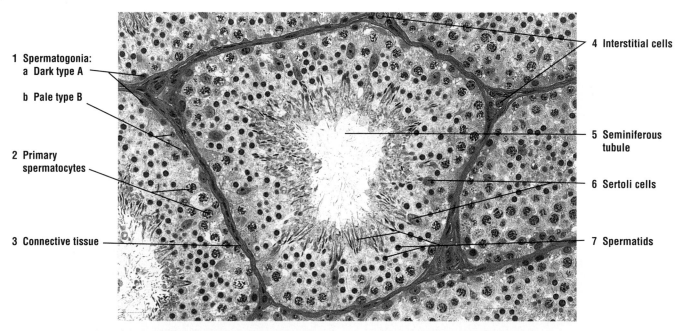

1 Spermatogonia:
  a Dark type A

  b Pale type B

2 Primary
  spermatocytes

3 Connective tissue

4 Interstitial cells

5 Seminiferous
  tubule

6 Sertoli cells

7 Spermatids

FIGURE 18.5 ■ Testis: seminiferous tubules (transverse section). Stain: hematoxylin and eosin (plastic section). ×80.

FIGURE 18.6 ■ Ductuli Efferentes and Tubules of Ductus Epididymis

The **ductuli efferentes (1)** or efferent ductules emerge from the mediastinum on the posterosuperior surface of the testis and connect the rete testis with the ductus epididymis. The ductuli efferentes are located in the **connective tissue (2, 12)** and form a portion of the head of the epididymis.

The lumen of the ductuli efferentes (1) exhibits an irregular contour because the lining epithelium consists of simple alternating groups of tall **ciliated** and shorter **nonciliated cells.** The basal surface of the tubules has a smooth contour. Located under the basement membrane is a thin layer of connective tissue (2) containing a thin **smooth muscle layer (5, 11).** As the ductuli efferentes (1) terminate in the ductus epididymis, the lumina are lined with **pseudostratified columnar epithelium (6, 8)** of the ductus epididymis (7).

The **ductus epididymis (3, 4)** is a long, convoluted tubule surrounded by connective tissue (2) and a thin smooth muscle layer (5, 11). A section through the ductus epididymis shows both **cross sections (3)** and **longitudinal sections (4).** Some parts of the ductus contain mature **sperm (7).**

The pseudostratified columnar epithelium (6, 8) consists of tall columnar **principal cells (9)** with long, nonmotile **stereocilia (8)** and small **basal cells (10).**

FIGURE 18.7 ■ Tubules of the Ductus Epididymis (Transverse Section)

This photomicrograph illustrates the tubules of the ductus epididymis, some of which are filled with **sperm (1).** The tubules of the ductus are lined with **pseudostratified epithelium (2).** The **principal cells (2a)** are tall columnar epithelium and are lined with **stereocilia (5),** the long, branching microvilli. The **basal cells (2b)** are small and spherical and situated near the base of the epithelium. A thin layer of **smooth muscle (3)** surrounds each tubule. Adjacent to the smooth muscle layer (3) are cells and fibers of the **connective tissue (4).**

1 Ductuli efferentes

2 Connective tissue

3 Cross sections of
ductus epididymis

4 Longitudinal sections
of ductus epididymis

5 Smooth muscle layer

6 Epithelium

7 Sperm

8 Pseudostratified
columnar epithelium
with stereocilia

9 Principal cells

10 Basal cells

11 Smooth muscle layer

12 Connective tissue

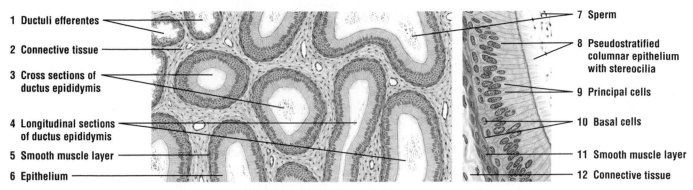

FIGURE 18.6 ■ Ductuli efferentes and tubules of the ductus epididymis. Stain: hematoxylin and eosin. Left side, low magnification; right side, high magnification.

1 Sperm

2 Pseudostratified
epithelium

a. Principal cells

b. Basal cells

3 Smooth muscle

4 Connective
tissue

5 Stereocilia

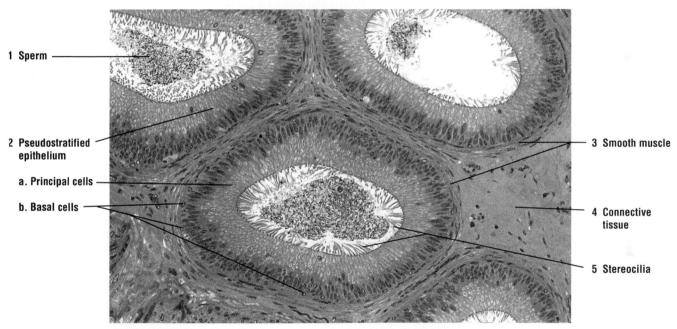

FIGURE 18.7 ■ Tubules of the ductus epididymis (transverse section). Stain: hematoxylin and eosin (plastic section). ×50.

FIGURE 18.8 ■ Ductus (Vas) Deferens (Transverse Section)

The ductus (vas) deferens exhibits a narrow and irregular lumen with **longitudinal mucosal folds (6),** a thin mucosa, a thick muscularis, and an adventitia.

The lumen of the ductus deferens is lined by **pseudostratified columnar epithelium (8)** with stereocilia. The epithelium of the ductus deferens is somewhat lower than in the ductus epididymis. The underlying thin **lamina propria (7)** consists of compact collagen fibers and a fine network of elastic fibers.

The thick muscularis consists of three smooth muscle layers: a thinner **inner longitudinal layer (1),** a thick **middle circular layer (2),** and a thinner **outer longitudinal layer (3).** The muscularis is surrounded by **adventitia (5)** in which are found abundant **blood vessels, venule** and **arteriole (4),** and nerves. The adventitia (5) of the ductus deferens merges with the connective tissue of the spermatic cord.

FIGURE 18.9 ■ Ampulla of the Ductus (Vas) Deferens (Transverse Section)

The terminal portion of the ductus deferens enlarges into an ampulla. The ampulla mainly differs from the ductus deferens in the structure of its mucosa.

The **lumen (3)** of the ampulla is larger than that of the ductus deferens. The mucosa also exhibits numerous irregular, branching **mucosal folds (4)** and deep **glandular diverticula** or **crypts (1)** located between the folds that extend to the surrounding muscle layer. The secretory epithelium that lines the lumen (3) and the glandular diverticula (1) is simple columnar or cuboidal. Below the epithelium is the **lamina propria (6).**

The smooth muscle layers in the muscularis are similar to those in the ductus deferens. These consist of a thin **inner longitudinal muscle layer (7),** a thick **middle circular muscle layer (8),** and a thin **outer longitudinal muscle layer (9).** Surrounding the ampulla is the connective tissue **adventitia (5).**

FUNCTIONAL CORRELATIONS

Ductuli Efferentes (Efferent Ductules)

The motility of cilia in the **ductuli efferentes** creates a current that assists in transporting the fluid and sperm from the seminiferous tubules to the **ductus epididymis.** In addition, contractility of the smooth muscle fibers that surround these tubules provides additional assistance to sperm transport. The nonciliated cuboidal cells that also line the ductuli efferentes absorb most of the testicular fluid that was produced in the seminiferous tubules by Sertoli cells.

Ductus Epididymis

The highly coiled ductus epididymis is the site for **accumulation, storage,** and further **maturation** of sperm. When sperm enter the epididymis, they are nonmotile and incapable of fertilizing an oocyte. However, about a week later in transit through the ductus epididymis, the sperm acquire motility. The **principal cells** in the ductus epididymis are lined with long branching microvilli, or **stereocilia,** that continue to absorb testicular fluid that was not absorbed in the ductuli efferentes during the passage of sperm from the testes. The principal cells in the epididymis also phagocytose the remaining residual bodies that were not removed by the Sertoli cells in the seminiferous tubules, as well as any abnormal or degenerating sperm cells. These cells also produce a glycoprotein that **inhibits capacitation** or the fertilizing ability of the sperm until they are deposited in the female reproductive tract.

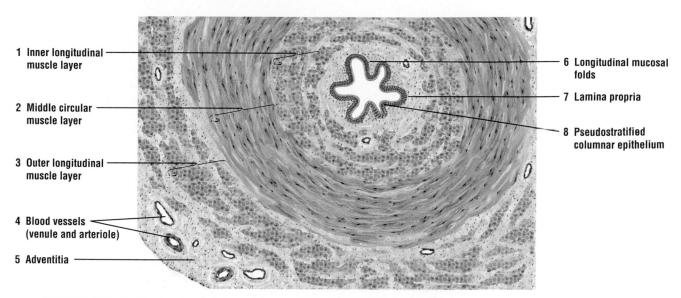

1 Inner longitudinal
  muscle layer

2 Middle circular
  muscle layer

3 Outer longitudinal
  muscle layer

4 Blood vessels
  (venule and arteriole)

5 Adventitia

6 Longitudinal mucosal
  folds

7 Lamina propria

8 Pseudostratified
  columnar epithelium

FIGURE 18.8 ■ Ductus (vas) deferens (transverse section). Stain: hematoxylin and eosin. Low magnification.

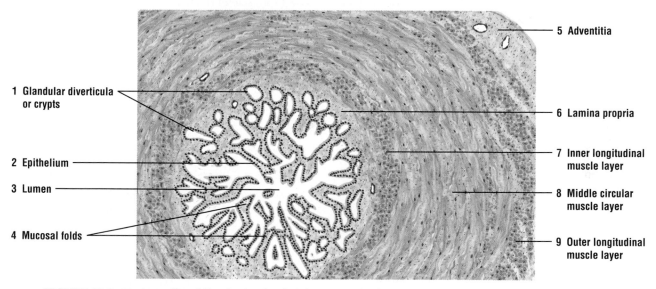

1 Glandular diverticula
  or crypts

2 Epithelium

3 Lumen

4 Mucosal folds

5 Adventitia

6 Lamina propria

7 Inner longitudinal
  muscle layer

8 Middle circular
  muscle layer

9 Outer longitudinal
  muscle layer

FIGURE 18.9 ■ Ampulla of the ductus (vas) deferens. Stain: hematoxylin and eosin. Low magnification.

CHAPTER 18 ■ **Summary**

The Male Reproductive System: Composition

- Consists of two testes that contain spermatogenic cells, which produce sperm
- Numerous excurrent ducts move sperm for storage and maturation into ductus epididymis
- During ejaculation, sperm leave system via ductus (vas) deferens and penile urethra
- Accessory glands include prostate, seminal vesicles, and bulbourethral glands

Scrotum

- Testes located outside of body in scrotum whose temperature is 2° to 3°C lower than body
- Lower temperature in scrotum a result of sweat evaporation and pampiniform plexus
- Countercurrent heat-exchange mechanism in veins cools arterial blood as it enters the testes

Testes

- Thick connective tissue tunica albuginea surrounds each testis and forms mediastinum testis
- Thin connective tissue septa from mediastinum testis separate testis into testicular lobules
- Testicular lobules contain coiled seminiferous tubules that are lined by germinal epithelium
- Germinal epithelium contains spermatogenic cells and Sertoli (supportive) cells
- Between seminiferous tubules are testosterone-secreting interstitial cells (of Leydig)

Spermatogenesis

- Includes mitotic divisions of spermatogenic cells to form type A stem cells
- Spermatogenic cells type B give rise to primary spermatocytes, the largest cells in tubules
- Primary spermatocytes give rise to smaller secondary spermatocytes
- Meiotic divisions of primary and secondary spermatocytes reduce number of chromosomes
- Secondary spermatocytes divide to form spermatids
- Spermatids do not divide and contain 23 single chromosomes (22+X or 22+Y)
- Developing sperm connected by intercellular bridges until released as mature sperm into tubules

Spermiogenesis

- Morphologic transformation of spermatid into sperm

- Size and shape of spermatid altered, with condensation of nuclear chromatin
- On anterior side, acrosome granules in vesicle spread over the condensing nucleus as acrosome
- Acrosome contains hydrolytic enzymes needed to penetrate cells that surround the oocyte
- On posterior side, flagellum (tail) forms with mitochondria aggregating at middle piece of sperm
- Residual cytoplasm shed from spermatids and phagocytosed by Sertoli cells
- Mature sperm consists of head, neck, middle piece, and principal piece

Excurrent Ducts

- Released sperm pass through straight tubules and rete testis to ductuli efferentes
- Ductuli efferentes emerge from mediastinum and conduct sperm to head of ductus epididymis
- Epithelium of ductuli efferentes uneven owing to ciliated and nonciliated cells in the lumina
- Cilia in ductuli efferentes move sperm and fluid from seminiferous tubules to ductus epididymis
- Nonciliated cells absorb much of the testicular fluid as it passes to ductus epididymis
- Ductus epididymis is continuous with ductus (vas) deferens that conducts sperm to penile urethra
- Smooth muscles around ductuli efferentes, ductus epididymis, and vas deferens contract to move sperm
- Pseudostratified epithelium with principal and basal cells lines ductuli efferentes and epididymis
- Stereocilia line the surface of cells in ductus epididymis and vas deferens
- Stereocilia absorb testicular fluid and the principal cells phagocytose residual cytoplasm
- Principal cells in ductus epididymis also produce glycoprotein that inhibits sperm capacitation

Sertoli Cells

- Physical support, protection, nutrition, and release of mature sperm into tubules
- Phagocytosis of residual cytoplasm of spermatids
- Secretion of ABP to concentrate testosterone in tubules and testicular fluid for sperm transport
- Secretion of hormone inhibin and anti-müllerian hormone

Blood-Testis Barrier

- Formed by tight junctions of adjacent Sertoli cells
- Separates seminiferous tubules in basal and adluminal compartments

- Protects developing sperm from autoimmune response and harmful materials

Male Hormones

- Spermatogenesis dependent on LH and FSH hormones produced by the pituitary gland
- LH binds to receptors on interstitial cells and stimulates testosterone secretion

- FSH stimulates Sertoli cells to produce ABP into seminiferous tubules to bind testosterone
- Testosterone in seminiferous tubules is vital for spermatogenesis and accessory gland function
- Sertoli cells produce inhibin, which inhibits FSH production from pituitary gland

SECTION 2 ■ Accessory Reproductive Glands

Seminal Vesicles, Prostate Gland, Bulbourethral Glands, and Penis

The accessory glands of the male reproductive system consist of paired **seminal vesicles,** paired **bulbourethral glands,** and a single **prostate gland.** These structures are directly associated with the male reproductive tract and produce numerous secretory products that mix with sperm to produce a fluid called **semen.** The penis serves as the copulatory organ, and the penile urethra serves as a common passageway for urine or semen.

The seminal vesicles are located posterior to the bladder and superior to the prostate gland. The excretory duct of each seminal vesicle joins the dilated terminal part of each ductus (vas) deferens, the **ampulla,** to form the **ejaculatory ducts.** The ejaculatory ducts enter and continue through the prostate gland to open into the **prostatic urethra.**

The prostate gland is located inferior to the neck of the bladder. The **urethra** exits the bladder and passes through the prostate gland as the **prostatic urethra.** In addition to the ejaculatory ducts, numerous excretory ducts from prostatic glands open into the prostatic urethra.

The bulbourethral glands are small, pea-sized glands located at the root of the **penis** and embedded in the skeletal muscles of the urogenital diaphragm; their excretory ducts terminate in the proximal portion of the **penile urethra.**

The **penis** consists of **erectile tissues,** the paired dorsal **corpora cavernosa** and a single ventral **corpus spongiosum** that expands distally into the **glans penis.** Because the penile urethra extends through the entire length of the corpus spongiosum, this portion of the penis is also called the **corpus cavernosum urethrae.** Each erectile body in the penis is surrounded by the connective tissue layer **tunica albuginea.**

The erectile tissues in the penis consist of irregular vascular spaces lined by vascular endothelium. The trabeculae between these spaces contain collagen and elastic fibers and smooth muscles. Blood enters the vascular spaces from the branches of the **dorsal artery** and **deep arteries of the penis** and is drained by peripheral veins.

FIGURE 18.10 ■ Prostate Gland and Prostatic Urethra

The prostate gland is an encapsulated organ situated inferior to the neck of the bladder. The urethra that leaves the bladder and passes through the prostate gland is called the **prostatic urethra (1)**. A **transitional epithelium (6)** lines the lumen of the crescent-shaped prostatic urethra (1). Most of the prostate gland consists of small, branched tubuloacinar **prostatic glands (5, 11)**. Some of the prostatic glands (5, 11) contain solid secretory aggregations called **prostatic concretions (11)** in their acini. The prostatic concretions (11) appear as small red dots in this illustration. A characteristic **fibromuscular stroma (10)** with **smooth muscle bundles (4),** mixed with collagen and elastic fibers, surrounds the prostatic glands (5, 11) and the prostatic urethra (1).

A longitudinal urethral crest of dense fibromuscular stroma without glands widens in the prostatic urethra (1) to form a smooth domelike structure called the **colliculus seminalis (7).** The colliculus seminalis (7) protrudes into and gives the prostatic urethra (1) a crescent shape. On each side of the colliculus seminalis (7) are the **prostatic sinuses (2).** Most excretory **ducts of prostatic glands (9)** open into the prostatic sinuses (2).

In the middle of the colliculus seminalis (7) is a cul-de-sac called the **utricle (8).** The utricle (8) often shows dilation at its distal end before it opens into the prostatic urethra (1). The thin mucous membrane of the utricle (8) is typically folded, and the epithelium is usually simple secretory or pseudostratified columnar type. Also, two **ejaculatory ducts (3)** open at the colliculus, one on each side of the utricle (8).

1 Prostatic urethra

2 Prostatic sinuses

3 Ejaculatory ducts

4 Smooth muscle bundles

5 Prostatic glands

6 Transitional epithelium

7 Colliculus seminalis

8 Utricle

9 Ducts of prostatic glands

10 Fibromuscular stroma

11 Prostatic glands with concretions

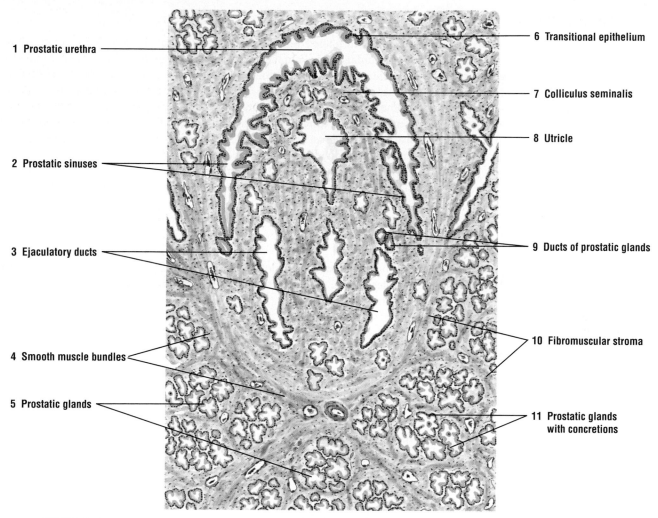

FIGURE 18.10 ■ Prostate gland and prostatic urethra. Stain: hematoxylin and eosin. Low magnification.

FIGURE 18.11 ■ Prostate Gland: Glandular Acini and Prostatic Concretions

A small section of the prostate gland from Figure 18.10 is illustrated at a higher magnification.

The size of the **glandular acini (1)** in the prostate gland is highly variable. The lumina of the acini are normally wide and typically irregular because of the protrusion of the epithelium-covered **connective tissue folds (10).** Some of the glandular acini (1) contain proteinaceous **prostatic secretions (9).** Other glandular acini (1) contain spherical **prostatic concretions (4, 6, 8)** that are formed by concentric layers of condensed prostatic secretions. The prostatic concretions (4, 6, 8) are characteristic features of the prostate gland acini. The number of prostatic concretions (4, 6, 8) increases with the age of the individual, and they may become calcified.

Although the **glandular epithelium (5)** is usually simple columnar or pseudostratified and the cells are light staining, there is considerable variation. In some regions, the epithelium may be squamous or cuboidal.

The **excretory ducts of the prostatic glands (2)** may often resemble the glandular acini (1). In the terminal portions of the ducts (2), the epithelium is usually columnar and stains darker before entering the urethra.

The **fibromuscular stroma (7)** is another characteristic feature of the prostate gland. **Smooth muscle bundles (3)** and the connective tissue fibers blend together in the stroma (7) and are distributed throughout the gland.

FIGURE 18.12 ■ Prostate Gland: Prostatic Glands With Prostatic Concretions

The parenchyma of the prostate gland consists of individual **prostatic glands (3)** that vary in size and shape. The glandular epithelium also varies from simple cuboidal or **columnar (2)** to pseudostratified epithelium. In older individuals, the secretory material of the prostatic glands (3) precipitates to form the characteristic dense-staining **prostatic concretions (1, 5).** The prostate gland is also characterized by the **fibromuscular stroma (4).** In this photomicrograph, the **smooth muscle fibers (4a)** in the fibromuscular stroma (4) are stained red and the **connective tissue fibers (4b)** stained blue.

1 Glandular acini

2 Excretory ducts of prostatic glands

3 Smooth muscle bundles

4 Prostatic concretion

5 Glandular epithelium

6 Prostatic concretion

7 Fibromuscular stroma

8 Prostatic concretion

9 Prostatic secretion

10 Connective tissue folds

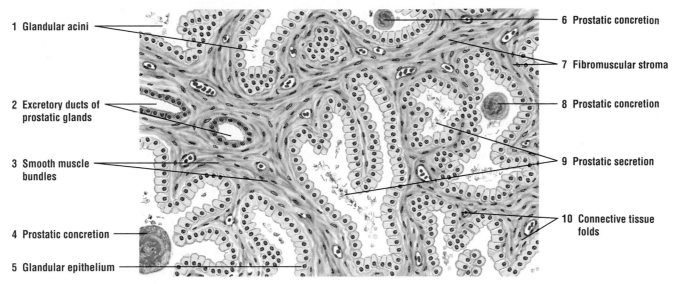

FIGURE 18.11 ■ Prostate gland: glandular acini and prostatic concretions. Stain: hematoxylin and eosin. Medium magnification.

1 Prostatic concretion

2 Columnar epithelium

3 Prostatic glands

4 Fibromuscular stroma:

  a. Smooth muscle fibers

  b. Connective tissue fibers

5 Prostatic concretion

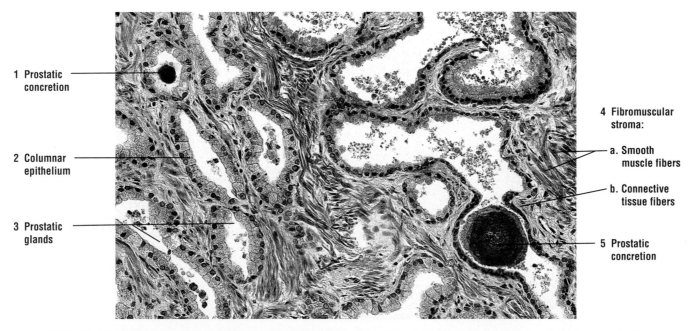

FIGURE 18.12 ■ Prostate gland: prostatic glands with prostatic concretions. Stain: Masson's trichrome. ×64.

FIGURE 18.13 ■ Seminal Vesicle

The paired seminal vesicles are elongated glands located on the posterior side of the bladder. The excretory duct from each seminal vesicle joins the ampulla of each ductus deferens to form the ejaculatory duct, which then runs through the prostate gland to open into the prostatic urethra.

The seminal vesicle exhibits highly convoluted and irregular lumina. A cross section through the gland illustrates the complexity of the **primary mucosal folds (1).** These folds branch into numerous **secondary mucosal folds (2),** which frequently anastomose and form irregular cavities, chambers, or **mucosal crypts (7).** The **lamina propria (6)** projects into and forms the core of the larger primary folds (1) and the smaller secondary folds (2). The folds extend far into the lumen of the seminal vesicle.

The glandular **epithelium (5)** of the seminal vesicles varies in appearance, but is usually low pseudostratified and low columnar or cuboidal.

The muscularis consists of an **inner circular muscle layer (3)** and an **outer longitudinal muscle layer (4).** This arrangement of the smooth muscles is often difficult to observe because of the complex folding of the mucosa. The **adventitia (8)** surrounds the muscularis and blends with the connective tissue.

FIGURE 18.14 ■ Bulbourethral Gland

The paired bulbourethral glands are compound tubuloacinar glands. The fibroelastic capsule that surrounds these glands contains **connective tissue (3),** smooth muscle fibers, and **skeletal muscle fibers (2, 7)** in the interlobular **connective tissue septum (5).** Because the bulbourethral glands are located in the urogenital diaphragm, the skeletal muscle fibers (2, 7) from the diaphragm are present in the glands. Connective tissue septa (5) from the capsule (3) divide the gland into several lobules.

The secretory units vary in structure and size and resemble mucous glands. The glands exhibit either **acinar secretory units (6)** or **tubular secretory units (1).** The secretory cells are cuboidal, low columnar or squamous, and light staining. The height of the epithelial cells depends on the functional state of the gland. The secretory product of the bulbourethral glands is primarily mucus.

Smaller **excretory ducts (4)** from the secretory units may be lined with secretory cells, whereas the larger excretory ducts exhibit pseudostratified or stratified columnar epithelium.

FUNCTIONAL CORRELATIONS: Accessory Male Reproductive Glands

The secretory products from the seminal vesicles, prostate gland, and bulbourethral glands mix with sperm and form **semen.** Semen provides the sperm with a liquid transport medium and nutrients. It also neutralizes the acidity of the male urethra and vaginal canal, and activates the sperm after ejaculation.

The **seminal vesicles** produce a yellowish, viscous fluid that contain high concentration of sperm-activating chemicals, such as **fructose,** the main carbohydrate component of semen. Fructose is metabolized by sperm and serves as the main **energy** source for sperm motility. Seminal vesicles produce most of the fluid found in semen.

The **prostate gland** produces a thin, watery, slightly acidic fluid, rich in citric acid, prostatic acid phosphatase, amylase, and prostate-specific antigen (PSA). The enzyme fibrinolysin in the fluid liquefies the congealed semen after ejaculation. PSA is very useful for diagnosis of prostatic cancer because its concentration often increases in the blood during malignancy.

The **bulbourethral glands** produce a clear, viscid, mucouslike secretion that, during erotic stimulation, is released and serves as a lubricant for the penile urethra. During ejaculation, secretions from the bulbourethral glands precede other components of the semen.

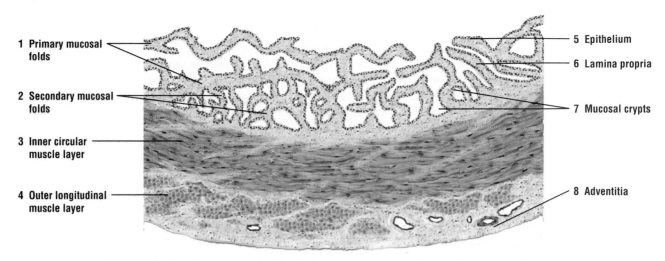

1 Primary mucosal folds

2 Secondary mucosal folds

3 Inner circular muscle layer

4 Outer longitudinal muscle layer

5 Epithelium

6 Lamina propria

7 Mucosal crypts

8 Adventitia

FIGURE 18.13 ■ Seminal vesicle. Stain: hematoxylin and eosin. Low magnification.

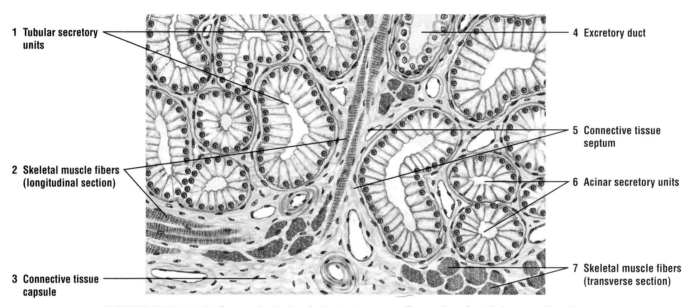

1 Tubular secretory units

2 Skeletal muscle fibers (longitudinal section)

3 Connective tissue capsule

4 Excretory duct

5 Connective tissue septum

6 Acinar secretory units

7 Skeletal muscle fibers (transverse section)

FIGURE 18.14 ■ Bulbourethral gland. Stain: hematoxylin and eosin. High magnification.

FIGURE 18.15 ■   Human Penis (Transverse Section)

A cross section of the human penis illustrates the two dorsal **corpora cavernosa (15)** (singular, corpus cavernosum) and a single ventral **corpus spongiosum (21)** that form the body of the organ. The **urethra (9)** passes through the entire length of the penis in the corpus spongiosum (21). A thick connective tissue capsule called the **tunica albuginea (4)** surrounds the corpora cavernosa (15) and forms a **median septum (17)** between the two bodies. A thinner **tunica albuginea (8)** with smooth muscle fibers and elastic fibers surrounds the corpus spongiosum (21).

All three cavernous bodies (15, 21) are surrounded by loose connective tissue called the **deep penile** (Buck's) **fascia (5, 16)**, which, in turn, is surrounded by the connective tissue of the **dermis (10)** located below the stratified squamous keratinized epithelium of the **epidermis (11)**. Strands of smooth muscle of the **dartos tunic (7)**, **nerves (2)**, **sebaceous glands (20)**, and peripheral blood vessels are located in the dermis (10).

Trabeculae (19) with collagenous, elastic, nerve, and smooth muscle fibers surround and form the core of the **cavernous sinuses** (veins) **(18, 22)** in the corpora cavernosa (15) and corpus spongiosum (21). The cavernous sinuses (18) of the corpora cavernosa (15) are lined with endothelium and receive the blood from the **dorsal arteries (1, 14)** and **deep arteries (3)** of the penis. The deep arteries (3) branch in the corpora cavernosa (15) and form the **helicine arteries (6)**, which empty directly into the cavernous sinuses (18). The cavernous sinuses (22) in the corpus spongiosum (21) receive their blood from the bulbourethral artery, a branch of the internal pudendal artery. Blood leaving the cavernous sinuses (18, 22) exits mainly through the **superficial vein (12)** and the **deep dorsal vein (13)**.

As the urethra (9) passes the base of the penis, it is lined with pseudostratified or stratified columnar epithelium. As the urethra exits the penis, the epithelium changes to stratified squamous. The urethra (9) also shows invaginations called urethral lacunae (of Morgagni) with mucous cells. Branched tubular urethral glands (of Littre) located below the epithelium open into these recesses. These glands are shown at higher magnification in Figure 18.16.

FIGURE 18.16 ■   Penile Urethra (Transverse Section)

The penile urethra extends the entire length of the penis and is surrounded by the **corpus spongiosum (9)**. This illustration shows a transverse section through the **lumen of the penile urethra (3)** and the surrounding corpus spongiosum (9). The lining of this portion of the urethra is a pseudostratified or stratified **columnar epithelium (2)**. A thin underlying **lamina propria (5)** merges with the surrounding connective tissue of the corpus spongiosum (9).

Numerous irregular outpockets or **urethral lacunae (4)** with mucous cells are found in the lumen of the penile urethra (3). The urethral lacunae (4) are connected with the branched mucous **urethral glands (of Littre) (6, 7)** located in the surrounding connective tissue of the corpus spongiosum (9) and found throughout the length of the penile urethra. The ducts from the urethral glands (6) open into the lumen of penile urethra (3).

The corpus spongiosum (9) consists of **cavernous sinuses (1, 10)** lined by endothelial cells and separated by connective tissue **trabeculae (8)** that contain smooth muscle fibers and collagen fibers. Numerous **blood vessels, arteriole and venule (11)**, supply the corpus spongiosum. The internal structure of the corpus spongiosum (9) is similar to that of the corpora cavernosa described in Figure 18.15.

1 Dorsal artery

2 Nerves

3 Deep arteries

4 Tunica albuginea

5 Deep penile fascia

6 Helicine arteries

7 Dartos tunic

8 Tunica albuginea

9 Urethra

10 Dermis

11 Epidermis

12 Superficial dorsal vein

13 Deep dorsal vein

14 Dorsal artery

15 Corpora cavernosa

16 Deep penile fascia

17 Median septum

18 Cavernous sinuses

19 Trabeculae

20 Sebaceous glands

21 Corpus spongiosum

22 Cavernous sinuses

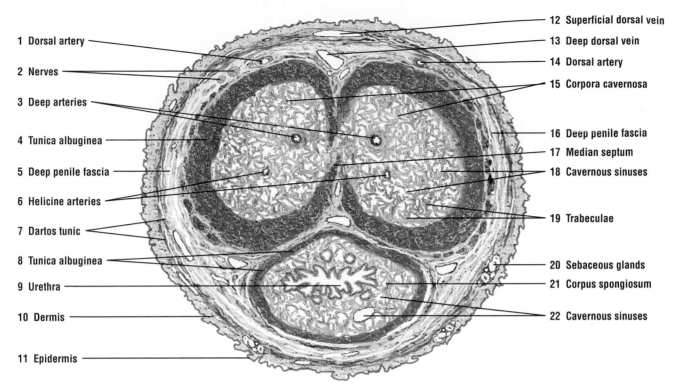

FIGURE 18.15 ■ Human penis (transverse section). Stain: hematoxylin and eosin. Low magnification.

1 Cavernous sinuses

2 Columnar epithelium

3 Lumen of penile urethra

4 Urethral lacunae

5 Lamina propria

6 Urethral glands (of Littre) and duct

7 Urethral gland (of Littre)

8 Trabeculae

9 Corpus spongiosum

10 Cavernous sinuses

11 Blood vessels (arteriole and venule)

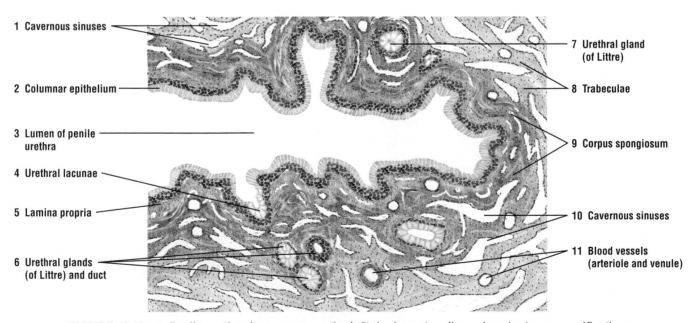

FIGURE 18.16 ■ Penile urethra (transverse section). Stain: hematoxylin and eosin. Low magnification.

CHAPTER 18 ■ Summary

Seminal Vesicles

- Located posterior to the bladder and superior to prostate gland
- Excretory ducts join with the ampulla of vas deferens to form ejaculatory ducts
- Ejaculatory ducts continue through prostate gland to open into prostatic urethra
- Produce fluid with sperm-activating fructose, the main energy source for sperm motility
- Produce most of the fluid found in semen

Prostate Gland

- Located inferior to the neck of the bladder
- Urethra exits bladder and passes through prostate as prostatic urethra
- Excretory ducts from prostatic glands enter the prostatic urethra
- Transitional epithelium lines the prostatic urethra
- Characterized by fibromuscular stroma and prostatic concretions in the glands
- Produces watery secretions with numerous chemicals, including prostate-specific antigen

Bulbourethral Glands

- Small glands located at root of penis and in skeletal muscle of urogenital diaphragm
- Excretory ducts enter the proximal part of penile urethra
- Produce mucouslike secretion that serves as lubricant for penile urethra

Penis

- Consists of erectile tissue or vascular spaces lined by endothelium
- Erectile corpora cavernosa is located on dorsal side and corpus spongiosum on ventral side
- Tunica albuginea surrounds the erectile bodies
- Dorsal artery and deep artery supply erectile bodies with blood

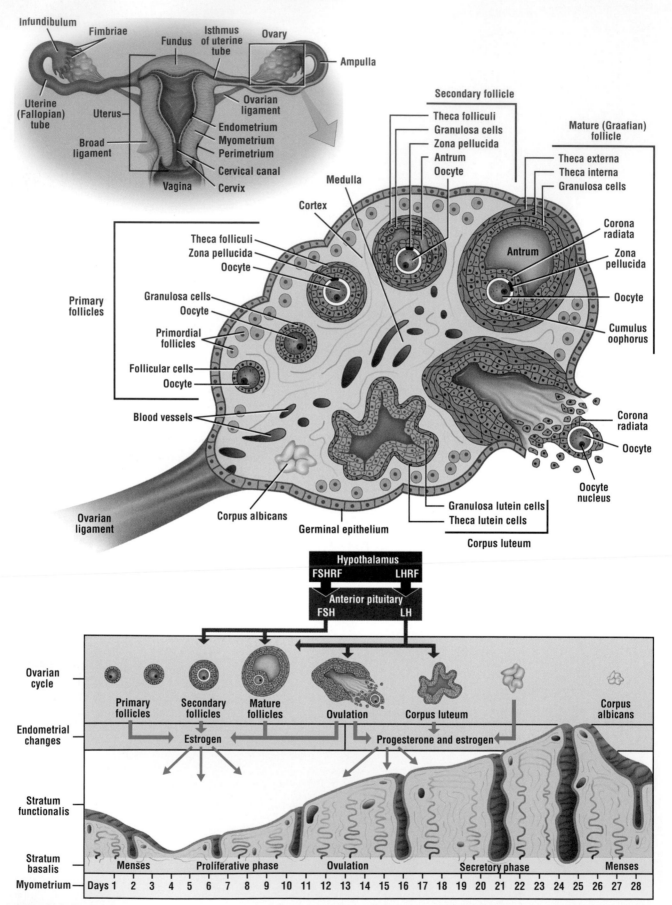

OVERVIEW FIGURE 19 ■ The anatomy of the female reproductive organs is presented in detail, with emphasis on the ovary and the sequence of changes during follicular development, culminating in ovulation and corpus luteum formation. In addition, the changes in the uterine wall during the menstrual cycle are correlated with pituitary hormones and ovarian functions.

438

Female Reproductive System

SECTION 1 ■ Overview of the Female Reproductive System

The human female reproductive system consists of paired internal **ovaries,** paired **uterine (fallopian) tubes,** and a single **uterus.** Inferior to the uterus and separated by the **cervix** is the **vagina.** Because **mammary glands** are associated with the female reproductive system, their histologic structure and function are discussed in th;is chapter.

During reproductive life, the human female reproductive organs exhibit cyclical monthly changes in both structure and function. These changes constitute the **menstrual cycle.** The appearance of the initial menstrual cycle in the maturing individual is **menarche.** When the cycles become irregular and eventually disappear, this phase is **menopause.**

The menstrual cycle is primarily controlled by two hormones secreted by the adenohypophysis of the pituitary gland, **follicle-stimulating hormone (FSH)** and **luteinizing hormone (LH),** and by two ovarian steroid hormones, **estrogen** and **progesterone.** The release of FSH and LH from the pituitary gland is controlled by releasing factors or hormones secreted by neurons in the hypothalamus, **FSH-releasing factor (hormone)** and **LH-releasing factor (hormone)** (see Overview Figure 19).

The individual organs of the female reproductive system perform numerous important functions, including secretion of female sex hormones (estrogen and progesterone) for development of female sexual characteristics, production of oocytes, providing suitable environment for fertilization of the oocytes in the uterine (fallopian) tube, transportation of the embryo to the uterus and its implantation, nutrition and development of the fetus during pregnancy, and nutrition of the newborn.

In humans, a mature ovarian follicle releases an immature egg called the oocyte into the uterine tube approximately every 28 days. The oocyte remains viable in the female reproductive tract for about 24 hours, after which the oocyte degenerates if it is not fertilized. The transformation or maturation of the immature oocyte into a mature egg or ovum occurs at the time of fertilization, when the sperm penetrates the oocyte.

Ovaries

Each ovary is a flattened, ovoid structure located deep in the pelvic cavity. One section of the ovary is attached to the **broad ligament** by a peritoneal fold called the **mesovarium** and another section to the uterine wall by an **ovarian ligament.** The ovarian surface is covered by a single layer of cells called the **germinal epithelium** that overlies the dense, irregular connective tissue **tunica albuginea.** Located below the tunica albuginea is the **cortex** of the ovary. Deep to the cortex is the highly vascularized, connective tissue core of the ovary, the **medulla.** There is no distinct boundary line between the cortex and medulla, and these two regions blend together.

During embryonic development, germ cells colonize the gonadal ridges, differentiate into **oogonia,** divide by mitosis, and then enter the first phase of **meiotic** division without completing it. They become arrested in this state of development and are now called the **primary oocytes.** **Primordial follicles** are also formed during fetal life and consist of a primary oocyte surrounded by a single layer of squamous follicular cells. Beginning at puberty and under the influence of pituitary hormones, the primordial follicles grow and enlarge to become **primary, secondary,** and the large **mature follicles,** which can span the cortex and extend deep into the medulla of the ovary. The cortex of an ovary is normally filled with numerous ovarian follicles in various stages of development.

In addition, the ovary may contain a large **corpus luteum** of an ovulated follicle and **corpus albicans** of a degenerated corpus luteum. Also, ovarian follicles in various stages of development (primordial, primary, secondary, and maturation) may undergo a process of degeneration called **atresia,** and the atretic degenerating cells are then phagocytosed by macrophages. Follicular atresia occurs before birth and continues throughout the reproductive period of the individual.

Uterine (Fallopian) Tubes

Each uterine tube is about 12 cm long and extends from the ovaries to the uterus. One end of the uterine tube penetrates and opens into the uterus; the other end opens into the peritoneal cavity near the ovary. The uterine tubes are normally divided into four continuous regions. The region closest to the ovary is the funnel-shaped **infundibulum.** Extending from the infundibulum are slender, fingerlike processes called **fimbriae** (singular, fimbria) located close to the ovary. Continuous with the infundibulum is the second region, the **ampulla,** the widest and longest portion. The **isthmus** is short and narrow, and joins each uterine tube to the uterus. The last portion of the uterine tube is the **interstitial (intramural) region.** It passes through the thick uterine wall to open into the uterine cavity.

Uterus

The human uterus is a pear-shaped organ with a thick muscular wall. The **body** or **corpus** forms the major portion of the uterus. The rounded upper portion of the uterus located above the entrance of uterine tubes is called the **fundus.** The lower, narrower, and terminal portion of the uterus located below the body or corpus is the **cervix.** The cervix protrudes and opens into the vagina.

The wall of the uterus is composed of three layers: an outer **perimetrium** lined by serosa or adventitia; a thick smooth muscle layer called the **myometrium;** and an inner **endometrium.** The endometrium is lined by simple epithelium that descends into a lamina propria to form numerous **uterine glands.**

The endometrium is normally subdivided into two functional layers, the luminal **stratum functionalis** and the basal **stratum basalis.** In a nonpregnant female, the superficial functionalis layer with the uterine glands and blood vessels is sloughed off or shed during **menstruation,** leaving intact the deeper basalis layer with the basal remnants of the uterine glands—the source of cells for regeneration of a new functionalis layer. The arterial supply to the endometrium plays an important role during the menstrual phase of the menstrual cycle.

Uterine arteries in the broad ligament give rise to the **arcuate arteries.** These arteries penetrate and assume a circumferential course in the myometrium of the uterus. Arcuate vessels give rise to **straight** and **spiral arteries** that supply the endometrium. The straight arteries are short and supply the basalis layer of the endometrium, whereas the spiral arteries are long and coiled and supply the surface or functionalis layer of endometrium. In contrast to the straight arteries, spiral arteries are highly sensitive to hormonal changes in the blood. Decreased blood levels of the ovarian hormones estrogen and progesterone during the menstrual cycle produces degeneration and shedding of stratum functionalis, resulting in menstruation.

FIGURE 19.1 ■ Ovary: Different Stages of Follicular Development (Panoramic View)

This low-power image illustrates a sagittal section of an ovary and all of the various forms of follicular development that would normally be seen in different functional periods of the ovary.

The ovary is covered by a single layer of low cuboidal or squamous cells called the **germinal epithelium (11)**, which is continuous with the **mesothelium (13)** of the visceral peritoneum. Beneath the germinal epithelium (11) is a dense, connective tissue layer called the **tunica albuginea (15)**.

The ovary has a peripheral **cortex (10)** and a central **medulla (8)**, in which are found numerous blood vessels, nerves, and lymphatics. In addition to the follicles, the cortex (10) contains fibrocytes with collagen and reticular fibers. The medulla (8) is a typical dense irregular connective tissue that is continuous with the **mesovarium (23)** ligament that suspends the ovary. Larger **blood vessels (8)** in the medulla (8) distribute smaller vessels to all parts of the ovarian cortex. The mesovarium (23) is covered by the germinal epithelium (11) and peritoneal mesothelium (13).

Numerous ovarian follicles, especially the smaller types, are seen in various stages of development in the stroma of the cortex (10). The most numerous follicles are the **primordial follicles (19)**, which are located in the periphery of the cortex (10) and inferior to the tunica albuginea (15). The primordial follicles (19) are the smallest and simplest in structure. They are surrounded by a single layer of squamous follicular cells. The primordial follicles (19) contain the immature and small primary oocyte, which gradually increases in size as the follicles develop into the primary, secondary, and mature follicles. Before ovulation of the mature follicle, all developing follicles contain a **primary oocyte (2, 12, 21)**.

Smaller follicles with cuboidal, columnar, or stratified cuboidal cells that surround the primary oocytes (12) are called **primary follicles (12)**. As the follicles increase in size, a fluid, called liquor folliculi (follicular liquid), begins to accumulate between the follicular cells, now called the **granulosa cells (5)**. The fluid areas eventually coalesce to form a fluid-filled cavity, called the **antrum (4, 20)**. Follicles with antral cavities are called **secondary (antral) follicles (21)**. These follicles (21) are larger and are situated deeper in the cortex (10). All larger follicles, including primary follicles (12), secondary follicles (21), and **mature follicles** exhibit a granulosa cell layer (5), a **theca interna (6)**, and an outer connective tissue layer, the **theca externa (7)**.

The largest ovarian follicle is the **mature follicle**. It exhibits the following structures: a large antrum (4) filled with liquor folliculi (follicular fluid); **cumulus oophorus (1)**, a mound on which the primary oocyte (2) is situated; a **corona radiata (3)**, a cell layer that is attached directly to the primary oocyte (2); **granulosa cells (5)** that surround the antrum (4); the inner layer theca interna (6), and the outer theca externa (7).

After ovulation, the large follicle collapses and transforms into a temporary endocrine organ, the **corpus luteum (16)**. The granulosa cells (5) of the follicle are transformed into light-staining **granulosa lutein cells (17)**, and the theca interna (6) cells become the darker-staining **theca lutein cells (18)** of the functioning corpus luteum (16). If fertilization and implantation do not occur, the corpus luteum (16) regresses, degenerates, and ultimately turns into a connective tissue scar called the **corpus albicans (9, 14)**. This illustration shows a recent larger corpus albicans (9), and an older smaller corpus albicans (14).

Most ovarian follicles do not attain maturity. Instead, they undergo degeneration (atresia) at all stages of follicular growth and become **atretic follicles (22)**, which eventually are replaced by the connective tissue.

FUNCTIONAL CORRELATIONS: Ovaries

Beginning at puberty and during the reproductive years of the individual, the ovaries exhibit structural and functional changes during each menstrual cycle, which lasts an average of 28 days. These changes involve growth of different follicles, maturation of follicles, completion of the first meiotic division, ovulation of a secondary oocyte from a mature, dominant follicle, and formation and degeneration of the corpus luteum. The pituitary hormones FSH and LH are primarily responsible for the development, maturation, and ovulation of ovarian follicles and production of hormones estrogen and progesterone.

The first half of the menstrual cycle lasts about 14 days and involves the growth of ovarian follicles. During follicular growth, the follicular cells possess FSH receptors. At this time, FSH is the principal circulating gonadotrophic hormone. FSH controls the growth and maturation of ovarian follicles, and initially stimulates the **theca interna cells** around the follicular peripheries to produce **androgenic steroid precursors.** The androgenic precursors diffuse into the follicles, where the **granulosa cells** of the follicles convert them into **estrogen.** As the follicles develop and mature, the circulating levels of estrogen in the blood rise. Increased levels of estrogen inhibit the release of FSH-releasing factor (hormone) from the hypothalamus and decrease the release of FSH from the pituitary gland. In addition, a hormone called **inhibin,** produced by granulosa cells in ovarian follicles, further inhibits the release of FSH from the pituitary gland.

At midcycle or shortly before ovulation, estrogen levels reach a peak. This peak causes a surge of LH hormone from the adenohypophysis of the pituitary gland. At this time, theca cells and granulosa cells in the follicles have LH receptors. There is also a concomitant smaller release of FSH hormone. Increased blood levels of both LH and FSH cause the following:

- Completion of the **first meiotic division** just before ovulation and liberation of a **secondary oocyte** into the uterine tube
- Final **maturation** of a mature ovarian follicle and **ovulation** (rupture) of a secondary oocyte at about the 14th day of the cycle
- Collapse of the ovulated follicle and the luteinization or modification of the granulosa lutein cells and theca lutein cells that surrounded the oocyte
- Transformation of the postovulatory mature follicle into the corpus luteum, a temporary endocrine organ

Final maturation or second meiotic division of the secondary oocyte occurs only when it is fertilized by a sperm. The liberated secondary oocyte remains viable in the female reproductive tract for about 24 hours before it begins to degenerate without completing the second meiotic division.

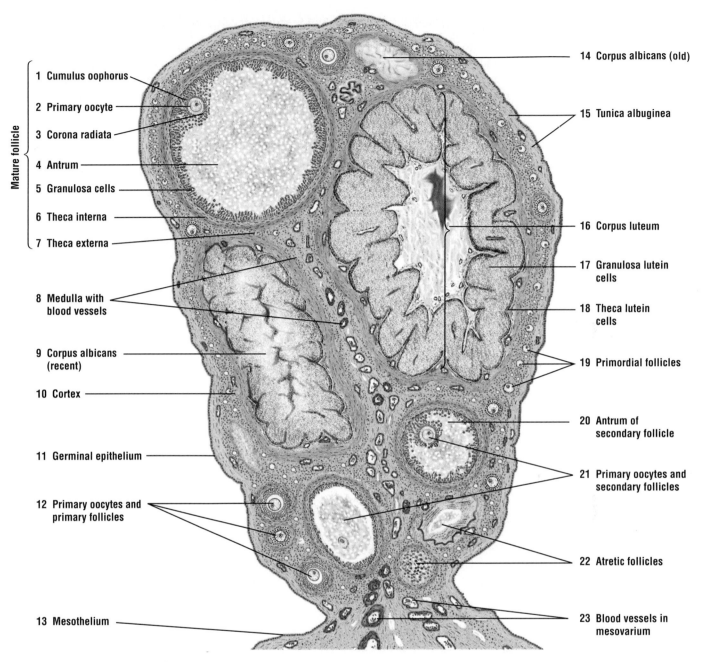

Mature follicle

1 Cumulus oophorus
2 Primary oocyte
3 Corona radiata
4 Antrum
5 Granulosa cells
6 Theca interna
7 Theca externa

8 Medulla with blood vessels

9 Corpus albicans (recent)

10 Cortex

11 Germinal epithelium

12 Primary oocytes and primary follicles

13 Mesothelium

14 Corpus albicans (old)

15 Tunica albuginea

16 Corpus luteum

17 Granulosa lutein cells

18 Theca lutein cells

19 Primordial follicles

20 Antrum of secondary follicle

21 Primary oocytes and secondary follicles

22 Atretic follicles

23 Blood vessels in mesovarium

FIGURE 19.1 ■ Ovary (panoramic view). Stain: hematoxylin and eosin. Low magnification.

FIGURE 19.2 ■ Ovary: Maturing Follicles and Initial Formation of Corpus Luteum

This photomicrograph shows a section of an ovary collected from a European mink. At the superior pole of the ovary is visible a large follicle shortly after ovulation and during the initial stages of corpus luteum formation. The follicular wall of the large mature follicle has collapsed on the **former antral cavity (1).** The folded granulosa cells that surround the antral cavity (1) are exhibiting a transformation into the **granulosa lutein cells (2).** Surrounding the granulosa lutein cells (2) on their periphery are the darker-staining **theca lutein cells (3),** which are the former theca interna cells of the mature follicle before ovulation.

Also visible in the ovarian section are other follicles in different stages of development. In the outer **cortex (11)** are seen **primary follicles (12, 14)** and larger **secondary follicles (8)** with enlarged **antral cavities (8).** In the middle of the ovary are three **mature follicles (4)** with large antral cavities. In one of these follicles (4) are visible the **primary oocyte (5),** the surrounding cells of the **corona radiata (13),** the **granulosa cells (6),** and the peripheral **theca interna cells (7).**

The ovary also exhibits an **atretic follicle (10)** in the cortex (11) and numerous **interstitial cells (9).** The interstitial cells (9) represent the remnants of theca interna cells that persist as individual cells or small groups of cells throughout the cortex following the follicular atresia.

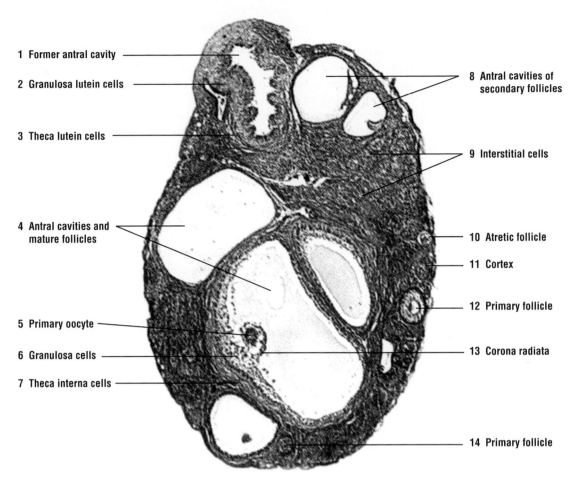

1 Former antral cavity

2 Granulosa lutein cells

3 Theca lutein cells

4 Antral cavities and
   mature follicles

5 Primary oocyte

6 Granulosa cells

7 Theca interna cells

8 Antral cavities of
   secondary follicles

9 Interstitial cells

10 Atretic follicle

11 Cortex

12 Primary follicle

13 Corona radiata

14 Primary follicle

FIGURE 19.2 ■ Ovary (European mink) (panoramic view). Mature follicles and the initial formation of the corpus luteum. Stain: hematoxylin and eosin. Low magnification. (The image is courtesy of Dr. Sergei Yakovlevich Amstislavsky, Institute of Cytology and Genetics, Russian Academy of Sciences, Siberian Division, Novosibirsk, Russia.)

FIGURE 19.3 ◼ Maturing Follicles and a Section of Corpus Luteum

This higher-power photomicrograph shows a peripheral fragment of an ovary section that was also collected from the European mink. The photomicrograph shows small and numerous developing **primordial follicles (6)** close to the periphery in the cortex of the ovary. Also visible among the developing primordial follicles (6) is a maturing follicle with a large liquid-filled **antrum (5)**. Pressed to one side of the follicle is a **primary oocyte surrounded by the corona radiata (4)**. Located on the periphery of the antrum (5) are **granulosa cells (3)** surrounded by the **theca interna cells (2)**.

Also visible in this section of the ovary are **granulosa lutein cells (7)** and peripheral **theca lutein cells (8)** of the formed corpus luteum. This ovary also exhibits a group of scattered **interstitial cells (1)**.

FIGURE 19.4 ◼ Ovary: Ovarian Cortex and Primary and Primordial Follicles

The ovarian surface is covered by a cuboidal **germinal epithelium (10)**. Located directly beneath the germinal epithelium (10) is a layer of dense connective tissue called the **tunica albuginea (16)**. Numerous **primordial follicles (14, 17)** are located in the cortex below the tunica albuginea (16). Each primordial follicle (14, 17) is surrounded by a single layer of squamous **follicular cells (17)**. As the follicles grow larger, the follicular cells (17) of the primordial follicles (14, 17) change to cuboidal or low columnar and the follicles are now called **primary follicles (4, 11)**. The developing oocytes (4, 13) also have a large eccentric **nucleus (7, 13)** with a conspicuous nucleolus.

In the growing or primary follicles (4, 11), the follicular cells proliferate by **mitosis (3)** and form layers of cuboidal cells called the **granulosa cells (8, 12)** that surround the primary oocytes (4, 13). A single layer of the granulosa cells that surround the oocyte forms the **corona radiata (5)**.

Between the corona radiata (5) and the oocyte appears the noncellular glycoprotein layer called the **zona pellucida (6)**. The stromal cells that surround the follicular cells now differentiate into the **theca interna (9)** layer that is located adjacent to the granulosa cells (8, 12). A thin basement membrane (not shown) separates the granulosa cells (8, 12) from the theca interna (9) cells.

Many primordial, developing, or mature follicles exhibit degeneration, die, and are lost through a process called atresia. A degenerating **atretic follicle (1)** is illustrated in the upper left corner of the illustration. Numerous blood vessels, such as a **capillary (2)**, surround the developing follicles and are found in the **connective tissue of the cortex (15)**.

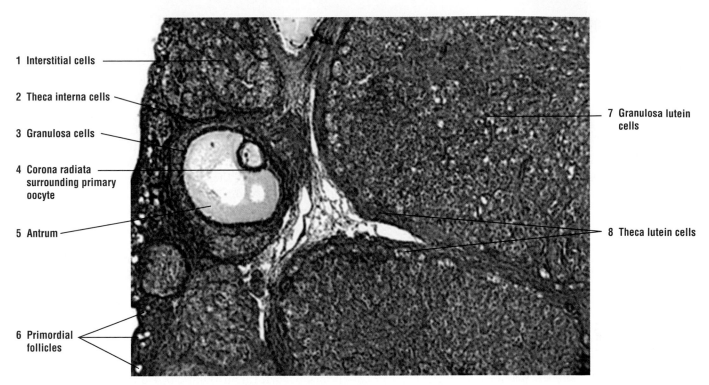

1 Interstitial cells

2 Theca interna cells

3 Granulosa cells

4 Corona radiata surrounding primary oocyte

5 Antrum

6 Primordial follicles

7 Granulosa lutein cells

8 Theca lutein cells

FIGURE 19.3 ■ Ovary (European mink) (panoramic view). Maturing follicles and corpus luteum. Stain: hematoxylin and eosin. Low magnification. (The image is courtesy of Dr. Sergei Yakovlevich Amstislavsky, Institute of Cytology and Genetics, Russian Academy of Sciences, Siberian Division, Novosibirsk, Russia.)

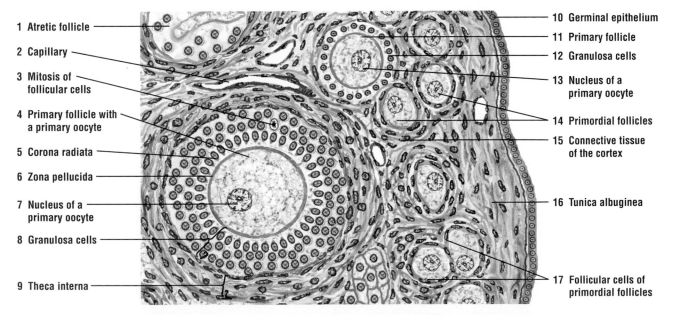

1 Atretic follicle

2 Capillary

3 Mitosis of follicular cells

4 Primary follicle with a primary oocyte

5 Corona radiata

6 Zona pellucida

7 Nucleus of a primary oocyte

8 Granulosa cells

9 Theca interna

10 Germinal epithelium

11 Primary follicle

12 Granulosa cells

13 Nucleus of a primary oocyte

14 Primordial follicles

15 Connective tissue of the cortex

16 Tunica albuginea

17 Follicular cells of primordial follicles

FIGURE 19.4 ■ Ovary: ovarian cortex and primordial and primary follicles. Stain: hematoxylin and eosin. Low magnification.

FIGURE 19.5 ■ Ovary: Primary Oocyte and Wall of a Mature Follicle

During growth of the follicles, fluid begins to accumulate between the granulosa cells that surround the oocyte, forming a fluid-filled cavity, the antrum. The follicle is called a secondary follicle when the antrum is present.

This figure illustrates the **cytoplasm** and **nucleus** of a **primary oocyte (3)** and the wall of a fluid-filled mature follicle. A local thickening of the **granulosa cells (5)** on one side of the follicle surrounds the primary oocyte (3) and projects into the **antrum (4, 7)** of the follicle. Here, the granulosa cells form a hillock or a mound called the **cumulus oophorus (8).** The single layer of granulosa cells (5) that are located immediately adjacent to the primary oocyte (3) forms the **corona radiata (1).** Between the corona radiata (1) and the cytoplasm of the primary oocyte (3) is a prominent, acidophilic-staining glycoprotein, the **zona pellucida (2).**

The granulosa cells (5) surround the antrum (4, 7) and secrete follicular fluid that fills the antrum cavity. Smaller isolated accumulations of the fluid also occur among the granulosa cells (5) as **intercellular follicular fluid (6, 9).**

The basal row of granulosa cells (5) rests on a thin **basement membrane (10)** that separates the granulosa cells (5) from the cells of the **theca interna (11),** an inner layer of vascularized, secretory cells of the follicle. Surrounding the cells of the theca interna (11) is the **theca externa (12)** layer that blends with the **connective tissue (13)** of the ovarian cortex.

FIGURE 19.6 ■ Ovary: Primordial and Primary Follicles

This photomicrograph shows different types of follicles in the cortex of an ovary. The immature **primordial follicles (2)** consist of a primary **oocyte (3)** surrounded by a layer of simple squamous **follicular cells (1, 7).** As the primordial follicles (2) grow to become **primary follicles (4),** the layer of simple squamous follicular cells around the oocyte changes to a cuboidal layer. In a larger **primary follicle (8),** the follicular cells have proliferated into a stratified layer around the oocyte called **granulosa cells (11).** A prominent layer of glycoprotein, the **zona pellucida (10),** develops between the granulosa cells (11) and the immature **oocyte (9).**

The cells around the developing follicles also organize into two distinct cell layers, the inner hormone-secreting **theca interna (12)** and the outer connective tissue layer **theca externa (13).** The theca interna (12) and theca externa (13) are separated from the granulosa cells (11) by a thin **basement membrane (6).** Surrounding the follicles in the cortex are cells and fibers of the **connective tissue (5).**

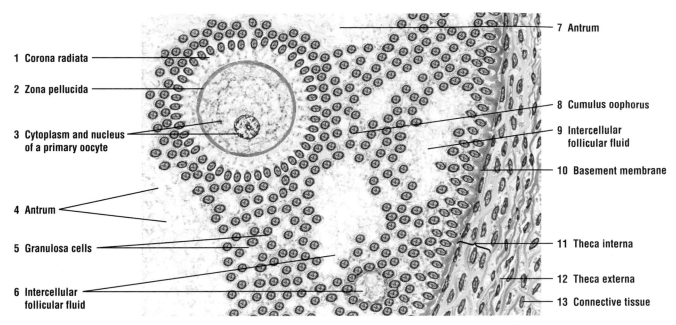

1 Corona radiata

2 Zona pellucida

3 Cytoplasm and nucleus of a primary oocyte

4 Antrum

5 Granulosa cells

6 Intercellular follicular fluid

7 Antrum

8 Cumulus oophorus

9 Intercellular follicular fluid

10 Basement membrane

11 Theca interna

12 Theca externa

13 Connective tissue

FIGURE 19.5 ■ Ovary: primary oocyte and wall of mature follicle. Stain: hematoxylin and eosin. High magnification.

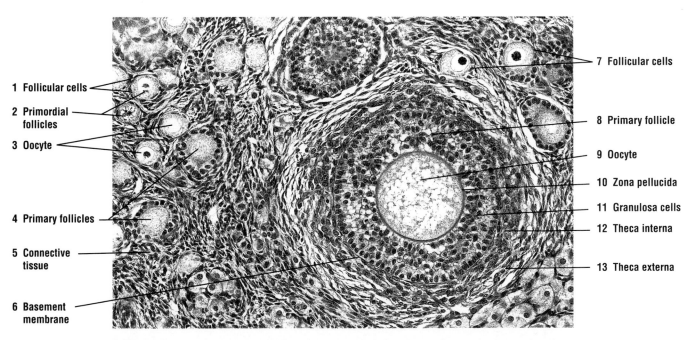

1 Follicular cells

2 Primordial follicles

3 Oocyte

4 Primary follicles

5 Connective tissue

6 Basement membrane

7 Follicular cells

8 Primary follicle

9 Oocyte

10 Zona pellucida

11 Granulosa cells

12 Theca interna

13 Theca externa

FIGURE 19.6 ■ Ovary: primordial and primary follicles. Stain: hematoxylin and eosin. ×64.

FIGURE 19.7 ■ Corpus Luteum (Panoramic View)

At a higher magnification, the corpus luteum is a collapsed and folded mass of glandular epithelium, primarily consisting of **theca lutein cells** (5) and **granulosa lutein cells** (6). Theca lutein cells (5) extend along the **connective tissue septa** (3) into the folds of the corpus luteum.

The **theca externa** (2) cells form a poorly defined capsule around the corpus luteum that also extends inward with the connective tissue septa (3) into folds.

The center of the corpus luteum or the **former follicular cavity** (9) contains remnants of follicular fluid, serum, blood cells, and loose **connective tissue with blood vessels** (7) from the theca externa that has proliferated and extended into the layers of the glandular epithelium. The connective tissue (7) also covers the inner surface of the granulosa lutein cells (6) and then spreads throughout the core of the corpus luteum. Some corpora lutea may contain a postovulatory **blood clot** (8) in the former follicular cavity (9).

The **connective tissue of the cortex** (1) that surrounds the corpus luteum contains numerous **blood vessels** (4).

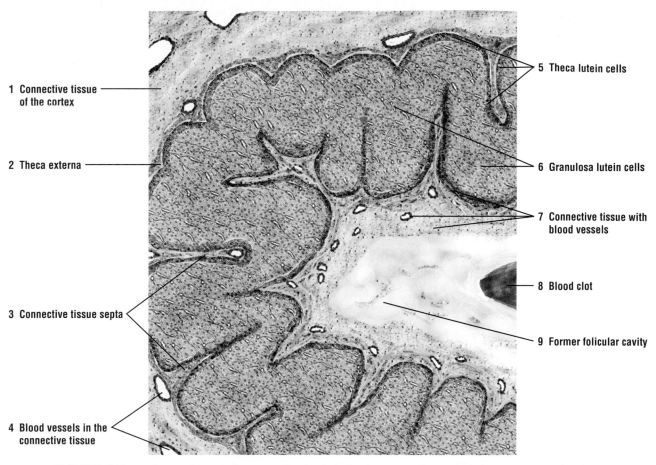

1 Connective tissue
   of the cortex

2 Theca externa

3 Connective tissue septa

4 Blood vessels in the
   connective tissue

5 Theca lutein cells

6 Granulosa lutein cells

7 Connective tissue with
   blood vessels

8 Blood clot

9 Former folicular cavity

FIGURE 19.7 ■ Corpus luteum (panoramic view). Stain: hematoxylin and eosin. Low magnification.

FIGURE 19.8 ■ Corpus Luteum: Theca Lutein Cells and Granulosa Lutein Cells

The **granulosa lutein cells (6)** represent the hypertrophied former granulosa cells of the mature follicle and constitute the highly folded mass of the corpus luteum. The granulosa lutein cells (6) are large, have large vesicular nuclei, and stain lightly owing to lipid inclusions. The **theca lutein cells (1, 7)** (the former theca interna cells) are located external to the granulosa lutein cells (6) on the periphery of the glandular epithelium. The theca lutein cells (1, 7) are smaller than the granulosa lutein cells (6), and their cytoplasm stains darker. Also, the nuclei of theca lutein cells (1, 7) are smaller and darker.

The **theca externa (2)** with numerous blood vessels, **venule and arteriole (4)** and **capillaries (5),** invades the granulosa lutein cells (6) and theca lutein cells (1, 7). A fine **connective tissue septum with fibrocytes (3)** penetrates the theca lutein cells (1, 7). The fibrocytes (3) in the septum between the theca lutein cells (1, 7) can be identified by their elongated and flattened appearance.

FUNCTIONAL CORRELATIONS: Corpus Luteum

After ovulation of a mature follicle and the liberation of a secondary oocyte into the infundibulum of the uterine tube, the wall of the ruptured follicle collapses and becomes highly folded. At this time, the ovary enters the **luteal phase.** During this phase, LH secretion induces hypertrophy and transformation of the granulosa cells and theca interna cells of the ovulated follicle into **granulosa lutein cells** and **theca lutein cells,** respectively. These changes transform the ovulated follicle into a temporary endocrine tissue, the corpus luteum. LH continues to stimulate and regulate the cells of the corpus lutein to secrete estrogen and large amounts of progesterone. High levels of estrogen and progesterone further stimulate the development of the **uterus** and mammary glands in anticipation of implantation of a fertilized egg and pregnancy.

Rising levels of estrogen and progesterone produced by the corpus luteum inhibit further release of FSH and LH, influencing both the neurons in the hypothalamus and gonadotrophs in the adenohypophysis. This effect prevents further ovulation.

If the ovulated secondary oocyte is not fertilized, the corpus luteum continues to secrete its hormones for about 12 days and begins to regress. After its regression, it is called the **corpus luteum of menstruation,** which eventually becomes a nonfunctional scar tissue called the **corpus albicans.** With the decreased functions of the corpus luteum, estrogen and progesterone levels decline, affecting the blood vessels in the endometrium of the uterus and resulting in the shedding of the stratum functionalis of the endometrium, followed by the menstrual flow.

As the corpus luteum ceases function, the inhibitory effects of estrogen and progesterone on the hypothalamus and pituitary gland cells are removed. As a result, FSH is again released from the adenohypophysis, initiating a new ovarian cycle of follicular development and maturation.

If fertilization of the oocyte and implantation of the embryo occurs, the corpus luteum increases in size and becomes the **corpus luteum of pregnancy.** The hormone **human chorionic gonadotropin (HCG)** secreted by the trophoblast cells of the implanting embryo continues to stimulate the corpus luteum and prevents its regression. The influence of HCG is similar to that produced by LH from the pituitary gland. As a result, the corpus luteum of pregnancy persists for several months. As the pregnancy progresses, the function of the corpus luteum is gradually taken over by the **placenta,** which begins to secrete sufficient amounts of estrogen and progesterone to maintain the pregnancy until parturition.

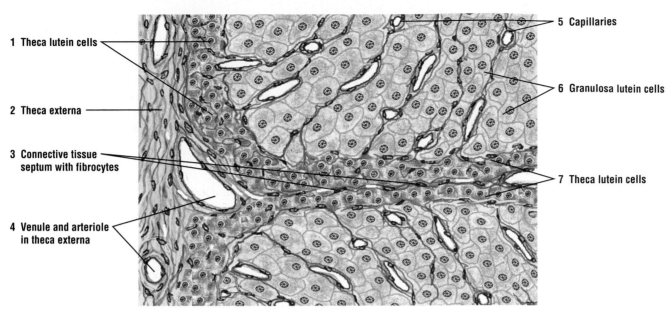

1 Theca lutein cells

2 Theca externa

3 Connective tissue septum with fibrocytes

4 Venule and arteriole in theca externa

5 Capillaries

6 Granulosa lutein cells

7 Theca lutein cells

FIGURE 19.8 ■ Corpus luteum: theca lutein cells and granulosa lutein cells Stain: hematoxylin and eosin. High magnification.

FIGURE 19.9 ■ Uterine Tube: Ampulla With the Mesosalpinx Ligament (Panoramic View, Transverse Section)

The paired, muscular uterine (fallopian) tubes extend from the proximity of the ovaries to the uterus. On one end, the infundibulum opens into the peritoneal cavity adjacent to the ovary. The other end penetrates the uterine wall to open into the interior of the uterus. The uterine tubes conduct the ovulated oocyte toward the uterus.

The ampulla is the longest part of the tube and is normally the site of fertilization. The mucosa of the ampulla exhibits the most extensive **mucosal folds (8).** These folds (8) form an irregular **lumen** in the **uterine tube (7)** that produces deep grooves between the folds (8). These folds become smaller as the uterine tube nears the uterus.

The mucosa of the uterine tube consists of simple columnar ciliated and nonciliated **epithelium (6)** that overlies the loose connective tissue **lamina propria (9).** The muscularis consists of two smooth muscle layers, an **inner circular layer (5)** and an **outer longitudinal layer (4).** The **interstitial connective tissue (10)** is abundant between the muscle layers, and, as a result, the smooth muscle layers (4, 5)—especially the outer layer (4)—are not distinct. Numerous **venules (3)** and **arterioles (2)** are visible in the interstitial connective tissue (10). The **serosa (11)** of the visceral peritoneum forms the outermost layer on the uterine tube, which is connected to the **mesosalpinx ligament (1)** of the superior margin of the broad ligament.

FIGURE 19.10 ■ Uterine Tube: Mucosal Folds

A higher magnification of the mucosal folds of the uterine tube shows that the lining epithelium consists of **ciliated cells (3)** and nonciliated **peg (secretory) cells (1).** The ciliated cells (3) are most numerous in the infundibulum and ampulla of the uterine tube. The beat of the cilia is directed toward the uterus. Under the epithelium is seen a prominent **basement membrane (2)** and the **lamina propria (4)** with numerous **blood vessels (5).** The lamina propria (4) is a cellular, loose connective tissue with fine collagen and reticular fibers.

During the early proliferative phase of the menstrual cycle and under the influence of estrogen, the ciliated cells (3) undergo hypertrophy, exhibit cilia growth, and become predominant. In addition, there is an increase in the secretory activity of the nonciliated peg cells (1). The epithelium of the uterine tube shows cyclic changes, and the proportion of ciliated and nonciliated cells varies with the stages of the menstrual cycle.

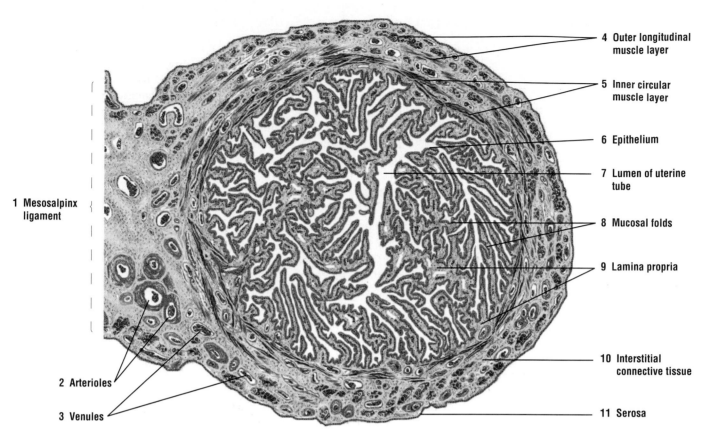

4 Outer longitudinal muscle layer

5 Inner circular muscle layer

6 Epithelium

7 Lumen of uterine tube

8 Mucosal folds

9 Lamina propria

10 Interstitial connective tissue

11 Serosa

1 Mesosalpinx ligament

2 Arterioles

3 Venules

FIGURE 19.9 ■ Uterine tube: ampulla with mesosalpinx ligament (panoramic view, transverse section). Stain: hematoxylin and eosin. Low magnification.

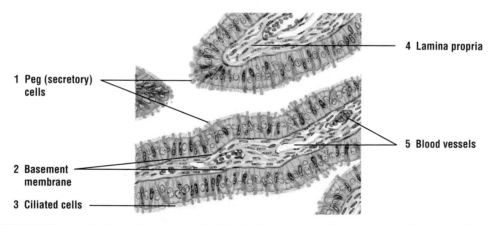

4 Lamina propria

1 Peg (secretory) cells

5 Blood vessels

2 Basement membrane

3 Ciliated cells

FIGURE 19.10 ■ Uterine tube: mucosal folds. Stain: hematoxylin and eosin. High magnification.

FIGURE 19.11 ■ Uterine Tube: Lining Epithelium

A higher-magnification photomicrograph illustrates a section of the uterine tube wall with complex mucosal folds that are lined by a **simple columnar epithelium (2).**

The luminal epithelium consists of two cell types, the **ciliated cells (5)** and the nonciliated **peg cells (6)** with apical bulges that extend above the cilia. A thin **basement membrane (1)** separates the luminal epithelium (2) from the underlying vascularized **connective tissue (4)** that forms the core of the mucosal folds. A portion of the **inner circular smooth muscle (3)** layer that surrounds the uterine tube is visible in the periphery on the left side of the illustration.

FUNCTIONAL CORRELATIONS: Uterine Tubes

The uterine tubes perform several important reproductive functions. Just before ovulation and rupture of the mature follicle, the fingerlike **fimbriae** of the infundibulum that are very close to the ovary sweep its surface to capture the released oocyte. This function is accomplished by gentle **peristaltic contractions** of smooth muscles in the uterine tube wall and fimbriae. In addition, the heavily ciliated cells on the fimbriae surface create a current toward the uterus that guides the oocyte into the infundibulum of the uterine tube. The cilia action and the muscular contractions in the wall of the uterine tube transport the captured oocyte or fertilized egg through the remaining regions of the uterine tube toward the uterus.

The uterine tubes also serve as the site of oocyte **fertilization,** which normally occurs in the upper region of the **ampulla.** The nonciliated or peg cells in the uterine tube are secretory and contribute important nutritive material for the oocyte, the initial development of the fertilized ovum, and the embryo. The uterine secretions also maintain the viability of sperm in the uterine tubes and allow them to undergo **capacitation,** a complex biochemical and structural process that activates the sperm and enables them to fertilize the released oocyte.

The epithelium in the uterine tubes exhibits changes that are associated with the ovarian cycle. The height of the uterine tube epithelium is at its maximum during the follicular phase, at which time the ovarian follicles are maturing and circulating levels of estrogen are high.

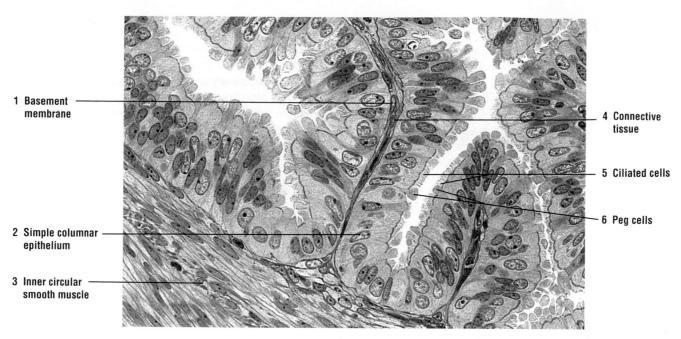

1 Basement
  membrane

4 Connective
  tissue

5 Ciliated cells

6 Peg cells

2 Simple columnar
  epithelium

3 Inner circular
  smooth muscle

FIGURE 19.11   ■   Uterine tube: lining epithelium. Stain: hematoxylin and eosin (plastic section). ×130.

FIGURE 19.12 ■ Uterus: Proliferative (Follicular) Phase

The surface of the **endometrium** is lined with a simple columnar **epithelium (1)** overlaying the thick **lamina propria (2).** The lining epithelium (1) extends down into the connective tissue of the lamina propria (2) and forms long, tubular **uterine glands (4).** In the proliferative phase, the uterine glands (4) are usually straight in the superficial portion of the endometrium, but may exhibit branching in the deeper regions near the myometrium. As a result, numerous uterine glands (4) are seen in cross section.

The wall of the uterus consists of three layers: the inner endometrium (1–4); a middle layer of smooth muscle **myometrium (5, 6);** and the outer serous membrane perimetrium (not illustrated). The endometrium is further subdivided into two zones or layers: a narrow, deep **basalis layer (8)** adjacent to the myometrium (5) and the **functionalis layer (7),** a wider, superficial layer above the basalis layer (8) that extends to the lumen of the uterus.

During the menstrual cycle, the endometrium exhibits morphologic changes that are directly correlated with ovarian function. The cyclic changes in a nonpregnant uterus are divided into three distinct phases: the proliferative (follicular) phase; the secretory (luteal) phase; and the menstrual phase.

In the proliferative phase of the cycle and under the influence of ovarian estrogen, the stratum functionalis (7) increases in thickness and the uterine glands (4) elongate and follow a straight course to the surface. Also, the **coiled (spiral) arteries (3)** (in cross section) are primarily seen in the deeper regions of the endometrium. The lamina propria (2) in the upper regions of the endometrium is cellular and resembles mesenchymal tissue. The connective tissue in the **basalis layer (8)** is more compact and appears darker in this illustration. The endometrium continues to develop during the proliferative phase as a result of the increasing levels of estrogen secreted by the developing ovarian follicles.

The endometrium is situated above the myometrium (5, 6), which consists of compact bundles of **smooth muscle (5, 6)** separated by thin strands of **interstitial connective tissue (9)** with numerous **blood vessels (10).** As a result, the muscle bundles are seen in cross, oblique, and longitudinal sections.

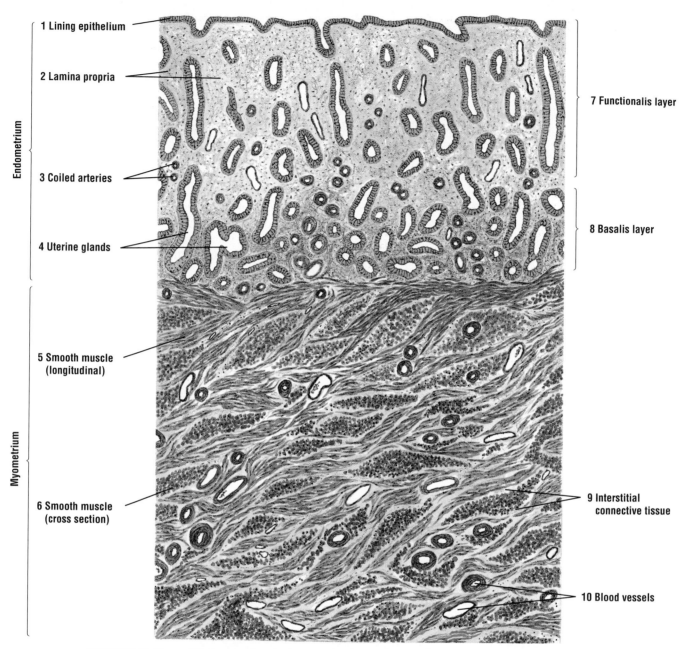

Endometrium

1 Lining epithelium

2 Lamina propria

3 Coiled arteries

4 Uterine glands

7 Functionalis layer

8 Basalis layer

Myometrium

5 Smooth muscle (longitudinal)

6 Smooth muscle (cross section)

9 Interstitial connective tissue

10 Blood vessels

FIGURE 19.12 ■ Uterine wall: proliferative (follicular) phase. Stain: hematoxylin and eosin. Low magnification.

FIGURE 19.13 ■ Uterus: Secretory (Luteal) Phase

The secretory (luteal) phase of the menstrual cycle is initiated after ovulation of the mature follicle. The additional changes in the endometrium are caused by the influence of both estrogen and progesterone that is secreted by the functioning corpus luteum. As a result, the **functionalis layer (1)** and **basalis layer (2)** of the endometrium become thicker owing to increased **glandular secretion (5)** and edema in the **lamina propria (6).**

The epithelium of the **uterine glands (5, 8)** undergoes hypertrophy (enlarges) as a result of increased accumulation of the secretory product (5, 8). The uterine glands (5, 8) also become highly coiled (tortuous), and their lumina become dilated with nutritive **secretory material (5)** rich in carbohydrates. The **coiled arteries (7)** continue to extend into the upper portion of the endometrium (functionalis layer) (1) and become prominent because of their thicker walls.

The alterations in the surface **columnar epithelium (4)**, uterine glands (5), and lamina propria (6) characterize the functionalis layer (1) of the endometrium during the secretory or luteal phase of the menstrual cycle. The basalis layer (2) exhibits minimal changes. Below the basalis layer is the **myometrium (3)** with **smooth muscle bundles (10),** sectioned in both longitudinal and transverse planes, and **blood vessels (9).**

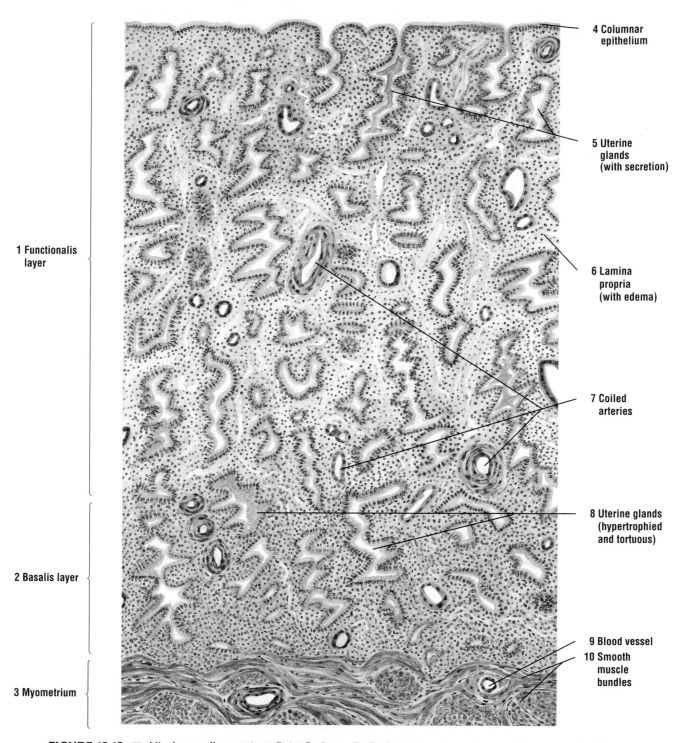

1 Functionalis
layer

2 Basalis layer

3 Myometrium

4 Columnar
epithelium

5 Uterine
glands
(with secretion)

6 Lamina
propria
(with edema)

7 Coiled
arteries

8 Uterine glands
(hypertrophied
and tortuous)

9 Blood vessel

10 Smooth
muscle
bundles

FIGURE 19.13 ■ Uterine wall: secretory (luteal) phase. Stain: hematoxylin and eosin. Low magnification.

FIGURE 19.14 ■ Uterine Wall (Endometrium): Secretory (Luteal) Phase

A low-power photomicrograph illustrates a section of the endometrium during the secretory (luteal) phase of the menstrual cycle. The thick and lighter area of the endometrium is the **stratum functionalis (1).** The darker and deeper endometrium is the **stratum basalis (2). The uterine glands (3)** during the secretory phase are coiled (tortuous) and secrete glycogen-rich nutrients into their lumina.

Surrounding the uterine glands (3) is the highly cellular **connective tissue (4).** The light, empty spaces in the connective tissue (4) layer are caused by increased edema in the endometrium. Below the stratum basalis (2) is the smooth muscle layer **myometrium (5)** of the uterine wall.

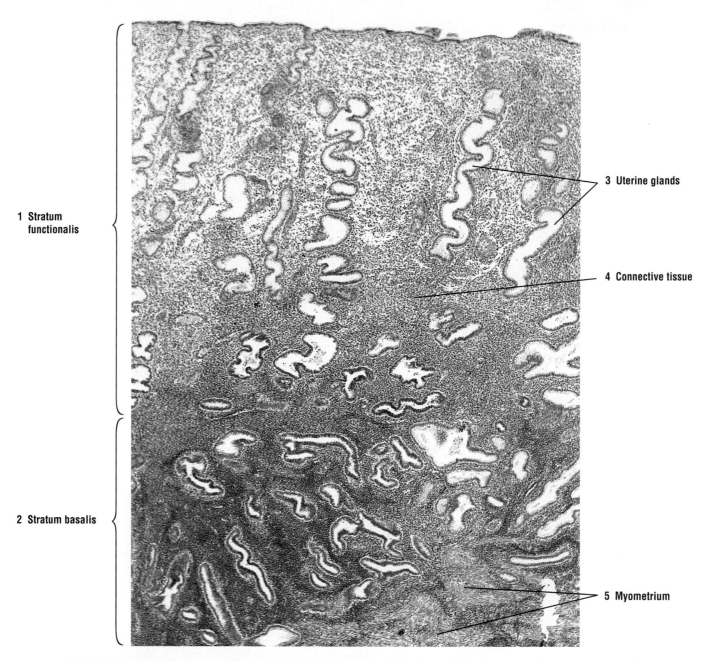

1 Stratum
  functionalis

2 Stratum basalis

3 Uterine glands

4 Connective tissue

5 Myometrium

FIGURE 19.14 ■ Uterine wall (endometrium): secretory (luteal) phase. Stain: hematoxylin and eosin. ×10.

FIGURE 19.15 ■ Uterus: Menstrual Phase

If fertilization of the ovum and implantation of the embryo do not occur, the uterus enters the menstrual phase, and much of the preparatory changes made for implantation in the endometrium are lost. During the menstrual phase, the **endometrium** in the **functionalis layer (1)** degenerates and is sloughed off. The shed endometrium contains fragments of disintegrated stroma, **blood clots (7)**, and uterine glands. Some of the intact **uterine glands (2)** are filled with **blood (6).** In the deeper layers of the endometrium, the **basalis layer (4),** the **bases of the uterine glands (9)** remain intact during the shedding of the functionalis layer and the menstrual flow.

The endometrial stroma of most of the functionalis layer contains aggregations of erythrocytes (7) that have been extruded from the torn and disintegrating blood vessels. In addition, the endometrial stroma exhibits infiltration of lymphocytes and neutrophils.

The basalis layer (4) of the endometrium remains unaffected during this phase. The distal (superficial) portions of the **coiled arteries (3, 8)** become necrotic, whereas the deeper parts of these vessels remain intact.

FUNCTIONAL CORRELATIONS: Uterus

During pregnancy, the uterus provides the site for **implantation** of the embryo, formation of the placenta, and a suitable environment for the development of the embryo and fetus. The endometrium also exhibits cyclical changes in its structure and function in response to the ovarian hormones **estrogen** and **progesterone.** The uterine changes are associated with impending implantation and nourishment of the developing organism. If fertilization of the oocyte and implantation of the embryo do not occur, blood vessels in the endometrium deteriorate and rupture, and the **functionalis layer** of endometrium is shed as part of the menstrual flow or discharge. With each menstrual cycle during the reproductive period of the individual, the endometrium passes through three phases, with each phase gradually passing into the next.

The **proliferative (preovulatory, follicular phase)** is characterized by rapid growth and development of the endometrium. The resurfacing and growth of the endometrium during the proliferative phase closely coincides with the rapid growth of **ovarian follicles** and their increased production of **estrogen.** This phase starts at the end of the menstrual phase, or about day 5, and continues to about day 14 of the cycle. Increased mitotic activity of the **lamina propria** and in remnants of the **uterine glands** in the **basalis layer** of the endometrium produces new cells that begin to cover the raw surface of the uterine mucosa that was denuded or shed during menstruation. The resurfacing of the mucosa produces a new functionalis layer of the endometrium. As the functionalis layer thickens, the uterine glands proliferate, lengthen, and become closely packed. The **spiral arteries** begin to grow toward the endometrial surface and begin to show light coiling.

The **secretory (postovulatory, luteal phase)** begins shortly after ovulation on about day 15 and continues to about day 28 of the cycle. This phase is dependent on the functional corpus luteum that was formed after ovulation and the secretion of **progesterone** and **estrogen** by the lutein cells (granulosa lutein and theca lutein cells). During the postovulatory phase, the endometrium thickens and accumulates fluid, becoming **edematous.** In addition, the uterine glands undergo hypertrophy and become tortuous, and their lumina become filled with secretions rich in **nutrients,** especially **glycoproteins** and **glycogen.** The spiral arteries in the endometrium also lengthen, become more coiled, and extend almost to the surface of the endometrium.

The **menstrual (menses) phase** of the cycle begins when the ovulated oocyte is not fertilized and no implantation occurs in the uterus. Reduced levels of circulating progesterone (and estrogen), as a result of the regressing corpus luteum, initiate this phase. Decreased levels of these hormones induce intermittent constrictions of the spiral arteries and interruption of blood flow to the functionalis layer of the endometrium, while the blood flow to the basalis layer remains uninterrupted. These constrictions deprive the functionalis layer of oxygenated blood and produce transitory **ischemia,** causing necrosis (death) of cells in the walls of blood vessels and degeneration of the functionalis layer in the endometrium. After extended periods of vascular constriction, the spiral arteries dilate, resulting in the rupture of their necrotic walls and hemorrhage (bleeding) into the stroma. The necrotic functionalis layer then detaches from the rest of the endometrium. Blood, uterine fluid, stromal cells, secretory material, and epithelial cells from the functionalis layer mix to form the **menstrual flow.**

The shedding of the functionalis layer of the endometrium continues until only the raw surface of the basalis layer is left. The remnants of uterine glands in the basalis layer serve as the source of cells for regenerating the next functionalis layer. Rapid proliferation of cells in the glands of the basalis layer, under the influence of rising estrogen levels during the proliferative phase, resurface and restore the lost endometrial layer and start the next phase of the menstrual cycle.

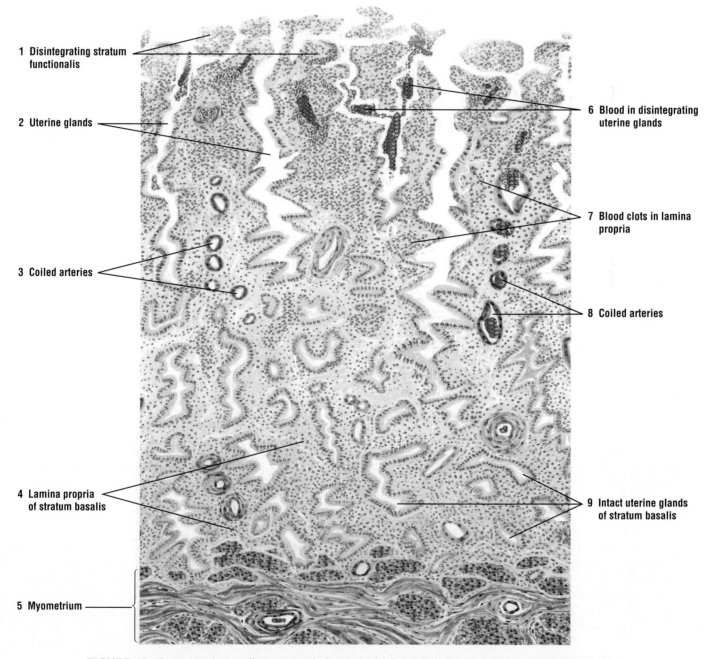

1 **Disintegrating stratum functionalis**

2 **Uterine glands**

3 **Coiled arteries**

4 **Lamina propria of stratum basalis**

5 **Myometrium**

6 **Blood in disintegrating uterine glands**

7 **Blood clots in lamina propria**

8 **Coiled arteries**

9 **Intact uterine glands of stratum basalis**

FIGURE 19.15 ■ Uterine wall: menstrual phase. Stain: hematoxylin and eosin. Low magnification.

CHAPTER 19 ■ Summary

SECTION 1 ■ Overview of the Female Reproductive System

Overview of Female Reproductive System

- Consists of paired ovaries, uterine tubes, and a single uterus
- Uterus separated from vagina by cervix
- Organs exhibit cyclical monthly changes in the form of menstrual cycle
- Start of first cycle is the menarche and ending of cycles is the menopause
- Cycles controlled by hormones FSH and LH, and ovarian estrogen and progesterone
- Immature oocyte released about every 28 days into uterine tube

Ovaries

- Germinal epithelium overlies connective tissue tunica albuginea
- Consist of an outer cortex and inner medulla, without distinct boundaries
- During embryonic development, oogonia divide by mitosis in gonadal ridges
- Oogonia enter first meiotic division and remain as primary oocytes in primordial follicles
- At puberty primordial follicles grow to become primary, secondary, and mature follicles
- Ovarian follicles can become atretic at any stage of development

Follicular Developments in Ovary

- Primordial follicles with primary oocyte are surrounded by squamous follicular cells
- Primary follicles exhibit simple cuboidal or stratified granulosa cell layers
- Secondary follicles exhibit liquid accumulations between granulosa cells or antrum
- Largest follicles are mature, span the cortex, and extend into medulla
- In maturing follicles, oocytes located on the mound cumulus oophorus
- Theca interna and theca externa visible in larger, developing follicles
- Primary oocytes are surrounded by zona pellucida and corona radiata cells in follicles
- FSH and LH responsible for development, maturation, and ovulation of follicles
- During first half of menstrual cycle and during follicular growth, FSH principal hormone
- FSH controls growth of follicles and stimulates estrogen production from follicles
- At midcycle estrogen levels peak and cause release of LH

- FSH and LH cause final maturation and ovulation of dominant, mature follicle
- At ovulation, first meiotic division is completed and secondary oocyte released
- Ovulation site on mature follicle is the thinned cell area called stigma
- Ovulated follicle collapses and becomes temporary corpus luteum
- Completion of second meiotic division occurs only when oocyte is fertilized by sperm
- Oocyte is viable for about 24 hours before it degenerates if not fertilized
- Interstitial cells in ovary are remnants of theca interna cells after follicular atresia

Corpus Luteum

- Forms after ovulation and liberation of secondary oocyte
- LH induces hypertrophy and luteinization of granulosa and theca interna cells
- LH causes liberation of estrogen and increased amounts of progesterone
- Without fertilization, is active for about 12 days before regression
- Regression eventually leads to connective scar tissue corpus albicans
- After regression, inhibitory effects of estrogen and progesterone are removed
- FSH and LH are again released to start new ovarian cycle
- If fertilization occurs, corpus luteum of pregnancy forms
- Human chorionic gonadotropin produced by trophoblasts stimulates corpus luteum
- Persists during pregnancy until placenta produces estrogen and progesterone

Uterine Tubes

- Extend from ovaries into the uterus and exhibit four continuous regions
- Infundibulum with fimbriae of the uterine tube located adjacent to the ovary
- Mucosa consists of extensive folds and forms irregular lumen
- Epithelium simple columnar with ciliated and nonciliated secretory (peg) cells
- Ciliated cells create a current toward uterus and become predominant in proliferative phase
- Secretory cells provide nutrition for oocyte, fertilized ovum, and developing embryo
- Uterine tube secretions maintain sperm and enhance capacitation of sperm
- Smooth muscles provide peristaltic contractions to help capture ovulated oocyte
- Epithelium exhibits changes associated with ovarian cycle

Uterus

- Consists of body, fundus, and cervix
- Wall consists of outer perimetrium, middle myometrium, and inner endometrium
- Endometrium divided into stratum functionalis and stratum basalis
- During monthly menstrual cycles, stratum functionalis is shed with menstrual flow
- Endometrium morphology responds to estrogen and progesterone and ovarian functions
- Proliferative phase starts at the end of menstrual phase after estrogen release
- Ovarian estrogen induces endometrial growth and formation of new stratum functionalis
- Secretory phase starts after ovulation and corpus luteum formation

- Estrogen and increased progesterone levels induce uterine gland secretion of nutrients
- Spiral arteries extend and reach surface of endometrium
- Menstrual phase starts when ovulated oocyte is not fertilized and no implantation occurs
- Spiral arteries highly sensitive to declining hormone levels and constrict intermittently
- Ischemia destroys walls of blood vessels and stratum functionalis
- Dilation of spiral arteries ruptures walls, detaches functionalis, and causes menstruation
- Stratum basalis remains intact and is not shed during menstruation
- Stratum basalis serves as the source of cells for regenerating new stratum functionalis

SECTION 2 ■ Cervix, Vagina, Placenta, and Mammary Glands

Cervix and Vagina

The cervix is located in the lower part of the uterus that projects into the vaginal canal as the **portio vaginalis.** A narrow **cervical canal** passes through the cervix. The opening of the cervical canal that directly communicates with the uterus is the **internal os** and, with the vagina, the **external os.** Unlike the functionalis layer of the uterine endometrium, the cervical mucosa undergoes only minimal changes during the menstrual cycle and is not shed during menstruation. The cervix contains numerous branched **cervical glands** that exhibit altered secretory activities during the different phases of the menstrual cycle. The amount and type of mucus secreted by the cervical glands change during the menstrual cycle as a result of different levels of ovarian hormones.

The **vagina** is a fibromuscular structure that extends from the cervix to the vestibule of the external genitalia. Its wall has numerous folds and consists of an inner **mucosa,** a middle **muscular layer,** and an outer connective tissue **adventitia.** The vagina does not have any glands in its wall and its lumen is lined by **stratified squamous epithelium.** Mucus produced by cells in the **cervical glands** lubricates the vaginal lumen. Loose fibroelastic connective tissue and a rich vasculature constitute the lamina propria that overlies the smooth muscle layers of the organ. Like the cervical epithelium, the vaginal lining is not shed during the menstrual flow.

Placenta

The **placenta** is a temporary organ that is formed when the developing embryo, now called a **blastocyst,** attaches to and implants in the endometrium of the uterus. The placenta consists of a **fetal portion,** formed by the **chorionic plate** and its **branching chorionic villi,** and a **maternal portion,** formed by the **decidua basalis** of the endometrium. Fetal and maternal blood come into close proximity in the villi of the placenta. Exchange of nutrients, electrolytes, hormones, antibodies, gaseous products, and waste metabolites takes place as the blood passes over the villi. Fetal blood enters the placenta through a pair of **umbilical arteries,** passes into the villi, and returns through a single **umbilical vein.**

Mammary Glands

The adult mammary gland is a compound **tubuloalveolar gland** that consists of about 20 lobes. All lobes are connected to **lactiferous ducts** that open at the **nipple.** The lobes are separated by connective tissue partitions and adipose tissue.

The resting or inactive mammary glands are small, consist primarily of **ducts,** and do not exhibit any developed or secretory alveoli. Inactive mammary glands also exhibit slight cyclic alterations during the course of the menstrual cycle. Under estrogenic stimulation, the secretory cells increase in height, lumina appear in the ducts, and a small amount of secretory material is accumulated.

FIGURE 19.16 ■ Cervix, Cervical Canal, and Vaginal Fornix (Longitudinal Section)

The cervix is the lower part of the uterus. This figure illustrates a longitudinal section through the cervix, the endocervix or **cervical canal (5)**, a portion of the **vaginal fornix (8)**, and the **vaginal wall (10)**.

The cervical canal (5) is lined with tall, mucus-secreting columnar **epithelium (2)** that is different from the uterine epithelium, with which it is continuous. The cervical epithelium also lines the highly branched and tubular **cervical glands (3)** that extend at an oblique angle to the cervical canal (5) into the **lamina propria (12)**. Some of the cervical glands may become occluded and develop into small **glandular cysts (4)**. The connective tissue in the lamina propria (12) of the cervix is more fibrous than in the uterus. Blood vessels, nerves, and occasional **lymphatic nodules (11)** may be seen.

The lower end of the cervix, the **os cervix (6)**, bulges into the lumen of the **vaginal canal (13)**. The columnar epithelium (2) of the cervical canal (5) abruptly changes to nonkeratinized stratified squamous epithelium to line the vaginal portion of the cervix called the **portio vaginalis (7)** and the external surface of the vaginal fornix (8). At the base of the fornix, the epithelium (7) of the vaginal cervix reflects back to become the **vaginal epithelium (9)** of the vaginal wall (10).

The smooth muscles of the **muscularis (1)** extend into the cervix but are not as compact as the muscles in the body of the uterus.

FUNCTIONAL CORRELATIONS: Cervix

The cervical mucosa does not undergo extensive changes during the menstrual cycle. However, the cervical glands exhibit functional changes that are related to sperm transport through the cervical canal. During the **proliferative phase** of the menstrual cycle, the secretion from the cervical glands is thin and watery. This type of secretion allows for easier passage of sperm through the cervix and into the uterus. During the **secretory (luteal) phase** of the menstrual cycle and increased progesterone secretions, as well as during pregnancy, the cervical gland secretions change and become highly viscous, forming a **mucus plug** in the cervical canal. The mucus plug is a protective measure that hinders the passage of sperm and microorganisms from the vagina into the body of the uterus. Thus, the cervical glands perform an important function in assisting fertilization of the oocyte and protection of the developing individual.

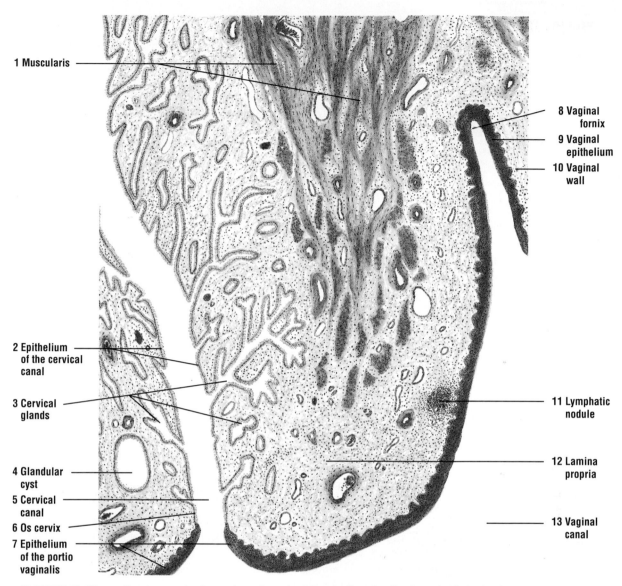

1 Muscularis

8 Vaginal fornix

9 Vaginal epithelium

10 Vaginal wall

2 Epithelium of the cervical canal

3 Cervical glands

11 Lymphatic nodule

4 Glandular cyst

5 Cervical canal

6 Os cervix

7 Epithelium of the portio vaginalis

12 Lamina propria

13 Vaginal canal

FIGURE 19.16 ■ Cervix, cervical canal, and vaginal fornix (longitudinal section). Stain: hematoxylin and eosin. Low magnification.

FIGURE 19.17 ■ Vagina (Longitudinal Section)

The vaginal mucosa is irregular and shows **mucosal folds (1)**. The surface epithelium of the vaginal canal is noncornified **stratified squamous (2)**. The underlying connective tissue **papillae (3)** are prominent and indent the epithelium.

The **lamina propria (7)** contains dense, irregular connective tissue with elastic fibers that extend into the muscularis layer as **interstitial fibers (10)**. Diffuse **lymphatic tissue (8)**, **lymphatic nodules (4)**, and small **blood vessels (9)** are in the lamina propria (7).

The muscularis of the vaginal wall consists predominantly of **longitudinal bundles (5a)** and oblique bundles of **smooth muscle (5)**. The **transverse bundles (5b)** of the smooth muscle are less numerous but more frequently found in the inner layers. The interstitial connective tissue (10) is rich in elastic fibers. **Blood vessels (11)** and nerve bundles are abundant in the **adventitia (6, 12)**.

FIGURE 19.18 ■ Glycogen in Human Vaginal Epithelium

Glycogen is a prominent component of the vaginal epithelium, except in the deepest layers, where it is minimal or absent. During the follicular phase of the menstrual cycle, glycogen accumulates in the vaginal epithelium, reaching its maximum level before ovulation. Glycogen can be demonstrated by iodine vapor or iodine solution in mineral oil (Mancini method); glycogen stains a reddish purple.

The vaginal specimens in illustrations (a) and (b) were fixed in absolute alcohol and formaldehyde. The amount of glycogen in the vaginal epithelium is illustrated during the **interfollicular phase (a)**. During the **follicular phase (b)**, glycogen content increases in the intermediate and superficial cell layers.

The tissue sample in illustration (c) is from the same specimen as in (b), but was fixed by the Altmann-Gersh method (freezing and drying in a vacuum). This method produces less tissue shrinkage and illustrates more glycogen and its diffuse distribution in the vaginal epithelium during the **follicular phase (c)**.

FUNCTIONAL CORRELATIONS: Vagina

The wall of the vagina consists of mucosa, a smooth muscle layer, and an adventitia. There are no glands in the vaginal mucosa. The surface of the vaginal canal is kept moist and lubricated by secretions produced by cervical glands.

The vaginal epithelium exhibits minimal changes during each menstrual cycle. During the proliferative (follicular) phase of the menstrual cycle and owing to increased estrogen stimulation, the vaginal epithelium increases in thickness. In addition, estrogen stimulates the vaginal cells to synthesize and accumulate increased amounts of **glycogen** as these cells migrate toward the vaginal lumen, into which they are shed or desquamated. Bacterial flora in the vagina metabolizes glycogen into **lactic acid.** Increased acidity in the vaginal canal protects the organ against microorganisms or pathogenic invasion.

Microscopic examination of cells collected (scraped) from the vaginal and cervical mucosae, called a **Pap smear,** provides highly valuable diagnostic information of clinical importance. Cervicovaginal Pap smears are routinely examined for early detection of pathologic changes in the epithelium of these organs that may lead to cervical cancer.

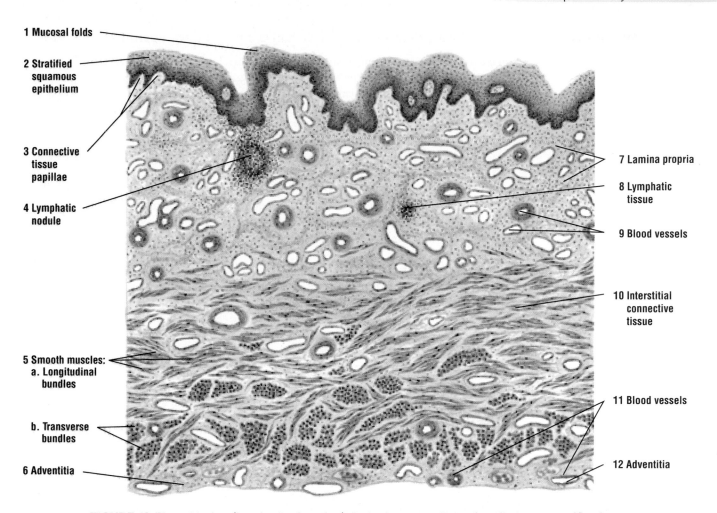

1 Mucosal folds

2 Stratified squamous epithelium

3 Connective tissue papillae

4 Lymphatic nodule

5 Smooth muscles:
   a. Longitudinal bundles

   b. Transverse bundles

6 Adventitia

7 Lamina propria

8 Lymphatic tissue

9 Blood vessels

10 Interstitial connective tissue

11 Blood vessels

12 Adventitia

FIGURE 19.17 ■ Vagina (longitudinal section). Stain: hematoxylin and eosin. Low magnification.

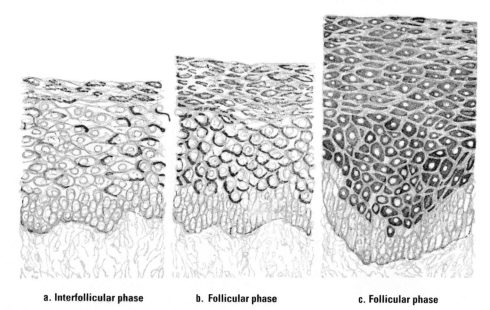

a. Interfollicular phase   b. Follicular phase   c. Follicular phase

FIGURE 19.18 ■ Glycogen in human vaginal epithelium. Stain: Mancini iodine technique. Medium magnification.

FIGURE 19.19 ■ Vaginal Exfoliate Cytology (Vaginal Smear) During Different Reproductive Phases

Vaginal exfoliate cytology (vaginal smear) is closely correlated with the ovarian cycle. The presence of certain cell types in the smear permits the recognition of the follicular activity during normal menstrual phases or after hormonal therapy. Also, exfoliate cytology together with cells from the endocervix provides a very important source of information for early detection of cervical or vaginal cancers.

This figure illustrates cells in vaginal smears obtained during different menstrual cycles, early pregnancy, and menopause. A combination of hematoxylin, orange G, and eosin azure facilitates the recognition of different cell types. In most phases, the surface squamous cells show small, dark-staining pyknotic nuclei and increased amount of cytoplasm.

Figure **a** illustrates vaginal cells collected during the **postmenstrual phase** (fifth day of the menstrual cycle). The **intermediate cells (1)** from the intermediate cell layers (precornified superficial vaginal cells) predominate. In addition, a few **superficial acidophilic (2)** cells and leukocytes are present.

Figure **b** represents a vaginal smear collected during the **ovulatory phase** (14th day) of the menstrual cycle. There is a scarcity of **intermediate cells (8)** and an absence of leukocytes. The large **superficial acidophilic cells (9)** characterize this phase. This smear characterizes the results of the high estrogenic stimulation normally observed before ovulation. The superficial acidophilic cells **(8)** mature with increased estrogen levels and become acidophilic. A similar type of smear is seen when a menopausal woman is treated with high doses of estrogen.

Figure **c** represents a vaginal smear collected during the **luteal (secretory) phase** and represents the effects of increased levels of progesterone. The large **intermediate cells (3)** with folded borders aggregate into clumps and characterize the smear. **Superficial acidophilic cells (4)** and leukocytes are scarce.

Figure **d** represents a vaginal smear taken during the **premenstrual phase.** This stage is characterized by a predominance of grouped **intermediate cells (10)** with folded borders, an increase in the number of the **neutrophils (11),** a scarcity of the **superficial acidophilic cells (12),** and an abundance of mucus.

Figure **e** illustrates a vaginal smear taken during **early pregnancy.** The cells exhibit dense groups or **conglomerations (5)** of predominantly **intermediate cells (6)** with folded borders. **Superficial acidophilic cells (7)** and neutrophils are scarce.

The vaginal smear collected during menopause in Figure **f** is different from all other phases. The **intermediate cells (13)** are scarce, whereas the predominant cells are the oval **basal cells (14).** Also, **neutrophils (15)** are in abundance. Menopausal smears are variable and depend on the stage of the menopause and the estrogen levels.

FUNCTIONAL CORRELATIONS: Cellular Characteristics of Vaginal Cytology (Smear)

The superficial **acidophilic cells** of the vaginal epithelium appear flat and irregular in outline, measuring about 35 to 65 µm in diameter, exhibit small pyknotic nuclei, and contain cytoplasm that is stained light red (acidophilic) or orange.

The **intermediate cells** are flat like the superficial cell, but are somewhat smaller, measuring 20 to 40 µm in diameter, and show a basophilic blue-green cytoplasm. The nuclei are somewhat larger than those of the superficial cells, and are often vesicular. The intermediate cells are also elongated with folded borders and elongated, eccentric nuclei.

The larger **basal cells** are from the basal layers of the vaginal epithelium. All basal cells are oval, measure from 12 to 15 µm in diameter, and exhibit large nuclei with prominent chromatin. Most of these cells exhibit basophilic staining.

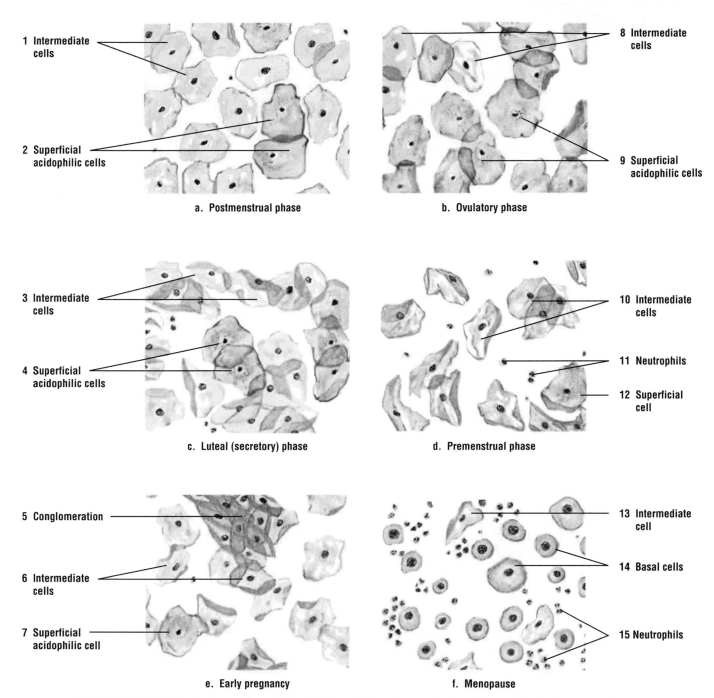

1 Intermediate cells

2 Superficial acidophilic cells

a. Postmenstrual phase

8 Intermediate cells

9 Superficial acidophilic cells

b. Ovulatory phase

3 Intermediate cells

4 Superficial acidophilic cells

c. Luteal (secretory) phase

10 Intermediate cells

11 Neutrophils

12 Superficial cell

d. Premenstrual phase

5 Conglomeration

6 Intermediate cells

7 Superficial acidophilic cell

e. Early pregnancy

13 Intermediate cell

14 Basal cells

15 Neutrophils

f. Menopause

FIGURE 19.19 ■ Vaginal smears collected during different reproductive phases. Stain: hematoxylin, orange G, and eosin azure. Medium magnification.

FIGURE 19.20 ■ Vagina: Surface Epithelium

This higher-magnification photomicrograph illustrates the vaginal epithelium and the underlying connective tissue. The surface epithelium is **stratified squamous nonkeratinized (1).** Most of the superficial cells in vaginal epithelium appear empty owing to increased accumulation of glycogen in their cytoplasm. During histologic preparation of the organ, the glycogen was extracted by chemicals.

The **lamina propria (2)** contains dense, irregular connective tissue. The lamina propria lacks glands but contains numerous **blood vessels (4)** and **lymphocytes (3).**

1 Stratified squamous
   nonkeratinized
   epithelium

3 Lymphocytes

2 Lamina propria

4 Blood vessels

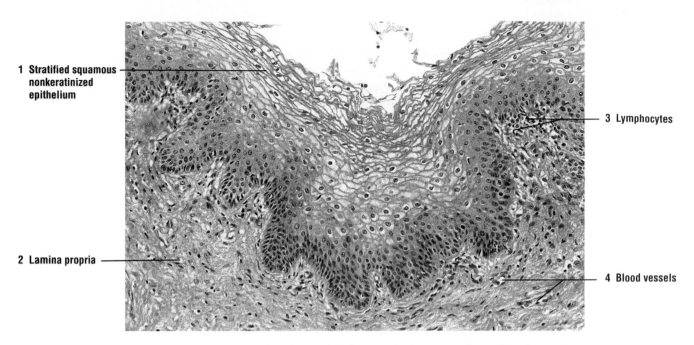

FIGURE 19.20 ■ Vaginal surface epithelium. Stain: hematoxylin and eosin. ×50.

FIGURE 19.21 ■ Human Placenta (Panoramic View)

The upper region of the figure illustrates the fetal portion of the placenta, which includes the **chorionic plate** (1) and the **chorionic villi** (2, 10, 12, 14). The maternal part of the placenta is the **decidua basalis** (15) of the endometrium that lies directly beneath the fetal placenta. The **amniotic surface** (8) is lined by **simple squamous epithelium** (8), below which is the **connective tissue** (1) of the chorion (1). Inferior to the connective tissue layer (1) are the **trophoblast cells** (9) of the chorion (1). The trophoblasts (9) and the underlying connective tissue (1) form the chorionic plate (1).

The **anchoring chorionic villi** (2, 14) arise from the chorionic plate (1), extend to the uterine wall, and attach to the **decidua basalis** (15). Numerous **floating villi (chorion frondosum)** (3, 10, 12), sectioned in various planes, extend in all directions from the anchoring villi (2). These villi "float" in the **intervillous space** (11), which is bathed in **maternal blood** (11).

The maternal portion of the placenta, the decidua basalis (15), contains anchoring villi (14), large **decidual cells** (5), and a typical connective tissue stroma. The decidua basalis (15) also contains the basal portions of the **uterine glands** (6). The **maternal blood vessels** (13) in the decidua basalis (15) are recognized by their size or by the presence of blood cells in their lumina. A **maternal blood vessel** (4) can be seen opening directly into the intervillous space (11).

A portion of the smooth muscle **myometrium** (7) of the uterine wall is visible in the left corner of the illustration.

1 Chorionic plate with
  connective tissue

2 Anchoring
  chorionic villi

3 Chorionic
  frondosum

4 Maternal blood
  vessel opening into
  intervillous space

5 Decidual cells

6 Basal uterine
  glands

7 Myometrium

8 Epithelium of
  amniotic surface

9 Trophoblasts

10 Floating
   chorionic villi

11 Intervillous space
   with maternal blood

12 Floating
   chorionic villi

13 Maternal blood
   vessels

14 Anchoring villi

15 Decidua basalis

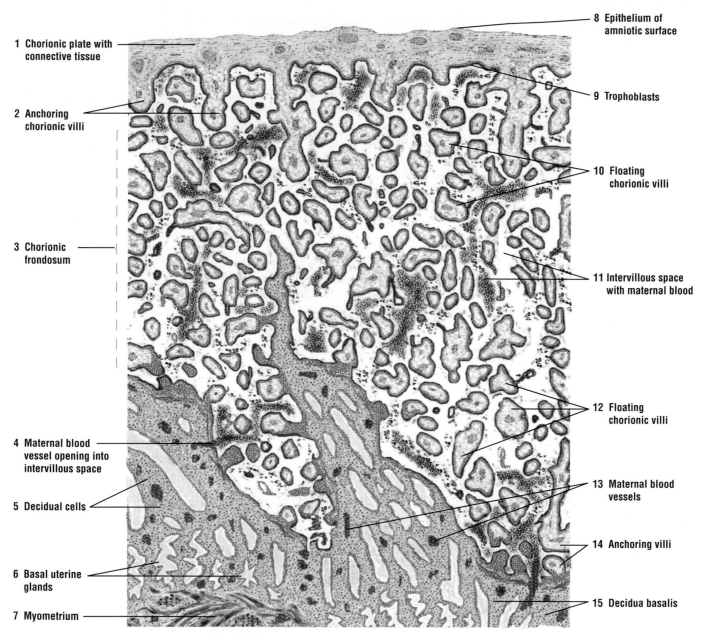

FIGURE 19.21 ■ Human placenta (panoramic view). Stain: hematoxylin and eosin. Low magnification.

FIGURE 19.22 ■ Chorionic Villi: Placenta During Early Pregnancy

The **chorionic villi (6)** from a placenta during early pregnancy are illustrated at a higher magnification. The trophoblast cells of the embryo give rise to the embryonic portion of the placenta. The chorionic villi (6) arise from the chorionic plate and become surrounded by the trophoblast epithelium that consists of an outer layer of the darker-staining **syncytiotrophoblasts (1, 10)** and an inner layer of lighter-staining **cytotrophoblasts (2, 9).**

The core of each chorionic villus (6) contains mesenchyme or embryonic connective tissue and contains two cell types, the fusiform **mesenchyme cells (8)** and the darker-staining **macrophage (Hofbauer cell) (4).** The **fetal blood vessels (3, 7),** branches of the umbilical arteries and veins, are located in the core of the chorionic villi (6) and contain fetal nucleated erythroblasts, although nonnucleated cells can also be seen. The **intervillous space (11)** is bathed by **maternal blood cells (5)** and nonnucleated erythrocytes.

FIGURE 19.23 ■ Chorionic Villi: Placenta at Term

The chorionic villi are illustrated from a placenta at term. In contrast to the chorionic villi in the placenta during pregnancy, the chorionic epithelium in the placenta at term is reduced to only a thin layer of **syncytiotrophoblasts (1).** The connective tissue in the villi is differentiated with more fibers and **fibroblasts (4),** and contains large, round **macrophages (Hofbauer cells) (5).** The villi also contain mature blood cells in the **fetal blood vessels (2)** that have increased in complexity during pregnancy. The **intervillous space (6)** is surrounded by **maternal blood cells (3).**

FUNCTIONAL CORRELATIONS: Placenta

The placenta is an organ that performs an important function in regulating the **exchange** of different substances between the maternal and fetal circulation during pregnancy. One side of the placenta is attached to the uterine wall, and on the other side it is attached to the fetus via the umbilical cord. Maternal blood enters the placenta through blood vessels located in the endometrium and is directed to the intervillous spaces, where it bathes the surface of the villi, which contain the fetal blood. Here, metabolic waste products, carbon dioxide, hormones, and water are passed from the fetal circulation to the maternal circulation. Oxygen, nutrients, vitamins, electrolytes, hormones, immunoglobulins (antibodies), metabolites, and other substances pass in the opposite direction. Maternal blood leaves the intervillous spaces through the endometrial veins.

The placenta also serves as a temporary—yet major—**endocrine organ** that produces numerous essential hormones for the maintenance of pregnancy. **Placental cells (syncytial trophoblasts)** secrete the hormone **chorionic gonadotropin** shortly after implantation of the fertilized ovum. In humans, chorionic gonadotropin appears in urine within 10 days of pregnancy, and its presence can be used to determine **pregnancy** with commercial kits. Chorionic gonadotropin hormone is similar to luteinizing hormone (LH) in structure and function, and it maintains the **corpus luteum** in the maternal ovary during the early stages of pregnancy. Chorionic gonadotropin also stimulates the corpus luteum to produce estrogen and progesterone, the two hormones that are essential for maintaining pregnancy. The placenta also secretes **chorionic somatomammotropin,** a glycoprotein hormone that exhibits both **lactogenic** and **growth-promoting** functions.

As pregnancy proceeds, the placenta gradually takes over production of estrogen and progesterone from the corpus luteum and produces sufficient amounts of progesterone to maintain the pregnancy until birth. The placenta also produces **relaxin,** a hormone that softens the fibrocartilage in the pubic symphysis to widen the pelvic canal for impending birth. In some mammals, the placenta also secretes **placental lactogen,** a hormone that promotes growth and development of the maternal mammary glands.

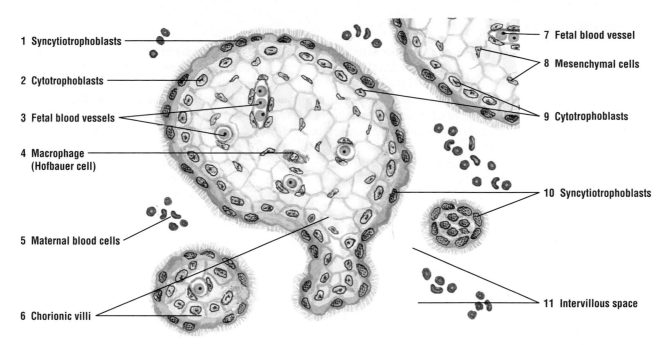

1 Syncytiotrophoblasts

2 Cytotrophoblasts

3 Fetal blood vessels

4 Macrophage
   (Hofbauer cell)

5 Maternal blood cells

6 Chorionic villi

7 Fetal blood vessel

8 Mesenchymal cells

9 Cytotrophoblasts

10 Syncytiotrophoblasts

11 Intervillous space

FIGURE 19.22 ◼ Chorionic villi: placenta during early pregnancy. Stain: hematoxylin and eosin. High magnification.

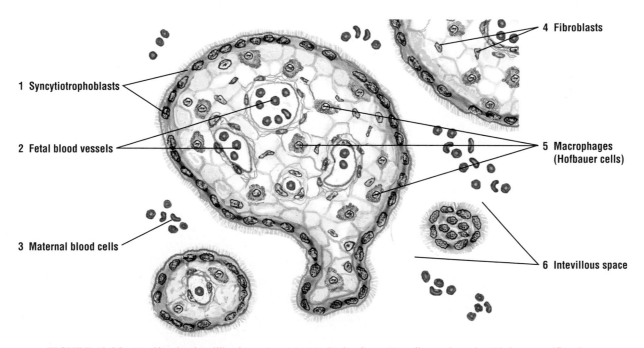

1 Syncytiotrophoblasts

2 Fetal blood vessels

3 Maternal blood cells

4 Fibroblasts

5 Macrophages
   (Hofbauer cells)

6 Intevillous space

FIGURE 19.23 ◼ Chorionic villi: placenta at term. Stain: hematoxylin and eosin. High magnification.

FIGURE 19.24 ■ Inactive Mammary Gland

The inactive mammary gland is characterized by an abundance of connective tissue and by a scarcity of the glandular elements. Some cyclic changes in the mammary gland may be seen during the menstrual cycles.

A glandular **lobule (1)** consists of small tubules or **intralobular ducts (4, 7)** lined with a cuboidal or a low columnar epithelium. At the base of the epithelium are the contractile **myoepithelial cells (6).** The larger **interlobular ducts (5)** surround the lobules (1) and the intralobular ducts (4, 7).

The intralobular ducts (4, 7) are surrounded by loose **intralobular connective tissue (3, 8)** that contains fibroblasts, lymphocytes, plasma cells, and eosinophils. Surrounding the lobules (1) is a dense **interlobular connective tissue (2, 10)** containing blood vessels, **venule** and **arteriole (9).**

The mammary gland consists of 15 to 25 lobes, each of which is an individual compound tubuloalveolar type of gland. Each lobe is separated by dense interlobar connective tissue. A lactiferous duct independently emerges from each lobe at the surface of the nipple.

FIGURE 19.25 ■ Mammary Gland During Proliferation and Early Pregnancy

In preparation for milk secretion (lactation), the mammary gland undergoes extensive structural changes. During the first half of the pregnancy, the intralobular ducts undergo rapid proliferation and form terminal buds that differentiate into **alveoli (2, 7).** At this stage, most of the alveoli are empty and it is difficult to distinguish between the small **intralobular excretory ducts (10)** and the alveoli (2, 7). The intralobular excretory ducts (10) appear more regular with a more distinct epithelial lining. The intralobular excretory ducts (10) and the alveoli (2, 7) are lined by two layers of cells, the luminal epithelium and a basal layer of flattened **myoepithelial cells (8).**

A loose **intralobular connective tissue (1, 9)** surrounds the alveoli (2, 7) and the ducts (10). A denser connective tissue with **adipose cells (6)** surrounds the individual lobules and forms **interlobular connective tissue septa (3).** The **interlobular excretory ducts (4, 11),** lined with taller columnar cells, course in the interlobular connective tissue septa (3) to join the larger **lactiferous duct (5)** that is usually lined with low pseudostratified columnar epithelium. Each lactiferous duct (5) collects the secretory product from the lobe and transports it to the nipple.

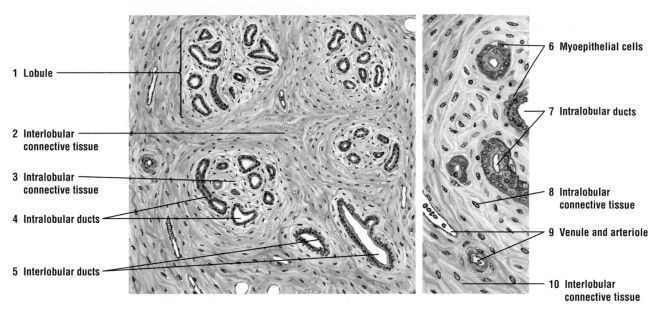

1 Lobule

2 Interlobular connective tissue

3 Intralobular connective tissue

4 Intralobular ducts

5 Interlobular ducts

6 Myoepithelial cells

7 Intralobular ducts

8 Intralobular connective tissue

9 Venule and arteriole

10 Interlobular connective tissue

FIGURE 19.24 ■ Inactive mammary gland. Stain: hematoxylin and eosin. Left side, medium magnification; right side, high magnification.

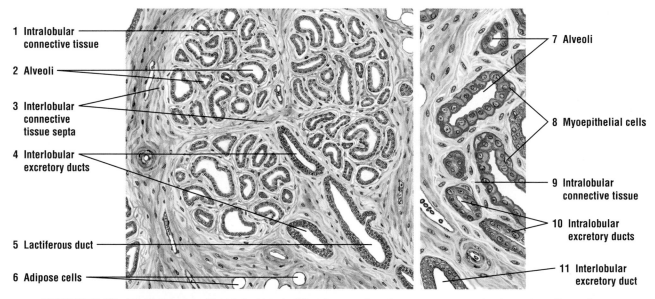

1 Intralobular connective tissue

2 Alveoli

3 Interlobular connective tissue septa

4 Interlobular excretory ducts

5 Lactiferous duct

6 Adipose cells

7 Alveoli

8 Myoepithelial cells

9 Intralobular connective tissue

10 Intralobular excretory ducts

11 Interlobular excretory duct

FIGURE 19.25 ■ Mammary gland during proliferation and early pregnancy. Stain: hematoxylin and eosin. Left side, medium magnification; right side, high magnification.

FIGURE 19.26 ■ Mammary Gland During Late Pregnancy

A small section of a mammary gland with lobules, connective tissue, and excretory ducts is illustrated at lower (left) and higher (right) magnification. During pregnancy, the glandular epithelium is prepared for lactation. The alveolar cells become secretory, and the **alveoli (2, 8)** and the **ducts (1, 7, 13)** enlarge. Some of the alveoli (2) contain a secretory product (2, upper leader). However, the secretion of milk by the mammary gland does not begin until after parturition (birth). Because the **intralobular excretory ducts** (1) of the mammary gland also contain secretory material, the distinction between alveoli and ducts is difficult.

As pregnancy progresses, the amount of **intralobular connective tissue (4, 11)** decreases, while the amount of **interlobular connective tissue (3, 9)** increases because of the enlargement of the glandular tissue. Surrounding the alveoli are flattened **myoepithelial cells (10, 12),** which are more visible in the higher magnification on the right. Located in the interlobular connective tissue (3, 9) are the **interlobular excretory ducts (7, 13), lactiferous ducts (14)** with secretory product in their lumina, various types of **blood vessels (5),** and **adipose cells (6).**

FIGURE 19.27 ■ Mammary Gland During Lactation

This illustration depicts a section of a lactating mammary gland at lower (left) and higher (right) magnification.

The lactating mammary gland contains a large number of distended **alveoli** filled with **secretions** and **vacuoles (2, 9).** The alveoli (2, 9) show irregular **branching patterns (3).** Because of the increased size of the glandular epithelium (alveoli), the **interlobular connective tissue septa (4)** is reduced.

During lactation, the histology of individual alveoli varies. Not all of the alveoli exhibit secretory activity. The active alveoli (2, 9) are lined with low epithelium and filled with milk that appears as eosinophilic (pink) material with large vacuoles of dissolved **fat droplets (2, 9).** Some alveoli accumulate secretory product in their **cytoplasm (8),** and their apices appear vacuolated because of the removal of fat during tissue preparation. Other alveoli appear **inactive (6, 11)** with empty lumina lined by a taller epithelium.

In the mammary gland, the myoepithelial cells (not illustrated) are present between the alveolar cells and the basal lamina. The contraction of myoepithelial cells expels milk from the alveoli into the excretory ducts. The **interlobular excretory ducts (5, 7)** are embedded in the connective tissue septa that contain **adipose cells (1, 12).**

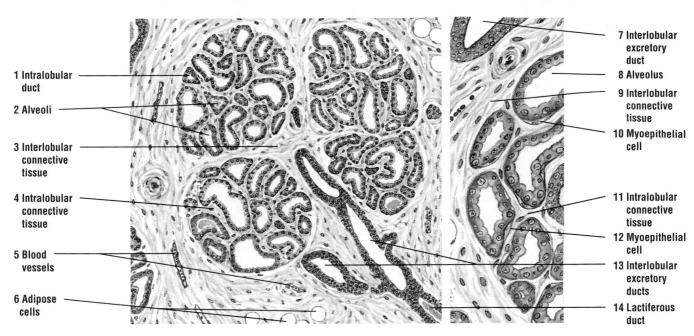

1 Intralobular duct
2 Alveoli
3 Interlobular connective tissue
4 Intralobular connective tissue
5 Blood vessels
6 Adipose cells
7 Interlobular excretory duct
8 Alveolus
9 Interlobular connective tissue
10 Myoepithelial cell
11 Intralobular connective tissue
12 Myoepithelial cell
13 Interlobular excretory ducts
14 Lactiferous duct

FIGURE 19.26 ■ Mammary gland during late pregnancy Stain: hematoxylin and eosin. Left side, medium magnification; right side, high magnification.

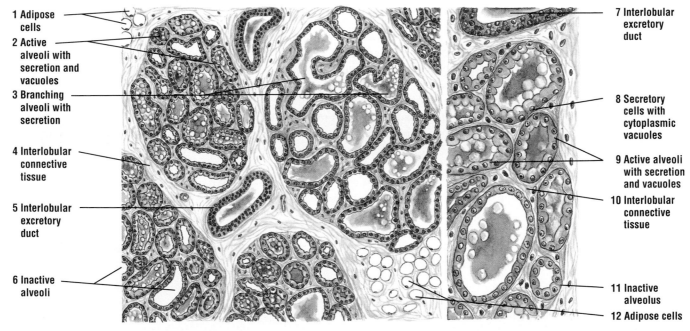

1 Adipose cells
2 Active alveoli with secretion and vacuoles
3 Branching alveoli with secretion
4 Interlobular connective tissue
5 Interlobular excretory duct
6 Inactive alveoli
7 Interlobular excretory duct
8 Secretory cells with cytoplasmic vacuoles
9 Active alveoli with secretion and vacuoles
10 Interlobular connective tissue
11 Inactive alveolus
12 Adipose cells

FIGURE 19.27 ■ Mammary gland during lactation. Stain: hematoxylin and eosin. Left side, medium magnification; right side, high magnification.

FIGURE 19.28 ■ Lactating Mammary Gland

This photomicrograph illustrates a lobule of a lactating mammary gland that is separated from the adjacent lactating lobule by a thin layer of **connective tissue (5).** The lactating mammary gland contains **alveoli (2, 3)** with the **secretory product (6)** milk and separated by thin connective tissue septa (5). Some of the alveoli (3) are single, whereas others are branching alveoli (2). All of the alveoli eventually drain into larger excretory ducts that eventually deliver the milk to the lactiferous ducts in the nipple. The mammary glands contain large amounts of **adipose tissue (1, 4)** during lactation.

FUNCTIONAL CORRELATIONS: Mammary Glands

Before puberty, the mammary glands are undeveloped and consist primarily of branched **lactiferous ducts** that open at the nipple. In males, the mammary glands remain undeveloped. In females, mammary glands enlarge during puberty because of stimulation by estrogen. As a result, adipose tissue and connective tissue accumulate and grow, and branching of the lactiferous ducts in the mammary glands increases.

During pregnancy, the mammary glands undergo increased growth owing to the continuous and prolonged stimulatory actions of estrogen and progesterone. These hormones are initially produced by the corpus luteum of the ovary and later by cells in the placenta. In addition, further growth of the mammary glands depends on the pituitary hormone **prolactin, placental lactogen,** and **adrenal corticoids.** These hormones stimulate the intralobular ducts of the mammary glands to rapidly proliferate, branch, and form numerous **alveoli.** The alveoli then undergo hypertrophy and become active sites of **milk production** during the lactation period. All alveoli become surrounded by contractile **myoepithelial cells.**

At the end of pregnancy, the alveoli initially produce fluid called **colostrum** that is rich in proteins, vitamins, minerals, and antibodies. Unlike milk, however, colostrum contains little lipid. Milk is not produced until a few days after parturition (birth). The hormones estrogen and progesterone from the corpus luteum and placenta suppress milk production.

After parturition and elimination of the placenta, the hormones that inhibited milk secretion are eliminated and the mammary glands begin active secretion of milk. As the pituitary hormone **prolactin** activates milk secretion, the production of colostrum ceases. During nursing of the newborn, tactile stimulation of the nipple by the suckling infant promotes further release of prolactin and prolonged milk production.

In addition, tactile stimulation of the nipple by the infant initiates the **milk ejection reflex** that causes the release of the hormone **oxytocin** from the neurohypophysis of the pituitary gland. Oxytocin causes the contraction of myoepithelial cells around the secretory alveoli and excretory ducts in the mammary glands, resulting in milk ejection from the mammary glands toward the nipple.

Decreased nursing and suckling by the infant soon results in the cessation of milk production and eventual regression of the mammary glands to an inactive state.

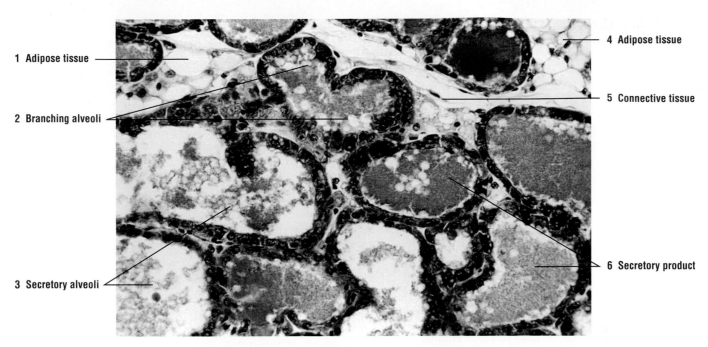

1 Adipose tissue

2 Branching alveoli

3 Secretory alveoli

4 Adipose tissue

5 Connective tissue

6 Secretory product

FIGURE 19.28 ■ Lactating mammary gland. Stain: hematoxylin and eosin. ×75.

CHAPTER 19 ■ Summary

SECTION 2 ■ Cervix, Vagina, Placenta, and Mammary Glands

Cervix

- Located between uterus and vagina, with cervical canal passing into uterus
- Undergoes minimal change during menstrual cycle
- Cervical glands exhibit altered secretory activities, depending on menstrual cycle
- During proliferative phase, secretion is watery to allow sperm passage into uterus
- During secretory phase, secretion is viscous, forms a plug, and protects uterus

Vagina

- Extends from cervix to external genitalia
- Does not have glands, is lined by stratified epithelium, and is lubricated by cervical glands
- Epithelium thickens after estrogenic stimulation, but is not shed during menstrual cycles
- Glycogen accumulates during proliferative phase and, after metabolism, becomes acidic
- Vaginal exfoliate cytology (vaginal smear) is closely correlated with the ovarian cycle
- Follicular activity can be determined by predominant cell type in the smear
- Smears of surface epithelium is highly valuable for detecting cervical or vaginal cancers

Placenta

- The fetal portion includes the chorionic plate and its villi
- Maternal part includes decidua basalis layer of endometrium
- Anchoring villi arise from chorionic plate and attach to decidua basalis
- Maternal blood enters intervillous space to bathe villi that contain fetal blood
- Regulates exchange of vital substances between maternal and fetal circulations
- Cells secrete hormone chorionic gonadotropin (hCG) shortly after pregnancy
- Human chorionic gonadotropin (hCG) appears in urine and is used for pregnancy tests
- hCG stimulates corpus luteum to secrete estrogen and progesterone, and other substances
- Takes over function of corpus luteum until birth

Mammary Glands

- Before puberty consist primarily of lactiferous ducts that open at the nipple
- Inactive glands contain connective tissue and ducts, surrounded by myoepithelial cells
- Estrogen and progesterone induce growth in females, forming tubuloalveolar glands
- Development also depends on prolactin, placental lactogen, and adrenal corticoids
- During pregnancy, ducts branch, enlarge and form terminal buds with alveoli
- Late in pregnancy, alveoli contain some secretory products, but not milk
- At end of pregnancy, alveolar secretion is colostrum, rich in proteins and antibodies
- During lactation, some alveoli are distended with secretory material containing more fat
- After placenta eliminated, prolactin activates milk secretion
- Suckling of nipple releases oxytocin, causing myoepithelial contraction and milk release

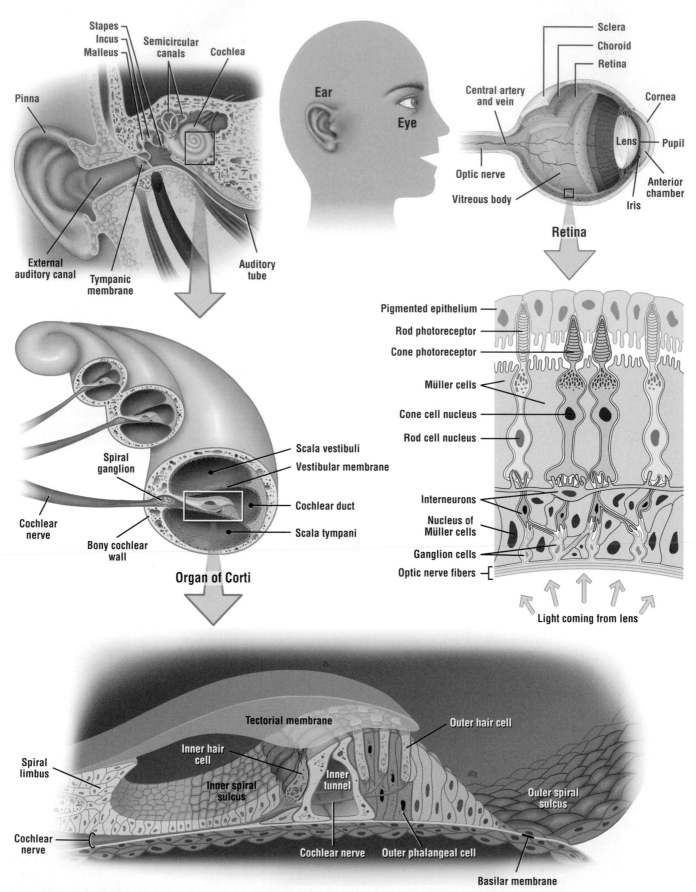

OVERVIEW FIGURE 20 ■ The internal structures of the eye and the ear are illustrated, with emphasis on the cells that constitute the photosensitive retina and the hearing organ of Corti.

Organs of Special Senses

The Visual System

In the visual system, the eye is a highly specialized organ for perception of form, light, and color. The eyes are located in protective cavities within the skull called **orbits.** Each eye contains a protective cover to maintain its shape, a lens for focusing, photosensitive cells that respond to light stimuli, and numerous cells that process visual information. The visual impulses from the photosensitive cells are then conveyed to the brain via the axons in the **optic nerve.**

Layers in the Eye

Each eyeball is surrounded by three distinct layers.

Sclera

The outer layer in the eye is the **sclera,** an opaque layer of dense connective tissue. The inner sclera is located adjacent to the choroid. It contains different types of connective tissue fibers and connective tissue cells, including macrophages and melanocytes. Anteriorly, the sclera is modified into a transparent **cornea,** through which light rays enter the eye.

Vascular Layer (uvea)

Internal to the sclera is the middle or vascular layer (**uvea**). This layer consists of three parts: a densely pigmented layer called the **choroid,** a **ciliary body,** and an **iris.** Located in the choroid are numerous blood vessels that nourish the photoreceptor cells in the retina and structures of the eyeball.

Retina

The innermost lining of the most posterior chamber of the eye is the **retina.** The posterior three quarters of the retina is a **photosensitive** region. It consists of **rods, cones,** and various **interneurons,** cells that are stimulated by and respond to light. The retina terminates in the anterior region of the eye called the **ora serrata,** which is the **nonphotosensitive** part of the retina. This region continues forward in the eye to line the inner part of the ciliary body and the posterior region of the iris.

Chambers in the Eye

The eye also contains three chambers.

The **anterior chamber** is a space located between the cornea, iris, and lens.

The **posterior chamber** is a small space situated between the iris, ciliary process, zonular fibers, and lens.

The **vitreous chamber** is a larger, posterior space that is situated behind the lens and zonular fibers, and surrounded by the retina.

The anterior and posterior chambers are filled with a watery fluid called the **aqueous humor.** This fluid is continually produced by the **ciliary process** located behind the iris. Aqueous humor circulates from the posterior chamber to the anterior chamber, where it is drained by veins. The vitreous chamber is filled with the gelatinous substance called the **vitreous body.**

Photosensitive Parts of the Eye

The photosensitive retina contains numerous cell types organized into numerous and distinct cell layers. The layer that is sensitive to light contains cells called **rods** and **cones.** These cells are stimulated by light rays that pass through the lens. Leaving the retina are **afferent** (sensory) **axons** (nerve fibers) that conduct light impulses from the retina via the **optic nerve** to the brain for visual interpretation.

The posterior region of the eye also contains a yellowish pigmented spot called the **macula lutea.** In the center of the macula lutea is a depression called the **fovea.** The fovea is devoid of photoreceptive rods and blood vessels. Instead, the fovea contains a dense concentration of photosensitive cones.

The Auditory System

The **auditory system** consists of three major parts: the external ear, the middle ear, and the inner ear.

The ear is a specialized organ that contains structures responsible for hearing, balance, and maintenance of equilibrium.

External Ear

The auricle or **pinna** of the **external ear** gathers sound waves and directs them through the **external auditory canal** interiorly to the eardrum or **tympanic membrane.**

Middle Ear

The **middle ear** is a small, air-filled cavity called the **tympanic cavity.** It is located in and protected by the temporal bone of the skull. The tympanic membrane separates the external auditory canal from the middle ear. Located in the middle ear are three very small bones, the **auditory ossicles** consisting of the **stapes, incus,** and **malleus;** also in the middle ear is the **auditory (eustachian) tube.** The cavity of the middle ear communicates with the nasopharynx region of the head via the auditory tube. The auditory tube allows for equalization of air pressure on both sides of the tympanic membrane during swallowing or blowing the nose.

Inner Ear

The inner ear lies deep in the temporal bone of the skull. It consists of small, communicating cavities and canals of different shapes. These cavities, the **semicircular canals, vestibule,** and **cochlea,** are collectively called the **osseous** or **bony labyrinth.** Located within the bony labyrinth is the **membranous labyrinth** that consists of a series of interconnected, thin-walled compartments filled with fluid.

Cochlea

The organ specialized for receiving and transmitting sound (hearing) is found in the inner ear in the structure called the cochlea. It is a spiral bony canal that resembles a snail's shell. The cochlea makes three turns on itself around a central bony pillar called the **modiolus.**

Interiorly, the cochlea is partitioned into three channels, the **vestibular duct (scala vestibuli), tympanic duct (scala tympani),** and **cochlear duct (scala media).** Located within the cochlear duct on the **basilar membrane** is the hearing **organ of Corti.** This organ consists of numerous auditory receptor cells or **hair cells** and several supporting cells that respond to different sound frequencies. The auditory stimuli (sounds) are carried away from the receptor cells via afferent axons of the **cochlear nerve** to the brain for interpretation.

Vestibular Functions

The organ of vestibular functions that is responsible for **balance** and **equilibrium** is found in the **utricle, saccule,** and three **semicircular canals.**

FIGURE 20.1 ■ Eyelid (Sagittal Section)

The exterior layer of the eyelid is composed of thin skin (left side). The **epidermis (4)** consists of stratified squamous epithelium with papillae. In the **dermis (6)** are **hair follicles (1, 3)** with associated **sebaceous glands (3)** and **sweat glands (5).**

The interior layer of the eyelid is a mucous membrane called the **palpebral conjunctiva (15).** It lies adjacent to the eyeball. The lining epithelium of the palpebral conjunctiva (15) is low stratified columnar with a few goblet cells. The stratified squamous epithelium (4) of the thin skin continues over the margin of the eyelid and then merges into the stratified columnar of the palpebral conjunctiva (15).

The thin lamina propria of the palpebral conjunctiva (15) contains both elastic and collagen fibers. Beneath the lamina propria is a plate of dense, collagenous connective tissue called the **tarsus (16)** in which are found large, specialized sebaceous glands called the **tarsal (meibomian) glands (17).** The secretory acini of the tarsal glands (17) open into a **central duct (19)** that runs parallel to the palpebral conjunctiva (15) and opens at the margin of the eyelid.

The free end of the eyelid contains **eyelashes (10)** that arise from large, long **hair follicles (9).** Associated with the eyelashes (10) are small **sebaceous glands (11).** Between the hair follicles (9) of the eyelashes (10) are large **sweat glands (of Moll) (18).**

The eyelid contains three sets of muscles: the palpebral portion of the skeletal muscle called the **orbicularis oculi (8);** the skeletal **ciliary muscle (of Riolan) (20)** in the region of the hair follicles (9), the eyelashes (10), and the tarsal glands (17); and smooth muscle called the **superior tarsal muscle (of Müller) (12)** in the upper eyelid.

The **connective tissue (7)** of the eyelid contains **adipose cells (2), blood vessels (14),** and **lymphatic tissue (13).**

FUNCTIONAL CORRELATIONS: Eye

Secretions (Tears)

Each eyeball is covered on its anterior surface with thin **eyelids** and fine hairs, **eyelashes,** located on the margins of eyelids. Eyelids and eyelashes protect the eyes from foreign objects and excessive light. Situated above each eye is a secretory **lacrimal gland** that continually produces **lacrimal secretions** or **tears.** Blinking spreads the lacrimal secretion across the outer surface of the eyeball and the inner surface of the eyelid. The lacrimal secretion contains mucus, salts, and the antibacterial enzyme **lysozyme.** Lacrimal secretions clean, protect, moisten, and lubricate the surface of the eye (conjunctiva and cornea).

The **tarsal glands** produce a secretion that forms an oily layer on the surface of the tear film. This functions in preventing the evaporation of the normal tear layer. The **sweat glands (of Moll)** produce and empty their secretions into the follicles of the eyelashes.

Aqueous Humor

Aqueous humor is the product of the **ciliary epithelium** of the eye. This watery fluid flows into the anterior and posterior chambers of the eye between the cornea and lens. Aqueous humor bathes the nonvascular **cornea** and **lens,** and also supplies them with nutrients and oxygen.

Vitreous Body

The vitreous chamber of the eye is located behind the lens and contains a gelatinous substance called the vitreous body, a transparent colorless gel that consists mainly of water. In addition, the vitreous body contains hyaluronic acid, very thin collagen fibers, glycosaminoglycans, and some proteins. The vitreous body transmits incoming light, is nonrefractive with respect to the lens, contributes to the intraocular pressure of the eyeball, and holds the retina in place against the pigmented layer of the eyeball.

Retina

The photosensitive retina contains three types of neurons, distributed in different layers: photoreceptive **rods** and **cones, bipolar cells,** and **ganglion cells.** The rods and cones are receptor neurons essential for vision. They synapse with the bipolar cells, which then connect the receptor neurons with the ganglion cells. The afferent axons that leave the ganglion cells converge posteriorly in the eye at the **optic papilla** (optic disk) and leave the eye as the **optic nerve.** The optic papilla is also called the **blind spot** because this area lacks photoreceptor cells and only contains axons.

Because the rods and cones are situated adjacent to the **choroid layer** of the retina, light rays must first pass through the ganglion and bipolar cell layers to reach and activate the photosensitive rods and cones. The **pigmented layer** of the choroid next to the retina absorbs light rays and prevents them from reflecting back through the retina.

Rods and Cones

The rods are highly sensitive to light and function best in dim or **low light,** such as at dusk or at night. In the dark, a visual pigment called **rhodopsin** is synthesized and accumulates in the rods. In contrast, the cones are less sensitive to low light, but respond best to **bright light.** Cones are also essential for high visual acuity and **color vision.** The cones are more sensitive to red, green, or blue regions of the color spectrums. The cones contain the visual pigment **iodopsin.** Absorption and interaction of light rays with these pigments cause transformations in the pigment molecules. This action excites the rods or cones and produces a nerve impulse for vision.

At the posterior region of the eye is a shallow depression in the retina where the blood vessels do not pass over the photosensitive cells. This thin region is called the **fovea** and in its center contains only cone cells. The visual axis of the eye passes through the fovea. As a result, light rays fall directly on and stimulate the tightly packed cones in the center of fovea. For this reason, the fovea in the eye produces the greatest **visual acuity** and the sharpest **color discrimination.**

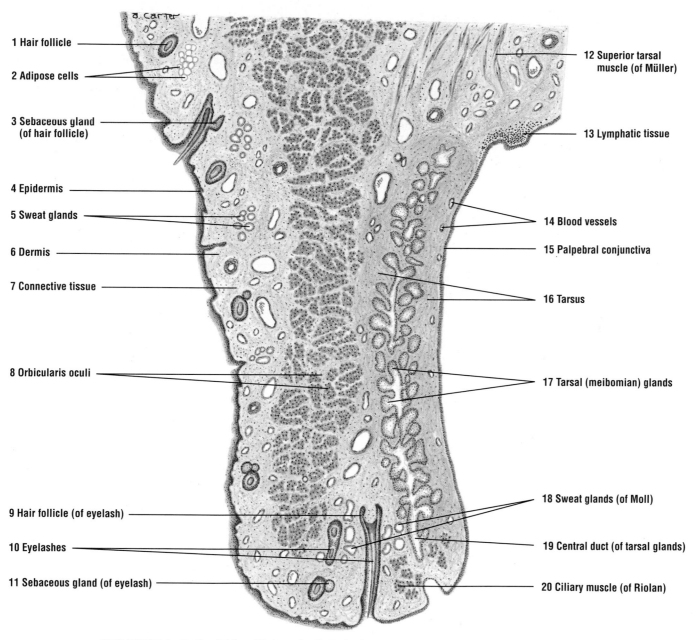

1 Hair follicle

2 Adipose cells

3 Sebaceous gland (of hair follicle)

4 Epidermis

5 Sweat glands

6 Dermis

7 Connective tissue

8 Orbicularis oculi

9 Hair follicle (of eyelash)

10 Eyelashes

11 Sebaceous gland (of eyelash)

12 Superior tarsal muscle (of Müller)

13 Lymphatic tissue

14 Blood vessels

15 Palpebral conjunctiva

16 Tarsus

17 Tarsal (meibomian) glands

18 Sweat glands (of Moll)

19 Central duct (of tarsal glands)

20 Ciliary muscle (of Riolan)

FIGURE 20.1 ■ Eyelid (sagittal section). Stain: hematoxylin and eosin. Low magnification.

FIGURE 20.2 ■ Lacrimal Gland

The lacrimal gland consists of several lobes that are separated into separate lobules by the **connective tissue (2)** septa that contain **nerves (4), adipose cells (6),** and **blood vessels (9).** The lacrimal gland is a serous compound gland that resembles the salivary glands in lobular structure and **tubuloalveolar acini (8)** that vary in size and shape. The well-developed **myoepithelial cells (1, 5)** surround the individual secretory acini (8) of the gland.

A small **intralobular excretory duct (7),** lined with simple cuboidal or columnar epithelium, is located between the tubuloalveolar acini (8). The larger **interlobular excretory duct (3)** is lined with two layers of low columnar cells or pseudostratified epithelium.

FIGURE 20.3 ■ Cornea (Transverse Section)

The cornea is a thick, transparent, nonvascular structure of the eye. The anterior surface of the cornea is covered with a **stratified squamous corneal epithelium (1)** that is nonkeratinized and consists of five or more cell layers. The basal cell layer is columnar and rests on a thin basement membrane that is supported by a thick, homogeneous **anterior limiting (Bowman's) membrane (4).** The underlying **corneal stroma (substantia propria) (2)** forms the body of the cornea. It consists of parallel bundles of **collagen fibers (5)** and layers of flat **fibroblasts (6).**

The **posterior limiting (Descemet's) membrane (7)** is a thick basement membrane that is located at the posterior portion of the corneal stroma (2). The posterior surface of the cornea that faces the anterior chamber of the eye is covered with a simple squamous epithelium called the **posterior epithelium (3),** which is also the corneal endothelium.

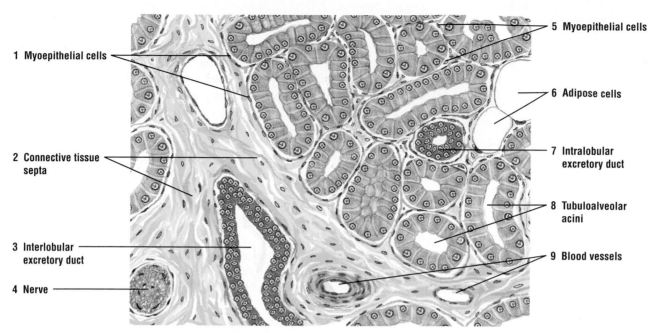

1 Myoepithelial cells

2 Connective tissue septa

3 Interlobular excretory duct

4 Nerve

5 Myoepithelial cells

6 Adipose cells

7 Intralobular excretory duct

8 Tubuloalveolar acini

9 Blood vessels

FIGURE 20.2 ■ Lacrimal gland. Stain: hematoxylin and eosin. Medium magnification.

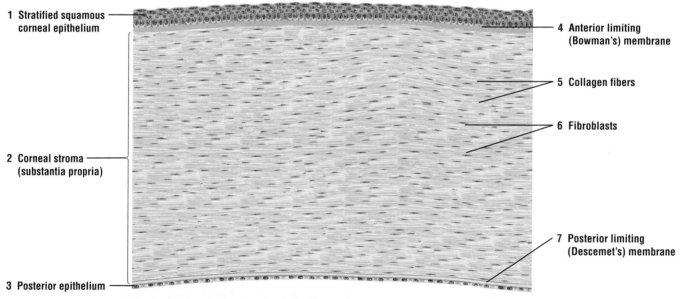

1 Stratified squamous corneal epithelium

2 Corneal stroma (substantia propria)

3 Posterior epithelium

4 Anterior limiting (Bowman's) membrane

5 Collagen fibers

6 Fibroblasts

7 Posterior limiting (Descemet's) membrane

FIGURE 20.3 ■ Cornea (transverse section). Stain: hematoxylin and eosin. Medium magnification.

FIGURE 20.4 ■ Whole Eye (Sagittal Section)

The eyeball is surrounded by three major concentric layers: an outer, tough fibrous connective tissue layer composed of the **sclera (18)** and **cornea (1)**; a middle layer or uvea composed of the highly vascular, pigmented **choroid (7)**, the **ciliary body (consisting of ciliary processes and ciliary muscle) (4, 14, 15)**, and the **iris (13)**; and the innermost layer composed of the photosensitive **retina (8)**.

The sclera (18) is a white, opaque, and tough connective tissue layer composed of densely woven collagen fibers. The sclera (18) maintains the rigidity of the eyeball and appears as the "white" of the eye. The junction between the cornea and sclera occurs at the transition area called the **limbus (12)**, located in the anterior region of the eye. In the posterior region of the eye, where the **optic nerve (10)** emerges from the ocular capsule, is the transition site between the sclera (18) of the eyeball and the connective tissue **dura mater (23)** of the central nervous system.

The choroid (7) and the ciliary body (4, 14, 15) are adjacent to the sclera (18). In a sagittal section of the eyeball, the ciliary body (4, 14, 15) appears triangular in shape and is composed of the smooth **ciliary muscle (14)** and the **ciliary processes (4, 15)**. The fibers in the ciliary muscle (14) exhibit longitudinal, circular, and radial arrangements. The folded and highly vascular extensions of the ciliary body constitute the ciliary processes (4, 15) that attach to the equator of the **lens (16)** by the suspensory ligament or **zonular fibers (5)** of the lens. Contraction of the ciliary muscle (14) reduces the tension on the zonular fibers (5) and allows the lens (16) to assume a convex shape.

The **iris (13)** partially covers the lens and is the colored portion of the eye. The circular and radial smooth muscle fibers form an opening in the iris called the **pupil (11)**.

The interior portion of the eye in front of the lens is subdivided into two compartments: the **anterior chamber (2)** located between the iris (13) and the cornea (1), and the **posterior chamber (3)** located between the iris (13) and the lens (16). Both the anterior (2) and posterior (3) chambers are filled with a watery fluid called the aqueous humor. The large posterior compartment in the eyeball located behind the lens is the **vitreous body (19)**. It is filled with a gelatinous material, the transparent vitreous humor.

Behind the ciliary body (4, 14, 15) is the **ora serrata (6, 17)**, the sharp, anteriormost boundary of the photosensitive portion of the retina (8). The retina (8) consists of numerous cell layers, one of which contains the light-sensitive cells, the rods and cones. Anterior to the ora serrata (6, 17) lies the nonphotosensitive portion of the retina that continues forward in the eyeball to form the inner lining of the ciliary body (4, 14, 15) and posterior part of the iris (13). The histology of the retina is presented in greater detail in Figures 20.6 and 20.7.

In the posterior wall of the eye is the **macula lutea (20)** and the **optic papilla (9)** or the optic disk. The macula lutea (20) is a small, yellow-pigmented spot, as seen through an ophthalmoscope, with a shallow central depression called the **fovea (20)**. The macula lutea (20) is the area of greatest visual acuity in the eye. The center of the fovea (20) is devoid of rod cells and blood vessels. Instead, the fovea has exclusively a high concentration of cone cells.

The optic papilla (9) is the region where the **optic nerve (10)** leaves the eyeball. The optic papilla (9) lacks the light-sensitive rods and the cones, and constitutes the "blind spot" of the eye.

The outer sclera (18) is adjacent to the orbital tissue and contains loose connective tissue, **adipose cells (21)** of the orbital fatty tissue, nerve fibers, **blood vessels (22)**, lymphatics, and glands.

FIGURE 20.5 ■ Posterior Eyeball: Sclera, Choroid, Optic Papilla, Optic Nerve, Retina, and Fovea (Panoramic View)

This higher-magnification illustration shows a section of the retina in the posterior region of the eyeball. Visible here are the pigmented **choroid (7)** with its numerous blood vessels, and the connective tissue layer **sclera (8)**. A distinct shallow depression in the retina represents the **fovea (5)**, which primarily consists of the light-sensitive **cones (6)**. In the rest of the retina are visible the **rods** and **cones (3)**, the different cell and fiber layers of the retina, and **fibers** of the **optic nerve (1)**. The optic nerve fibers (1) converge in the posterior region of the eyeball to form the **optic papilla (2)** and the **optic nerve (4)**, which exits the eyeball.

The specific cell and fiber layers that constitute the rest of photosensitive retina are illustrated and described at a higher magnification in Figures 20.6 and 20.7.

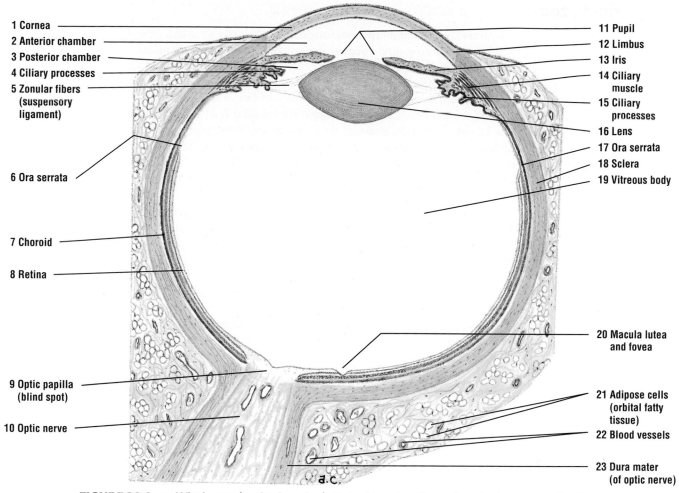

1 Cornea
2 Anterior chamber
3 Posterior chamber
4 Ciliary processes
5 Zonular fibers (suspensory ligament)
6 Ora serrata
7 Choroid
8 Retina
9 Optic papilla (blind spot)
10 Optic nerve

11 Pupil
12 Limbus
13 Iris
14 Ciliary muscle
15 Ciliary processes
16 Lens
17 Ora serrata
18 Sclera
19 Vitreous body
20 Macula lutea and fovea
21 Adipose cells (orbital fatty tissue)
22 Blood vessels
23 Dura mater (of optic nerve)

FIGURE 20.4 ■ Whole eye (sagittal section). Stain: hematoxylin and eosin. Low magnification.

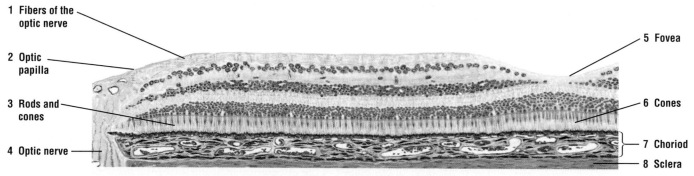

1 Fibers of the optic nerve
2 Optic papilla
3 Rods and cones
4 Optic nerve

5 Fovea
6 Cones
7 Choriod
8 Sclera

FIGURE 20.5 ■ Posterior eyeball: sclera, choroid, optic papilla, optic nerve, retina, and fovea (panoramic view). Stain: hematoxylin and eosin. Medium magnification.

FIGURE 20.6 ■ Layers of the Choroid and Retina (Detail)

The inner layer of the connective tissue **sclera (10)** is located adjacent to the choroid. The choroid is subdivided into several layers: the **suprachoroid lamina with melanocytes (11)**, the **vascular layer (1)**, the **choriocapillary layer (12)**, and the transparent limiting membrane, or glassy (Bruch's) membrane.

The suprachoroid lamina (11) consists of fine collagen fibers, a network of elastic fibers, fibroblasts, and numerous melanocytes. The vascular layer (1) of the choroid contains medium-sized and large **blood vessels (1).** In the loose connective tissue between the blood vessels (1) are large flat **melanocytes (2)** that impart a dark color to this layer. The choriocapillary layer (11) contains a network of capillaries with large lumina. The innermost layer of the choroid, the glassy (Bruch's) membrane, lies adjacent to the **pigment epithelium cells (3)** of the retina and separates the choroid and retina (see Figure 20.7).

The outermost layer of the retina contains the pigment epithelium cells (3). The basement membrane of the pigment epithelium cells (3) forms the innermost layer of the glassy (Bruch's) membrane of the choroid. The cuboidal pigment epithelium cells (3) contain melanin (pigment) granules in their cytoplasm.

Adjacent to the pigment epithelium cells (3) is a photosensitive layer of slender **rods (4)** and thicker **cones (5).** These cells are situated next to the **outer limiting membrane (6)** that is formed by the processes of supportive neuroglial cells called Müller's cells.

The **outer nuclear layer (13)** contains the **nuclei of rods (4, 7)** and **cones (5, 7)** and the outer processes of Müller's cells. In the **outer plexiform layer (14)** are found the axons of rods and cones (4, 5) that synapse with the dendrites of bipolar cells and horizontal cells that connect the rods (4) and cones (5) to the **ganglion cell layer (8).** The **inner nuclear layer (15)** contains the nuclei of bipolar, horizontal, amacrine, and neuroglial Müller's cells. The horizontal and amacrine cells are association cells. In the **inner plexiform layer (16),** the axons of bipolar cells synapse with the dendrites of the ganglion (8) and amacrine cells.

The ganglion cell layer (8) contains the cell bodies of ganglion cells and neuroglial cells. The dendrites from the ganglion cells synapse in the inner plexiform layer (16).

The **optic nerve fiber layer (17)** contains the axons of the ganglion cells (8) and the inner fibers of Müller's cells. Axons of ganglion cells (8) converge toward the optic disk and form the optic nerve fiber layer (17). The terminations of the inner fibers of Müller's cells expand to form the **inner limiting membrane (9)** of the retina.

Blood vessels of the retina course in the optic nerve fiber layer (17) and penetrate as far as the inner nuclear layer (15). Numerous blood vessels in various planes of section can be seen in this layer (unlabeled).

FIGURE 20.7 ■ Eye: Layers of Retina and Choroid (Detail)

A high-power photomicrograph illustrates the layers of the photosensitive retina. The **choroid (1)** is a vascular outer layer with loose connective tissue and pigmented melanocytes. The choroid (1) layer is situated adjacent to the outermost retinal layer, the single-cell, **pigment epithelium (2)** layer. The light-sensitive **rods and cones (3)** form the next layer, which is separated from the dense **outer nuclear layer (4)** by a thin **outer limiting membrane (5).** Deep to the outer nuclear layer (4) is a clear area of synaptic connections. This is the **outer plexiform layer (6).**

The dense layer of cell bodies of the integrating neurons forms the **inner nuclear layer (7),** which is adjacent to the clear **inner plexiform layer (8).** In the inner plexiform layer (8), the axons of the integrating neurons form synaptic connections with axons of the neurons that form the optic tract. The cell bodies of the optic tract neurons form the **ganglion cell layer (9),** and their afferent axons form the light-staining **optic nerve fiber layer (10).** The innermost layer of the retina is the inner **limiting membrane (11),** which separates the retina from the vitreous body of the eyeball.

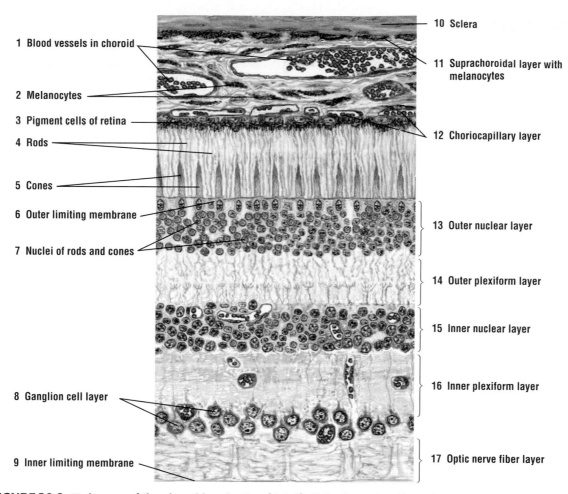

1 Blood vessels in choroid
2 Melanocytes
3 Pigment cells of retina
4 Rods
5 Cones
6 Outer limiting membrane
7 Nuclei of rods and cones
8 Ganglion cell layer
9 Inner limiting membrane

10 Sclera
11 Suprachoroidal layer with melanocytes
12 Choriocapillary layer
13 Outer nuclear layer
14 Outer plexiform layer
15 Inner nuclear layer
16 Inner plexiform layer
17 Optic nerve fiber layer

FIGURE 20.6 ▪ Layers of the choroid and retina (detail). Stain: hematoxylin and eosin. High magnification.

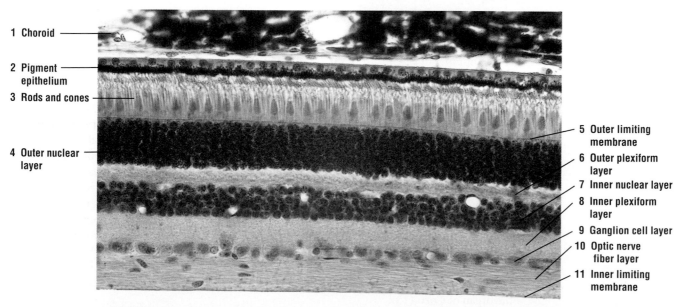

1 Choroid
2 Pigment epithelium
3 Rods and cones
4 Outer nuclear layer

5 Outer limiting membrane
6 Outer plexiform layer
7 Inner nuclear layer
8 Inner plexiform layer
9 Ganglion cell layer
10 Optic nerve fiber layer
11 Inner limiting membrane

FIGURE 20.7 ▪ Eye: layers of retina and choroid. Stain: Masson's trichrome. ×100.

FIGURE 20.8 ■ Inner Ear: Cochlea (Vertical Section)

This low-magnification image illustrates the labyrinthine characteristics of the inner ear. The **osseous or bony labyrinth** of the **cochlea (14, 16)** spirals around a central axis of a spongy bone called the **modiolus (15).** Located within the modiolus (15) are the **spiral ganglia (7),** which are composed of numerous bipolar afferent or sensory neurons (7). The dendrites from these bipolar neurons (7) extend to and innervate the hair cells that are located in the hearing apparatus called the **organ of Corti (12).** The axons from these afferent neurons join and form the **cochlear nerve (13),** which is located in the modiolus (15).

The osseous labyrinth (14, 16) of the inner ear is divided into two major cavities by the **osseous (bony) spiral lamina (6)** and the **basilar membrane (9).** The osseous spiral lamina (6) projects from the modiolus (15) about halfway into the lumen of the cochlear canal. The basilar membrane (9) continues from the osseous spiral lamina (6) to the **spiral ligament (11),** which is a thickening of the connective tissue of the periosteum on the **outer bony wall** of the **cochlear canal (8).**

The cochlear canal (8) is subdivided into two large compartments, the lower **tympanic duct (scala tympani) (4)** and the upper **vestibular duct (scala vestibuli) (2).** The separate tympanic duct (4) and vestibular duct (2) continue in a spiral course to the apex of the cochlea, where they communicate through a small opening called the **helicotrema (1).**

The **vestibular (Reissner's) membrane (5)** separates the vestibular duct (2) from the **cochlear duct (scala media) (3)** and forms the roof of the cochlear duct (3). The vestibular membrane (5) attaches to the spiral ligament (11) in the outer bony wall of the cochlear canal (8). The sensory cells for sound detection are located in the organ of Corti (12), which rests on the basilar membrane (9) of the cochlear duct (3). A **tectorial membrane (10)** overlies the cells in the organ of Corti (12) (see also Figure 20.9).

FIGURE 20.9 ■ Inner Ear: Cochlear Duct (Scala Media) and the Hearing Organ of Corti

This illustration shows in more detail the **cochlear duct (scala media) (9),** the hearing **organ of Corti (13),** and its associated cells at higher magnification.

The outer wall of the cochlear duct (9) is formed by a vascular area called the **stria vascularis (15).** The stratified epithelium covering the stria vascularis (15) contains an intraepithelial capillary network that was formed from the blood vessels that supply the connective tissue in the **spiral ligament (17).** The spiral ligament (17) contains collagen fibers, pigmented fibroblasts, and numerous blood vessels.

The roof of the cochlear duct (9) is formed by a thin **vestibular (Reissner's) membrane (6),** which separates the cochlear duct (9) from the **vestibular duct (scala vestibuli) (7).** The vestibular membrane (6) extends from the spiral ligament (17) in the outer wall of the cochlear duct (9) that is located at the upper extent of the stria vascularis (15) to the thickened periosteum of the **osseous spiral lamina (2)** near the **spiral limbus (1).**

The spiral limbus (1) is a thickened mass of periosteal connective tissue of the osseous spiral lamina (2) that extends into and forms the floor of the cochlear duct (9). The spiral limbus (1) is covered by an **epithelium (5)** that appears columnar and is supported by a lateral extension of the osseous spiral lamina (2). The lateral extracellular extension of the spiral limbus epithelium (5) beyond the spiral limbus (1) forms the **tectorial membrane (10),** which overlies the **inner spiral tunnel (8)** and a portion of the organ of Corti (13).

The **basilar membrane (16)** is a vascularized connective tissue that forms the lower wall of the cochlear duct (9). The organ of Corti (13) rests on the fibers of the basilar membrane (16) and consists of the sensory **outer hair cells (11),** supporting cells, associated inner spiral tunnel (8) and an **inner tunnel (12).**

The afferent fibers of **the cochlear nerve (4)** from the bipolar cells located in the **spiral ganglion (3)** course through the osseous spiral lamina (2) and synapse with outer hair cells (11) in the organ of Corti (13).

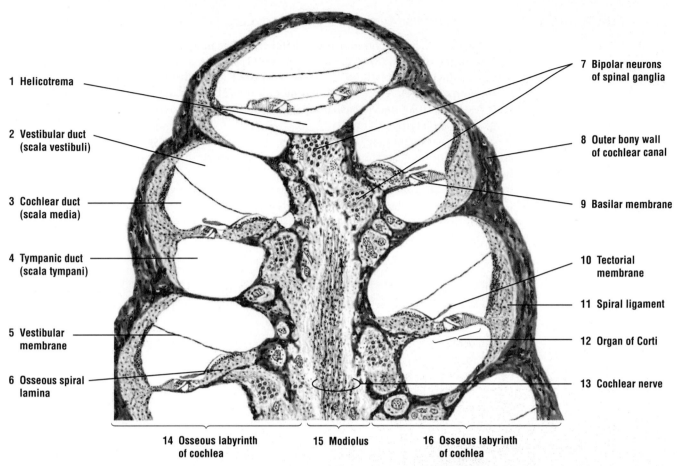

1 Helicotrema

2 Vestibular duct
(scala vestibuli)

3 Cochlear duct
(scala media)

4 Tympanic duct
(scala tympani)

5 Vestibular
membrane

6 Osseous spiral
lamina

7 Bipolar neurons
of spinal ganglia

8 Outer bony wall
of cochlear canal

9 Basilar membrane

10 Tectorial
membrane

11 Spiral ligament

12 Organ of Corti

13 Cochlear nerve

14 Osseous labyrinth
of cochlea

15 Modiolus

16 Osseous labyrinth
of cochlea

FIGURE 20.8 ■ Inner ear: cochlea (vertical section). Stain: hematoxylin and eosin. Low magnification.

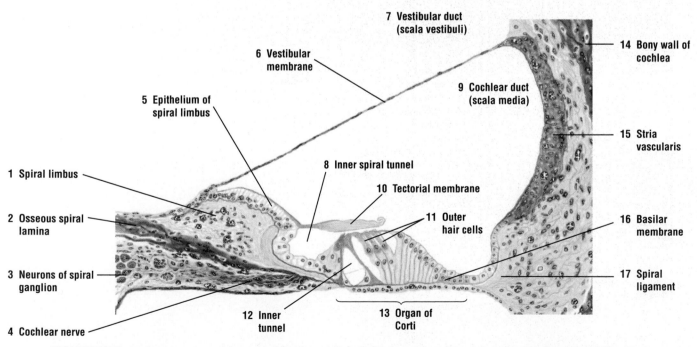

7 Vestibular duct
(scala vestibuli)

6 Vestibular
membrane

5 Epithelium of
spiral limbus

8 Inner spiral tunnel

10 Tectorial membrane

11 Outer
hair cells

1 Spiral limbus

2 Osseous spiral
lamina

3 Neurons of spiral
ganglion

4 Cochlear nerve

12 Inner
tunnel

13 Organ of
Corti

9 Cochlear duct
(scala media)

14 Bony wall of
cochlea

15 Stria
vascularis

16 Basilar
membrane

17 Spiral
ligament

FIGURE 20.9 ■ Inner ear: cochlear duct (scala media). Stain: hematoxylin and eosin. Medium magnification.

FIGURE 20.10 ■ Inner Ear: Cochlear Duct and the Organ of Corti

A higher-magnification photomicrograph illustrates the inner ear with the cochlear canal and the hearing **organ of Corti (8)** in the **bony cochlea (1, 9).** The cochlear canal is subdivided into the vestibular duct (**scala vestibuli**) **(10), cochlear duct** (scala media) **(3),** and the tympanic duct (**scala tympani**) **(14).** A thin, **vestibular membrane (2)** separates the cochlear duct (3) from the scala vestibuli (10). A thicker **basilar membrane (7)** separates the cochlear duct (3) from the tympanic duct (scala tympani) (14).

The basilar membrane (7) extends from the connective tissue **spiral ligament (6)** to a thickened **spiral limbus (11).** The basilar membrane (7) supports the organ of Corti (8) with its sensory **hair cells (5)** and supportive cells. Extending from the spiral limbus (11) is the **tectorial membrane (4).** The tectorial membrane (4) covers a portion of the organ of Corti (8) and the hair cells (5). The sensory bipolar **spiral ganglion cells (13)** are located in the bony cochlea (1, 9). The afferent axons from the spiral ganglion cells (13) pass through the **osseous spiral lamina (12)** to the organ of Corti (8) where their dendrites synapse with the hair cells (5) in the organ of Corti (8).

FUNCTIONAL CORRELATIONS: Inner Ear

Cochlea

The cochlea of the inner ear contains the auditory **organ of Corti.** Sound waves that enter the ear and pass through the **external auditory canal** vibrate the **tympanic membrane.** The vibrations activate the three bony **ossicles** (stapes, incus, and malleus) in the middle ear, which then transmit these vibrations across the air-filled **middle ear** or **tympanic cavity** to the fluid-filled **inner ear.** The sounds vibrate the **basilar membrane** on which is located the **organ of Corti.** The vibrations stimulate sensitive **hair cells** in the organ of Corti and convert the mechanical vibrations into **nerve impulses.**

Impulses for sound pass along the afferent axons of bipolar **ganglion cells** located in the **spiral ganglia** of the inner ear. The axons from the spiral ganglia join and form the **auditory or cochlear nerve,** which carries the impulses from the sensitive cells in the organ of Corti to the brain for sound interpretation.

Vestibular Apparatus

The vestibular apparatus consists of the **utricle, saccule,** and **semicircular canals.** These sensitive organs respond to linear or angular accelerations or movements of the head. Sensory inputs from the vestibular apparatus initiate the very complex neural pathways that activate specific skeletal muscles that correct balance and equilibrium, and restore the body to its normal position.

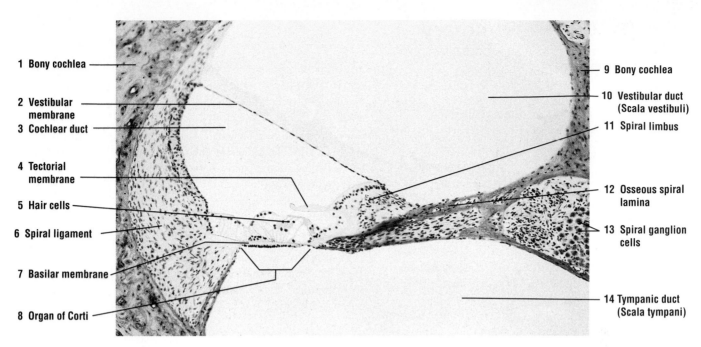

1 Bony cochlea

2 Vestibular membrane

3 Cochlear duct

4 Tectorial membrane

5 Hair cells

6 Spiral ligament

7 Basilar membrane

8 Organ of Corti

9 Bony cochlea

10 Vestibular duct (Scala vestibuli)

11 Spiral limbus

12 Osseous spiral lamina

13 Spiral ganglion cells

14 Tympanic duct (Scala tympani)

FIGURE 20.10 ■ Inner ear: cochlear duct and the organ of Corti. Stain: hematoxylin and eosin. ×30.

CHAPTER 20 ■ Summary

Organs of Special Senses

Visual System

- Eyes are located in protective orbits in the skull
- Visual images are conveyed from eye to brain via optic nerves

Layers in the Eye

- Sclera is the outer layer of eye and is composed of dense connective tissue
- Internal to sclera is middle or vascular layer uvea that nourishes retina and the eyeball
- Uvea consists of pigmented choroid, ciliary body, and iris
- Retina is the innermost lining of eye; posterior three quarters of retina is photosensitive
- Retina terminates anteriorly at ora serrata, which is nonphotosensitive part of retina

The Whole Eye

- Sclera maintains rigidity of eyeball and is the white of the eye
- Anteriorly, sclera is modified into transparent cornea, through which light enters eye
- Choroid and ciliary body are adjacent to sclera
- Ciliary processes from ciliary body attach lens by suspensory ligament or zonular fibers
- Iris partially covers the lens and is the colored part of the eye
- Radial smooth muscle forms an opening in the iris called the pupil

Chambers of the Eye

- Anterior chamber located between cornea, iris, and lens
- Posterior chamber is small space between iris, ciliary process, zonular fibers, and lens
- Vitreous chamber is a large posterior space behind lens and zonular fibers, surrounded by retina

Photosensitive Parts of the Eye

- Rods and cones in the retina are sensitive to light
- Afferent axons leave retina and conduct impulses from eye to brain for interpretation

Secretions (Tears)

- Each eyeball is covered with an eyelid, which contains sebaceous glands and sweat glands (of Moll)
- Above each eyeball is the lacrimal gland, which produces lacrimal secretions or tears
- Myoepithelial cells surround secretory acini in lacrimal gland
- Tears contain mucus, salts, and antibacterial enzyme lysozyme

- Sebaceous (tarsal) gland secretions form an oily layer on surface of tear film

Aqueous Humor

- Produced by ciliary epithelium of the eye and fills both the anterior and posterior chambers
- Bathes nonvascular cornea and lens; supplies them with nutrients and oxygen

Vitreous Body

- Vitreous chamber located behind lens and contains gelatinous substance called vitreous body
- Transmits incoming light, is nonrefractive, and contributes to intraocular pressure of eyeball
- Holds retina in place against pigmented layer of the eyeball

Retina

- Contains three types of neurons, distributed in different layers
- Rods and cones are receptor neurons essential for vision that synapse with bipolar cells
- Bipolar cells connect to ganglion cells, from which axons converge posteriorly at optic papilla
- Area of optic papilla contains only axons of optic nerve and is the blind spot
- Light rays pass through all cell layers to activate rods and cones
- Pigmented layer of choroid next to retina absorbs light and prevent reflection

Choroid

- Divided into suprachoroid lamina, vascular layer, and choriocapillary layer
- Suprachoroid contains connective tissue fibers and numerous melanocytes
- Vascular layer contains numerous blood vessels and melanocytes
- Choriocapillary layer contains capillaries with large lumina
- Innermost layer of choroid is glassy membrane and lies adjacent to pigment cells
- Pigment cells separate choroid from retina

Rods and Cones

- Rods highly sensitive to light, function in low light, and synthesize visual pigment rhodopsin
- Cones sensitive to bright light; essential for visual acuity and color vision
- Cones most sensitive to red, green, or blue color spectrums and contain visual pigment iodopsin
- Interaction of light with visual pigments transforms their molecules and excites rods and cones

- Posterior region in retina contains a pigmented spot called macula lutea with depression called fovea
- Fovea is devoid of rods and blood vessels, and contains photosensitive cones
- Fovea produces greatest visual acuity and sharpest color discrimination

Auditory System

- Ear is specialized for hearing, balance, and maintenance of equilibrium

External Ear

- Auricle or pinna gathers sound waves and directs them through external auditory canal
- Sound waves reach eardrum or tympanic membrane

Middle Ear

- Contains small, air-filled cavity called tympanic cavity in temporal bone of skull
- Tympanic membrane separates external auditory canal from middle ear
- Contains three very small bones, the auditory ossicles: stapes, incus, and malleus
- Contains auditory (eustachian) tube that communicates with nasopharynx
- Auditory tube equalizes air pressure on both sides of tympanic membrane

Inner Ear

- Lies deep in the temporal bone of the skull
- Consists of semicircular canals, vestibule, and cochlea, which is called bony labyrinth
- In bony labyrinth is the membranous labyrinth, a series of compartments filled with fluid

Cochlea

- Located in inner ear; receives and transmits sound
- A spiral canal that makes three turns around central bony pillar called modiolus
- Embedded in modiolus is the spiral ganglion composed of bipolar afferent neurons
- Interiorly partitioned into vestibular duct (scala vestibuli) typanic duct (scala tympani), and cochlear duct (scala media)
- Cochlear duct contains receptor or hair cells in the hearing organ of Corti
- Sound waves vibrate tympanic membrane, which activates the bony ossicles in the middle ear
- Bony ossicles transmit vibrations to inner ear and vibrate basilar membrane
- Organ of Corti is located on basilar membrane; vibrations stimulate hair cells in the organ
- Hair cells in the organ of Corti convert mechanical vibrations into nerve impulses
- Impulses pass along afferent nerves in spiral ganglia of inner ear to cochlear nerve and brain

Page numbers in *italics* denote figures.